Freedman
*Frohman, B.
Gaffney, E.
Gale
*Ganchrow, M.
Garner
Garrick, J.
*Gasior, R.
*Gau, F.
*Geer, T.
Geetter, A.
Geisterfer
*Gensler, S.
Geoghegan, M.
Gerbas, J.
Geshchke, D.
Gettleman, N.
*Getzen, L.
Gianetti
Gibson, P.
*Gielchinsky, I.
Giffen
*Gillespie, J.
*Gillis, S.
Given, J.
Glass
Goffinet, D.
*Goldstein, M.
*Gonzales, P.
*Goodman, A.
Goodson
*Gordon, F.
Gordon, L.
*Gorman, J.
*Graff, C.
*Graham, P.
*Grant, R.
*Green, D.
Gregg
Grey
Gribben
Grismore
*Guernsey, J.
*Guillory, J.
*Gustafson, G.
*Gutierrez, V.
Gutman

Haakon, R.
Haas
Habna
*Hagan, D.
Hakahamimi, L.
Halgrimson, C.
Hall
Halpern
Halverson, C.
*Hamaker, W.
*Hanna, E.
Hanneher
Hansen
Harmon, B.
Harris
Harrison
*Harshaw, D.
*Hasl, R.
*Hassinger, J.
*Hauser, R.
*Hayes, T.
*Healey, E.
Heimlich
*Heller, C.
*Hendron, T.
Henning
Henrichsen
*Herrington, P.
*Hewitt, R.
*Heymann, R.
*Hill, J.
*Hirsch, E.
*Hix, W.
Hoberock, T.
Hockmuth, R.
Horton
*Howard, E.
*Hudson, T.
Hue
Hueman
Hughes
*Hunt, R.
*Hutton, J.
*Ibach, J.
*Jabaley, M.
*James, P.
*Jaques, D.

*Jar...
Ja...
Je...
Johnson
Jones, E.
Jorgensen, M.
Kadiver, H.
Kameron
Katz
Keeler, W.
*Keggi, K.
*Kelly, G.
Kelsh
King, D.
*King, E.
Kissack, A.
*Klein, M.
Kolvek, O.
*Komorn, H.
Kotch, P.
Krause, J.
Kretchmer, P.
Kubly, M.
Kuhn
*Kurrus, F.
*Lanier, T.
*LaPlante, E.
LaPointe, D.
*LaRaja, R.
Larson, J.
Latom
Lau
*Lavenson, G.
*Lawler, M.
*Lawson, D.
*Leacock, F.
*Lebowitz, M.
Lee
*Lehman, R.
*Lemoine, J.
*Lemons, R.
*Lenio, P.
Lesham
Lesta
*Levin, H.
*Levitsky, S.
Lewis, D.

...M.
...ppa, F.
Lisac
Llewellyn
Lloyd
*Lockhart, J.
Loew, O.
Long, R.
*Lowery, C.
*Lucero, J.
*Luehers, J.
Lynch
Lyons, C.
Mackey
*Madura, J.
*Major, J.
*Marrash, S.
Martin
*Matloff, D.
*McAnlis, J.
*McCallom, L.
McClean
*McClure, J.
McCowan
McCurdy, W.
McGert
McKay, D.
*McKee, W.
*McMahon, D.
*McNabney, W.
*McNamara, J.
McRoberts
*Meads, E.
*Meeks, L.
*Meisner, B.
*Mellolyl
*Mengoli, L.
Meredith
*Messersmith, J.
Middendorf
*Miller, R.
Mittleman, M.
Mobley, H.
*Modie, P.
Monroe
Monsen, D.

---

* Signifies individuals who made specific personal contributions to the Registry.

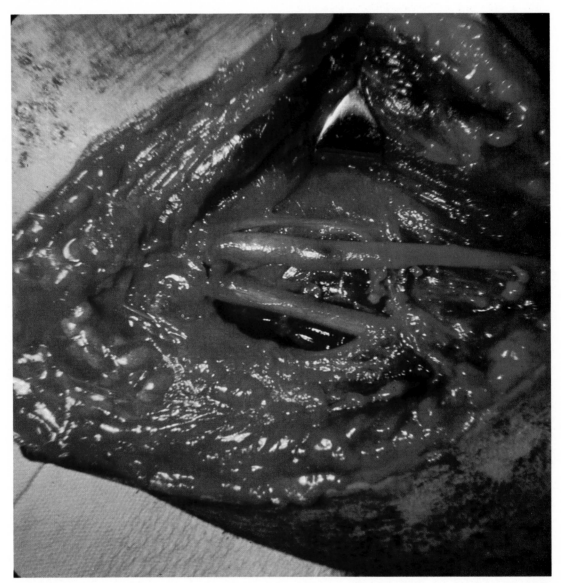

Contusion of the brachial artery caused by high velocity cavitational effect, with the bullet not actually striking the artery. In addition to the adventitial hemorrhage, the intima was disrupted and thrombosis of the brachial artery occurred approximately three hours after wounding. The brachial artery is distended with blood to the left, cephalad, and constricted right, toward the hand, where blood flow was prevented by the thrombus at the site of injury. (NMR, 2nd Surgical Hospital, An Khe, Republic of Vietnam, 1966.)

NORMAN M. RICH, M.D.

COL, MC, USA
Chief, Peripheral Vascular Surgery Service,
Walter Reed Army Medical Center;
Professor and Chairman of Department of Surgery
at the Uniformed Services University of
the Health Sciences, Washington, D.C.

FRANK C. SPENCER, M.D.

George David Stewart Professor of Surgery
and Chairman of the Department of Surgery,
New York University School of Medicine,
New York, New York

Vascular Trauma

W. B. SAUNDERS COMPANY
Philadelphia, London, Toronto   1978

W. B. Saunders Company: West Washington Square
                          Philadelphia, PA   19105

                          1 St. Anne's Road
                          Eastbourne, East Sussex BN21 3UN, England

                          1 Goldthorne Avenue
                          Toronto, Ontario M8Z 5T9, Canada

Vascular Trauma   ISBN   0-7216-7580-8

Last digit is the print number: 9   8   7   6   5   4   3   2   1

To those who served in Southeast Asia
(1965–1972)

PREFACE

Although vascular surgery has reached a level of refinement similar to the other surgical specialties, many questions continue to challenge and stimulate surgeons around the world. Alexis Carrel was awarded the Nobel Prize for Medicine in 1912, based in large part on his pioneering efforts in vascular surgery. However, approximately 40 years passed before it was demonstrated during the Korean Conflict that vascular repair could be accomplished routinely and successfully, even under adverse conditions. Discovery of antibiotics and development of blood banking programs obviously contributed to the success in managing vascular injuries during the Korean Conflict, as contrasted to the earlier experiences during World War I and World War II. Yet as of this date, a glaring deficiency remains: discovery of the "ideal conduit" for segmental arterial and venous replacement continues to elude vascular surgeons. Other areas of question, and even controversy, include the value of venous repair, methods of immobilization of fractures associated with vascular injuries, performance of fasciotomies, and management of infected vascular repairs.

In the sixteenth century, Ambroise Paré, recognized as one of the early pioneers of surgery, first documented that major advancements in surgery occurred under battlefield conditions, when surgeons were faced with large numbers of injured patients during a relatively short period of time. The truth of his observation has been underscored during the armed conflicts of the twentieth century.

Whether trauma results from warfare or from civilian tragedies—such as automobile accidents, industrial casualties, and urban violence—physicians and paramedical personnel are frequently required to manage injured arteries and veins. Because of the unique aspect of recent American involvement in Southeast Asia, it was apparent from the beginning that information gained from treating combat victims who sustained vascular trauma would be valuable to both military and civilian surgeons. The Vietnam Vascular Registry was organized at Walter Reed Army Medical Center in 1966 to document and analyze the data obtained from study of these injuries and to provide long-term follow-up so that the ultimate fate of various types of blood vessel repair might be ascertained. Appropriately, considerable emphasis in this book is accorded to the experiences of some 600 young American surgeons who between 1965 and 1972 performed vascular repairs on thousands of American combat casualties in Southeast Asia. Through the Vascular Clinic and the Vascular Fellowship Training Program at Walter Reed Army Medical Center, it has been possible to obtain long-term results on approximately 1500 of the 7500 former combat casualties included in the study. Other results have been generated by mailed questionnaires and by personal communication and cooperative exchange with physicians throughout the world. Historical development and relevant aspects of managing civilian vascular injuries have been included to show the many similarities and the essential differences between the civilian and military experiences.

The requirement for a book of this scope is obvious in our society, where blood vessel injuries remain a significant problem and indeed are increasing in incidence. The book has been organized to provide general information in the first 10 chapters and specific discussion of important areas of injury in the remaining chapters. We have endeavored to assist those with a general background, while at the same time analyzing the challenging problems that might be faced by a surgeon with special interest and experience in vascular surgery.

It is impossible to acknowledge personally the contributions of the hundreds of individuals who helped make this book a reality through their guidance and support. It is important, nevertheless, to emphasize the extraordinary assistance of W. B. Saunders Company. Mr. Robert Rowan, Mr. John Hanley, and Ms. Marie Low provided the senior leadership. Mr. Grant Lashbrook and Mr. Herbert Powell were among a number of department heads who supervised an outstanding staff. Busy surgeons not only appreciate such support; they also realize that without it a book of this scope could never be written. Mr. Gary Lees of Johns Hopkins University contributed excellent artwork to our effort. We remain grateful to the many individuals who cannot be named specifically.

We trust that this text will assist in establishing the best care possible for those unfortunate enough to experience vascular trauma.

NORMAN M. RICH AND FRANK C. SPENCER

FOREWORD

From time immemorial, hungry or suspicious cavemen, frustrated and jealous lovers, violent criminals, and, more recently, industrial machinery and automobiles have inflicted serious and often irreparable injury on the human body and soul, both of which are ill adapted to cope with much of this stress. But warfare with its mass casualties has always been the most pertinent stimulus for the management of injuries, vascular ones in particular.

It is often presumed that technical skill and experience in vascular repair are the only important factors in obtaining the best possible results. But the present, highly significant contribution of the authors indicates two other reasons for the spectacular advances obtained in this field. Collection, analysis and registration of all vascular injuries, started at the Walter Reed Army Medical Center in 1966 as the Vietnam Vascular Registry, have helped countless surgeons throughout the world to be aware of the latest and most successful methods of vascular repair.

This was not always so. Who else but Susruta in ancient India (500 B.C.?) knew that one could ligate blood vessels with fibers of plants or hair? The Egyptians used cautery in 3000 B.C. to control hemorrhage; for many centuries this was forgotten. Celsus, who advocated ligatures in the first century A.D., was utterly ignored. Five centuries later his was one of the first medical books to see print, containing his message. Carrel and Guthrie's arterial anastomoses and organ transplants did not receive clinical application for 50 years.

The other factor decisive in improving the results of vascular reconstruction and decreasing the incidence of amputations is the shortening of the time lag between wounding and appropriate care. In World War II the time lag exceeded 12 hours in most injuries; during the Korean Conflict the average time lag was 9 hours; in Vietnam this shortened to 1 to 2 hours. Looking back from the helicopter transport in Vietnam to the horse cart in World War I arriving on the Balkan front from Salonika to Belgrade through narrow mountain roads, harassed by guerrilla troops watching from the mountain tops, I still hear the creaky wheels of the wagon and the neighing of horses and still smell the stench of the gangrenous limbs. This time lag and the conviction of German Army surgeons on the western front that all war wounds were infected and not fit for vascular repair resulted in the absence of arterial reconstruction during World War I, even though it had been occasionally performed in civilian practice.

The reader of this opus will find detailed description and documentation of vascular reconstruction, including that of major veins. The latter were ligated in World Wars I and II. The impact of this material should be and already has been felt in our ever-growing emergency services of civilian hospitals. The civilian time lag is being daily improved by the ever-expanding ambulance service to Trauma Hospitals. The model to follow is here.

GEZA DE TAKATS

FOREWORD

Acute injuries of major vessels constitute an important therapeutic problem, representing, as they do, a serious threat to life and limb. In times of war, these injuries assume even greater significance and therefore provide further impetus for studying the problem and devising effective treatment. With the ever-increasing number of vehicular accidents and violent crimes and the common use of arterial cannulation, such injuries are being seen more frequently in civilian practice as well.

Only in the past several decades, however, has an acceptable method of primary surgical repair of arterial injuries evolved, even though more than 200 years ago W. S. Lambert reported successful repair of a lacerated brachial artery (extract from a letter from W. S. Lambert, surgeon at Newcastle-upon-Tyne, to Dr. Hunter. *In* Medical Observations and Inquiries by a Society of Physicians in London. Vol. 2. 1972, p. 360). In the ensuing years, a number of surgeons pioneered in the surgical treatment of acute arterial injuries, and considerable progress was made in this endeavor between World War I and World War II. The general principles formulated from experience in previous wars, especially World War I, yielded limited application and did not lead to effective therapy. It was not until the Korean War that application of the general principles derived from experience in the previous wars, particularly the rapid advances in vascular surgery following World War II, yielded successful therapeutic results.

Norman Rich and Frank Spencer have had broad experience in the development of methods of treatment of vascular injuries and their application, especially during the Korean and Vietnam Wars. This book provides a comprehensive consideration of the subject of vascular injuries, including a thorough review of the history and useful information about the incidence and nature of these injuries. Although the genesis of the book was experiences obtained on the battlefield, data from war have been supplemented by data from civilian practice. Thus this volume will be useful to military and civilian surgeons alike.

MICHAEL E. DEBAKEY, M.D.

FOREWORD

The Korean War provided a timely milieu for the development of vascular surgery. The problems and challenges of vascular trauma encountered during World War II were still fresh in the minds of many. The De Bakey and Simeone studies of arterial injuries inflicted in battle and the documented experiences with traumatic arteriovenous fistulas and aneurysms of Elkins, Freeman, Shumacker and others all provided a fertile source of references for further progress in vascular surgery.

Also in the interval between World War II and the Korean War, the growing interest and research in vascular surgery, the development of the Potts vascular clamps, the appearance of new antibiotics and the introduction of graft preservation techniques all additionally served as important factors in advancing this field of surgery.

Early in the Korean War, Brigadier General Sam F. Seeley, Chief of the Department of Surgery at Walter Reed General Hospital, requested that the Army Surgeon General designate Walter Reed General Hospital as a vascular center. His request was granted, and as a result, army patients with vascular injuries from Korea were directed to the center. There the decision was made to attempt reconstructive and reparative surgery for arteriovenous fistulas and aneurysms rather than to continue the obliterative and excisional techniques commonly used for such lesions during World War II. The results were so successful that soon major veins involved in fistulas also were repaired along with the arteries. Some 215 traumatic vascular lesions were operated upon without loss of a single limb.

Because of these overwhelmingly positive results, great interest arose in applying this experience to acute vascular injuries in the battlefield, especially in light of developments in rapid helicopter evacuation of patients. Colonel William S. Stone, Commandant of the Army Medical Service Graduate School (now the Walter Reed Army Institute of Research), had the foresight to support surgical research teams in Korea. The study of acute vascular injuries was only one of the problems chosen for investigation.

For the vascular patient, many questions had to be answered. Would clots in distal vessels be a problem? What hazards would be imposed by infection? Should wounds be closed completely? When should fasciotomy be performed? Should anticoagulants be used? How long after arterial injury might it be feasible to salvage extremities? Could major veins safely be repaired in acute injuries? How soon would it be safe to evacuate the postoperative vascular patient from forward hospitals?

While members of the Army's Surgical Research Team were studying the repair of acute arterial injuries, Dr. Frank Spencer of the Navy was similarly

xiii

occupied in a nearby Marine hospital. As a result of combined efforts in Korea, 304 acute arterial injuries were studied, with a limb loss of 13 per cent in 269 major arterial repairs, compared to the approximate 50 per cent limb loss following injuries to major arteries in World War II.

Dr. Rich, with his interest in trauma, gained a wealth of experience in the repair of acute vascular injuries in the Vietnam Conflict. Both authors, with experience in battlefield as well as civilian vascular injuries plus their rich background in other types of vascular surgery, speak authoritatively in this book. It contains a wealth of historical, statistical and clinical information.

CARL W. HUGHES, M.D.

CONTENTS

CHAPTER 1

HISTORICAL ASPECTS OF VASCULAR TRAUMA

The advances in vascular surgery are typical of those in other fields of medicine and surgery. Each step is discovered and recorded only to be rediscovered by other individuals who failed to read and profit by the experience of others.

Carl W. Hughes, 1961

Although the first crude arteriorrhaphy was performed more than 200 years ago, only in the past 20 years has vascular surgery become widely practiced with the anticipation of consistently obtaining good results. Historically, it is of particular interest that by the turn of this century, extensive experimental work and some early clinical applications had occurred, employing most of the techniques of vascular surgery in use today. In retrospect it is almost astonishing that it took nearly 50 years before the work of early pioneers such as Murphy, Goyanes, Carrel, Guthrie and Lexer was widely accepted and applied in the treatment of vascular injuries.

Since the days of Ambroise Paré in the mid-sixteenth century, major advances in the surgery of trauma have occurred during the times of armed conflict, when it was necessary to treat large numbers of severely injured patients often under conditions far from ideal. This has been especially true with vascular injuries.

Although German surgeons accomplished some arterial repairs in the early part of World War I, it was not until the Korean Conflict in the early 1950s that ligation of major arteries was abandoned as the standard treatment for arterial trauma. The results of ligation of major arteries following trauma were clearly recorded in the classic manuscript by DeBakey and Simeone (1946), who found only 81 repairs in 2471 arterial injuries among American troops in World War II. All but three of the arterial repairs were performed by lateral suture. Ligation was followed by gangrene and amputation in nearly one-half of the cases. The pessimistic conclusion reached by many was expressed by Sir James Learmonth, who said that there was little place for definitive arterial repair in the combat wound.

Within a few years, however, in the Korean Conflict, the possibility of successfully repairing arterial injuries was conclusively established, stemming especially from the work of Hughes, Howard, Jahnke and Spencer. Hughes in 1958 emphasized the significance of this contribution in a review of the Korean experience, finding that the over-all amputation rate was lowered to about 13 per cent, compared to the approximately 49 per cent amputation rate that followed ligation in World War II.

During the Vietnam hostilities, more than 500 young American surgeons, representing most of the major surgical training programs in the United States, have treated more than 7500 vascular injuries. Rich and Hughes (1969) reported the preliminary statistics from the Vietnam Vascular Registry, established in 1966 at Walter Reed General Hospital to document and follow all servicemen who sustained vascular trauma in Vietnam. The interim Registry report, encompassing 1000 major acute arterial injuries, showed little change from the overall statistics presented in the preliminary report (Rich et al., 1970A). Considering all major extremity arteries, the amputation rate remained near 13 per cent. Although high velocity missiles created more soft tissue destruction in injuries seen in Vietnam, the combination of a stable hospital environment and rapid evacuation of casualties, similar to that in Korea, made successful repair possible. Injuries of the popliteal artery, however, have remained an enigma, with an amputation rate remaining near 30 per cent.

In the past 20 years, civilian experience with vascular trauma has developed rapidly under conditions much more favorable than those of warfare. As might be predicted, several series have reported results that are significantly better than those achieved with military casualties in Korea and Vietnam.

INITIAL CONTROL OF HEMORRHAGE

The control of hemorrhage following injury has been of prime concern to man since his beginning. Methods have included various animal and vegetable tissues, hot irons, boiling pitch, cold instruments, styptics, bandaging and compression. These methods were described in a historical review by Schwartz in 1958. Celsus was the first to record an accurate account of the use of ligature for hemostasis in 25 A.D. During the first three centuries, Galen, Heliodorus, Rufus of Ephsus and Archigenes advocated ligation or compression of a bleeding vessel to control hemorrhage.

Ancient methods of hemostasis used by Egyptians about 1600 B.C. are described in the Ebers' papyrus, discovered by Ebers at Luxor in 1873 (Schwartz, 1958). Styptics prepared from mineral or vegetable matter were popular, including lead sulphate, antimony and copper sulphate. Several hundred years later, copper sulphate again became popular during the Middle Ages in Europe and was known as the hemostatic "button." In ancient India, compression, cold, elevation and hot oil were used to control hemorrhage, while the Chinese about 1000 B.C. used tight bandaging and styptics.

The writings of Celsus provide most of the knowledge of methods of hemostasis in the first and second centuries A.D. (Schwartz, 1958). The prevailing surgical practice when amputation was done for gangrene was to amputate at the line of demarcation to prevent hemorrhage. Archigenes, in the first century A.D., was apparently the first to advocate amputating above the line of demarcation for tumors and gangrene, using ligature of the artery to control hemorrhage.

Rufus of Ephesus (first century A.D.) noted that an artery would continue to bleed when partly severed, but when completely severed it would contract and stop bleeding within a short period of time. Galen, the leading physician of Rome in the second century A.D., advised placing a finger on the orifice of a bleeding superficial vessel for a period of time to initiate the formation of a thrombus and the cessation of bleeding. He noted, however, that if the vessel were deeper, it was important to determine whether the bleeding was coming from an artery or a vein. If a vein, pressure or a styptic usually sufficed, but ligation with linen was recommended for an arterial injury. Herophilus, the Greek physician and anatomist of the third century B.C., described the difference between veins and arteries as follows: "Veins were weak and thin-walled, containing only blood, whereas arteries were thick-walled, containing air 'pneuma' and blood."

Following the initial contributions of Celsus, Galen and their contemporaries, the use of ligature was essentially forgotten for almost 1200 years. Throughout the Middle Ages cautery was used almost exclusively to control hemorrhage. Jerome of Brunswick (Hieronymus Brunschwig), an Alsatian army surgeon, actually preceded Paré in describing the use of ligatures as the best way to stop hemorrhage (Schwartz, 1958). His recommendations were recorded in a textbook published in 1497 and provided a detailed account of the treatment of gunshot wounds. Ambroise Paré, with a wide experience in the surgery of trauma, especially on the battlefield, firmly established the use of ligature for control of hemorrhage from open blood vessels. In 1552 he startled the surgical world by amputating a leg above the line of demarcation, repeating the demonstration of Archigenes 1400 years earlier. The vessels were ligated with linen, leaving the ends long. Paré also developed the "bec de corbin," ancestor of the modern hemostat, to grasp the vessel prior to ligating it (Fig. 1–1). Previously, vessels had been grasped with hooks, tenaculums or the assistant's fingers.

In the seventeenth century Harvey's monumental contribution describing the circulation of the blood greatly aided the understanding of vascular injuries. Historical aspects of arteriovenous fistulas are discussed in Chapter 9. Although Rufus of Ephesus apparently discussed arteriovenous communications in the first century A.D., it was not until 1757 that William Hunter first described the arteriovenous fistula as a pathological entity. The historical development of the treatment of false aneurysms is discussed in Chapter 10. As early as the second century A.D., Antyllus described the physical findings and management by proximal and distal ligation.

The development of the tourniquet was another advance that played an important role in the control of hemorrhage. Tight

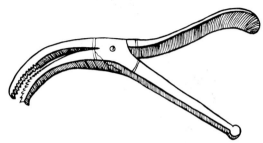

Figure 1–1. Artist's concept of the *bec de corbin,* developed by Paré and Scultetus in the mid-sixteenth century. It was used to grasp the vessel prior to ligating it. (Schwartz, A. M., Surgery, *44*:604, 1958.)

bandages had been applied since antiquity, but subsequent development of the tourniquet was slow. Finally, in 1674 a military surgeon named Morel introduced a stick into the bandage and twisted it until arterial flow stopped (Schwartz, 1958). The screw tourniquet came into use shortly thereafter. This method of temporary control of hemorrhage encouraged more frequent use of the ligature, which required time for its application. In 1873 Freidrich von Esmarch, a student of Langenbeck, introduced his elastic tourniquet bandage for first aid use on the battlefield. Previously it was thought that such compression would irreversibly injure vessels. His discovery permitted surgeons to operate electively on extremities in a dry, bloodless field.

In addition to the control of hemorrhage at the time of injury, the second major area of concern for centuries was the prevention of secondary hemorrhage. Because of its great frequency, styptics, compression and pressure were used for several centuries after ligation of injured vessels became possible. Undoubtedly the high rate of secondary hemorrhage after ligation was due to infection of the wound. Although John Hunter demonstrated the value of proximal ligation for control of a false aneurysm in 1757, failure to control secondary hemorrhage resulted in the use of ligature only for secondary bleeding from the amputation stump. Subsequently, Bell (1801) and Guthrie (1815) performed ligation both proximal and distal to the arterial wound with better results than those previously obtained.

Some of the first clear records of ligation of major arteries were written in the nineteenth century and are of particular interest. The first successful ligation of the common carotid artery for hemorrhage was performed in 1803 by Fleming, but was not reported until 14 years later by Coley (1817), because Fleming died a short time after the operation was performed. A servant aboard the HMS Tonnant attempted suicide by slashing his throat. When Fleming saw the patient, it appeared that he had exsanguinated. There was no pulse at the wrist and the pupils were dilated. It was possible to ligate two superior thyroid arteries and one internal jugular vein. A laceration of the outer and muscular layers of the carotid artery was noted, as well as a laceration of the trachea between the thyroid and cricoid cartilages. This allowed drainage from the wound to enter the trachea, provoking violent seizures of coughing, although the patient seemed to be improving. Approximately one week following the injury, Fleming recorded:

"On the evening of the 17th, during a violent paroxysm of coughing, the artery burst, and my poor patient was, in an instant, deluged with blood!"

The dilemma of the surgeon is appreciated by the following statement:

In this dreadful situation I concluded that there was but one step to take, with any prospect of success; mainly, to cut-down upon, and tie the carotid artery below the wound. I had never heard of such an operation being performed; but conceived that its effects might be less formidable, in this case, than in a person not reduced by hemorrhage.

The wound rapidly healed following ligation of the carotid artery and the patient recovered.

Ellis (1845) reported the astonishing experience of successful ligation of both carotid arteries in a 21 year old patient who sustained a gunshot wound of the neck while he was setting a trap in the woods on October 21, 1844, near Grand Rapids, Michigan, when he was unfortunately mistaken for a bear by a companion. Approximately one week later, Ellis had to ligate the patient's left carotid artery because of hemorrhage. An appreciation of the surgeon's problem can be gained by Ellis' description of the operation:

We placed him on a table, and with the assistance of Dr. Platt and a student, I ligatured the left carotid artery, below the omohyoideus muscle; an operation attended with a good deal of difficulty, owing to the swollen state of the parts, the necessity of keeping up pressure, the bad position of the parts owing to the necessity of keeping the mouth in a certain position to prevent his being strangulated by the blood, and the necessity of operating by candle light.

There was recurrent hemorrhage on the eleventh day after the accident and right carotid artery pressure helped control the blood loss. It was, therefore, necessary to ligate also the right carotid artery four and one-half days after the left carotid artery had been ligated. Ellis remarked:

"For convenience, we had him in the sitting posture during the operation; when we tightened the ligature, no disagreeable effects followed; no fainting; no bad feeling about the head; and all the perceptible change was a slight paleness, a cessation of pulsation in both temporal arteries, and of the hemorrhage."

The patient recovered rapidly with good wound healing and returned to normal daily activity. There was no perceptible pulsation in either superficial temporal artery.

The importance of collateral circulation in preserving viability of the limb after ligation was well understood for centuries. The fact that time was necessary for establishment of this collateral circulation was recognized. Halsted (1912) reported cure of an iliofemoral aneurysm by application of an aluminum band to the proximal artery without seriously affecting the circulation or function of the lower extremity. The importance of asepsis had now been recognized, and the frequency of secondary hemorrhage and gangrene following ligation promptly decreased. Subsequently, Halsted (1914) demonstrated the role of collateral circulation by gradually completely occluding the aorta and other large arteries in dogs by means of silver or aluminum bands which were gradually tightened over a period of time.

EARLY VASCULAR SURGERY

About two centuries after Paré established the use of the ligature, the first direct repair of an injured artery was accomplished. This event, almost 230 years ago, is credited as the first documented vascular repair. Hallowell, acting on a suggestion by Lambert in 1759, repaired a wound of the brachial artery by placing a pin through the arterial walls and holding the edges in apposition by applying a suture in a figure-of-eight fashion about the pin (Fig. 1–2). This technique (known as the farrier's stitch) had been utilized by veterinarians, but had fallen into disrepute following unsuccessful

Figure 1–2. The first arterial repair performed by Hallowell, acting on a suggestion by Lambert in 1759. The technique, known as the farrier's (veterinarian's) stitch, was followed in repairing the brachial artery by placing a pin through the arterial walls and holding the edges in apposition with a suture in a figure-of-eight fashion about the pin. (Drawn from the original description by Mr. Lambert, Med. Obser. and Inq., 2:360, 1762.)

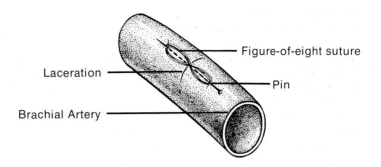

experiments. Table 1–1 outlines early vascular techniques.

Unfortunately, others could not duplicate Hallowell's successful experience, almost surely because of the multiple problems of infection and lack of anesthesia. There was one report by Broca (1762) of a successful suture of a longitudinal incision in an artery. However, according to Shumacker (1969), an additional 127 years passed following the Hallowell-Lambert arterial repair before a second instance of arterial repair by lateral suture of an artery in man was reported, by Postemski in 1886.

With the combined developments of anesthesia and asepsis, several reports of attempts to repair arteries appeared in the latter part of the nineteenth century. The work of Jassinowsky, who is credited in 1889 for experimentally proving that arterial wounds could be sutured with preservation of the lumen, was later judged by Murphy in 1897 as the best experimental work published at that time. In 1865 Henry Lee of London attempted repair of arterial lacerations without suture (Shumacker, 1969). Glück in 1883 reported 19 experiments with arterial suture, but all ex-

TABLE 1–1. VASCULAR REPAIR PRIOR TO 1900*

TECHNIQUE	YEAR	SURGEON
Pin and thread	1759	Hallowell
Small ivory clamps	1881	Glück
Fine needles and silk	1889	Jassinowski
Continuous suture	1890	Burci
Invagination	1896	Murphy
Suture all layers	1899	Dörfler

*Adapted from Guthrie, G. C., Blood Vessel Surgery and Its Application. Longmans, Green and Co., New York, 1912.

periments failed because of bleeding from the holes made by the suture needles. He also devised aluminum and ivory clamps to unite longitudinal incisions in a vessel, and it was recorded that the ivory clamps succeeded in one experiment on the femoral artery of a large dog. Von Horoch of Vienna reported six experiments, including one end-to-end union, in 1887, all of which thrombosed. In 1889, Bruci sutured six longitudinal arteriotomies in dogs; the procedure was successful in four. In 1890 Muscatello successfully sutured a partial transection of the abdominal aorta in a dog. In 1894 Heidenhain closed by catgut suture a 1 cm opening in the axillary artery made accidentally while removing adherent carcinomatous glands. The patient recovered without any circulatory disturbance. In 1883, Israel, in a discussion of a paper by Glück, described closing a laceration in the common iliac artery created during an operation for perityphlitic abscess. The closure was accomplished by five silk sutures. However, Murphy (1897) did not believe it could be possible from his personal observations to have success in this type of arterial repair. In 1896 Sabanyeff successfully closed small openings in the femoral artery with sutures.

The classic studies of J. B. Murphy of Chicago (1897) contributed greatly to the development of arterial repair and culminated in the first successful end-to-end anastomosis of an artery in 1896. Previously, Murphy had carefully reviewed earlier clinical and experimental studies of arterial repair and had evaluated different techniques extensively in laboratory studies. Murphy attempted to determine experimentally how much artery could be removed and still allow an anastomosis. He found that 1 inch of calf's carotid artery could be removed and the ends still approximated by invagination suture technique because of the elasticity of the artery. He concluded that arterial repair could be done with safety when no more than three-fourths of an inch of an artery had been removed, except in certain locations such as the popliteal fossa or the axillary space where the limb could be moved to relieve tension on the repair. He also concluded that when more than one-half of the artery was destroyed, it was better to perform an end-to-end anastomosis by invagination rather than to attempt repair of the laceration. This repair was done by introducing sutures into the proximal artery, including only the two outer coats, and using three sutures to invaginate the proximal artery into the distal one, reinforcing the closure with an interrupted suture (Fig. 1–3). In 1896 Murphy was unable to find a similar recorded case involving the suture of an artery after complete division, and he consequently reported his experience (1897) and carried out a number of experiments to determine the feasibility of his procedure. Murphy's patient was a 29 year old male shot twice, with one bullet entering the femoral triangle. The patient was admitted to Cook County Hospital in Chicago on September 19, 1896, approximately two hours after wounding. There was no hemorrhage or increased pulsation noted at the time. Murphy first saw the patient 15 days later, October 4, 1896, and found a large bruit surrounding the site of injury. Distal pulses were barely perceptible. Two days later, when demonstrating this patient to students, a thrill was also detected. An operative repair was decided upon. Because of the historical significance, the operation report is quoted:

Operation, October 7, 1896. An incision five inches long was made from Poupart's ligament along the course of the femoral artery. The artery was readily exposed about one inch above Poupart's ligament; it was separated from its sheath and a provisional ligature thrown about it but not tied. A careful dissection was then made down along the wall of the vessel to the pulsating clot. The artery was exposed to one inch below the point and a ligature thrown around it but not tied: a careful dissection was made upward to the point of the clot. The artery

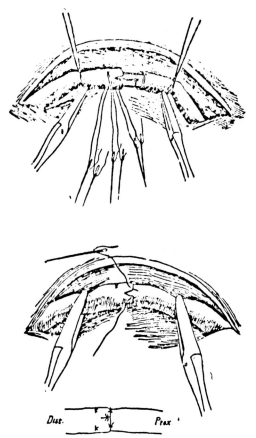

Figure 1–3. The first successful clinical end-to-end anastomosis of an artery was performed in 1896. Sutures were placed in the proximal artery, including only the few outer coats, and three sutures were used to invaginate the proximal artery into the distal one; the closure was reinforced with an interrupted suture. (Murphy, J. B., Med. Record, *51*:73, 1897.)

was then closed above and below with gentle compression clamps and was elevated, at which time there was a profuse hemorrhage from an opening in the vein. A cavity, about the size of a filbert, was found posterior to the artery communicating with its caliber, the aneurysmal pocket. A small aneurysmal sac about the same size was found on the anterior surface of the artery over the point of perforation. The hemorrhage from the vein was very profuse and was controlled by digital compression. It was found that one-eighth of an inch of the arterial wall on the outer side of the opening remained, and on the inner side of the perforation only a band of one-sixteenth of an inch of adventitia was intact. The bullet had passed through the center of the artery, carried away all of its wall except the strands described above, and passed downward and backward making a large hole in the vein in its posterior and external side just above the junction of the vena profunda. Great difficulty was experienced in controlling the hemorrhage from the vein. After dissecting the vein above and below the point of laceration and placing a temporary ligature on the vena profunda, the hemorrhage was controlled so that the vein could be sutured. At the point of suture the vein was greatly diminished in size, but when the clamps were removed it dilated about one-third the normal diameter or one-third the diameter of the vein above and below. There was no bleeding from the vein when the clamps were removed. Our attention was then turned to the artery. Two inches of it had been exposed and freed from all surroundings. The opening in the artery was three-eighths of an inch in length; one-half inch was resected and the proximal was invaginated into the distal for one-third of an inch with four double needle threads which penetrated all of the walls of the artery. The adventitia was peeled off the invaginated portion for a distance of one-third of an inch: a row of sutures was placed around the edge of the overlapping distal end, the sutures penetrating only the media of the proximal portion; the adventitia was then brought over the end of the union and sutured. The clamps were removed. Not a drop of blood escaped at the line of suture. Pulsation was immediately restored in the artery below the line of approximation and it could be felt feebly in the posterior tibial and dorsalis pedis pulses. The sheath and connective tissue around the artery were then approximated at the position of the suture with catgut, so as to support the wall of the artery. The whole cavity was washed out with a five per cent solution of carbolic acid and the edges of the wound were accurately approximated with silk worm-gut sutures. No drainage. The time of the operation was approximately two and one-half hours, most of the time being consumed in suturing the vein. The artery was easily secured and sutured, and the hemorrhage from it readily controlled. The patient was placed in bed with the leg elevated and wrapped in cotton.

The anatomic location of the injuries, the gross pathology involved and the repair for Murphy's historically successful arterial anastomosis are shown in Figure 1–4. Murphy mentioned that a pulsation could be felt in the dorsalis pedis artery four days following the operation. The patient had no edema and no disturbance of his circulation during the reported three months of observation.

Subsequently, Murphy (1897) reviewed the results of ligature of large arteries be-fore the turn of the century. He found that the abdominal aorta had been ligated 10 times with only one patient surviving for 10 days. Lidell reported only 16 recoveries after ligation of the common iliac artery 68 times, a mortality of 77 per cent. Balance and Edmunds reported a 40 per cent mortality following ligation of a femoral artery aneurysm in 31 patients. Billroth reported secondary hemorrhage from 50 per cent of large arteries ligated in continuity. Wyeth collected 106 cases of carotid artery aneurysms treated by proximal ligation, with a mortality rate of 35 per cent.

In 1897 Murphy summarized techniques he considered necessary for arterial suture. They bear a close resemblance to principles generally followed today:

1. Complete asepsis.
2. Exposure of the vessel with as little injury as possible.
3. Temporary suppression of the blood current.
4. Control of the vessel while applying the suture.
5. Accurate approximation of the walls.
6. Perfect hemostasis by pressure after the clamps are taken off.
7. Toilet of the wound.

Murphy also reported that Billroth, Schede, Braun, Schmidt and others had successfully sutured wounds in veins. He personally had used five silk sutures to close an opening three-eighths of an inch long in the common jugular vein.

Several significant accomplishments occurred in vascular surgery within the next few years. Matas (1903) described his technique with endoaneurysmorrhaphy for aneurysm, a technique which remained the standard technique for aneurysms for over 40 years. In 1906 Carrel and Guthrie performed classic experimental studies over a period of time with many significant results. These included direct suture repair of arteries, vein transplantation, and transplantation of blood vessels as well as organs and limbs (Fig. 1–5). In 1912 Guthrie independently published his continuing work on vascular surgery. Following Murphy's successful case in 1896, the next successful repair of an arterial defect came 10 years later when Goyanes used a vein graft to bridge an arterial defect in 1906. Working in Madrid, Goyanes excised a popliteal

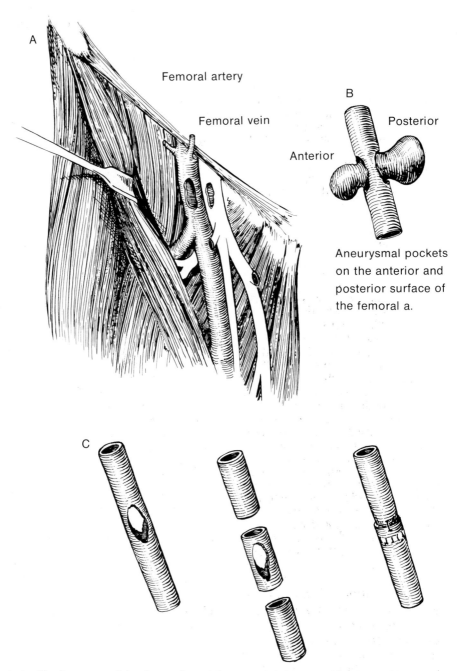

Figure 1–4. The first successful end-to-end arterial anastomosis in man by Murphy in 1896. (A) The anatomic location of the injury. (B) The close pathology involved. (C) Degree of destruction, portion resected and appearance after invagination of femoral artery. (Redrawn from Murphy, J. B., Med. Record, *51*:73, 1897.)

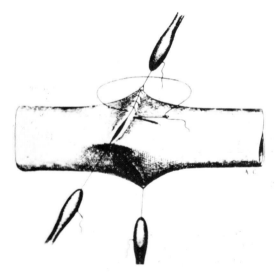

Figure 1–5. The triangulation method of suturing vessels. Initially conceived in 1902 by Carrel, this method was used by Carrel and Guthrie in their monumental contributions in the direct suture repair of arteries, vein transplants and transplantation of blood vessels and organs. (Courtesy the New York Academy of Medicine Library.)

artery aneurysm and used the accompanying popliteal vein to restore continuity (Fig. 1–6). He used the suture technique developed by Carrel and Guthrie of triangulating the arterial orifice with three sutures, followed by continuous suture between each of the three areas. A year later in Germany, Lexer (1907) first used the saphenous vein as an arterial substitute to restore continuity after excision of an aneurysm of the axillary artery. In his 1969 review, Shumacker commented that within the first few years of this century the triangulation stitch of Carrel (1902), the quadrangulation method of Frouin (1908), and the Mourin modification (1914) (Fig. 1–7) had developed.

By 1910 Stich reported over 100 cases of arterial reconstruction by lateral suture. His review also included 46 repairs by end-to-end anastomosis or by insertion of a vein graft (Nolan, 1968). It is curious with this promising start that over 30 years elapsed before vascular surgery was widely employed. A high failure rate, usually by thrombosis, attended early attempts at repair, and few surgeons were convinced that repair of an artery was worthwhile. Matas (1913) stated that vascular injuries, particularly arteriovenous aneurysms, had become a conspicuous feature of modern

military surgery, and he felt that this class of injury must command the closest attention of the modern military surgeon:

A most timely and valuable contribution to the surgery of blood vessels resulted from wounds in war.... Unusual opportunities for the observation of vascular wounds inflicted with modern military weapons...based on material fresh from the field of action, and fully confirmed the belief that this last war, waged in close proximity to well equipped surgical centers, would also offer an unusual opportunity for the study of the most advanced methods of treating injuries of blood vessels.

In 1913 Soubbotitch described the experience of Serbian military surgeons during the Serbo-Turkish and Serbo-Bulgarian Wars. Seventy-seven false aneurysms and arteriovenous fistulas were treated. There were 45 ligations, but 32 vessels were repaired, including 19 arteriorrhaphies, 13 venorrhaphies and 15 end-to-end anastomoses (11 arteries and four veins). It is impressive that infection and

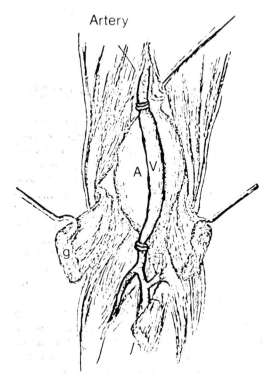

Figure 1–6. The first successful repair of an arterial defect utilizing a vein graft. Using the triangulation technique of Carrel with endothelial coaptation, a segment of the adjacent popliteal vein was used to repair the popliteal artery. (Goyanes, D. J., El Siglo Med., *53*:561, 1906.)

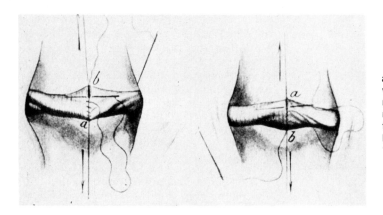

Figure 1–7. The original triangulation stitch of Carrel in 1902 was modified to a quadrangulation method by Frouin in 1908. Another modification, as shown here, was that of Mourin in 1914. (From Moure, P., Les Greffes Artérielles, 1914.)

secondary hemorrhage were avoided. Matas (1915), in discussing Soubbotitch's report, emphasized that a notable feature was the suture (circular and lateral repair) of blood vessels and the fact that it had been utilized more frequently in the Balkan conflict than in previous wars. He also noted that judging by Soubbotitch's statistics, the success obtained by surgeons in the Serbian Army Hospital in Belgrade far surpassed those obtained by other military surgeons in previous wars, with the exception perhaps of the remarkably favorable results in the Japanese Reserve Hospitals reported by Kikuzi.

WORLD WAR I EXPERIENCE

During the early part of World War I, with the new techniques of vascular surgery well established, the German surgeons attempted repair of acutely injured arteries, and were successful in more than 100 cases (Nolan, 1968). During the first nine months of World War I, low velocity missiles caused arterial trauma of a limited extent. In 1915, however, the widespread use of high explosives and high velocity bullets, combined with mass casualties and slow evacuation of the wounded, made arterial repair impractical.

Bernheim (1920) went to France with the specific intent of repairing arterial injuries. Despite extensive prior experience and equipment, however, he concluded that attempts at vascular repair were unwise. He wrote:

Opportunities for carrying out the more modern procedures for repair or reconstruction of damaged blood vessels were conspicuous by their absence during the recent military activities. ...Not that blood vessels were immune from injury; not that gaping arteries and veins and vicariously united vessels did not cry out for relief by fine suture or anastomosis. They did, most eloquently, and in great numbers, but he would have been a foolhardy man who would have essayed sutures of arterial or venous trunks in the presence of such infections as were the rule in practically all of the battle wounded.

The great frequency of infection with secondary hemorrhage virtually precluded arterial repair. In addition, there were inadequate statistics about the frequency of gangrene following ligation, and initial reports subsequently proved to be unduly optimistic. Poole (1927), in the Medical Department History of World War I, remarked that if gangrene were a danger following arterial ligation, primary suture should be performed and the patient watched very carefully.

Despite the discouragement of managing acute arterial injuries in World War I, fairly frequent repair of false aneurysms and arteriovenous fistulas was carried out by many surgeons. These cases were treated after the acute period of injury, when collateral circulation had developed with the passage of time and assured viability of extremities. Matas (1921) recorded that the majority of these repairs consisted of arteriorrhaphy by lateral or circular suture, with excision of the sac or endoaneurysmorrhaphy.

Makins (1919), who served in World War I as a British surgeon, recommended ligating the concomitant vein when it was necessary to ligate a major artery. He thought that this reduced the frequency of gangrene. This hypothesis was debated for over 20 years before it was finally abandoned.

WORLD WAR II EXPERIENCE

Experiences with vascular surgery in World War II are well recorded in the review by DeBakey and Simeone (1946), analyzing 2471 arterial injuries. Almost all were treated by ligation, with a subsequent amputation rate near 49 per cent. There were only 81 repairs attempted, 78 by lateral suture and three by end-to-end anastomosis, with an amputation rate of approximately 35 per cent. The use of vein grafts was even more disappointing: they were attempted in 40 cases with an amputation rate of nearly 58 per cent.

The controversial question of ligation of the concomitant vein remained, though few observers were convinced that the procedure enhanced circulation. The varying opinions were summarized by Linton in 1949.

A refreshing exception to the dismal World War II experience in regard to ligation and gangrene was the case operated upon by Dr. Allen M. Boyden: an acute arteriovenous fistula of the femoral vessels repaired shortly after D-Day in Normandy. The following comments are taken from his field notes about 26 years later (Boyden, 1970) and emphasize the value of adequate records, even in military combat:

High explosive wound left groin, 14 June 1944, at 2200 hours. Acute arteriovenous aneurysm femoral artery.
Preoperative blood pressure 140–70; pulse 104.
Operation: 16 June 1944, nitrous oxide and oxygen.
Operation: 1910 to 22 hours.
One unit of blood transfused during the operation.
Arteriovenous aneurysms isolated near junction with profunda femoris artery.
Considerable hemorrhage.
Openings in both artery and vein were sutured with fine silk.
Postoperative blood pressure 120–68; pulse 118.
Circulation of the extremity remained intact until evacuation.

As this case demonstrated Boyden's interest in vascular surgery, the Consulting Surgeon for the First Army presented him with one-half of the latter's supply of vascular instruments and material. This supply consisted of two sets of Blakemore tubes, two bulldog forceps and a 2 cc ampule of heparin!

The conclusion that ligation was the treatment of choice for injured arteries was summarized by DeBakey and Simeone in 1946:

It is clear that no procedure other than ligation is applicable to the majority of vascular injuries which come under the military surgeons' observation. It is not a procedure of choice. It is a procedure of stern necessity, for the basic purpose of controlling hemorrhage, as well as because of the location, type, size and character of most battle injuries of the arteries.

In retrospect it should be remembered that the average time lag between wounding and surgical treatment was over 10 hours in World War II, virtually precluding successful arterial repair in most patients. Of historical interest is the nonsuture method of arterial repair used during World War II (Figs. 1–8 and 1–9).

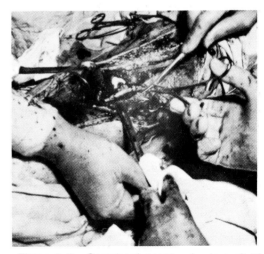

Figure 1–8. Completed unsutured vein graft of the popliteal artery which was complicated by a severe compound fracture of the tibia. This was representative of 40 cases utilizing the double-tube graft technique in World War II as advocated by Blakemore, Lord and Stefko in 1942. (DeBakey, M. E., and Simeone, F. A., *Ann. Surg.*, *123*:534, 1946.)

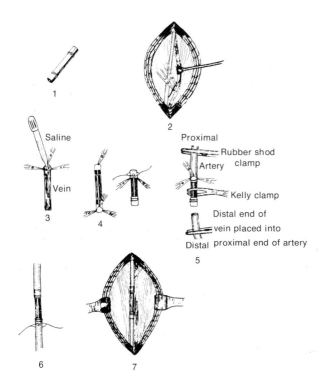

Figure 1–9. The various steps of a non-suture method of bridging arterial defects designed during World War II. (1) The Vitallium tube with its two ridges (sometimes grooves). (2) The exposed femoral artery and vein with the vein retracted and clamps placed on a branch. (3) The removed segment of vein is irrigated with saline solution. (4) The vein has been pushed through the inside of the Vitallium tube, and the two ends everted over the ends of the tube held in place with one or two ligatures of fine silk. (5) Distal end of the segment of vein is placed into the proximal end of the artery and held there by two ligatures of fine silk. (6) The snug ligature near the end of the Vitallium tube is tied to provide apposition of the artery and vein. (7) The completed operation, showing the bridging of a 2-cm. gap in the femoral artery. (Modified description of the original drawings from Blakemore, A. H., Lord, J. W., Jr., and Stefko, P. L., Surgery, *12*:488, 1942.)

EXPERIENCES DURING THE KOREAN CONFLICT

The successful repair of arterial injuries in the Korean Conflict, in pleasant contrast to the experiences of World War II, was due to several factors. There had been substantial progress in the techniques of vascular surgery, accompanied by improvements in anesthesia, blood transfusion, and antibiotics. Perhaps of greatest importance was rapid evacuation of wounded men, often by helicopter, permitting their transport from time of wounding to surgical care often within one to two hours (Fig. 1–10). In addition, a thorough understanding of the importance of débridement, delayed primary closure and antibiotics greatly decreased the hazards of infection.

Initially in the Korean Conflict, attempts at arterial repair were disappointing. During one report of experiences at a surgical hospital for eight months between September 1951 and April 1952, only 11 of 40 attempted arterial repairs were thought to be successful (Hughes, 1959). Only 6 of 29 end-to-end anastomoses were considered initially successful, and all six venous grafts failed. In another report from a similar period of time, only 4 of 18 attempted repairs were considered successful. Warren (1952) emphasized that an aggressive approach was needed, with the establishment of a research team headed by a surgeon experienced in vascular grafting. Surgical research teams were established in the Army, and there was improvement in results of vascular repairs by 1952. Significant reports were published by Jahnke and Seeley (1953), Hughes (1955, 1958), and Inui, Shannon and Howard (1955). Similar work in the Navy was done with the U.S. Marines during 1952 and 1953 by Spencer and Grewe (1955). These surgeons worked in specialized research groups under fairly stabilized conditions, considering that they were in a combat zone (Fig. 1–11). Brigadier General Sam Seeley, who was Chief of the Department of Surgery at Walter Reed Army Hospital in 1950, had the foresight to establish Walter Reed Army Hospital as a vascular surgery center, and this made it possible for patients with vascular injuries to be returned there for later study (Fig.

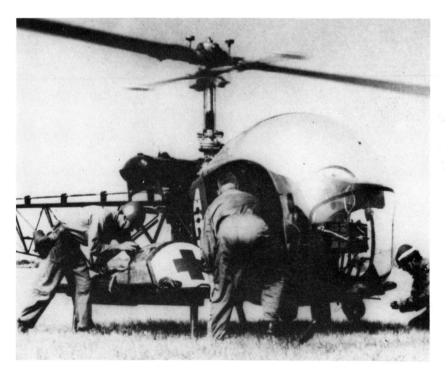

Figure 1–10. Helicopter evacuation of the wounded during the Korean Conflict helped reduce the lag time between injury and definitive surgical care. Continued improvement in Vietnam in helicopter evacuation of the wounded allowed some patients with vascular trauma to reach a definitive surgical center within 15 to 30 minutes. (U.S. Army photograph.)

1–12). In a total experience with 304 arterial injuries, 269 were repaired and 35 ligated (Hughes, 1958). The over-all amputation rate was 13 per cent, a marked contrast to that of about 49 per cent in World War II. Because amputation rate is only one method of determining ultimate success or failure in arterial repair, it is important to emphasize that Jahnke (1958) revealed that, in addition to the lowered rate of limb loss, limbs functioned normally when arterial repair was successful.

Figure 1–11. Postoperative ward in a *mobile army surgical hospital* (MASH) shows some of the conditions at the time of the Korean Conflict when it was demonstrated that arterial repair could be successful, even under battlefield conditions. (Hughes, C. W., Milit. Med., *124:* 30, 1959.)

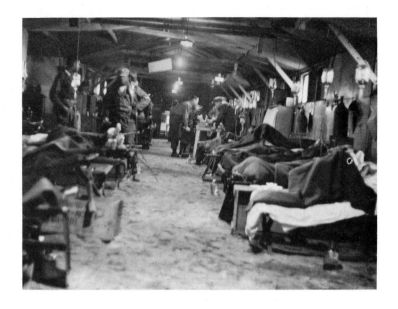

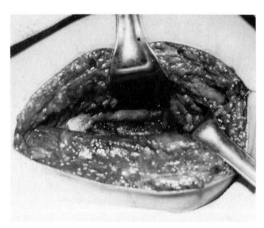

Figure 1–12. An autogenous greater saphenous vein graft was utilized in 1952 at Walter Reed General Hospital to repair a traumatized proximal popliteal artery. Each anastomosis is an everting type with intima-to-intima held by everting mattress sutures. (Rich, N. M., and Hughes, C. W., Bull. Amer. Coll. Surg., *57*:35, 1972.)

EXPERIENCE IN VIETNAM

In Vietnam the time lag between injury and treatment was reduced even further by the almost routine evacuation by helicopter combined with the widespread availability of surgeons experienced in vascular surgery. In one study of 750 patients with missile wounds in Vietnam, 95 per cent of the patients reached the hospital by helicopter (Rich, 1968) (Fig. 1–13). This prompt evacuation, however, similarly created an adverse effect on the overall results, for patients with severe injuries from high velocity missiles survived only long enough to reach the hospital. During initial care they expired. These patients would never have reached the hospital alive in previous military conflicts.

In the initial Vietnam studies, between October 1, 1965, and June 30, 1966, there were 177 known vascular injuries in American casualties, excluding those with traumatic amputation (Heaton et al., 1966). One hundred and sixteen operations were performed on 106 patients with 108 injuries (Table 1–2). These results included the personal experience of one of us (NMR) at the 2nd Surgical Hospital. The results reported included a short term follow-up of approximately 7 to 10 days in Vietnam. In Vietnam, amputations were required for only 9 of the 108 vascular injuries: a rate of about 8 per cent. Subsequently, more de-

tailed analysis from the Vietnam Vascular Registry (Rich and Hughes, 1969; Rich et al., 1970A) found the amputation rate of approximately 13 per cent identical to that of the Korean Conflict. Almost all amputations were performed within the first month after wounding.

The Vietnam Vascular Registry was established at Walter Reed General Hospital in 1966 to document and analyze all vascular injuries treated in Army Hospitals in Vietnam. A preliminary report (Rich and Hughes, 1969) involved the complete follow-up of 500 patients who sustained 718 vascular injuries (Table 1–3). Although vascular repairs on Vietnamese and allied military personnel were not included, the Registry effort was soon expanded to include all American service personnel, rather than limiting the effort to soldiers.

Fisher (1967) collected 154 acute arterial injuries in Vietnam covering the 1965–1966 period. There were 108 arterial injuries with significant information for the initial review from Army hospitals. In 1967, Chandler and Knapp reported results in managing acute vascular injuries in the U.S. Navy hospitals in Vietnam. These patients were not included in the initial Vietnam Vascular Registry report; but after 1967 an attempt was made to include all

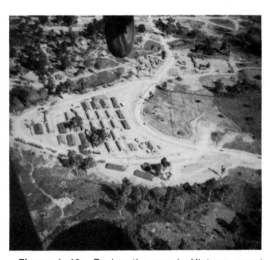

Figure 1–13. During the war in Vietnam, most patients were rapidly treated in fixed installations. An early example is the 2nd Surgical Hospital at An Khe in January, 1966. Ninety-five per cent of the wounded reached a hospital by helicopter. (Rich, N. M., *in* Georgiade, N. G. (Ed.), Plastic and Maxillofacial Trauma Symposium. Vol. 1. The C. V. Mosby Co., St. Louis, 1969.)

TABLE 1–2. EARLY EXPERIENCE WITH VASCULAR SURGERY IN VIETNAM
108 ARTERIAL INJURIES AT ARMY HOSPITALS*
(1 October 1965 to 30 June 1966)

	Type of Repair							Results		
									No Amputation	
Artery	Number of Injuries	Anasto-mosis	Vein Graft	Lateral Repair	Throm-bectomy	Pros Graft	Total Repairs	Pulse Present	Pulse Absent	Amp
Common carotid	7	1	3	3	0	0	7	7	0	0
Axillary	9	3	4	2	0	0	9	8	1	0
Brachial	33	15	11	9	1	0	36	29	3	1
Innominate	1	1	0	0	0	0	1	1	0	0
Subclavian	1	0	0	1	0	0	1	1	0	0
External iliac	4	2	1	0	0	1	4	4	0	0
Common femoral	7	3	4	1	0	0	8	7	0	0
Superficial femoral	30	21	3	6	0	0	30	26	1	3
Popliteal	16	7	7	5	1	0	20	10	1	5
Total	108	53	33	27	2	1	116	93	6	9

*Including 2nd Surg, 3rd Surg, 85th Evac, 91st Evac, 3rd Field and 8th Field Hospitals.
†Modified from Heaton, L. D., Hughes, C. W., Rosegay, H., Fisher, G. W., and Feighny, R. E., Military surgical practices of the United States Army in Viet Nam. Curr. Probl. Surg., November, 1966.

military personnel sustaining vascular trauma in Vietnam. This included active duty members of the United States Armed Forces treated at approximately 25 Army hospitals, six Navy hospitals and one Air Force hospital.

As with any registry, success of the Vietnam Vascular Registry has depended upon the cooperation of hundreds of individuals within the military and civilian communities. In the initial report from the Registry, the names of 20 surgeons who had done more than five vascular repairs were included (Rich and Hughes, 1969), and these are listed below:

Chimene, D.	Levitsky, S.
Dynan, J.	Mengoli, L.
Flynn, C.	Novack, T.
Frohman, B.	Rich, N.
Geoghegan, L.	Ricks, K.
Glass, L.	Snyder, L.
Hamaker, W.	Turney, S.
Hughes, J.	Walker, E.
Krouse, J.	Waltzer, A.
Kurrus, F.	Williams, G.

TABLE 1–3. MANAGEMENT OF ARTERIAL TRAUMA IN VIETNAM CASUALTIES
PRELIMINARY REPORT FROM THE VIETNAM VASCULAR REGISTRY*

Artery	**End-to-End Anastomosis**	**Vein Graft**	**Lateral Suture**	**Prosthetic Graft**	**Throm-bectomy**	**Ligation**
Common carotid	2	6 (2)	3		(2)	1
Internal carotid			2			1
Subclavian	1					
Axillary	6 (3)	12 (3)	2 (3)	(1)	(3)	(1)
Brachial	57 (8)	32 (10)	2 (1)		1 (9)	1 (2)
Aorta			3 (1)			
Renal						1
Iliac	1	1		1 (1)	(1)	(1)
Common femoral	4 (2)	11 (1)	4 (1)	1 (2)	(2)	(4)
Superficial femoral	63 (5)	37 (14)	7 (7)	(4)	2 (6)	(4)
Popliteal	31 (5)	28 (13)	6 (4)		(10)	2 (4)
Total	165 (23)	127 (43)	29 (17)	2 (8)	3 (33)	6 (16)

*Modified from Rich, N. M., and Hughes, C. W., Surgery, 65:218, 1969.
†Numbers in parenthesis represent additional procedures performed after the initial repair in Vietnam and repair of major arterial injuries not initially treated in Vietnam.

As can be seen by the list of more than 500 surgeons within the front and back covers of this book, many surgeons in every training program in the United States have contributed to the generally good results obtained in Vietnam.

The following is the list of Surgical Consultants representing the Army in Vietnam who were helpful in obtaining the initial documentation of many vascular injuries in Vietnam:

>LTC George W. Fisher, MC
>LTC Alphonse C. Gomez, MC
>LTC Gene V. Aaby, MC
>COL Arthur M. Cohen, MC
>COL James P. Geiger, MC
>LTC Stuart S. Roberts, MC

Hundreds of individuals in addition to the surgeons already cited have been directly contacted through the Registry. The cooperative effort that has been obtained has not only provided long term follow-up information for the individual surgeon, but it has also given the names of additional patients who have previously been missed, and more additional specific information has been added where needed regarding individual patients. A major success in the Registry effort was obtained at the American College of Surgeons' Clinical Congress in Chicago in 1970, where 110 surgeons who had previously performed arterial repairs in Vietnam signed in at the Vietnam Vascular Registry exhibit. The exhibit attempted to represent some of the activities and presented some of the interim results of the combined effort of all of the surgeons (Fig. 1–14).

In addition to the reports from the Registry, which will be cited throughout the following chapters, additional individual surgeons who have documented their experience in Vietnam include Levitsky and associates (1968), Gorman (1968, 1969), Williams (1968), Hewitt and associates (1969A, 1969B), Bizer (1969), Mengoli (1969), Fitchett and associates (1969), Tassi and Davies (1969), Gielchinsky and McNamara (1970), Cohen and associates (1969, 1970) and McNamara and associates (1973).

The fact that significant problems continue to confront the surgeon managing combat vascular injuries is emphasized by the report by Cohen and co-workers (1969), which evaluated a six month period of experience in Vietnam. The following list represents some of the major remaining problems.

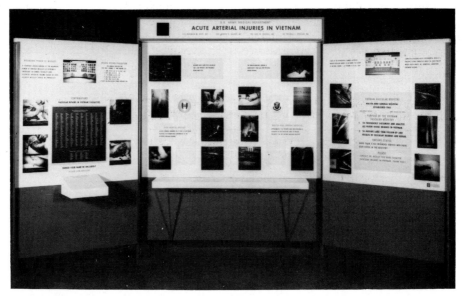

Figure 1–14. This exhibit representing the management of acute arterial trauma in Vietnam was presented from material in the Vietnam Vascular Registry to the Clinical Congress of the American College of Surgeons in Chicago in 1970. At least 110 surgeons who had previously performed arterial repairs in Vietnam visited the exhibit. (A.F.I.P. photograph.)

Purpose of the Vietnam Vascular Registry

1. TO THOROUGHLY DOCUMENT AND ANALYZE ALL BLOOD VESSEL INJURIES IN VIETNAM.

2. TO PROVIDE LONG TERM FOLLOW-UP AND RESULTS OF VASCULAR INJURIES AND REPAIRS.

In the Event of Further Evaluation or Treatment Please Notify

PERIPHERAL VASCULAR SURG NORMAN M. RICH, M.D.
WALTER REED GEN. HOSPITAL   LTC   MC   USA
WASHINGTON, D. C. 20012   CH. PERIP. VASCULAR SURG.

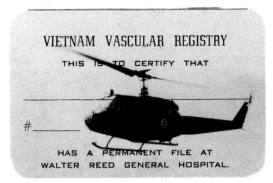

VIETNAM VASCULAR REGISTRY

THIS IS TO CERTIFY THAT

#_____

HAS A PERMANENT FILE AT
WALTER REED GENERAL HOSPITAL.

Figure 1–15. Identification card sent to armed forces personnel who were wounded in Vietnam. This card was issued in an attempt to identify participation in the Registry and with the hope that additional long-term follow-up information will be generated. (W. R. G. H.)*

1. Arterial injuries associated with massive damage to soft tissues.
2. Major venous obstruction.
3. Repeated vascular operations with a viable limb.
4. Associated unstable fractures.
5. Inadequate tissue débridement.
6. Calf wounds with small vessel injury.

Through the Vietnam Vascular Registry, identification cards have been sent to the majority of the patients whose names and records are included in the long term follow-up (Fig. 1–15). The response from the individual patients through this media has been extremely encouraging, and the typical response that is frequently received is that the patients appreciate the fact that "someone still cares." Nearly 1500 patients have been evaluated by one of the authors (NMR) in the Peripheral Vascular Surgery

*All photographs marked W. R. G. H. in this book are from the personal file of one of the authors (N. M. R.).

Clinic and Registry at Walter Reed Army Medical Center over the past ten years. Preliminary plans are presently being made to maintain an extended long term follow-up. This will be important in determining the long term results of the repairs and in determining the incidence of such problems as the early development of arteriosclerosis in the repair site of these young men. Personal contact has been made through the Registry with approximately 300 other surgeons who have performed vascular repairs in Vietnam, and the support of these surgeons has been solicited in helping with this long term follow-up project.

CIVILIAN EXPERIENCE

The frequency of arterial injuries in civilian life has increased greatly in the past decade. This is due to more automobile accidents, the appalling increase of gunshot and stab wounds, and the increasing use of therapeutic and diagnostic techniques involving the cannulation of major arteries.

As recently as 1950, most general surgeons had little experience or confidence in techniques of arterial repair. The experiences in the Korean Conflict, combined with the widespread teaching of techniques of vascular surgery in surgical residencies, resulted in a great increase in frequency of arterial repair between 1950 and 1960. This is well illustrated in the report by Ferguson and co-authors in 1961 of experiences with 200 arterial injuries treated in Atlanta over the ten year period beginning in 1950. The proportion of patients treated by arterial repair increased from less than 10 per cent in 1950 to more than 80 per cent in 1959 (Fig. 1–16). In the latter part of the study, ligation was done only for injuries of minor arteries, such as the radial or ulnar, or certain visceral arteries. The mortality rate was reduced by one-third and the amputation rate by one-half when two consecutive five year periods were compared (Fig. 1–17). The rate of success of arterial repair improved from 36 to 90 per cent.

In 1964 Patman and associates reported experiences with 271 repairs of arterial injuries in Dallas. In the past decade a series

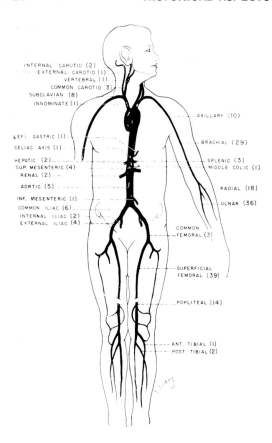

Figure 1–16. The increase in the repair of acute arterial injuries with the concomitant decrease in ligation is emphasized above by a civilian study covering a 10-year period in Atlanta for 200 patients with arterial injuries. Arterial repair was used in less than 10 per cent of the repairs in 1950 and in more than 80 per cent in 1959, and ligation in the latter part of this study was reserved for minor arteries. (Ferguson, I. A., Sr., Byrd, W. M., and McAfee, D. K., Ann. Surg., *153*:980, 1961.)

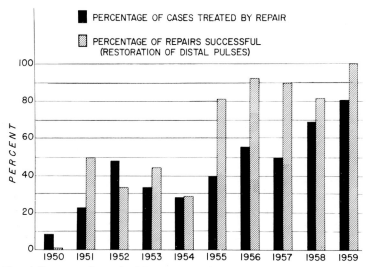

Figure 1–17. The civilian experience in Atlanta comparing two consecutive five-year periods shows the increase in incidence of injury and the marked improvement of successful repair from 36 per cent to 90 per cent. There was also an associated reduction in the mortality rate by one-third and amputation rate by one-half. (Ferguson, I. A., Sr., Byrd, W. M., and McAfee, D. K., Ann. Surg., *153*:980, 1961.)

of reports from large urban centers throughout the United States have appeared, all documenting the effectiveness of current techniques of arterial repair. Reference will be made to these reports in specific discussions in the following chapters. Two large recent series are those of Drapanas and colleagues (1970) from New Orleans, which included 226 arterial injuries; and the cumulative report by Perry and associates from Dallas (1971), which included 508 arterial injuries.

Smith and coworkers (1974) reported a survey of 268 patients in Detroit with 285 penetrating wounds of the limbs and neck. There were 127 peripheral arterial injuries identified. Cheek and co-authors (1975) reviewed 200 operative cases of major vascular injuries in Memphis which included 155 arterial injuries. Kelly and Eiseman (1975) from Denver found 116 arterial injuries among 175 injuries to major named vessels in 143 patients. Hardy and associates (1975) reviewed 360 arterial injuries in 353 patients in Jackson. Bole and colleagues (1976) reported 126 arterial injuries in 122 patients in New York City during 1968–1973.

CHAPTER 2

ETIOLOGY, INCIDENCE AND CLINICAL PATHOLOGY

Currently accepted principles regarding management of acute vascular injuries are largely based on military experience.

Drapanas, T., et al., 1970

Vascular injuries in large numbers are usually seen only during military conflicts. As a result, most data are from four major wars of this century, World Wars I and II, Korea and Vietnam. In the past 15 to 20 years, however, there have been an increasing number of significant reports of arterial injuries from civilian trauma, re-flecting not only the increasing frequency of civilian trauma but also the improved methods of treatment as a result of widespread training in vascular surgery in surgical residency programs.

Military and civilian vascular injuries differ in several respects. Military injuries occur almost exclusively in young males

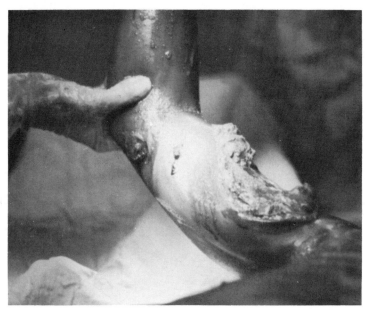

Figure 2–1. Typical high velocity missile wound which caused extensive soft tissue destruction as well as vascular trauma (2nd Surgical Hospital in Vietnam in 1966). The relatively small two entrance wounds above the elbow of the right arm caused by 7.62 mm bullets are contrasted by the much larger proximal exit wound. (Rich, N. M., J. Cardiovas. Surg., *11*:368, 1970.)

MILITARY INJURIES

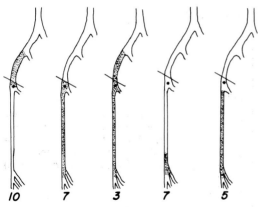

Figure 2–2. Site of thrombus in 32 patients who developed acute vascular insufficiency of a lower extremity following percutaneous femoral angiography. (Yellin, A. E., and Shore, E. H., Surgery, *73:* 772, 1973.)

free from chronic arterial disease and are often due to high velocity missiles which cause extensive soft tissue destruction and disruption of collateral circulation (Fig. 2–1). Although more frequent in young males, civilian trauma may occur in any age group. It is being seen more often in the arteriosclerotic patient, especially following diagnostic procedures involving peripheral arteries, such as angiography or cardiac catheterization (Figs. 2–2 and 2–3). Usually, civilian trauma is from low velocity missiles or stab wounds with little associated soft tissue destruction.

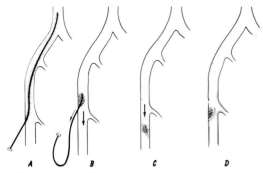

Figure 2–3. The mechanisms of arterial occlusion following percutaneous angiography: (A) Thrombus forming on outer wall of intra-arterial catheter. (B) Catheter withdrawn, thrombus stripped off, adhering to puncture site and occluding the arterial lumen. (C) Dislodgement and distal embolization of thrombus. (D) Intimal injury at puncture site with plaque elevation at subintimal dissection. (Yellin, A. E., and Shore, E. H., Surgery, 73:772, 1973.)

Incidence. Vascular trauma in World War I was well summarized by Makins (1919), in World War II by DeBakey and Simeone (1946), and in the Korean Conflict by Hughes (1958). Vascular injuries occurred in about 1 per cent of battle casualties in World War II (Fig. 2–4) and have ranged in different military conflicts of the past 120 years from as low as 0.07 per cent in the American Civil War to as high as 2.4 per cent in both the Russo-Japanese War (DeBakey and Simeone, 1946) and the Korean Conflict (Hughes, 1958). In Vietnam, one analysis of 200,000 combat wounded, including many minor injuries, found 4000 vascular injuries, a frequency of 2 per cent (Rich et al., 1970A). Other specific series reported an even higher frequency. Thomas (1972) reported 3.35 per cent among 2000 patients treated at the First Marine Medical Battalion from January to October, 1967, and Geer (1972) found a 9.4 per cent frequency among 2373 casualties requiring treatment in the operating room at the 27th Surgical Hospital from April, 1968, to May, 1971.

Table 2–1 outlines the incidence of various arterial injuries in World Wars I and II. The experience was similar during the Korean Conflict, in which major extremity vessels were most frequently injured (Table 2–2). The frequency distribution of various types of vascular injury was studied in the preliminary report from the Vietnam Vascular Registry, a study of 500 patients (Rich and Hughes, 1969). There was a total of 718 vascular injuries in the 500 patients, indicating the frequency of multiple wounds. The 718 injuries included 365 major arterial injuries, 194 major venous injuries and 159 minor arterial injuries (Table 2–3). Approximately 94 per cent of the major arterial injuries, 342 of 365, occurred in the extremities (Table 2–4). This included about 60 per cent in the lower extremities and approximately 34 per cent in the upper extremities. Only 4 per cent occurred in the neck, and the remaining few arterial injuries were in the thoracic and abdominal cavities. This frequency distribution was confirmed in the 1970 interim analysis of 1000 acute major

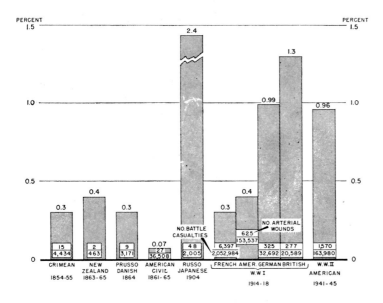

Figure 2–4. Incidence of arterial wounds among battle casualties in various wars. (DeBakey, M. E., and Simeone, F. A., Ann. Surg., *123*:534, 1946.)

TABLE 2–1. INCIDENCE OF ARTERIAL INJURIES IN COMBAT

Artery	British World War I (Makins, 1919)		American World War II (DeBakey and Simeone, 1946)*	
	Total	Per Cent	Total	Per Cent
Aorta	5	0.4	3	0.12
Carotid	128	10.7	10	0.40
External carotid			3	0.12
Renal			2	0.10
Vertebral	3	0.2		
Subclavian	45	3.7	21	0.85
Axillary	108	9.0	74	0.30
Brachial (total)	200	16.7	601	24.32
Above profunda			97	3.92
Below profunda			209	8.45
Radial-ulnar	59	4.9		
Radial			99	4.00
Ulnar			69	2.79
Radial and ulnar			28	1.13
Common iliac	1	0.1	13	0.52
External iliac	4	0.3	30	1.21
Internal iliac	1	0.1	1	0.04
Femoral (total)	366	30.5	517	20.92
Above profunda			106	4.28
Below profunda			177	7.16
Profunda			27	1.09
Popliteal	144	12.0	502	20.31
Anterior tibial	26	2.2	129	5.22
Posterior tibial	97	8.1	265	10.72
Anterior and posterior tibial	7	0.6	91	3.68
Peroneal	4	0.3	7	0.28
Anterior tibial and peroneal	1	0.1	5	0.20
Both tibial and peroneal			1	0.04
Total	1202†		2471	

*Modified from DeBakey, M. E., and Simeone, F. A., Ann. Surg., *123*:534, 1946.

†This total differs from the number of 1191 cases from Makins' master table because 11 vessels of the leg were added from a detailed table printed in the text.

TABLE 2–2. MAJOR ACUTE ARTERIAL INJURIES KOREAN CONFLICT*

ARTERY	NUMBER	PER CENT
Carotid	11	3.6
Subclavian	3	1.0
Axillary	20	6.6
Brachial	89	29.3
Iliac	7	2.3
Femoral	95	31.2
Popliteal	79	26.0
Total	304	100.0

*Modified from Hughes, C. W., Ann. Surg., *147*: 555, 1958.

arterial injuries in Vietnam (Table 2–5). In this group the superficial femoral artery was the most commonly injured—about 31 per cent of the total. The brachial artery was injured in 28 per cent, and the popliteal in nearly 22 per cent. The high localization of injuries to the extremities is partly due to the fact that penetrating injuries of the thorax or abdomen with high velocity missiles are often fatal.

Etiology. Most vascular trauma in Vietnam resulted from fragmenting missiles, such as artillery, rockets, grenades and booby traps. There were, however, more injuries from high velocity bullets than in previous wars because of the large number of jungle skirmishes by small units in direct contact. In the 1970 analysis of 1000 major acute arterial injuries, fragments caused about 60 per cent of the injuries, and bullets

caused approximately 35 per cent (Table 2–6). Blunt trauma accounted for only 1 per cent, usually from vehicular or helicopter accidents. In at least 12 instances, puncture wounds from the primitive punji stick caused an arterial injury (Fig. 2–5). These were analyzed among a large series of 342 punji stick wounds treated at the 2nd Surgical Hospital by one of the authors (NMR) (Shepard et al., 1967).

The development of the high velocity M-16 weapon introduced a different category of injury. Massive tissue destruction far exceeded that from previous military weapons firing a bullet of equal or even

TABLE 2–3. VIETNAM VASCULAR REGISTRY PRELIMINARY REPORT*

Location of Injury	PATIENTS Number	Per Cent
A. Completed Follow-up of Registered Patients		
Major arterial injuries	344	68.8
Minor arterial injuries	128	25.6
Major venous injuries	28	5.6
Total	500	100.0
B. Vessel Involvement Among the 500 Patients		
Major arterial injuries	365	50.8
Major venous injuries	194	27.1
Minor arterial injuries	159	22.1
Total	718	100.0

*Modified from Rich, N. M. and Hughes, C. W., Surgery, *65*:218, 1969.

TABLE 2–4. LOCATION OF MAJOR ACUTE ARTERIAL INJURIES VIETNAM VASCULAR REGISTRY PRELIMINARY REPORT*

Site	Artery	TOTAL TO EACH Number	Site	Per Cent
Neck	Common carotid	12	15	4.1
	Internal carotid	3		
Thorax	Subclavian	1	1	0.3
Upper extremity	Axillary	22	125	34.2
	Brachial	103		
Abdomen	Aorta	3	7	1.9
	Renal	1		
	Iliac	3		
Lower extremity	Common femoral	24	217	59.5
	Superficial femoral	116		
	Popliteal	77		
Total		365	365	100.0

*Modified from Rich, N. M., and Hughes, C. W., Surgery, *65*:218, 1969.

TABLE 2-5. LOCATION OF 1000 ACUTE MAJOR ARTERIAL INJURIES
VIETNAM VASCULAR REGISTRY PRELIMINARY REPORT*

Site	Artery	Number	Per Cent
Neck	Carotid	50	5.0
Chest	Innominate	3	
	Subclavian	8	1.1
Upper extremity	Axillary	59	
	Brachial	283	34.2
Abdomen and pelvis	Abdominal aorta	3	
	Common iliac	9	2.9
	External iliac	17	
Lower extremity	Common femoral	46	
	Superficial femoral	305	56.8
	Popliteal	217	
Total		1000	100.0

*Modified from Rich, N. M., Baugh, J. H., and Hughes, C. W., J. Trauma, *10*:359, 1970.

larger size. This can be demonstrated by comparing the size of the entrance and exit wound caused by different missiles. With a .45 caliber bullet wound, entrance and exit wounds are similar in size, about 1.5 cm (Fig. 2–6). With the M-16 wound, however, the entrance wound is of similar size (Fig. 2–7) to that of the .45 caliber bullet, but causes a markedly larger exit wound, about 6 by 10 cm with extensive tissue destruction (Fig. 2–8). Experimental studies of high velocity wounds shows that a temporary cavity can be created nearly 30 times as large as the permanent residual tract. This temporary cavitational effect injures tissues far beyond the actual path of the missile (see Chap. 3).

The following case report illustrates arterial thrombosis from temporary cavitational effect (Rich, et al., 1971 B):

TABLE 2-6. ETIOLOGY OF 1000 MAJOR
ACUTE ARTERIAL INJURIES
VIETNAM VASCULAR REGISTRY*

Agent	Number	Per Cent
Fragment	601	60.1
Bullet	345	34.5
Blunt	11	1.1
Punji stick	4	0.4
Miscellaneous	6	0.6
Questionable	33	3.3
Total	1000	100.0

*Modified from Rich, N. M., Baugh, J. H., and Hughes, C. W., J. Trauma, *10*:359, 1970.

A 20 year old soldier sustained multiple M-16 gunshot wounds of the abdomen, right thigh and right arm. He arrived at the 2nd Surgical Hospital (MA), An Khe, Republic of Vietnam, by helicopter evacuation approximately two hours after wounding.

After rapid assessment of his injuries, necessary resuscitative measures were instituted

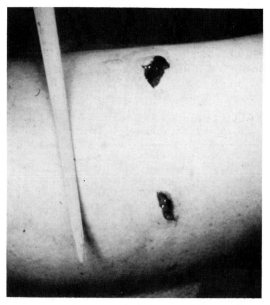

Figure 2–5. There have been at least 12 vascular injuries caused by trauma from the primitive punji stick in Vietnam. This photograph taken at the 2nd Surgical Hospital in Vietnam in 1966 shows a typical through-and-through punji stick wound of the leg. (Rich, N. M., Milit. Med., *133*:9, 1968.)

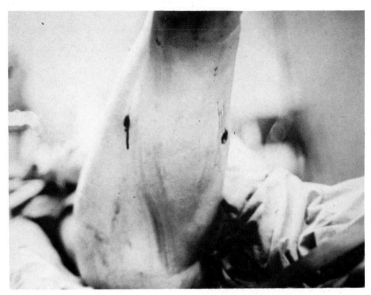

Figure 2-6. Both the entrance and exit wounds measured approximately 1.5 cm for this .45 caliber gunshot wound of the posterior thigh treated at the 2nd Surgical Hospital in Vietnam in 1966. (Rich, N. M., Milit. Med., *133*:9, 1968.)

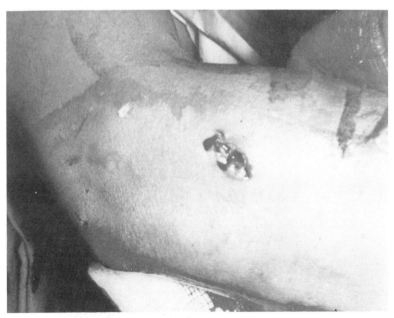

Figure 2-7. The entrance wound from an M-16 missile fired from approximately 30 feet is located on the lateral aspect of the right forearm and measures approximately the same size as the .45 caliber wounds shown in Figure 2-6. (Dimond, F. C., Jr., and Rich, N. M., J. Trauma, 7:619, 1967. Copyright 1967, The Williams & Wilkins Co., Baltimore.)

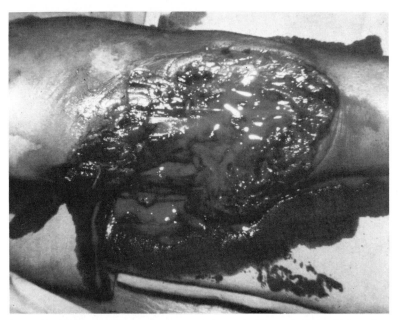

Figure 2–8. In contrast to the small entrance wound shown in Figure 2–7, the M-16 exit wound measures approximately 6 by 10 cm and shows massive tissue destruction on the volar surface of the forearm. (Dimond, F. C., Jr., and Rich, N. M., J. Trauma, 7:619, 1967. Copyright 1967, The Williams & Wilkins Co., Baltimore.)

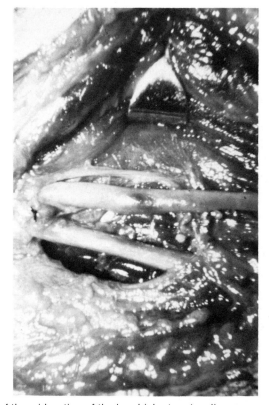

Figure 2–9. Contusion of the midportion of the brachial artery (median nerve seen below it) was caused by the temporary cavitational effect of a high velocity M-16 bullet. The lack of arterial flow beyond the contused segment can be appreciated by the smaller size of the artery. (Rich, N. M., Amato, J. J., and Billy, L. J., Surg. Digest, 6:12, 1971.)

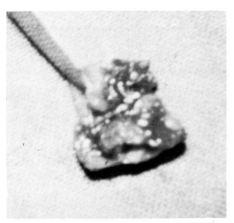

Figure 2–10. The excised segment of the brachial artery demonstrated in Figure 2–9 shows organized thrombus, at the area of intimal disruption, which occluded the lumen. This resulted from the temporary cavitational effect of the high velocity bullet which did not actually strike the brachial artery. (Rich, N. M., Amato, J. J., and Billy, L. J., Surg. Digest, 6: 12, 1971.)

and exploratory celiotomy was performed. Although the patient had a palpable right radial pulse when admitted to the emergency area, by the time of débridement of the wound of the right upper extremity approximately three hours later, this pulse had disappeared. Despite significant soft tissue destruction it was evident by the entrance and exit wounds and the permanent missile tract that the M-16 bullet had not directly struck the brachial artery. The effect of the temporary cavitation of the high velocity missile was realized when the brachial artery was found to be contused (Fig. 2–9). It was evident that the proximal artery was full and bounding with no pulsation in the collapsed brachial artery distal to the contused segment. After adequate débridement of the damaged artery, an end-to-end anastomosis was possible.

A longitudinal incision through the involved segment revealed disruption of the intima, subintimal hematoma and intraluminal thrombus (Fig. 2–10). Microscopic findings substantiated the clinical impression of gross disruption of the intima and media with thrombus formation.

CIVILIAN VASCULAR INJURIES

Incidence and Etiology. Several differences exist between civilian and military vascular injuries. First, military injuries are characteristically in young persons without arterial disease. They frequently result from high velocity missiles with extensive soft tissue destruction, often with injuries of multiple organ systems, and in circumstances where surgical treatment is less than ideal. Civilian injuries, however, are usually from wounds associated with minimal soft tissue destruction. Prompt treatment and excellent hospital facilities are usually available. Although young civilians are commonly injured, there is also a significant percentage of older patients, who often have pre-existing arterial disease. In addition, there are frequent injuries from blunt trauma, such as automobile or industrial accidents, and fractures of long bones. Finally, an increasing number of vascular injuries are being seen as a complication of diagnostic procedures involving cannulation of peripheral arteries, as in angiography or cardiac catheterization. In the following paragraphs a brief narrative summary of significant reports of the past decade is given to indicate the type and frequency of vascular injury most commonly reported.

One of the first large series of civilian arterial trauma was reported by Morris and associates in 1957. They described a series of 136 patients with acute arterial injuries treated over a period of seven years at Baylor University affiliated hospitals in Houston (Fig. 2–11). Sixty-eight injuries, one-half of the group, involved the upper extremities, and 47 injuries (about 35 per cent) involved the lower extremities. There were 10 injuries of either the abdominal or thoracic aorta and 11 of the carotid artery. One hundred and twenty of the patients, 88 per cent, were male, and most of the injuries were caused by acts of violence. Primary arterial repair was possible in a high percentage of these patients.

In 1961 Ferguson and co-workers reported from Grady Memorial Hospital in Atlanta 200 arterial injuries treated over a period of ten years (Fig. 1–16). The superficial femoral artery was injured most frequently—39 cases, or nearly 20 per cent of the total group. However, 54 of the 200 cases were injuries of minor arteries such as the radial or ulnar arteries. As in Houston, most resulted from acts of violence (Table 2–7). Automobile, industrial and domestic accidents accounted for most of the remaining injuries.

In 1963 Smith and associates described

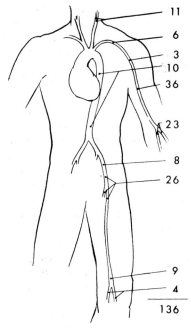

11
6
3
10
36
23
8
26
9
4
136

Figure 2–11. Anatomic locations of arterial injuries in the civilian experience in Houston. In addition to the fact that nearly one-half of the injuries involved the brachial and femoral arteries, exactly 50 per cent of the injuries also involved arteries supplying the upper extremity. (Morris, G. C., Jr., Creech, O., Jr., and DeBakey, M. E., Amer. J. Surg., 93:565, 1957.)

experiences with 59 patients with 61 vascular injuries in Detroit, including both acute and chronic arterial injuries (Table 2–8). They properly emphasized that a careful distinction must be made between results with acute and chronic lesions. Collateral circulation has usually developed when a chronic lesion is treated and the problem of soft tissue destruction is not present. Acts of violence, gunshot and stab wounds, caused 18 arterial injuries—44 per cent of the penetrating lesions (Table 2–9). Their

patients included a total of 10 industrial injuries, as well as eight iatrogenic injuries resulting either from surgical operations or diagnostic procedures. These eight included three injuries of the external iliac artery during inguinal herniorrhaphy, three arterial injuries following diagnostic arterial catheterization, one injury of the internal iliac artery during removal of a herniated intravertebral disc, and one arteriovenous fistula developing after a mass suture ligature of the renal pedicle during nephrectomy.

In 1968 Dillard and co-authors described the treatment of 85 arterial injuries in St. Louis over a period of eight years beginning in 1958 (Table 2–10). Eighty-one per cent of the injuries involved an extremity. Penetrating injuries from knives or glass caused 35 of the injuries, 31 resulted from gunshot wounds and 19 were caused by blunt trauma or crushing injuries (Table 2–11).

A somewhat different group of cases was reported from Europe by Vollmar in 1968. In an analysis of 85,000 injured patients treated in the Heidelburg University Surgery Clinic between 1953 and 1966,

TABLE 2–7. TYPE OF WOUND CAUSING ARTERIAL INJURY*
Grady Memorial Hospital, Atlanta, Georgia
January 1, 1950–December 31, 1959

| | NUMBER | |
TYPE	CASES	PER CENT
Lacerations and stab wounds	100	50.0
Pistol and rifle	67	33.5
Shotgun	24	12.0
Blunt injury	9	4.5
Total	200	100.0

*Modified from Ferguson, I. A., Byrd, W. M., and McAfee, D. K., Ann. Surg., *153*:980, 1961.

TABLE 2–8. CIVILIAN ARTERIAL TRAUMA IN DETROIT
61 ARTERIAL INJURIES*

| | 28 EARLY LESIONS | | | | | 33 LATE LESIONS | | |
Type of Trauma	Laceration	Transsection	Thrombosis	Spasm	Type of Trauma	A-V Fistula	False Aneurysm	True Aneurysm
Penetrating injuries	10	6	2	—	Penetrating injuries	17	8	—
Nonpenetrating injuries	2	2	4	2	Nonpenetrating injuries	4	1	3
Total	12	8	6	2	Total	21	9	3

*Modified from Smith, R. F., Szilagyi, D. E., and Pfeifer, J. R., Arch. Surg., *86*:825, 1963.

TABLE 2-9. ETIOLOGICAL FACTORS CAUSING 61 ARTERIAL INJURIES
59 PATIENTS IN A CIVILIAN SERIES IN DETROIT*

42 PENETRATING INJURIES	PER CENT	19 NONPENETRATING INJURIES	PER CENT
Gunshot.....................13	21.3	Industrial.......................11	18.0
Industrial.................10	16.4	Auto................................ 4	6.6
Iatrogenic................. 8	13.1	Athletic........................... 2	3.3
Household................. 6	9.8	Household...................... 2	3.3
Stab........................ 5	8.2		

*Modified from Smith, R. F., Szilagyi, D. E., and Pfeifer, J. R., Arch. Surg., *86*:825, 1963.

TABLE 2-10. DISTRIBUTION OF ARTERIAL INJURIES IN ST. LOUIS* 1958–1966

ARTERY	NUMBER	PER CENT
Axillary artery	6	7.1
Brachial artery	26	30.6
Subclavian artery	4	4.7
Thoracic aorta	8	9.4
Abdominal aorta and branches	8	9.4
Iliac artery	2	2.3
Common femoral artery	7	8.2
Superficial femoral artery	14	16.5
Popliteal artery	10	11.8
Total	85	100.0

*Modified from Dillard, B. M., Nelson, D. L., and Norman, H. G., Jr., Surgery, *63*:391, 1968.

there were only 172 arterial lesions, an incidence of 0.3 per cent. In marked contrast to the American experience, only 1 per cent of the injuries was due to gunshot wounds. Most patients were injured in industrial accidents (Table 2–12). Approximately one-fourth resulted from simple domestic accidents. Twelve resulted from automobile accidents. It was significant in this group that 41 per cent of the total series resulted from blunt trauma (Table 2–13).

In 1968 Saletta and Freeark described experiences with 57 patients with partially severed major peripheral arteries treated in Chicago (Table 2–14). The majority of the injuries resulted from physical violence from gunshot wounds or knives.

In 1964 Patman and associates described experiences with 256 patients, with a total of 271 arterial injuries, treated at the Parkland Memorial Hospital in Dallas over a 12 year period starting in July, 1949. As in other American series, most resulted from acts of violence, and only a few resulted

from industrial or automobile accidents. Multiple arterial injuries occurred in 6 per cent of the group. Although chronic lesions from trauma were included, it was noteworthy that these were few—only six arteriovenous fistulas and 12 false aneurysms among the entire group of 256 patients.

At Charity Hospital in New Orleans, 226 patients with arterial injuries were treated between 1942 and 1969 (Drapanas et al., 1970) (Fig. 2–12). Of the 226 patients, 173 were major arterial injuries and 53 were minor. The most frequently injured arteries were the brachial (39 injuries) and the superficial femoral (31 injuries). There was an unusually large number (23) of aortic injuries involving the thoracic or abdominal aorta.

In 1971 Perry and associates reported an

TABLE 2-11. ETIOLOGY AND ANATOMIC DISTRIBUTION OF 85 ARTERIAL INJURIES* ST. LOUIS, 1958–1966

A. KNIFE OR GLASS PENETRATING INJURIES

Upper extremities	15
Thoracic aorta	3
Abdominal aorta and branches	5
Lower extremities	12
Total	35(41.2%)

B. PENETRATING GUNSHOT INJURIES

Upper extremities	13
Thoracic aorta	2
Abdominal aorta and branches	2
Lower extremities	14
Total	31(36.5%)

C. BLUNT TRAUMA OR CRUSH INJURIES

Upper extremities	8
Thoracic aorta	3
Abdominal aorta and branches	3
Lower extremities	5
Total	19(22.3%)

*Modified from Dillard, B. M., Nelson, D. L., and Norman, H. G., Jr., Surgery, *63*:391, 1968.

TABLE 2–12. TYPE OF ACCIDENT RESPONSIBLE FOR 169 PATIENTS WITH ARTERIAL INJURIES HEIDELBERG UNIVERSITY SURGICAL CLINIC* 1953–1966

ETIOLOGY	NUMBER	PER CENT
Industrial accident	59	35
Domestic accident	44	26
Suicide	32	19
Traffic	24	14
Iatrogenic	10	6
Total	169	100

*Modified from Vollmar, J., *in* Hiertonn, T., and Rybeck, B., Traumatic Arterial Lesions. Försvaretes Forskningsanstalt, Stockholm, 1968.

TABLE 2–13. NATURE OF 197 ARTERIAL LESIONS IN 168 PATIENTS HEIDELBERG UNIVERSITY,* SURGICAL CLINIC 1953–1966

	TYPE	NUMBER	PER CENT	
Sharp-penetrating	Cut	95	48	⎫
	Stab	19	10	⎬ 59
	Shot	3	1	⎭
Blunt	Closed	22	11	⎫ 41
	Open	58	30	⎭

*Modified from Vollmar, J., *in* Hiertonn, T., and Rybeck, B., Traumatic Arterial Lesions. Försvaretes Forskningsanstalt, Stockholm, 1968.

additional series of 259 arterial injuries from Dallas. About 55 per cent of these were associated with gunshot wounds (Table 2–15). Combined with the 1964 report (Patman et al.), there were a total of 508 injuries (Table 2–16). These included 442 injuries of arteries in the extremities, representing 87 per cent of the total. There were also 42 cervical arterial injuries and 24 visceral arterial injuries.

Moore and co-workers in 1971 reported 250 vascular injuries treated in Galveston, 45 per cent of which occurred in the extremities (Table 2–17). In this series, 40 per cent of the cases involved either the chest, abdomen, or head and neck, a percentage higher than that in other reports. The injuries resulted from either gunshot or stab wounds in 60 per cent of the group (Table 2–18). Thirteen per cent resulted from blunt trauma, and iatrogenic injuries were responsible for 10 per cent. Among the 25 iatrogenic injuries, there were 16 acute arterial thromboses resulting from a total of more than 3000 cardiovascular radiographic procedures, a frequency less than 1 per cent (Table 2–19). Kelly and Eiseman (1975) reported 43 per cent of 143 patients in Denver with vascular injuries sustained gunshot wounds. The brachial artery was injured most often,

TABLE 2–14. LOCATION AND CAUSE OF INJURY IN 57 PATIENTS WITH PARTIALLY SEVERED ARTERIES*

LOCATION AND ARTERY	NUMBER	Gunshot	Knife	Glass	Blunt	Other
				ETIOLOGY		
Head and neck						
Temporal	3			1	2	
Internal carotid	2	2				
External carotid	2	1	1			
Vertebral	1		1			
Lingual	1		1			
Upper extremity						
Axillary	6	2	3	1		
Brachial	5	1	4			
Innominate	1	1				
Subclavian	1		1			
Lower extremity						
Femoral	15	11	3			1(needle)
Common femoral	6	3	1	1		1(needle)
Popliteal	6	6				
External iliac	4	3	1			
Deep femoral	2	1	1			
Anterior tibial	1			1		
Posterior tibial	1					1(tin can)
Tibioperoneal	1	1				

*Modified from Saletta, J. D., and Freeark, R. J., Arch. Surg., *97*:198, 1968.

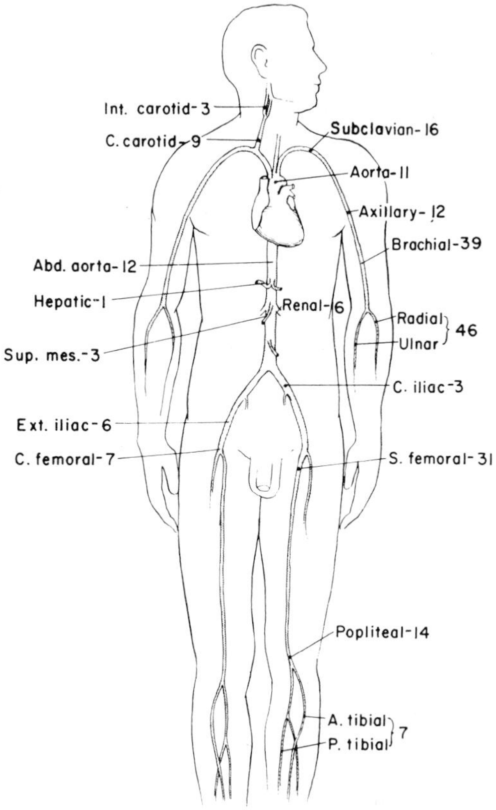

Figure 2–12. Distribution of 226 acute civilian arterial injuries covering a 30-year period in New Orleans starting in 1942. Eighty per cent of the injuries involve arteries to the extremities. (Drapanas, T., Hewitt, R. L., Weichert, R. F., and Smith, A.D., Ann. Surg., *172*:351, 1970.)

TABLE 2–15. CAUSE AND TYPE OF INJURY CIVILIAN ARTERIAL TRAUMA IN DALLAS*

CAUSE	NUMBER	PER CENT	ARTERIAL INJURY	NUMBER	PER CENT
Gunshot wound	143	55.2	Laceration	133	51.4
Edged instruments	92	35.5	Transection	99	38.2
Blunt trauma	24	9.3	Puncture	18	6.9
Total	259	100.0	Contusion	7	2.7
			Spasm	2	0.8
			Total	259	100.0

*Modified from Perry, M. O., Thal, E. R., and Shires, G. T., Ann. Surg., *173*:403, 1971.

TABLE 2–16. DISTRIBUTION OF CIVILIAN ARTERIAL INJURIES IN DALLAS*
508 ARTERIAL INJURIES

EXTREMITY(87.0%)		CERVICAL(8.3%)		VISCERAL(4.7%)	
Aorta	26	Common carotid	24	Celiac	2
Innominate	1	Internal carotid	8	Splenic	2
Subclavian	23	External carotid	6	Superior mesenteric	7
Axillary	38	Vertebral	4	Renal	9
Brachial	78	Total	42	Hepatic	4
Radial	58			Total	24
Ulnar	39				
Common iliac	20				
External iliac	11				
Hypogastric	7				
Common femoral	11				
Superficial femoral	93				
Profunda femoral	8				
Popliteal	17				
Tibial	12				
Total	442				

*Modified from Perry, M. O., Thal, E. R., and Shires, G. T., Ann. Surg., *173*:403, 1971.

TABLE 2–17. LOCATION OF VASCULAR TRAUMA IN 250 CIVILIAN INJURIES*
Galveston, Texas, 1960–1970

LOCATION	PER CENT
Head and neck	10
Thoracic outlet	16
Chest	15
Abdomen	14
Extremities	45
Total	100

*Modified from Moore, C. H., Wolman, F. J., Brown, R. W., and Derrick, J. R., Am. J. Surg., *122*:576, 1971.

37 times. Hardy and coworkers (1975) in Jackson recorded 192 arterial injuries from firearms (155 gunshot and 37 shotgun), 91 stab wounds and lacerations, 48 injuries from blunt trauma, and 20 iatrogenic injuries. Their series included 36 aortic injuries. However, approximately two-thirds involved extremity vessels.

TABLE 2–18. CAUSE OF 250 CIVILIAN VASCULAR INJURIES*
Galveston, Texas, 1960–1970

TYPE	PER CENT
Gunshot	39.0
Stab	25.0
Blunt	13.0
Iatrogenic	10.0
Other	13.0
Total	100.0

*Modified from Moore, C. H., Wolma, F. J., Brown, R. W., and Derrick, J. R., Am. J. Surg., *122*:576, 1971.

The specific site of arterial injury is important. All of the cited series emphasize the predominance of extremity arterial injuries. On the other hand, arterial injuries in the thorax or abdomen may be more difficult to diagnose or may present additional problems in management. There has been a relatively high mortality rate associated with arterial injuries at the base of the neck as a result of uncontrollable hemorrhage and cerebral ischemia. In 1964 Pate and Wilson described experiences with 21 patients with arterial injuries at the base of the neck treated at the City of Memphis Hospital over a 12 year period. As would be expected, there was a significant percentage of permanent, crippling neurologic injuries. The interesting observation was made that 93 per cent of the patients who were stabbed were injured on the left side, suggesting that most of the assailants were right-handed. Details of recent reports are found in Chapters 12 and 13.

Little has been published about intra-abdominal vascular injuries, perhaps because most victims died of exsanguinating hemorrhage. In 1968 Perdue and Smith reported a group of 90 patients, with 126 separate injuries, treated in Atlanta over a period of 10 years beginning in 1956. Most injuries resulted from low velocity bullet wounds. Five were injured with a shotgun and 14 were stab wounds. Nonpenetrating trauma occurred in six patients. Additional reports from recent series are described in Chapters 19 and 20.

TABLE 2–19. 25 CASES OF IATROGENIC VASCULAR INJURIES*
Galveston, Texas, 1960–1970

PROCEDURE	INJURY	TREATMENT	NUMBER
Central venous catheterization	thrombosis	thrombectomy	16
Lumbar laminectomy	arteriovenous fistula	repair of fistula	3
Osteotomy of hip	arteriovenous fistula	repair of fistula	1
Renal hemodialysis arteriovenous shunts	false aneurysm	resection of aneurysm	2
Pelvic irradiation	femoral artery rupture	aortofemoral bypass	1
Fracture of humerus closed reduction	Volkmann's ischemia	open reduction; free artery and fasciotomy	1
Subclavian catheterization	arteriovenous fistula	repair of fistula	1
Total			25

*Modified from Moore, C. H., Wolma, F. J., Brown, R. W., and Derrick, J. R., Am. J. Surg., *122*:576, 1971.

Iatrogenic Injuries. Of historical interest is the fact that one of the first hospital-incurred vascular injuries was well described nearly 80 years ago. Murphy (1897) reported that Heidenhain used a catgut suture to close a 1 cm laceration of the axillary artery, accidentally injured during removal of adherent carcinomatous glands on May 28, 1894. The patient made a good recovery with no disturbance of the circulation in the extremity.

In recent years several reports have described arterial injuries complicating the removal of a herniated nucleus pulposus; usually the injury involves the common iliac artery. One of the first detailed reports of this complication was made by Seeley and associates (1954). The injury resulted from the anatomic location of the iliac vessels on the anterior surface of the lumbar vertebrae, especially at the intervertebral spaces between the fourth and fifth lumbar vertebrae and between the fifth lumbar and first sacral ribs. In addition to the anatomic susceptibility to injury, the use of a pituitary rongeur for removal of the intervertebral discs was found to predispose to this type of injury (Fig. 2–13). At least eight such cases have been seen at Walter Reed General Hospital over a period of 25 years.

Arteriovenous fistulas have occurred at numerous sites after ligation in continuity of an artery and a vein, such as a renal artery and vein following nephrectomy, the splenic artery and vein following splenectomy, or the superior thyroid artery and vein following thyroid lobectomy. In 1968 Dillard and co-authors described an arterial injury developing from a Kirschner wire placed through the popliteal artery while applying skeletal traction for a femoral fracture. Saletta and Freeark (1972) described injury of the profunda femoris artery caused by a drill point during an orthopedic procedure. Injuries of the femoral artery and vein have occurred during inguinal herniorrhaphy, especially during attempts to control hemorrhage with deep, blindly inserted sutures. A series of 11 iatrogenic injuries were reported by Lord and associates in 1958 (Table 2–20). Although retrograde dissection of an iliac artery and the aorta has been uncommon, Kay and associates (1966) have emphasized this catastrophic complication of cannula-

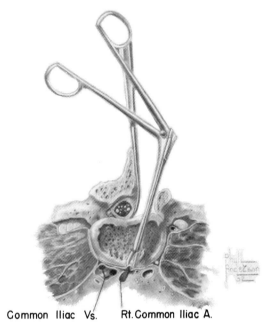

Common Iliac Vs.   Rt. Common Iliac A.

Figure 2–13. Manner in which the common iliac artery can be injured while using an angled pituitary rongeur at the intervertebral space between L4 and L5 during removal of a herniated nucleus pulposus. (Seeley, S. F., Hughes, C. W., and Jahnke, E. J., Jr., *Surgery, 35*:421, 1954.)

tion and perfusion of the common femoral artery in open heart surgery (see Chap. 22).

Vascular injuries following angiographic procedures have increased in number with the rapid development of precise techniques of angiography. The actual incidence of these injuries has decreased somewhat with the availability of skilled vascular radiologists, specifically trained for angiography, but the increasing utilization of such diagnostic techniques has resulted in an over-all increase in the total number of cases seen. Complications include hemorrhage, hematoma formation, false aneurysm, arteriovenous fistula, subintimal dissection, (with and without thrombus), distal embolization of thrombi material, and breakage of a guide wire or catheter.

In 1971 Bolasny and Killen reviewed the frequency and management of arterial injuries following angiography at Vanderbilt University over a period of two and one-half years, starting in January of 1968. Almost 4000 angiographic procedures were performed, following which there were 33 vascular injuries requiring surgical

TABLE 2–20. MAJOR VASCULAR INJURY DURING ELECTIVE OPERATIVE PROCEDURES*

CASE	AGE	SEX	DATE	OPERATION	ARTERY INJURED	MANAGEMENT	PULSES	RESULT
Injuries to the Axillary, Carotid and Subclavian Arteries								
1	42 yr.	F	1949	radical mastectomy	axillary	end-to-end anastomosis	yes	recovery
3	37 yr.	F	1956	Z-plasty contracture of axilla	axillary	end-to-end anastomosis	yes	recovery
4	22 mo.	F	1955	emergency tracheostomy	common carotid	ligation	no	died 2 days later from aspir. pneumonia
5	66 yr.	M	1956	radical neck dissection	common carotid	ligation and preservation of carotid bifurcation	in both int. and ext. branches	recovery
7	64 yr.	M	1953	radical neck dissection	subclavian	ligation	no	recovery
Injuries to the Iliac and Femoral Arteries								
2	37 yr.	F	1955	posthysterectomy bleeding	common iliac	ligation at aortic bifurcation, end-to-side, left-to-right common iliac artery	yes	recovery
6	48 yr.	F	1951	anterior resection	common iliac	ligation	no	2 yr. postop., good
10	21 yr.	F	1955	varicose vein ligation	common femoral	delayed bypass vein graft	yes	recovery
11	29 yr.	M	1949	right inguinal hernia	common femoral	end-to-end anastomosis	yes	recovery

*Modified from Lord, J. W., Jr., Stone, P. W., Cloutier, W. A., and Breidenbach, L., Arch. Surg., 77:282, 1958.

TABLE 2–21. ARTERIAL INJURY RESULTING FROM 3934 ANGIOGRAPHIC PROCEDURES: 0.8 PER CENT INCIDENCE* Vanderbilt University Medical Center, 1 Jan. 1968–1 July 1970

COMPLICATIONS	CASES	PER CENT
Thrombosis at site of entry	26	78.8
Femoral..........................18		
Axillary........................... 3		
Brachial........................... 5		
Intimal dissection with occlusion	3	9.1
Arteriovenous fistula	2	6.1
Embolus from puncture site	1	3.0
Perforation with hemorrhage	1	3.0
Total	33	100.0

*Modified from Bolasny, B. L., and Killen, D. A., Ann. Surg., *174*:962, 1971.

intervention, a frequency of 0.8 per cent (Table 2–21). Twenty-six of 33 complications were thrombosis at the site of catheterization. Sixteen involved the femoral artery, three the axillary, and five the brachial. In three instances there was extensive dissection of the intima in association with thrombosis (Fig. 2–14). Two patients developed arteriovenous fistulas and one had a distal embolus from the puncture site in the femoral artery. Almost none of the arterial injuries resulted simply from the needle puncture, and in only one case did injury occur from uncomplicated passage of a single arterial catheter. Most injuries occurred when manipulation of the catheter was "difficult" or multiple catheters were inserted. Complications were more frequent with arteries with atherosclerotic plaques. Spasm alone did not cause serious problems in any patient. Among numerous other recent papers describing complications associated with angiographic procedures is the 1973 report by Brener and Couch from Boston. They reported a thrombosis rate of 13 per cent in using the brachial route for angiocardiographic catheterization (Table 2–22). Their over-all complication rate was 6 per cent when the femoral route was used, and 28 per cent when the brachial route was used.

Blunt Trauma. Although an arterial injury can occur with almost any type of fracture or dislocation, it is surprising that such an injury does not occur more fre-

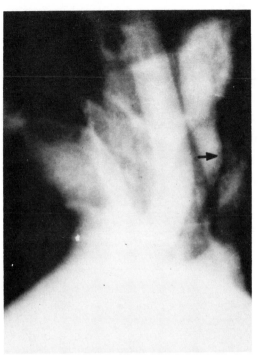

Figure 2–14. Arch aortogram in a patient with angiographic dissection of the left subclavian artery shows an intimal dissection caused by transfemoral selective arteriography. View is of the origin of the arch vessels. Arrow indicates intimal "septum" in the first portion of the left subclavian artery. (Bolasny, B. L., and Killen, D. A., Ann. Surg., *174*:962, 1971.)

quently. The usual injury is contusion with spasm and subsequent thrombosis, rather than laceration or transection (Collins and Jacobs, 1961; Makin et al., 1966). Such injuries commonly have been overlooked in the past, confusing the signs of acute arterial insufficiency with soft tissue trauma, hemorrhage and "arterial spasm." The

TABLE 2–22. INCIDENCE OF ANGIOGRAPHIC CATHETER COMPLICATIONS*

COMPLICATIONS	FEMORAL (223 PATIENTS)	BRACHIAL (96 PATIENTS)
Thrombosis	2 (1%)	12 (13%)
Stenosis	–	14 (15%)
Embolus	7 (3%)	–
False aneurysm	4 (2%)	–
Total	13 (6%)	26 (28%)

*Modified from Brener, B. J., and Couch, M. P., Am. J. Surg., *125*:521, 1973.

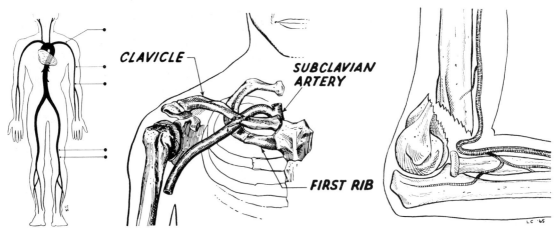

Figure 2–15. Artist's concept of some of the fractures and dislocations that are associated with arterial injuries. (Klingensmith, W., Oles, P., and Martinez, H.: Am. J. Surg., *110*:849, 1965.)

availability of angiography has greatly facilitated the management of such problems; the question of arterial injury in a patient with a fracture can be resolved simply by performing an angiogram. Fractures of the mid-shaft of the femur may lacerate the superficial femoral artery (Kirkup, 1963), while fractures of the distal tibia and fibula may lacerate the posterior and anterior tibial arteries (Miller, 1957). Pelvic fractures have traumatized the iliac arteries, while medial angulation of the radial fragments of a fracture of the neck of the humerus may lacerate the axillary or brachial artery (Hughes, 1958B). Figure 2–15 illustrates different fractures and dislocations associated with arterial injuries.

Dislocation of the knee has frequently been associated with injury of the popliteal artery, often leading to amputation. In one series of 22 dislocated knees, the popliteal artery was injured in 13 patients, an incidence of nearly 60 per cent (Kennedy, 1959). Similarly, Hoover, reporting from the Mayo Clinic in 1961, found nine popliteal artery occlusions associated with 14 knee dislocations. Less commonly, dislocation of the elbow has injured the brachial or radial arteries. Anterior dislocation of the shoulder has injured the axillary artery (McKenzie and Sinclair, 1958). Trauma to the axillary artery may be compounded by trauma to the subscapular and humeral circumflex branches; this may make the injury more serious by

destroying important collateral pathways for arterial flow to the upper extremity. Fractures of the clavicle may injure the

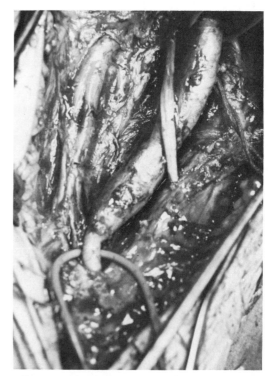

Figure 2–16. Axillary artery aneurysm secondary to crutch trauma, from a series of eight aneurysms at the Massachusetts General Hospital between 1965 and 1971, reported by Abbott and Darling (1973). (Courtesy Dr. William M. Abbott.)

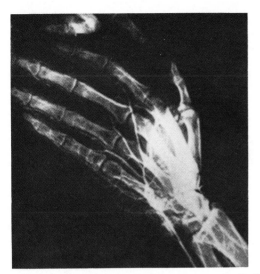

Figure 2–17. Chronic repetitive trauma resulted in a symptomatic hand in this 19-year-old handball player. Angiography revealed occlusive lesions in the digital arteries of the index and middle fingers. The deep palmar arch appeared to be uninvolved. Cervical dorsal sympathectomy resulted in partial relief of his symptoms. (Whelan, T. J., Jr., and Baugh, J. H.: Year Book Medical Publishers, Inc., Chicago, 1967.)

players (Whelan and Baugh, 1967). In baseball players, the syndrome has developed in the index finger of the catching hand, where the major force of the baseball is received. Although signs of ischemia may become marked, amputations have not been necessary. In baseball pitchers, thrombosis of the axillary artery has developed, apparently a result of the motion of the throwing arm from a position of exaggerated hyperabduction through a wide downward arc with great force. The two possibilities of injury are a tear of the intima from repeated stretching or twisting; and compression from hypertrophy of the pectoralis minor tendon, causing repetitive trauma to the artery (Whelan and Baugh, 1967) (Fig. 2–17).

The importance of complete angiography in these unusual instances of arterial trauma has been emphasized in recent years. Aneurysms of the ulnar artery in the wrist or palm, which without angiographic investigation would have gone undetected, have been found to be responsible for distal emboli.

CLINICAL PATHOLOGY

The types of arterial injury which can occur can be conveniently divided into five groups: lacerations, transections, contusions, spasm and arteriovenous fistulas (Fig. 2–18). In almost every series reported, laceration or transection accounts for 85 to 90 per cent of the total injuries seen.

A *laceration* varies from a simple puncture wound to almost complete transection of the arterial wall. *Transection* varies from simple division of the artery to actual loss of substance from a high velocity bullet, often with injury of the ends of the divided artery. *Contusion* ranges from a trivial hematoma in the adventitia to diffuse fragmentation and hematomas throughout the arterial wall. In the most severe form there is fracture of the intima, subsequent prolapse into the lumen and eventual thrombosis. *Spasm* is a definite entity that can occur in the absence of any organic injury, but it is extremely rare. It can be demonstrated simply in the laboratory by repetitively stretching an artery. This initiates a sustained contraction of "spasm" of the con-

subclavian artery, the subclavian vein and the brachial plexus.

The types of blunt trauma which may in unusual instances injure an artery are almost endless. Gibson (1962) described injury from direct blunt force. Instances of intimal dissection, prolapse and eventual thrombosis were reported by Elliott in 1956 and by Moore in 1958. Ngu and Konstan (1965) reported the case of a woman who developed traumatic dissection of the abdominal aorta following blunt trauma from a surfboard.

Lesions of the axillary artery have resulted from long term use of crutches (Rob and Standeven, 1956). In 1973 Abott and Darling added eight cases of axillary artery aneurysm secondary to crutch trauma from the Massachusetts General Hospital between 1965 and 1971 to a review of the English literature which contained only eleven cases of arterial thrombosis and two cases of arterial aneurysms (Fig. 2–16). Chronic use of vibratory tools, such as an air hammer, has caused thrombosis of the distal arteries (Barker and Hines, 1944; de Takats, 1959). A similar complication has been seen in baseball and handball

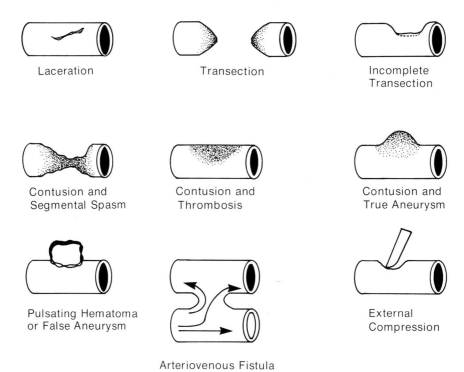

Laceration

Transection

Incomplete
Transection

Contusion and
Segmental Spasm

Contusion and
Thrombosis

Contusion and
True Aneurysm

Pulsating Hematoma
or False Aneurysm

External
Compression

Arteriovenous Fistula

Figure 2–18. Common types of arterial trauma. Lacerations and transections account for the vast majority of arterial injuries. Transections may be associated with avulsions with missing segments of artery. External compression can be caused by displaced bone from comminuted fractures.

centric bands of smooth muscle in the media of the arterial wall. When it occurs, it is important to appreciate that spasm is a mechanical myogenic response and not a *neurogenic* response that is typically seen in smaller arterial tributaries under the influence of the sympathetic nervous system. *Arteriovenous fistulas* classically occur with a fortuitous injury of concomitant artery and vein, but the over-all frequency of their occurrence is small. False aneurysms evolve from lacerations of an artery temporarily sealed by blood clot. Eventually the thrombus liquefies and the lesion begins to expand. Often only with the appearance of an expanding lesion is the presence of an arterial injury first recognized.

In considering the significance of arterial injuries, a careful distinction must be made between acute and chronic lesions. With an acute arterial injury, collateral circulation is often impaired and the ischemic insult compounded. In chronic lesions, however, collateral circulation is not only intact but is also often increased as a result of im-

pairment of blood flow resulting from the original arterial injury. This, of course, was the original basis for delaying treatment of arteriovenous fistulas for two to three months: it had been demonstrated repeatedly that after this period of time the development of collateral circulation permitted ligation of the involved artery without fear of gangrene. Although the importance of this distinction between acute and chronic lesions is now well recognized, probably one of the reasons that arterial ligation was accepted so widely in World War II was the unduly optimistic picture reported from World War I by Makins (1919), who included both acute and chronic lesions in his description of arterial injuries treated by ligation.

Normally, lacerations and transections result from penetrating injuries, and contusions or spasm result from nonpenetrating trauma. However, the surrounding cavitational effect from the high velocity missile may cause contusion or spasm, even though the missile does not touch the artery.

Conversely, bony fragments from a fracture caused by blunt trauma may perforate or even transect an artery.

A characteristic feature of lacerations, in contrast to transections, is that hemorrhage may be more severe because the edges of the arterial wound gape; the artery cannot retract and contract and facilitate the formation of thrombus. In 1942 Holman demonstrated in the laboratory that a tangential wound of the right femoral artery resulted in exsanguination within 20 minutes, while complete division of the femoral artery resulted in hemorrhage for five minutes. In the latter instance bleeding stopped spontaneously as the transected artery retracted, with survival of the animal. Also characteristic of lacerations, as opposed to transections, is the fact that a distal pulse may remain intact, making diagnosis of an arterial injury much more difficult.

Among the 136 patients reported by Morris and co-workers (1957), there were 56 lacerations and 71 transections (Table 2–23). Contusion was infrequent and spasm was recognized in only three patients. Similarly, in the 200 injuries reported by Ferguson and co-authors (1961) in Atlanta, almost all were lacerations or transections. Only 5 per cent resulted from blunt trauma. Patman and co-workers (1964) in Dallas found that more than 90 per cent of the arterial injuries in their series were either lacerations or transections (Table 2–24). Also, in the large series reported by Drapanas and associates (1970) in New Orleans, over 85 per cent of the injuries were either lacerations or transections (Table 2–25). Fracture of the intima with thrombosis was seen in 10 per cent, and

acute arteriovenous fistula in 3.5 per cent. Hardy and colleagues (1975) in Jackson recorded 111 lacerations and 140 injuries with perforation, transection and loss of arterial substance.

In recent years it has become well established that the diagnosis for arterial contusion or spasm almost always requires surgical exploration. Before this concept was developed an erroneous diagnosis of spasm frequently resulted in loss of the extremity. Even at surgery, external examination of a contracted artery may suggest spasm, but when the artery is opened, fracture of the intima with prolapse is found. Hence, blunt trauma to an artery may induce spasm, cause a localized innocuous hematoma or fracture the intima which subsequently prolapses and causes thrombosis. Historically, one of the earliest documentations of fracture of the intima with prolapse was made by Pick in 1873. He reported a case of partial rupture of the

TABLE 2–24. EXTENT OF ARTERIAL TRAUMA IN 271 CIVILIAN ARTERIAL INJURIES DALLAS, 1 JULY 1949–1 JULY 1969*

TYPE OF INJURY	NUMBER	PER CENT
Laceration	139	51.3
Incomplete transections	33	12.2
Complete transections	80	29.5
Contusions	14	5.2
Spasm	5	1.8
Total	271	100.0

*Modified from Patman, R. D., Poulos, E., and Shires, G. T., Surg. Gynec. & Obstet., *118*:725, 1964.

TABLE 2–23. TYPE OF ACUTE ARTERIAL INJURIES IN CIVILIAN PRACTICE, HOUSTON, PRIOR TO 31 JULY 1956*

	NUMBER	PER CENT
Transection	71	52.2
Laceration	56	41.2
Contusion	6	4.4
Spasm	3	2.2
Total	136	100.0

*Modified from Morris, G. C., Jr., Creech, O., Jr., and DeBakey, M. E., Am. J. Surg., *93*:565, 1957.

TABLE 2–25. TYPES OF ARTERIAL INJURIES* New Orleans, 1942–1969

ARTERIAL LESION	NUMBER	PER CENT
Penetration or perforation	77	33.9
Transection	59	26.0
Laceration	56	25.2
Fracture of intima; thrombosis	24	10.6
Arteriovenous fistula	8	3.5
False aneurysm	2	0.8
Total	226	100.0

*Modified from Drapanas, T., Hewitt, R. L., Weichert, R. F., and Smith, A. D., Ann. Surg., *172*:351, 1970.

common femoral artery by violent stretching, and reviewed two other cases in the Museum at St. George's Hospital in London. The following quote is from Pick (1873):

The left axillary artery showed a laceration of its two internal coats, which had been dissected from the external coat for about half an inch, turned down into the cavity of the vessel, so as to block it up. A red coagulum of blood was lodged above the inverted portion of the internal coat.

In 1962 Gryska reported a patient shot in the left thigh with a .22 caliber missile. At surgery the superficial femoral artery was pulseless, but intact. Spasm appeared the most likely diagnosis until an arteriotomy showed occlusion from a tear of the intima with prolapse and thrombosis. The traumatized area was excised and continuity restored with an end-to-end anastomosis.

The microscopic changes with an arterial injury from a high velocity missile have been of particular interest, since it is known that the artery is injured for a distance beyond the site of gross injury. Jahnke and Seeley (1953), reporting from their Korean experience, described fragmentation of the internal elastic membrane, prolapse of the media, tears of the intima and localized thrombi. A recommendation evolved that an artery should be debrided for almost 1 cm beyond the site of gross injury. Additional experience, nevertheless, revealed that this recommendation was generally erroneous. From Vietnam more than 100 arterial segments were carefully studied (Rich et al., 1969C). Microscopic changes similar to those reported by Jahnke and Seeley were consistently found (Fig. 2–19). However, these changes often extended for more than 1 cm from the point of injury into the grossly normal appearing artery. Similar changes could also be found in experimental studies of arterial injuries, and these changes extended even beyond 2 cm into what grossly appeared to be normal artery (Amato et al., 1970). Fortunately, clinical experience revealed that the presence of these microscopic changes does not compromise arterial repair significantly. Since débriding 1 cm of artery often leaves residual sites of microscopic injury, the policy of limiting débridement to the site of gross injury has been found to be the simplest and safest procedure.

Unusual types of arterial injury include those of external compression. In 1970, Mandelbaum and Kalsbeck reported an extrinsic compression of the internal carotid artery from hemorrhagic lymphadenopathy (see Chap. 11). In 1969 Isaacs and associates reported a 10 year old child with recurrent neurological deficits for seven

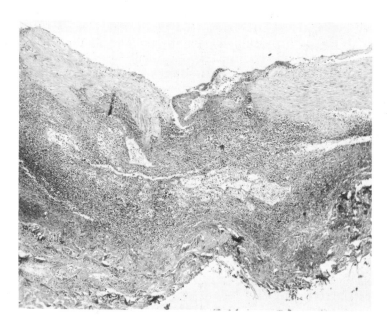

Figure 2–19. This photomicrograph of an H & E stained cross-section of a popliteal artery ×90 shows multiple disruptions with hemorrhage and fibrin deposition on the internal surface. There is focal disruption of the media and marked perivascular hemorrhage from some disruption of the perivascular tissue. This was from an area of the artery which appeared grossly normal. (Rich, N. M., Manion, W. C., and Hughes, C. W., J. Trauma, 9:279, 1969. Copyright 1969, The Williams & Wilkins Co., Baltimore.)

Figure 2–20. Cross-section of a normal artery on the left demonstrates the three layers of the artery wall: adventitia on the outside; media, containing muscle and elastic fibers; and intima, a thin, smooth, inner lining. The heavy arrow on the upper left of the diagram indicates the point of trauma. On the right, an arteriosclerotic vessel is shown with the thicker adventitia. The media has a thinning of muscle with a large atheromatous plaque that stains dark with a fat stain. Bleeding takes place readily in this area and creates a preformed space within the wall. The elastic fibers are frayed and fragmented, and the intima is thickened. The lumen of the vessel is narrowed and deformed in its "eccentric" position. (de Takats, G., and Fowler, E. F., *Trauma.* Matthew Bender and Co., Inc., Albany, 1963.)

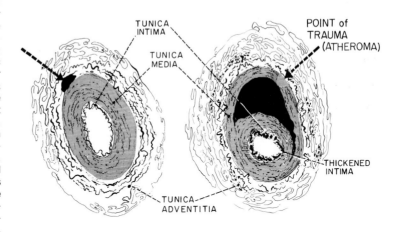

THE RESPONSE OF A NORMAL AND ARTERIO-SCLEROTIC ARTERY TO TRAUMA.

years after cervical trauma. At operation, adherent lymph nodes with perivascular scarring had constricted the internal carotid artery near its origin. The constriction was surgically relieved. In 1967 Davie and Coxe reported the case of a three year old child with hemiplegia and cervical lymph node adenopathy. At operation a single large lymph node was removed from the area of the carotid bifurcation, and a fresh thrombus was removed from the internal carotid artery. An almost identical case involving a 12 year old boy was reported by Poulyane in 1957, and a similar case involving a 13 year old boy was reported by Petit-Dutaillis in 1949.

In older patients with blunt trauma, the presence of atherosclerotic plaques complicates the pattern of arterial trauma. Hemorrhage into a plaque may precipitate thrombosis. However, thrombosis also spontaneously occurs with peripheral arteriosclerosis, and it is therefore often un-

certain whether or not the trauma caused the thrombosis unless surgical exploration demonstrates hemorrhage into a plaque (Fig. 2–20). Such a case was reported by de Takats and Fowler in 1963. A 55 year old patient with classic intermittent claudication slipped on a staircase, and the leg subsequently became severely ischemic. An arteriogram one week later showed complete occlusion of the superficial femoral artery. At operation, an old atheromatous plaque was found in the superficial femoral, with a superimposed fresh thrombus.

The extent of arterial trauma secondary to radiation therapy is not completely understood. However, it is generally believed that only smaller vessels are usually affected. Frequent observations have been made, nevertheless, that there seems to be an increase in the friable nature of the vena cava during a retroperitoneal node dissection following radiation for pelvic carcinoma.

CHAPTER 3

EXPERIMENTAL ARTERIAL TRAUMA

Primary damage and wounding results from direct crushing of tissue in front of the moving missile and from stretching and tearing in a wide range around the missile path. The stretching results from the formation of a large temporary cavity behind the missile which leaves a region of extravasated blood on collapse. The cavity formation is explosive in character and a comparison is drawn between a shot into tissue and an underwater explosion.

Harvey, E. N., Korr, I. M., Oster, G., and McMillen, J. H., 1947

Experimental effort has been expended by a small number of individuals in an attempt to better understand the wounding power of missiles, particularly during the last 50 years. This knowledge is of paramount importance before one can gain a full appreciation of the various etiologies of arterial trauma and the resultant degree of damage. As stated in the above quote, the temporary cavitational effect of a missile has an extremely important adverse effect on tissues, including arteries. This can best be demonstrated experimentally. The effort is warranted in view of an alarming increase in the number of gunshot wounds, including those involving arterial trauma, even in civilian experience.

In this chapter, there will be a brief review of some of the historical developments in wound ballistics. This will include notation referable to arterial wounds, and recent experimental efforts will be highlighted. The future value of continued experimental work in wound ballistics related to vascular trauma will be underscored.

HISTORY

Early developments in the treatment of gunshot wounds were reviewed and documented by Billroth in 1859. He credited the historian Villiani with the first mention of the use of gunpowder in warfare in 1338. Roger Bacon in 1242 had described an explosive mixture of saltpeter, charcoal and sulfur; however, the use of this mixture for propelling missiles was apparently not known until the next century. Billroth cited what he thought was the oldest work on surgery written in German, which contained a short chapter on gunshot wounds written in 1497 by Hieronymus Brunschwig of Strassburg. He also noted, nevertheless, that Pfolspeundt had written a few words in 1460 regarding gunshot wounds.

In the early nineteenth century, numerous authors attempted to explain many of the aspects of hemorrhage and vascular injury caused by missiles. Huguier in 1848, during the street fighting in Paris, first observed the bursting effect of high velocity missiles on soft tissues.

That low velocity missiles could push blood vessels aside as the missile traversed tissue was known in the nineteenth century. In his report for the Surgeon General to the Secretary of War, La Garde in 1893 reviewed the subject of gunshot injuries by fully jacketed military rounds in times of war. It was not until his subsequent report in 1916, however, that he provided further definition of the effect of a high velocity projectile on an artery:

As we have stated elsewhere injury to blood-vessels turns out to be one of the chief characteristic lesions of the new bullet. The projectile cuts the side of a vessel, or scoops out a hole in a large vessel, like a cutting instrument, leaving a band on each side of the openings. The cut edges are not lacerated and external hemorrhage or more frequently internal hemorrhage takes place at once. In the body cavities the hemorrhage is alarmingly fatal. In limbs or parts where the vessel is well supported by surrounding tissue, aneurysm is apt to follow. Vessels are no longer pushed aside as they were by the older lower-velocity bullets.

Wilson in 1921 provided further definition of the temporary cavitational effect of missiles. He described damage in large vessels by "explosive wounds" which caused stretching of the artery and resulted in intimal tears. There was some confusion, however, when Harvey and co-workers in 1947 stated that blood vessels and nerves when indirectly struck appeared grossly unharmed within the temporary cavity, and they felt that this was because of the elastic nature of the vessels. Puckett and co-authors (1946), on the other hand, showed that impairment of conduction in the sciatic nerves of cats resulted from near misses of high velocity missiles. Krauss (1957) demonstrated that there were significantly damaged striated muscle fibers within the muscle tissue which had been displaced within the temporary cavity caused by a high velocity missile. An important aspect of arterial trauma is its relationship to the high velocity missile with its associated temporary cavitational effect. This is true whether the missile actually strikes the artery or whether there has been a "near miss." Although the major interest in high velocity missile injuries has been among military surgeons in the past, these wounds are of equal importance to any surgeon who encounters this type of injury due to hunting accidents, civilian disorders or urban violence.

BALLISTICS

The term "ballistics" is derived from the Greek word meaning "to hurl." Ballistics is the study of the motion of projectiles. There are three divisions of ballistics: (1) interior ballistics, which is the study of the motion of the bullet within the gun; (2) exterior ballistics, which is the study of the flight of the bullet from the muzzle to the target (Fig. 3–1); and (3) terminal ballistics, which is the study of the motion of the bullet as it strikes the target and the motion of the bullet within the target. In dealing with the wounds involving tissues, the motion of the bullet within the tissues is termed "wound ballistics" (Fig. 3–2).

The following formula has been used to determine the wounding power of a missile, in which kinetic energy is equal to the mass of the missile times the velocity squared divided by two times the gravitational pull:

$$KE = \frac{M \times V^2}{2g}$$

It is more important to measure the velocity of the missile as it strikes the tissue, or the impact velocity, than the velocity of the missile at the time that it is fired from various weapons, or the muzzle velocity. The character of the tissue struck is also important in determining the wounding power of missiles. The air-filled lung tissue offers more resiliency than more solid organs such as the liver. Our recent experimental work on vascular trauma included the contrasting damage in various tissues caused by high and low velocity missiles (Figs. 3–3 to 3–7) (Amato et al., 1974).

Text continued on page 50

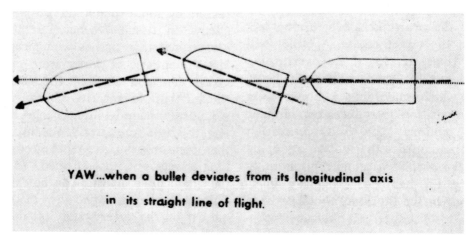

YAW...when a bullet deviates from its longitudinal axis in its straight line of flight.

A

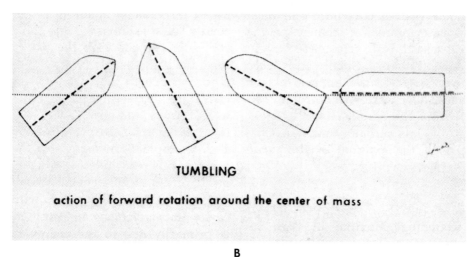

TUMBLING

action of forward rotation around the center of mass

B

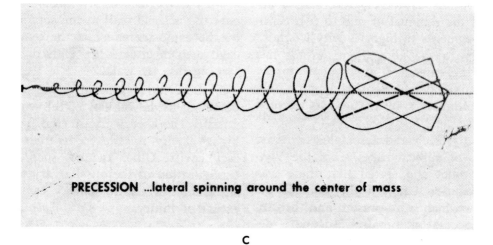

PRECESSION ...lateral spinning around the center of mass

C

Figure 3–1. *Legend on opposite page.*

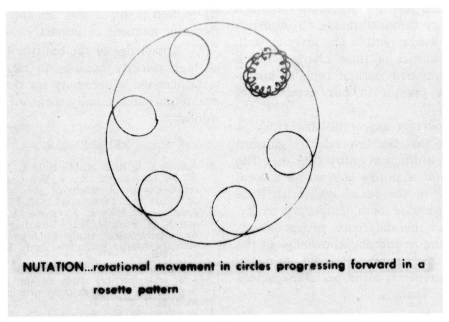

D

Figure 3–1. In exterior ballistics, various motions of the missile occur, as shown above. The missile is affected by yaw, tumbling, precession, and nutation. (Amato, J. J., and Rich, N. M., J. Cardiovasc. Surg., *13*:147, 1972.)

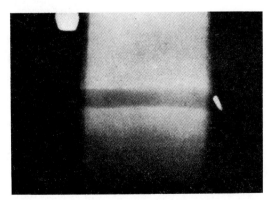

Figure 3–2. In terminal ballistics, specifically in wound ballistics, motion of the missile within the target can be demonstrated. The tumbling of an M–16 bullet is obvious after it perforates a block of 20 per cent gelatin used to simulate muscle tissue. (Amato, J. J., and Rich, N. M., J. Cardiovasc. Surg., *13*:147, 1972.)

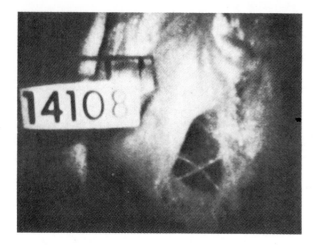

Figure 3–3. This high speed photograph demonstrates the temporary cavitational formation within muscle tissue caused by a high velocity missile. The photograph was taken within millimicroseconds after impact of the missile and demonstrates a cavity much larger than the residual tract that will remain. (Amato, J. J., Billy, L. J., Lawson, N. S., and Rich, N. M., Am. J. Surg., *127*:454, 1974.)

Figure 3–4. A venogram of the liver in an experimental model demonstrates the large temporary cavity of the solid organ (see Fig. 3–5) in a high velocity missile injury. (Amato, J. J., Billy, L. J., Lawson, N. S., and Rich, N. M., Am. J. Surg., *127*:454, 1974.)

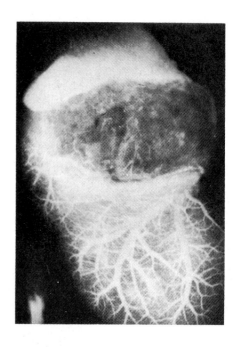

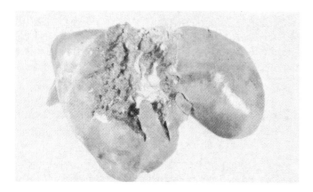

Figure 3–5. The relatively massive permanent missile tract within the liver tissue caused by a missile fired at 3000 feet per second is obvious in this experimental model (see Fig. 3–4). The dense liver tissue, not having as much elastic tissue as muscle, shows more massive disruption than that seen in muscle or in other organs such as the more resilient lung tissue. (Amato, J. J., Billy, L. J., Lawson, N. S., and Rich, N. M., Am. J. Surg., *127*:454, 1974.)

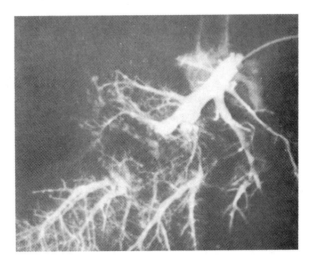

Figure 3–6. This pulmonary angiogram demonstrates a temporary cavity formed in lung parenchyma after injury by a high velocity bullet. The residual tract is smaller than in the more solid liver. (Amato, J. J., Billy, L. J., Lawson, N. S., and Rich, N. M., Am. J. Surg., *127*: 454, 1974.)

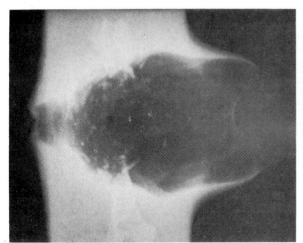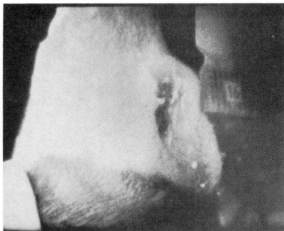

Figure 3–7. In the experimental model on the left, fragmentation of the bone within the temporary cavity caused by the high velocity bullet can be seen. The relatively large exit wound is seen on the right. Fragments of the bone can be seen exiting the wound as secondary missiles. Within the wound these missiles can also cause vascular trauma. (Amato, J. J., Billy, L. J., Lawson, N. S., and Rich, N. M., Am. J. Surg., *127*:454, 1974.)

MORE RECENT EXPERIMENTAL EFFORT

Miller and Welch (1949) after World War II performed important experimental work involving a series of experiments on dogs to obtain clinical data on survival of extremities subjected to varying periods of acute ischemia under standard conditions. They found that there was a salvage rate of 50 per cent of limbs ischemic for 12 to 18 hours, and 20 per cent of those ischemic for more than 24 hours. They felt that this would also give encouragement for the possibility of recovery of human extremities with severed arteries when treatment had been delayed beyond the accepted optimum time of six to eight hours. For periods of ischemia ranging from one to six hours, there was a 90 per cent survival.

Moore and associates (1954), in their review of the literature on the subject of gunshot wounds of major arteries, noted that reports covered only clinical experience. They could find no specific reports of experimental studies related to arterial trauma. They organized an experimental study to determine the extent of trauma to the thoracic and abdominal aortas of dogs by low velocity missiles. They emphasized that the significant feature of all of the injuries, regardless of the apparent involvement, was that the microscopic injury never extended further than 3 mm beyond the obvious gross wound. The following conclusions were cited from their experimental work regarding the nature and extent of arterial trauma: (1) resultant injury in normotensive vessels exposed to air was much greater in gross extent than that in normotensive vessels injured while surrounded by saline solution or body tissue; (2) hypotensive vessels were injured to a much greater gross extent than were normotensive vessels under the same conditions; (3) hypertensive vessels tended to spread extensively in a longitudinal direction, as contrasted with smaller stellate defects of the normal vessels under the same conditions; (4) regardless of the position of the injury, extent of intimal damage always exceeded the apparent external extent of damage; (5) in no instance in any of the groups studied

A

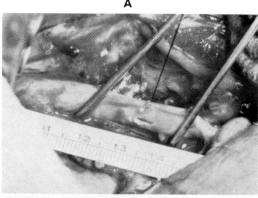

B

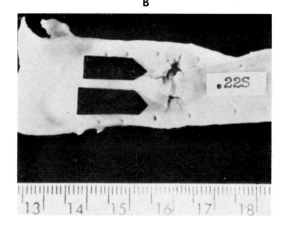

Figure 3–8. (A) This operative view of the abdominal aortic gunshot wound of a dog shows the relatively minimal injury caused by a .177 caliber missile. (B) Internal view of a wound (anterior wound at upper arrow) caused by a .22 caliber short missile fired through a canine thoracic aorta. Intimal damage was greater than external damage; however, it did not extend further than 3 mm beyond the gross wound. (C) Aortogram shows patency at the repair site (arrow) obtained 153 days after resection of 2 cm of thoracic aorta necessitated by the .22 caliber short missile wound with end-to-end anastomosis used for the repair. (Moore, H. G., Nyhus, L. M., Kanar, E. A., and Harkins, H. N., Surg. Gynecol. Obstet., *98*:129, 1954.)

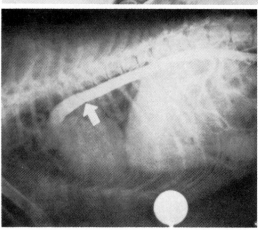

C

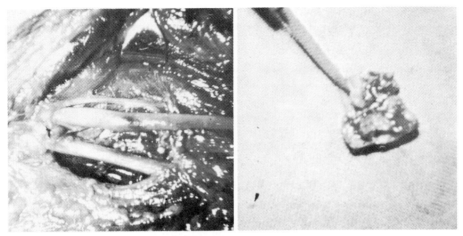

Figure 3–9. The photograph on the left illustrates contusion of the brachial artery (arrow) with the median nerve seen below, which was caused by the temporary cavitational effect of the high velocity M–16 bullet. The absence of arterial flow beyond the contusion can be appreciated by the smaller size of the artery. The photograph to the right shows the excised segment of brachial artery which has been opened to show the organized thrombus which occluded the lumen. The thrombus organized at an area of intimal disruption which was caused by the temporary cavitational effect of the high velocity M–16 bullet, although the bullet did not actually strike the brachial artery. (Rich, N. M., Amato, J. J., and Billy, L. J., Surg. Digest, 6:12, 1971.)

did microscopic damage extend more than 3 mm beyond the gross intimal damage.

Although Moore and associates (1954) cited the ingenious group of experiments reported from Princeton University on the mechanism of wounding by high velocity missiles in the 1940's, they also noted that the work of Harvey and others in 1945 and 1947 gave no specific reference to arterial trauma. Figure 3–8 demonstrates some of the gross arterial injuries produced in the experiments by Moore and associates (1954). They were also able to obtain angiograms to demonstrate the successful repairs following arterial trauma.

Because of the clinical experience documented in the Vietnam Vascular Registry (Fig. 3–9), it was possible to design a number of experiments at the Biomedical Department of the Biophysics Laboratory at the United States Edgewood Arsenal at Edgewood, Maryland (Amato et al., 1970, 1971, 1974; Rich et al, 1971B; Amato and Rich, 1972) (Fig. 3–10). In vitro studies were designed to visualize adequately the motion of vessels after wounding. The femoral arteries were removed from dogs and filled with safranin dye or Hypaque and imbedded in 20 per cent gelatin, which simulated normal muscle tissue. The me-

Figure 3–10. This photograph emphasizes the maximum temporary cavity in muscle caused by a high velocity missile passing through the hind limb of an experimental canine model. Angiographically demonstrated, the femoral artery is markedly stretched and compressed against the outer wall of the temporary cavity. (Amato, J. J., Billy, L. J., Lawson, N. S., and Rich, N. M., Am. J. Surg., *127*:454, 1974.)

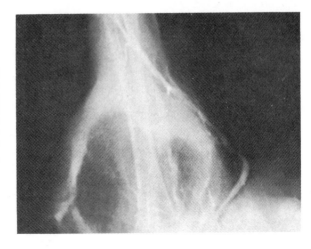

chanical phases of wounding were visualized through the translucent gelatin. High speed motion picture photography was utilized, with a graphic capability of representing the injury at 27,000 frames per second. In vivo studies were also carried out in the anesthetized canine models. In order to study the pathophysiology of ballistic injuries to blood vessels, three series of experiments were conducted. The purpose of these studies was to photographically document the mechanism of injury of blood vessels by high, intermediate and low velocity missiles and to describe the extent of microscopic trauma to the blood vessels. A high speed photographic camera taking from 3750 to 4500 frames per second was used, which was designed particularly for short-lived events. This capability could be extended to high speed motion pictures with up to 30,000 pictures per second. Angiograms were taken with the Felexetron 300 megawatt x-ray system, which is capable of producing a pulse of 0.1 microseconds duration delivering up to 1000 amps of 30 KV of anode potential.

IN VIVO STUDIES

The femoral arteries of ten anesthetized dogs were exposed bilaterally by medial skin flaps. The distal and proximal segments of these arteries were gently mobi-

lized to obtain distal and proximal control; however, the central portion of the artery was left undisturbed. The animal was placed in a supine position with the limb suspended and the artery sighted upon for missile firing (Fig. 3–11). This series made it possible to obtain high speed photographic documentation of vascular injury as various arteries were struck by 0.25 inch steel spheres weighing 16 grains with a velocity of 1000, 2000 or 3000 feet per second. The sphere was used in all initial experiments to obtain standard control in similar wounds. There was no appreciable deviation in flight of the missile; the mode of injury and presented area of the mass of the missile were constant. Only the velocity of the missile varied. A series of animals was used in which polyethylene tubes were introduced into the abdominal aorta through an abdominal incision. The catheters were inserted into the left and right iliac arteries and secured in place. The catheters were filled with 3 per cent heparinized solution. At the time of injury at calculated intervals, 90 per cent Hypaque was injected into the arteries, and x-rays were taken. Angiograms, shown in Figure 3–12, helped to emphasize the impressive formation of the temporary cavity: (1) the artery at the moment of impact of the 16 grain sphere traveling at 3000 feet per second; (2) the artery immediately after impact, with the 16 grain sphere neatly shear-

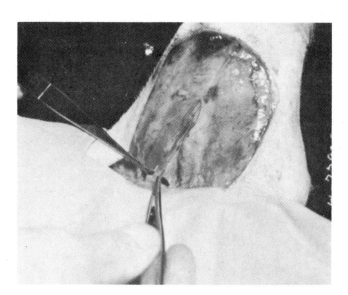

Figure 3–11. This operative photograph shows the suspended hind limb of the canine model with the femoral artery demonstrated in situ after the skin flap was reflected medially. (Amato, J. J., Rich, N. M., Billy, L. J., Gruber, R. P., and Lawson, N. S., J. Trauma, *11*:412, 1971. Copyright 1971, The Williams & Wilkins Company, Baltimore.)

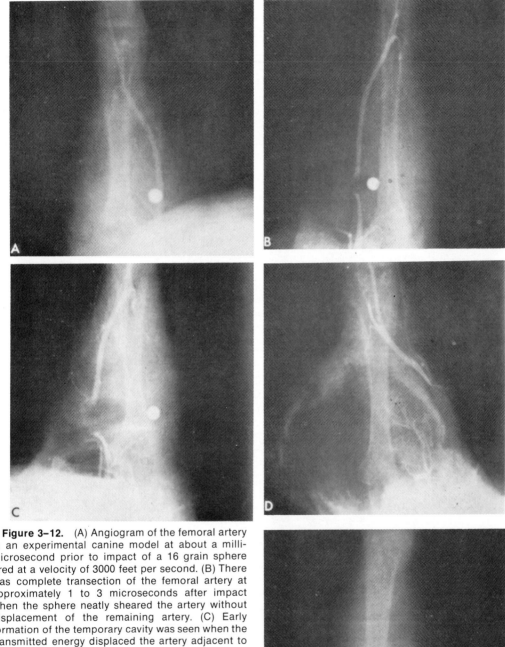

Figure 3–12. (A) Angiogram of the femoral artery in an experimental canine model at about a milli-microsecond prior to impact of a 16 grain sphere fired at a velocity of 3000 feet per second. (B) There was complete transection of the femoral artery at approximately 1 to 3 microseconds after impact when the sphere neatly sheared the artery without displacement of the remaining artery. (C) Early formation of the temporary cavity was seen when the transmitted energy displaced the artery adjacent to the missile tract. (D) Maximum formation of the temporary cavity can approximate 30 times the size of the residual tract. Note the striking compression of the distorted femoral artery displaced against the wall of the undulating temporary cavity. (E) The relatively small permanent tract as shown above may be the only visible damage apparent to the surgeon at the time of débridement following a high velocity missile wound. (Amato, J. J., Rich, N. M., Billy, L. J., Gruber, R. P., and Lawson, N. S., J. Trauma, *11*:412, 1971. Copyright 1971, The Williams & Wilkins Company, Baltimore.)

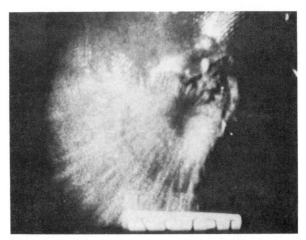

Figure 3–13.   The phenomenon of tail splashing is demonstrated within a few millimicroseconds after impact of the missile with tissue, as seen in the above experimental photograph. (Amato, J. J., Billy, L. J., Lawson, N. S., and Rich, N. M., Am. J. Surg., *127*:454, 1974.)

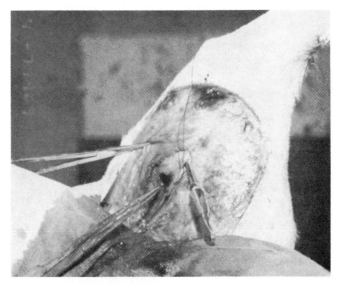

Figure 3–14.   In the in vivo models, it was difficult to visualize the extent of damage to the femoral artery. The above operative photograph demonstrates the permanent cavity after injury with a 16 grain sphere traveling at 3000 feet per second; however, the high velocity missile created more damage than can be appreciated. (Amato, J. J., Rich, N. M., Billy, L. J., Gruber, R. P., and Lawson, N. S., J. Trauma, *11*:412, 1971, Copyright 1971, The Williams & Wilkins Company, Baltimore.)

ing the artery; (3) the early formation of a temporary cavity; (4) the temporary cavity in its greatest diameter; and (5) the residual permanent cavity.

High speed photography demonstrated the extent of wounding in this series. The phenomenon of tail splash was well visualized as the missile struck the tissues (Fig. 3–13). The undulating motion of the tissues associated with the formation of the temporary cavity was demonstrated. Specific injury to the artery, however, was not clear because of the blood vessel's movement, which was obscured by the muscle mass immediately behind it (Fig. 3–14). There was angiographic documentation of the events of high velocity missile damage, as contrasted with those of low velocity missile damage. It was felt that further visualization of direct arterial trauma was warranted by studies in vitro.

IN VITRO STUDIES

Segments of femoral arteries were removed from 14 anesthetized dogs. The segments measured 6 to 9 cm in length and were filled with either Hypaque or safranin dye. Segments were ligated at both ends and suspended in 20 per cent gelatin solution, and the solution was allowed to gel. This preparation isolated the artery and allowed motion of the artery, as affected by missiles at various velocities, to be photographed. The translucent gelatin allowed adequate lighting for the events and enabled visualization of all phases of wounding. Also, the 20 per cent gelatin solution simulated muscle tissue. High speed photographic films and angiograms of the various events were then obtained to distinctively show the mechanism of injury at various velocities. At the low velocity of 1000 feet per second, the blood vessel was struck by the sphere, the sphere slowly pushed the blood vessel ahead (Fig. 3–15), and finally the sphere penetrated the blood vessel, dividing it in two, with the ends of the blood vessel returning to their original vertical position. At 2000 feet per second, there was a cutting of the blood vessel, with the formation of a small temporary cavity. Injury at 3000 feet per second, however,

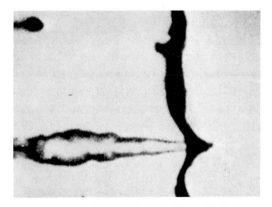

Figure 3–15. A femoral artery filled with Hypaque and suspended in 20 per cent gelatin was stretched forward before being severed by a low velocity 16 grain sphere traveling at 1000 feet per second. (Rich, N. M., Amato, J. J., and Billy, L. J., Surg. Digest, 6:12, 1971.)

involved the suspended vessel being neatly sheared by the missile, followed by the development of a relatively large temporary cavity, which corresponded to previous documentation that the cavity reached approximately 30 times the volume of the permanent tract left by the missile (Fig. 3–16). Because the diameters of the canine vessels were relatively small (3 mm to 5 mm), larger vessels from freshly slaughtered calves were obtained. The latter arteries are comparable in size to the human femoral artery. The in vitro studies were repeated and showed the same mechanism of injury at 1000, 2000 and 3000 feet per second.

In some of the experiments a high velocity M–16 bullet was utilized instead of the 16 grain sphere. Similar wounding results were obtained (Fig. 3–17). However, tumbling of the elongated missile within the gelatin was documented.

An interesting phenomenon was demonstrated with the angiograms in the in vitro studies. This involved the injury to the artery with a "near miss" of the missile. The missile passed near the vessel, but it did not actually strike it (Fig. 3–18). Although the missile path was close to the vessel, there was no motion in the vessel. However, the vessel was literally torn apart by the stretching of the tissues during the formation of the temporary cavity. The original experiments performed with a 16 grain sphere fired at 3000 feet per second

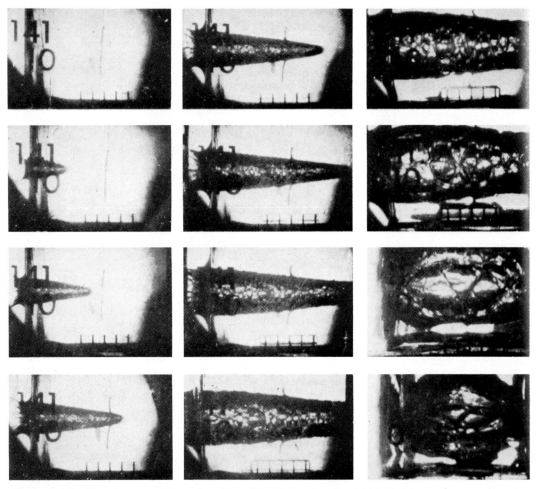

Figure 3–16. The above sequence of rapid motion picture frames at 27,000 pictures per second shows, moving from the top left to the lower right, injury to a blood vessel filled with Hypaque suspended in 20 per cent gelatin when it was struck directly by a high velocity missile, a 16 grain sphere traveling at 3000 feet per second. The formation of the temporary cavity and its effect on the ends of the blood vessel are obvious. (Amato, J. J., Billy, L. J., Gruber, R. P., Lawson, N. S., and Rich, N. M. Arch. Surg., *101*:167, 1970.)

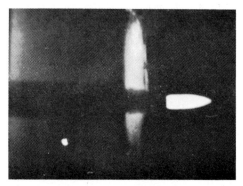

Figure 3–17. The high velocity M–16 bullet neatly sheared a calf's artery filled with Hypaque and suspended in 20 per cent gelatin. The severed ends of the artery were not displaced until subsequent formation of the temporary cavity. (Rich, N. M., Amato, J. J., and Billy, L. J., Surg. Digest, *6*:12, 1971.)

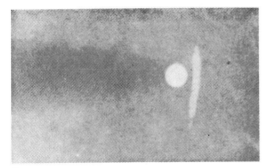

A

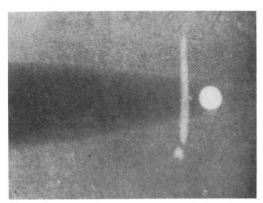

B

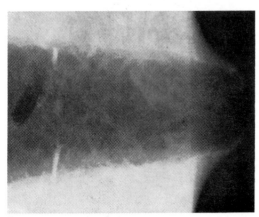

C

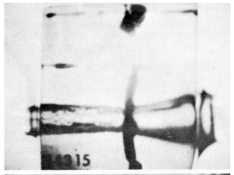

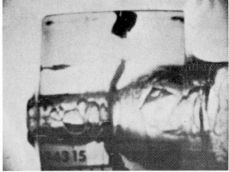

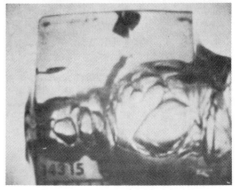

Figure 3–18. (A) and (B) In a "near miss" by a 16 grain sphere traveling at 3000 feet per second, there is no motion or deformation of the artery as the missile passes close to the artery, which has been filled with contrast media and suspended in 20 per cent gelatin. (C) The "near miss" affects the blood vessel by its high velocity temporary cavitational formation. The vessel was literally torn apart by the stretching of the tissues during the formation of the temporary cavity. (Amato, J. J., Billy, L. J., Gruber, R. P., Lawson, N. S., and Rich, N. M., Arch. Surg., *101*:167, 1970.)

Figure 3–19. An M–16 bullet traveling at 3250 feet per second passed through 20 per cent gelatin in a "near miss" of a calf's artery filled with contrast media. There was no displacement of the suspended artery. However, as the temporary cavity formed after passage of the bullet through the block, there was stretching and compression of the artery against the cavity wall. Within millimicroseconds after impact, maximum formation of the temporary cavity showed marked displacement, stretching and compression of the femoral artery. (Rich, N. M., Amato, J. J., and Billy, L. J., Surg. Digest, *6*:12, 1971.)

past a canine femoral artery suspended in 20 per cent gelatin were repeated using an M–16 missile and a larger calf's artery. The latter results were similar to the former (Fig. 3–19).

MICROSCOPIC ARTERIAL DAMAGE

In another set of experiments, the femoral arteries of ten anesthetized dogs were exposed by medial skin flaps, with distal and proximal control achieved by loosely placed silk ties. The skin flaps were approximated after the artery was sighted and then injured by steel spheres traveling at 1000, 2000 and 3000 feet per second in different models. At 30 minutes to two hours following injury, segments of the injured vessel measuring approximately 20

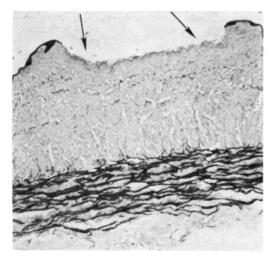

A

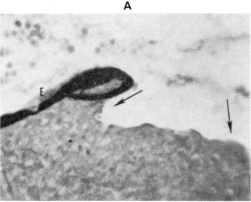

B

Figure 3–20. (A) The above arterial segment was adjacent to a complete disruption of the artery from a 16 grain sphere traveling at 1000 feet per second. Note the large area of discontinuity in the internal elastic lamina (arrows). (Verhoeff-van Gieson stain, reduced from × 220.) (B) Higher magnification of the arterial segment shows the margin of the large break in the internal elastic lamina. Endothelium (E) is intact over the internal elastic lamina, but it is lost over the part of the large break (arrows). (Verhoeff-van Gieson stain, reduced from × 220.) (Amato, J. J., Billy, L. J., Gruber, R. P., Lawson, N. S., and Rich, N. M., Arch. Surg., *101*:167, 1970. Copyright 1970, American Medical Association.)

TABLE 3–1. COMPARISON OF MEAN NUMBER OF LARGE BREAKS PER MILLIMETER AND VELOCITY OF IMPINGING MISSILE*

VELOCITY (FT/SEC)	HIT	MEAN (LARGE BREAKS PER MM)
1000	Direct	0.61
2000	Direct	0.70
3000	Direct	0.93
1000	Indirect	0.25
3000	Indirect	0.64

*Amato, J. J., Billy, L. J., Gruber, R. P., Lawson, N. S., and Rich, N. M., Arch. Surg., *101*:167, 1970. Copyright 1970, American Medical Association.

cm on each side of the gross trauma were excised. Therefore, 40 mm of artery, which was not directly injured, was excised nearest the center of the wound tract. The tissues were fixed in 10 per cent formaldehyde, dehydrated, paraffin-imbedded, and stained with various stains. A pathologist,

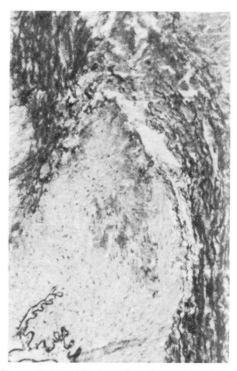

Figure 3–21. Missile-induced vascular trauma also causes changes in the media, as shown above. This arterial segment reveals partial herniation of the media through the damaged adventitia. (Verhoeff-van Gieson stain, reduced from × 220.) (Amato, J. J., Billy, L. J., Gruber, R. P., Lawson, N. S., and Rich, N. M., Arch. Surg., *101*:167, 1970. Copyright 1970, American Medical Association.)

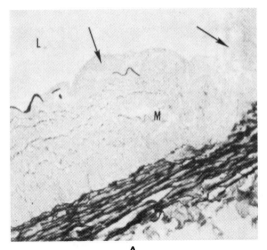

A

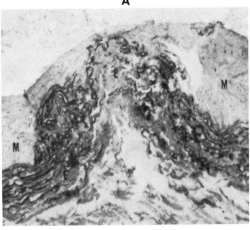

B

Figure 3–22. (A) This arterial segment from a vessel subjected to a "near miss" of 10 mm by a 16 grain sphere traveling at 3000 feet per second shows large areas of discontinuity in the internal elastic lamina. The arterial media (M) is in direct continuity with the vessel lumen (L). Early thrombus is present in the region of the large breaks (arrows). Media and external elastic layers are partially fragmented. (Verhoeff-van Gieson stain, reduced from × 220.) (B) This is a portion of an artery subjected to a "near miss" at 1000 feet per second. There is fragmentation and disruption of the external elastic layer (E) and overlying media (M). There is no endothelium or internal elastic lamina remaining. (Verhoeff-van Gieson stain, reduced from × 220.) (Amato, J. J., Billy, L. J., Gruber, R. P., Lawson, N. S., and Rich, N. M., Arch. Surg., *101*:167, 1970. Copyright 1970, American Medical Association.)

without knowledge of the wounding velocity, reviewed the slides. Histologic changes were evident in all layers of the arteries and at all velocities. The intima contained breaks which involved the internal elastic membrane (Fig. 3–20). Measurement of the number of breaks in the intima demonstrated a direct correlation between the ve-

locity of the sphere and the mean incidence of large breaks (Table 3–1). The formation of microthrombi also increased with the higher velocity of the sphere. The media showed evidence of hemorrhage, disruption and early exudate formation (Fig. 3–21). Periadvential hemorrhage was also noted. Microscopic intimal damage was noted throughout the entire length of the excised arterial segment. These results corroborated the clinical experience in Vietnam, as described in more detail in Chapter 2. Similar microscopic changes were seen in the "near miss" group, as well as in those in whom there was direct severing of the artery by the missile. Figure 3–22 demonstrates similar pathologic findings.

CORRELATION OF EXPERIMENTAL AND CLINICAL VASCULAR TRAUMA

The mechanical disruption of arteries by high velocity missiles has presented additional problems in arterial repair. Controversy regarding the extent of arterial trauma and the significance of this trauma to the eventual success of the arterial repair stimulated additional experimental work based on clinical impressions from both the Korean and Vietnam experience. Some of this effort has been documented earlier in this chapter, and other information can be found throughout the book, particularly in Chapter 2.

Many misconceptions regarding wound ballistics have been corrected through experimental research. Even a lower velocity missile creates a temporary cavity, as shown in Figure 3–23. Nevertheless the wounding power of high velocity missiles, in comparison to that of lower velocity missiles, is greatly accentuated by the additional energy in the larger temporary cavity. Within microseconds after impact, the missile transfers energy to the tissues struck. Herget (1956) emphasizd that high internal pressures and shock waves as high as 100 atmospheres (1500 pounds per square inch) exist in the temporary cavity as the tissue along the wound tract expands after the high velocity missile passes through it.

Under the auspices of the International Commission of the Red Cross, a series of

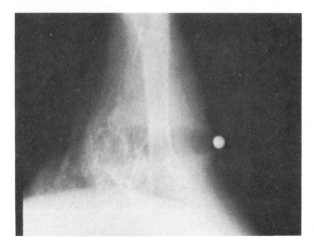

Figure 3–23. A 16 grain sphere traveling at 1000 feet per second through the suspended hind limb of a canine model demonstrates that there is even a small temporary cavity formed in muscle by a low velocity missile. (Amato, J. J., Billy, L. J., Lawson, N. S., and Rich, N. M., Am. J. Surg., *127*:454, 1974.)

meetings have been held by many interested nations to discuss the possibility of prohibition of certain weapons used in warfare (Rich, 1975B). Included in the weapons systems which have been criticized are those which fire high velocity bullets. In 1974 in Sweden, Rybeck and associates conducted an interesting series of five experiments to determine the hemodynamic effects of energy absorption following missile wounding. Among their results is a graphic demonstration of the increased arterial flow in the injured limb compared to that in the opposite uninjured limb (Fig. 3–24).

Experimental vascular trauma continues to challenge the interested investigator.

Some might say this is only a problem for military medicine. However, with the increasing number of gunshot wounds in our cities, including those caused by high velocity missiles, this information also has practical value in our civilian community. Despite the international prohibition at the turn of this century, the "dumdum" bullet is again being used. It is no longer used on the battlefield; however, numerous law enforcement agencies in the United States have reinstituted, or are considering reinstitution of, its use. Yet very little is understood regarding either the experimental or the clinical aspects of the wounding power of this missile.

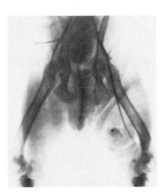 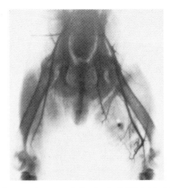 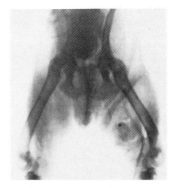

Figure 3–24.   These angiograms of a canine model, started 10 minutes after missile wounding (the entrance wound is marked), show the marked increase in arterial flow in the injured leg on the dog's left side, compared to the contralateral side, as judged by the rapid transit of contrast media. Note in *c* the earlier venous filling. (Rybeck, B., Acta Chir. Scand., Suppl. 450, 1974.)

CHAPTER 4

CLINICAL EVALUATION OF VASCULAR INJURIES

With most patients the history and physical examination will establish or exclude the presence of an arterial injury. However, it is especially important to realize that in some instances there are few or no clinical signs. With any penetrating wound near a major artery, a high index of suspicion must be maintained. Angiography, when feasible, is of increasing value in such instances. An alternate approach of exploring most wounds near a major artery has been followed by some groups and should be con- sidered when angiography is not possible. However, such an approach with military injuries, often with numerous penetrating wounds, is impractical.

Extremity arterial injuries are the most frequent arterial injuries in both civilian and military experience (Table 4–1). Since multiple injuries often occur with arterial injuries, priorities in diagnostic studies and treatment must be established accordingly. With life-threatening injuries of the abdomen or thorax, investigation of a pos-

TABLE 4–1. VIETNAM VASCULAR REGISTRY PRELIMINARY REPORT*

SITE	ARTERY	NUMBER	TOTAL TO EACH SITE	PER CENT
Neck	Common carotid	12	15	4.1
	Internal carotid	3		
Thorax	Subclavian	1	1	0.3
Upper extremity	Axillary	22	125	34.2
	Brachial	103		
Abdomen	Aorta	3	7	1.9
	Renal	1		
	Iliac	3		
Lower extremity	Common femoral	24	217	59.5
	Superficial femoral	116		
	Popliteal	77		
Total		365	365	100.0

*Rich, N. M., and Hughes, C. W., Surgery, 65:218, 1969.

sible arterial injury in an extremity must be postponed until the more serious injuries are treated.

The diagnosis and management of venous injuries are discussed in Chapter 8.

HISTORY

An adequate history of events occurring at the time of injury can be very helpful. If shock, neurological injury or other problems make the patient unable to give an accurate history, an attempt should be made to obtain information from anyone else present when the injury occurred. Particular attention should be given to the amount of blood loss, the patient's color, and the pulsations. Degree of blood loss may be estimated from gross description, development of collapse or shock, necessity for a tourniquet, or infusion of intravenous fluids. A history of bright red blood spurting from a wound is, of course, most significant. This becomes particularly useful with penetrating injuries which on first inspection appear relatively minor. With tangential arterial injuries in which peripheral pulses remain normal, the history of bright blood spurting from a wound at the time of injury may be the best diagnostic clue available.

In their extensive report of experiences with vascular injuries in Dallas, Patman and associates (1964) stated that surgical exploration was usually performed on patients with a history of significant bleeding, even when the wound appeared superficial and peripheral pulses were intact. A certain number of negative explorations were performed, but at that time the hazard of missing an arterial injury was considered more serious than a negative exploration. At times, however, even this approach may not be quite so simple. An example is a patient seen in a situation such as Vietnam with 100 or more fragment wounds over a great proportion of the body surface. It is practically impossible to consider exploring every major artery adjacent to one of the fragments. In this situation, a small percentage of arteriovenous fistulas and false aneurysms found at a later time will have to be accepted.

PHYSICAL EXAMINATION

General Examination. Arterial injuries are often associated with injuries of multiple organ systems and varying degrees of shock. Both of these factors make initial physical examination of the peripheral arterial circulation difficult, and often it is impossible to decide whether or not an arterial injury is present until shock has been corrected by infusion of fluids and peripheral pulses have become palpable. Shock of varying degree was seen with many arterial injuries in Vietnam. In reports of civilian arterial injuries it has also been frequent. In 1961 Ferguson and co-workers reported that 88 of 200 patients (44 per cent) seen in Atlanta arrived in profound shock, requiring an average of 2600 ml of blood. Similarly, Drapanas and co-authors (1970), reporting on 226 patients seen over a 30 year period in New Orleans, found shock in 56 per cent, as defined by a systolic blood pressure below 80 mm Hg. Almost identical findings were reported by Patman and associates in Dallas (1964), where shock occurred in 48 per cent of 256 patients with arterial injuries.

Abdominal, thoracic and head injuries frequently occur with arterial injuries of the extremities. These are often life-threatening, and decision about the presence of an arterial injury often has to be postponed until the more urgent injury is treated. In the extremity, concomitant injury of the adjacent vein, nerve or bone is frequent. In the interim Vietnam analysis of 1000 acute major arterial injuries (Rich et al., 1970A), associated nerve injuries were found in 42.4 per cent of the patients, venous in-

TABLE 4–2. CONCOMITANT INJURIES WITH 1000 ACUTE MAJOR ARTERIAL INJURIES
VIETNAM VASCULAR REGISTRY*

STRUCTURE	PATIENTS	PER CENT
Nerve	424	42.4
Vein	377	37.7
Bone	285	28.5

*Modified from Rich, N. M., Baugh, J. H., and Hughes, C. W., J. Trauma, *10:*359, 1970.

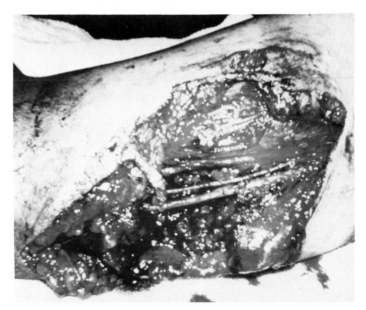

Figure 4-1. Extent of associated injuries frequently found with major arterial trauma. In addition to the severe trauma of the right brachial artery, there is also massive soft tissue destruction with trauma to the associated nerves, veins and bone. (Rich, N. M., Baugh, J. H., and Hughes, C. W., J. Trauma, *10*:359, 1970. Copyright 1970, The Williams & Wilkins Co., Baltimore.)

juries in 37.7 per cent and fractures in 28.5 per cent (Table 4-2). The associated injuries were particularly frequent in the axillary and popliteal areas (Fig. 4-1). Frequency of concomitant injuries has been similar in civilian trauma. Morris and associates (1957) found that approximately 62 per cent of 136 patients had associated injuries (Table 4-3). Similar findings were reported by Ferguson and co-authors (1961) (Table 4-4), by Patman and associates (1964) (Table 4-5) and by Drapanas and colleagues (1970).

Examination of the Wound. In examining the wound, particular attention should be given to the type of bleeding present, location and direction of the wound, surrounding hematoma, and the presence of a thrill or bruit. A wound spurting bright red blood, of course, immediately establishes the diagnosis. However, often bleeding has ceased, though a suspicious hematoma may be present. Drapanas and colleagues (1970) specifically noted that only 13.5 per cent of their 226 patients had active bleeding at the time of admission. A large, firm hematoma surrounding the wound, often with ill-defined margins, strongly suggests an

TABLE 4-3. ASSOCIATED INJURIES IN 84 CASES OF ACUTE ARTERIAL INJURY
61.8 PER CENT OF 136 INJURIES IN HOUSTON PRIOR TO 31 JULY 1956*

Injury to adjacent nerves	33
Injury to major veins	22
Injury to adjacent tendons	18
Fracture of adjacent bone	13
Abdominal injury	11
Extensive soft tissue injury	9
Thoracic injury	8
Fractures of other bones	7
Other injuries	6
Dislocation of adjacent joints	2
Total	129

*Modified from Morris, C. G., Jr., Creech, O., Jr., and DeBakey, M. E., Am. J. Surg., *93*:565, 1957.

TABLE 4-4. INCIDENCE OF ASSOCIATED INJURIES*
200 ACUTE ARTERIAL INJURIES GRADY MEMORIAL HOSPITAL, ATLANTA, GEORGIA, 1 JANUARY 1950 – 31 DECEMBER 1959

Veins	93	Lung	8
Nerves	55	Stomach	6
Tendons	38	Kidney	5
Bones	21	Diaphragm	5
Small intestine	14	Spleen	4
Colon	12	Duodenum	2
Liver	9	Pancreas	2

*Modified from Ferguson, I. A., Sr., Byrd, W. M., and McAfee, D. K., Ann. Surg., *153*:980, 1961.

TABLE 4–5. INCIDENCE OF ASSOCIATED INJURIES IN SURVIVING PATIENTS CIVILIAN ARTERIAL INJURIES IN DALLAS*

ASSOCIATED INJURIES	NUMBER OF INJURIES
Veins, associated	130
Other veins	30
Nerves	42
Muscles, severe	51
Bones, fractures	26
Small intestine	23
Hemothorax	16
Pneumothorax	17
Liver	8
Stomach	6
Pancreas	3
Colon	10
Diaphragm	4
Spleen	5
Kidney	5
Ureter	2
Trachea	3
Esophagus	3
Thoracic duct	3
Gallbladder	2
Bile ducts	2
Closed head injury	2
Uterus	1
Total	384 [sic]

*Patman, R. D., Paulos, E., and Shires, G. T., Surg. Gynec. Obstet., *118*:725, 1964.

arterial injury (Fig. 4–2). The hematoma is firm because of the pressure with which the blood has been expelled from the artery. The margins are vague because the hematoma lies beneath the fascia which eventually tamponades and stops the bleeding. Saletta and Freeark (1968) found a significant hematoma in 37 of 57 patients (65 per cent) with tangential arterial injuries. In six of these 37, a definite pulsation was present in the hematoma. Mufti and co-workers (1970) described significant hematoma formation as the sole manifestation of arterial injury in eight patients among 28 with proven arterial injuries of the extremities.

Feeling a thrill over the hematoma is unusual, occurring only with the comparatively infrequent arteriovenous fistula. However, a systolic bruit is frequently audible with tangential injuries that lacerate but that do not transect the artery. Saletta and Freeark (1968) found a bruit in nearly 50 per cent of 28 patients with tangential

injuries. In the large series by Drapanas and co-workers (1970) including all types of arterial injury, a bruit was found in only 8.4 per cent of the group. With the unusual lesion of acute arteriovenous fistula, a continuous murmur rather than a systolic bruit is present and immediately establishes the diagnosis.

Examination of the Extremity Distal to the Wound. Several characteristic findings promptly develop when an extremity becomes acutely ischemic from interruption of the arterial circulation, whether from trauma, embolism, or thrombosis. These have repeatedly been categorized as the "five P's":

1. Absence of peripheral pulses
2. Pallor
3. Pain
4. Paresthesia (or anesthesia)
5. Paralysis

The importance of these clinical findings is repeatedly emphasized in different chapters in this book. The most significant are the neurological signs of paresthesia and paralysis, because of all tissues in the extremities, peripheral nerves are the most sensitive to anoxia. If neurological function is intact, there is virtually no risk of gangrene; conversely, with loss of neurological function gangrene is very probable unless circulation is significantly improved within six to eight hours. When there are concomitant peripheral nerve injuries, the use of neurological function as an index to severity of anoxia is restricted. However, the deficit due to peripheral nerve injuries is segmental, whereas the neurological deficit from anoxia is more diffuse, with a uniform, stockinglike distribution in the peripheral extremity.

The significance of the inability to feel a distal pulse is a serious question. The pulse may be missing for several reasons: shock, intense vasospasm, pre-existing arterial disease, congenital absence, or an arterial injury. The influence of hypotension and vasospasm can be determined after blood pressure has been restored by infusion of fluids and vasospasm corrected; this is indicated by reappearance of other distal pulses, along with full veins and warm extremities. Continued inability to feel a pulse once this has occurred is suspicious. Absence of a pulse from pre-existing ar-

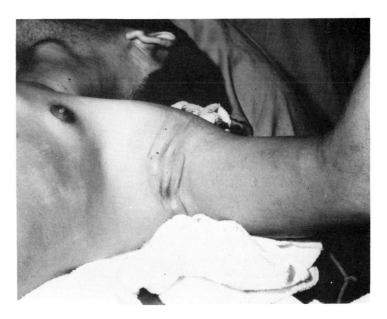

Figure 4–2. The finding of a large, tense hematoma, such as this axillary hematoma, should alert the examiner to the probability of an arterial injury. (Rich, N. M., Hobson, R. W., II, and Collins, G. J., Jr., Am. J. Surg., *130*: 712, 1975.)

terial disease becomes an increasingly likely possibility in patients over 50 to 60 years of age. A history of claudication and signs of chronic tissue ischemia such as rubor, loss of digital hair, or thickening of the nails indicate the possibility of chronic arterial disease. Comparison of the two extremities is often helpful. Congenital absence of a pulse is unusual. The posterior tibial is almost never congenitally absent, but the dorsalis pedis has been reported absent in between 5 and 10 per cent of the normal population.

A warning repeatedly given by several experienced observers is that it is hazardous to attribute absence of a pulse to "spasm." Discrete spasm to such a degree that flow of blood is stopped can occur and can be readily demonstrated in the experimental laboratory, but clinically it is a rare occurrence. Spasm implies a muscular contraction occurring in the absence of anatomical injury. It has been recognized most commonly in children with supracondylar fractures of the elbow in which the adjacent brachial artery seems unusually susceptible. In other areas of the body it is most rare. Usually the diagnosis is a contusion of the artery with fracture of the intima, which in turn gradually prolapses into the lumen and precipitates thrombosis. This sequence of events most commonly occurs with closed injuries of the extremity, such as a fracture

of the femur with displacement of bone and development of a large hematoma. The diagnosis of spasm should always be considered tentatively incorrect, to be proved only by angiography or by surgical exploration.

When pulses are present rather than absent, the likelihood of overlooking an arterial injury is great, although the risk of ischemic injury to the extremity is not present. Pulses remain either normal, or decreased in intensity, when a tangential injury lacerates but does not sever the artery. If circumstances permit the surrounding hematoma to seal the laceration, peripheral flow of blood may continue, either normally or restricted in volume. Drapanas and coauthors (1970) reported that 33 of 128 patients (27.3 per cent) had pulses detected distal to the injury. Perry and colleagues (1971) reported from Dallas that, between 1950 and 1961, 69 patients were seen with pulses detected distal to the site of injury. Forty of these were thought to have normal pulses, while in 29 the pulses were considered decreased. In a more recent report, 22 of 225 patients, about 10 per cent, had pulses detected distal to the injury.

The neurological signs of ischemia, paresthesia and paralysis appear when ischemia is severe. This will vary with the size of the artery injured; the degree to which collateral circulation is impaired, usually determined by the amount of soft tissue injury present; and the severity of hypotension. With the extensive soft tissue injuries that often occurred in Vietnam, neurological signs were frequent. In civilian trauma, often with minimal soft tissue injury, these findings are less common. Drapanas and associates (1970) found serious signs of ischemia in only 24.1 per cent of their patients.

As mentioned previously, the degree of ischemia varies with the size of the artery injured and the effectiveness of collateral circulation. This has been simply expressed in several reports by noting the frequency with which gangrene develops if the injured artery is ligated. A listing of the gravity of arterial injuries, ranging from the most critical to the least critical, was prepared by Whelan and Baugh (1967), who established this list from the World War II experience documented by DeBakey and Simeone (1946):

1. Femoral artery
2. Popliteal artery
3. Combination of anterior and posterior tibial arteries
4. Brachial artery (above the deep brachial artery)
5. Superficial femoral artery
6. Iliac artery
7. Axillary artery
8. Brachial artery (below the deep brachial artery)

The range is wide, for gangrene develops in 70 to 80 per cent of patients if the common femoral artery is ligated, but gangrene develops in only 10 to 15 per cent of patients if the brachial artery is ligated distal to the origin of the deep brachial artery.

SPECIAL DIAGNOSTIC CONSIDERATIONS

Variation in Types of Injury. In deciding whether an arterial injury is present, it is important to realize that several types of injury can occur. The most common is the most obvious: transection of the artery with immediate loss of pulses and signs of peripheral ischemia. As mentioned before, the converse exists with a tangential laceration sealed by a clot, because there is little or no detectable impairment of peripheral circulation. Contusion with eventual thrombosis is particularly deceptive because arterial circulation may initially be normal or only slightly impaired, but prolapse of a detached flap of intima into the lumen may gradually increase with progressive accumulation of superimposed thrombus until occlusion is complete several hours after the initial injury. This phenomenon can be detected only by serial evaluation. As mentioned previously, true spasm is rare and is not an acceptable diagnosis without arteriography or actual surgical exploration. An arteriovenous fistula can be recognized simply from the classic continuous murmur, but the overall frequency is rare and its clinical significance in diagnosis is not great.

Confusion of an Arterial Injury with an Abscess. A classic error, recorded again and again from ancient times to the present, is confusion of the enlarging hematoma of a false aneurysm with an abscess. The usual history is that of a penetrating wound with hemorrhage that spontaneously ceases as a hematoma develops, but peripheral pulses remain intact. What has occurred is a tangential injury sealed by a clot surrounding the artery. Within days or weeks the inner lining of the hematoma, communicating with the lumen of the artery, liquefies and the hematoma begins to pulsate and enlarge. It is now a classic false aneurysm, once termed a "pulsating hematoma." The course is then relentlessly progressive as arterial pressure leads to further enlargement with compression and even destruction of peripheral nerves, intense pain, and progressive enlargement until the aneurysm either ruptures through the skin or into an adjacent body cavity.

If the diagnosis has originally been missed, the clinical picture is that of a painful wound which is swollen, warm and tender. With the classic findings of inflammation, redness, heat, swelling and pain, the unwary have often made the erroneous diagnosis of an abscess and proceeded to incise the mass for drainage. The resulting catastrophic hemorrhage has been recorded repeatedly in past surgical reports. Fortunately, with increasing familiarity with this clinical picture, such a calamity is now rare.

Secondary Hemorrhage. In past wars when infection was common because of inadequate débridement, nonutilization of delayed primary wound closure, and lack

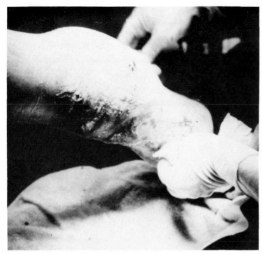

Figure 4–3. Although secondary hemorrhage from undetected arterial injuries is not seen as frequently now as in past wars, this patient had to be rushed to the operating room approximately three weeks following wounding because of hemorrhage from an infected wound. (W.R.G.H.)

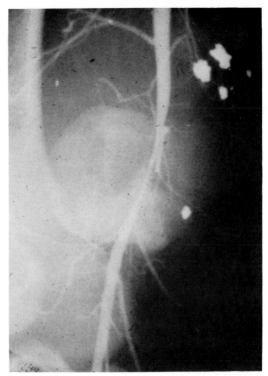

Figure 4–4. Same patient as shown in Figure 4–3. An angiogram performed in the operating room revealed that the hemorrhage was coming from an infected false aneurysm of the proximal popliteal artery. Although the angiography was not essential, it did localize the site of a single arterial injury. (W.R.G.H.)

of antibiotics, a frequent occurrence was secondary hemorrhage from undetected arterial injuries. The usual story was that of a penetrating wound: days or even weeks following injury there would be spontaneous episodes of small amounts of bright red bleeding which would spontaneously cease (Fig. 4–3). In World War II in the China-Burma theater, Freeman (1945) dramatically recorded several such experiences in which hemorrhage developed between the 10th and 16th days and, sometimes, as late as three months. Some exsanguinated in a hospital ward during the middle of the night beneath a cast applied for a fracture. With modern débridement, delayed primary wound closure, and antibiotics, such events are now rare. However, the appearance of bright red bleeding from a wound remains a grave

Figure 4–5. Same patient as shown in Figures 4–3 and 4–4. This small, longitudinal, arterial defect (arrow) was found upon exploration of an infected wound which developed spontaneous hemorrhage. (W.R.G.H.)

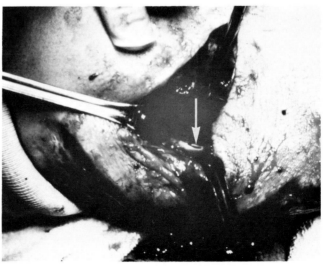

sign. The bleeding may seem trivial—only a small amount which spontaneously ceases. However, this almost always heralds a catastrophic hemorrhage. In most instances the appearance of such bleeding is an indication for either immediate surgical exploration of the wound or arteriography (Figs. 4–4 and 4–5).

Multiple Arterial Injuries. With multiple penetrating wounds, especially those due to exploding devices and multiple fragments, the possibility of multiple injuries of a peripheral artery exists. Attention, of course, will be focused upon the most proximal injury where the circulation is interrupted. The distal injury may become evident only when repair of the proximal lesion fails to restore peripheral pulses. Patman and associates (1964) found such multiple injuries in 14 of 256 patients. Thirteen of these had two injuries, while one had three discrete arterial injuries. Although the data are incomplete, multiple arterial injuries have also been found in a small percentage of the Vietnam combat casualties.

LABORATORY STUDIES

Radiographic Procedures. Roentgenograms, taken in two planes, should be performed routinely to detect fractures and foreign bodies and possibly to outline the course of the wound (Fig. 4–6). Wounds from fragmenting missiles may be readily displayed by demonstrating multiple fragments along the course of the wound.

Unusual instances of missile embolization periodically occur when a missile stops within a large artery or vein and is subsequently embolized in the circulatory system. In the venous system it migrates proximally, ultimately to the pulmonary artery (Fig. 4–7), while in the arterial system it migrates distally (Fig. 4–8).

Angiography is becoming an increasingly valuable procedure, especially in cases of civilian trauma where modern angiographic facilities are frequently available. Great progress has been made in angiography in recent years with the development of safer radiopaque media, selective angiography, and experienced vascular radiologists using percutaneous puncture techniques for introduction of catheters for selective angiography. These techniques are useful in preoperative studies, during operation, and in postoperative evaluation (Fig. 4–9).

A number of clinical problems can best be resolved with an angiogram. Continued absence of pulses after correction of shock is one example. Multiple penetrating wounds, such as those from shotgun pellets, is another. Penetrating injuries of body cavities, the chest or abdomen, can be investigated via angiography when circumstances permit. The familiar problem of a penetrating wound near an artery, a suspicious hematoma, but intact pulses may best be assessed with an angiogram, especially if surgical exploration has to be postponed. The question of arterial injury associated with a closed fracture of the femur in an elderly patient with absent pulses is similarly best resolved by arteriography rather than by surgical exploration.

Although the role of angiography in studying vascular trauma has progressively increased and undoubtedly will continue to do so, several recent publications have expressed varying opinions about its value. In Vietnam it was not widely used because most wounds were large open ones with massive tissue destruction, requiring immediate operation and making angiography superfluous. Also, there was a lack of facilities. As mentioned before, however, these facilities are becoming more common in civilian practice. When the diagnosis is obvious, preoperative angiography is of course superfluous and may use time better spent in expeditious repair of the injured vessel. However, operative angiography, when available, is a useful adjunct following repair and may detect distal thrombi, unrecognized arterial disease, or an injury distal to the site of the primary injury.

Freeark, in several publications, has championed the use of arteriography in the trauma patient. In 1969 he reported that house staff commonly performed carotid and femoral angiography by percutaneous puncture, often doing 100 such procedures a month. No major complications from angiography were observed in the previous year. In 1972 Saletta and Freeark described percutaneous angiogra-

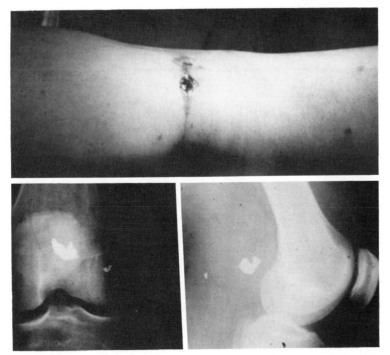

Figure 4–6. The location of a wound in the popliteal fossa, and roentgenograms taken in two planes showing a foreign body adjacent to neurovascular structures, provide additional information in determining the probability of major arterial trauma. (Rich, N. M., *in* Dale, W. A., (Ed.), Management for Arterial Occlusive Disease. Year Book Medical Publishers, Inc., Chicago, 1971.)

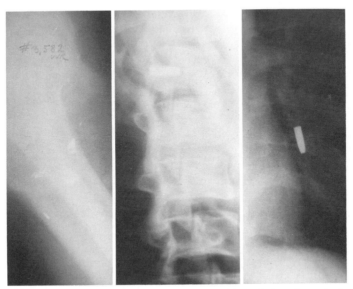

Figure 4–7. Although unusual, missile embolization can provide a challenging set of circumstances. This patient was originally shot in the right hip; the missile entered the major venous return to the heart and finally ended in the left pulmonary artery. (W.R.G.H.)

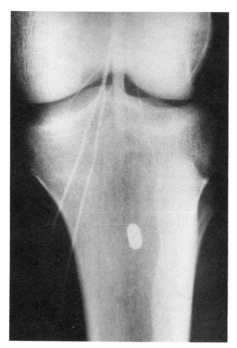

Figure 4–8. Missile embolization must also be considered as a possibility (see Fig. 4–7) in a patient who has sustained a penetrating wound of the thorax who subsequently develops ischemia in the lower extremities. This missile embolized distally after penetrating the thoracic aorta. (Dillard, B. M., and Staple, T. W., Arch. Surg. *98*:326, 1969. Copyright 1969, American Medical Association.)

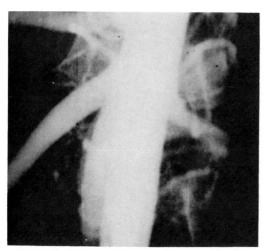

Figure 4–9. Angiography has been extremely valuable in selected situations, particularly in blunt trauma, in confirming the clinical suspicion of major arterial trauma, such as this occlusion of the left renal artery in a young adult male who had fallen 30 feet from a tower one month earlier and subsequently developed hypertension. (W.R.G.H.)

phy in all patients with lower extremity trauma with diminished pulses, suspicious bruits, large hematomas or recurrent hemorrhage (Table 4–6). They also found it helpful in locating the exact site of arterial injury before surgically exploring a large hematoma. Again, no significant complications were encountered. Also, false positive angiograms had not occurred. An earlier report by Lumpkin and colleagues (1958) (Fig. 4–10) emphasized that angiography had been used too little. They used it specifically when the diagnosis was uncertain, and also to localize the injury before surgical exploration. They did note that two patients with partially severed major lower extremity arteries also had palpable distal pulses with normal skin temperature. Table 4–7 outlines the angiographic findings and their correlation with the arterial pathology; these findings are also compared to the physical evaluation.

Gaspar and associates (1968) similarly recommended arteriography when signs of arterial injury were indefinite, especially in cases of blunt trauma and fracture. However, they did find that the arteriogram was not always diagnostic, for extravasation of contrast material did not always occur with vascular injuries, apparently because the site of injury had been sealed by a clot. Pessimism about angiography was again expressed by Patman and colleagues (1964),

TABLE 4–6. CLINICAL FINDINGS SUGGESTING ARTERIAL INJURY IN 57 PATIENTS WITH PARTIALLY SEVERED ARTERIES*

	FINDINGS	**EVALUATED**	**PER CENT**
Hemorrhagic shock	13	57	23
Local hematoma Nonpulsatile, 31 Pulsating, 6	37	57	65
Pulse deficit Diminished, 8 Absent, 18	26	46	57†
Bruit (systolic or continuous)	15	28	54†
Positive angiogram	22	22	100†

*From Saletta, J. D., and Freeark, R. J., Arch. Surg., 97:198, 1968. Copyright 1968, American Medical Association.

†Expressed as percentage of patients examined.

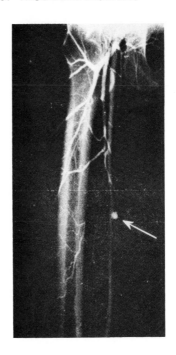

Figure 4–10. This arteriogram demonstrates a laceration of the superficial femoral artery, incurred by a knife. The wound was not bleeding, and posterior tibial and dorsalis pedis pulses were normal, as might be anticipated by the continuity of the arterial stream demonstrated. Exploration confirmed the radiographic findings with an 80 per cent transection of the superficial femoral artery. (Lumpkin, M. B., Logan, W. D., Couves, C. M., and Howard, J. M., Ann. Surg., *147*:353, 1958.)

who believed that the time invested could be better employed in the operating room. They also noted that some injuries were not detected by angiography because extravasation of contrast material did not occur.

Wholey and Bocher (1967) emphasized the great value of arteriography with closed injuries with fractures. Early detection of traumatic contusion and thrombosis was possible with fractures of the femur, permitting surgical correction much earlier than had previously been possible.

In the management of closed injuries, undoubtedly angiography should be used more frequently. In such instances surgical exploration is unnecessary and may be harmful unless an arterial injury is present. However, in the case of a penetrating wound where surgical exploration is required anyway, arteriography may only delay repair

TABLE 4–7. PENETRATING ARTERIAL TRAUMA*

ARTERY INJURED	MODE OF INJURY	PATHOLOGY	ARTERIOGRAPHIC FINDING	DISTAL PULSE	SKIN TEMPERATURE	HEMATOMA
Superficial femoral	knife	80% transection	extraluminal extravasation	present	normal	slight
Anterior and posterior tibial	bullet	transection	complete block	absent	cool	massive
Popliteal	shotgun	compression from hematoma	extrinsic compression	absent	cool	moderate
Popliteal	knife	partial severance	extraluminal extravasation	present	normal	moderate
Popliteal	shotgun	spasm	complete block	absent	cool	moderate

*Modified from Lumpkin, M. B., Logan, W. D., Couves, C. M., and Howard, J. M., Ann. Surg., *147*:353, 1958.

TABLE 4–8. PRINCIPAL PHYSICAL AND ARTERIOGRAPHIC FINDINGS IN 114 CASES OF PERIPHERAL VASCULAR TRAUMA TO AN EXTREMITY*

| | | | | PRINCIPAL ARTERIOGRAPHIC FINDINGS | | | | |
PRINCIPAL PHYSICAL FINDING	PATIENTS	NEGATIVE	SPASM	Pseudo-aneurysm	Intimal Tear	Arterio-venous Fistula	OCCLUSION	SURGICAL INTER-VENTION
Normal	85	80	4	1				
Neurological deficit only	10	7		1	1		1	3
Weak distal pulses	4	1		2			1	2
Absent pulse	7	2					5	2
Bruit	3			1		2		3
Expanding hematoma	4			1	2		1	3
Active bleeding	1					1		1
Total	114	90	4	6	3	3	8	14

*Modified from McDonald, E. J., Jr., Goodman, P. C., and Winestock, D. P., Radiology, *116*:45, 1975.

and is possibly superfluous. With closed injuries, the use of angiography may prevent an unnecessary exploration or may indicate the need for an operation to forestall gangrene.

Freeark (1969) has emphasized the use of angiography for penetrating injuries of the abdomen, thorax, neck and jaw. In these areas, hemorrhage, shock and injuries of other vital structures frequently conceal major vascular injuries later found on surgical exploration. When circumstances permit, angiography by the selective catheter technique can readily disclose the precise vascular injury beforehand. As emphasized in Chapter 18, such an approach has been crucial with traumatic rupture of the thoracic aorta from deceleration injuries in automobile accidents. Fu (1972) has provided additional details and many angiographic examples of the value of angiography in evaluating patients who sustained trauma. McDonald and associates (1975) correlated the presence or absence of physical signs of vascular injury with the arteriographic findings in 114 cases of penetrating and blunt injury to the extremity (Table 4–8).

The Doppler Ultrasonic Flow Detector. In Vietnam, use of the Doppler principle for ultrasonic detection of flow when pulses were absent was found clinically valuable (Table 4–9). The Doppler effect was described in 1842 by the German physicist Christian Doppler. It is based on the principle that the frequency of sound is changed by fluid in motion. From this principle, ultrasonic probes have been developed to measure velocity of blood flow in peripheral

arteries and veins. The transcutaneous ultrasonic flow detector is battery operated and easily used in either the operating room or at the patient's bedside. When the probe is temporarily applied to the skin, the piezoelectric crystal in the probe emits an ultrasound frequency which is reflected back from the underlying tissue and interpreted by a second crystal in the probe (Fig. 4–11). Any flow beneath the transistor is heard as a sound through the attached earphone, since the flow of blood changes the frequency of the sound. The pitch of the sound is related to the velocity of flow. It is hoped that future experiences with ultrasonic

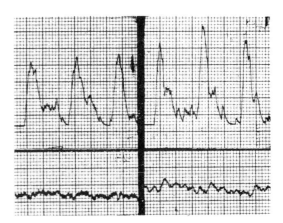

Figure 4–11. The value of the ultrasonic flow detector in conditions in which peripheral pulses are not palpable. The upper Doppler tracings show pulsatile flow in the dorsalis pedis arteries at a time when the lower plethysmogram tracings were essentially in a straight line. (Lavenson, G. S., Jr., Rich, N. M., and Baugh, J. H., Amer. J. Surg., *120*:522, 1970.)

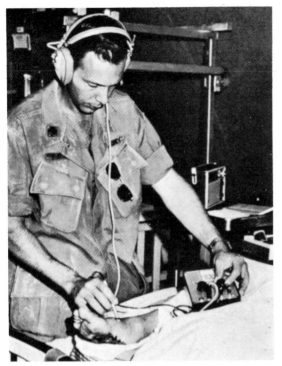

Figure 4–12. Use of the ultrasonic flow detector (Doppler) at the 24th Evacuation Hospital in Vietnam in 1969 during the study reported by Lavenson and co-workers (1971). (In discussion of Rich, N. M., *in* Dale, W. A. (Ed.), Management for Arterial Occlusive Disease. Year Book Medical Publishers, Inc., Chicago, 1971.)

measurements will permit a better quantitation of the degree of flow present.

One of the earliest reports using the ultrasonic flow detector was made in 1963 by Watson and Rushmer, who used a probe to detect flow of blood through the intact skin of human subjects. At Walter Reed Army Medical Center, the ultrasonic flow detector has been found to be of increasing value. The initial experience was reported by Lavenson and colleagues (1970). This experience was continued in Vietnam to assess distal flow when pulses did not return after arterial repair and the viability of the limb was uncertain (Lavenson et al., 1971) (Fig. 4–12). Their results are shown in Table 4–9. In 21 extremities without distal pulses, either after arterial repair or following disruption of a vascular repair, distal flow sounds were audible in 11. All proved to have a viable extremity. Conversely, in 10 extremities without audible distal flow, six that were not revascularized subsequently required amputation for gangrene.

In Vietnam this information was of particular value with the difficult clinical problem of wound infection leading to disruption of the arterial repair. In such instances safely delaying vascular reconstruction was of particular value, permitting time for control of the infection. If serious ischemia was present, the only alternative to amputation was to attempt another vascular reconstruction, even though seriously jeopardized by the presence of infection. On the other hand, delaying repair when the extremity was viable permitted control of infection and a much more effective vascular reconstruction at a later date.

Miscellaneous Studies. Oscillometry has been periodically used in the past, usually when pulses were not palpable (Linton, 1949). Although periodically reported by

TABLE 4–9. CORRELATION OF ULTRASONIC FLOW DETECTOR FINDINGS OF LIMB VIABILITY*
VIETNAM EXPERIENCE

	NUMBER OF EXTREMITIES	AMPUTATION	NO AMPUTATION
After repair			
Pulses palpable	74	1†	73
Pulses impalpable, flow audible	4	1†	3
Pulses impalpable, flow inaudible	7	3	4‡
After ligation			
Flow audible	7	0	7
Flow inaudible	3	3	0

*Modified from Lavenson, G. S., Jr., Rich, N. M., and Strandness, D. E., Arch. Surg., *103*:644, 1971.
†Extremity was viable; amputation was required because of extensive tissue damage and infection.
‡Reoperation was performed.

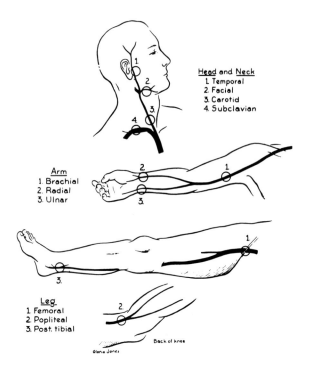

Head and Neck
1. Temporal
2. Facial
3. Carotid
4. Subclavian

Arm
1. Brachial
2. Radial
3. Ulnar

Leg
1. Femoral
2. Popliteal
3. Post. tibial

Back of knee

Gloria Jones

Figure 4–13. Palpation of peripheral pulses at the sites diagrammed here not only give an indication of the rate and rhythm or establish the diminution or absence of a pulse, but also reveal the quality of the arterial wall as being either soft and compressible or hard, nodular and rigid. Calcification in the artery may give a feeling similar to that of the trachea. Absence of palpable pulses does not entirely rule out patency of the vessel because there may be a nonpulsatile flow in the artery. In addition, narrowing of the artery produces turbulence that may be palpated as a thrill or heard with a stethoscope as a bruit. (Modified from de Takats, G., Med. Clin. North Am., *46*:647, 1962.)

different observers, it has never found widespread use possibly because the procedure is somewhat cumbersome and lacks precision. It is hoped that the Doppler ultrasonic technique will be clinically more useful.

Venous filling time has been long recorded as an index of arterial flow to an extremity. This is measured by elevating the lower extremity above the level of the heart and inflating a blood pressure cuff on the thigh to about 60 mm Hg. This permits arterial inflow but obstructs venous return. The limb is then placed back in a horizontal position and the time required for filling of veins of the dorsum of the foot noted. They may fill within 5 to 10 seconds, but a filling time as long as 40 seconds may exist with adequate circulation. Filling times as long as 60 to 120 seconds indicate progressive degrees of arterial insufficiency. The test is a traditional one, often quoted in the past, but is actually not of much clinical value and is gradually falling into disuse.

Finally, it should be re-emphasized that the recognition of an arterial injury is predominantly clinical, with a continued alertness for the variation in the clinical pattern that occurs with different types of arterial injury. Serial evaluation of an extremity, noting adequacy of peripheral flow and investigating promptly any suspicious signs, especially those of impaired neurological function, is the soundest clinical approach. Laboratory studies are valuable adjuncts, but under no circumstances should they displace the primary role of bedside evaluation and decision. de Takats (1963) emphasized the predominant role of clinical evaluation (Fig. 4–13):

There are a great many other research tools, which have been described....their elaborate and wordy use in reports simply argue for the learning, wisdom, and expensive equipment of the examiner, but do not further contribute to the problem on hand.

CHAPTER 5

MANAGEMENT OF ACUTE ARTERIAL INJURIES

The ligature of the main vessels of an extremity for control of haemorrhage seriously jeopardizes the life of that extremity, but this danger may be averted in many instances by suture, provided a certain degree of care be exercised in this attempt by the operator.

Major Charles Goodman, M.C., U.S.A.
B.E.F. France, 1918.

This chapter describes most of the general principles underlying the care of arterial injuries. In subsequent chapters considering specific arterial injuries, these principles are often repeated for emphasis and also to indicate their application to specific anatomic regions. However, the basic concepts are applicable to a varying degree with almost any type of arterial injury.

These general principles may be conveniently grouped into three categories: preoperative factors, operative factors and postoperative factors. For clarity and emphasis, these may be tabulated as follows:

I. Preoperative factors
  A. Control of hemorrhage
  B. Resuscitation from shock
  C. Minimizing time lag from injury to arterial repair
II. Operative factors
  A. Débridement of injured tissues and irrigation to minimize infection
  B. Arterial repair
    1. Débridement of injured artery
    2. Removal of distal thrombi
    3. Arterial reconstruction without stenosis or tension
    4. Soft tissue coverage

  C. Management of associated injuries (vein, bone, nerve, soft tissue)
III. Postoperative considerations
  A. Patency of arterial repair
  B. Muscle necrosis
  C. Wound infection

Although there is general agreement among experienced vascular surgeons concerning the above principles, there remain several areas of uncertainty for future investigation. These include the extent of débridement of an injured artery, which depends upon the type of wounding agent (knife wound, low velocity missile or high velocity missile); the best management of a contused artery or of an artery in severe spasm; the indications and contraindications for either lateral suture or lateral suture with patch graft reconstruction; the degree of tension acceptable for an end-to-end anastomosis as opposed to insertion of a vascular graft; the type of graft used; the management of associated fractures; and management of concomitant venous injuries (Fig. 5–1).

In the Korean Conflict, most arterial repairs were performed by a small group of surgeons trained in vascular surgery

75

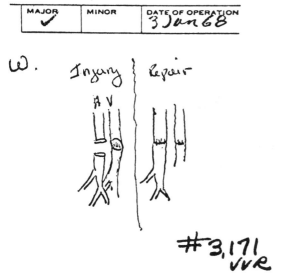

Figure 5–1. Concise documentation of all vascular injuries and associated trauma is extremely important. Often the nondescriptive word "repaired," as used for venous and nerve injuries, might be completely omitted from the description. Simple line drawings which augment a brief description of the operation, such as these done by Joseph J. McNamara, M.D., at the 24th Evacuation Hospital in Vietnam in 1968, not only graphically represent the trauma to the popliteal artery and vein but also detail the end-to-end anastomosis of both vessels.

who were in specialized units. By contrast, in Vietnam large numbers of surgeons have successfully repaired injured arteries. Rich and Hughes (1969) found that at least 159 surgeons were involved in treating 500 patients, and only 20 surgeons were identified who performed more than five major arterial repairs each. In subsequent follow-up through the Registry, the number of surgeons performing vascular repairs in Vietnam has been found to be more than 500. Although this information is not ideal, it clearly indicates that the general principles of vascular surgery have been successfully carried out by young general surgeons from a wide variety of training programs.

Since most injuries are in patients whose arteries are free of intrinsic arterial disease, a general guideline in arterial repair is that if repair can be performed within six to eight hours from the time of injury, a successful result should be obtained in over 95 per cent of the patients. Failure to achieve this high success rate indicates some defect in management which can be cor-

rected by proper education and training. It is not only erroneous but also deceptive to assume that failures are due to other causes, such as the injury itself or associated factors. This simple fact has been established by experiences of several groups in the past 10 years. With the increasing frequency of trauma in civilian life, strong emphasis should be given to this guideline, because arterial repairs must often be made by surgeons whose experience with vascular surgery may not be extensive.

PREOPERATIVE CONSIDERATIONS

CONTROL OF HEMORRHAGE

Hemorrhage in many instances can be temporarily stopped by simple digital pressure. Occasionally, but not often, clamps may be correctly applied to the visible lacerated artery. This must be done with caution, however, because the blind introduction of clamps may cause irreversible injury to the adjacent nerves and also needlessly injure adjacent segments of normal artery.

The majority of arterial injuries can be controlled by judicious packing of the extremity with a sufficient amount of gauze. Depending upon the location and size of the wound, the necessary amount of gauze may vary from a few inches to several feet. Once the wound has been snugly filled with gauze, a pressure dressing can be applied. The gauze is then compressed between the overlying skin and the underlying bone, effectively compressing the artery. If sufficient gauze packing is used, this method will control hemorrhage in the majority of wounds.

Rarely, a tourniquet is necessary. This is fortunate, because there are several dangers with the use of a tourniquet. When a tourniquet is used, the limbs should be carefully padded beneath the tourniquet, and preferably a pneumatic type of tourniquet should be employed. A narrow, constricting tourniquet can cause irreversible injury to underlying nerves, even though the arterial repair is successfully performed. If a tourniquet is not applied tightly enough, venous return is interrupted

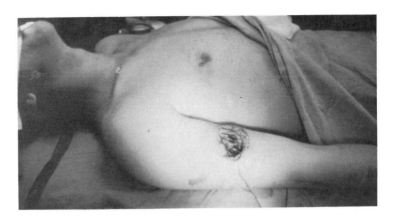

Figure 5-2. Placement of a tourniquet proximal to this injury of the right arm created massive hemorrhage from a severed cephalic vein. The arterial inflow was not occluded, and the venous return was obstructed by the tourniquet. Hemorrhage ceased when the tourniquet was released. (Rich, N. M., J. Cardiovasc. Surg., *11*:368, 1970.)

but arterial inflow continues, resulting in increased hemorrhage from the wound (Fig. 5-2). An additional disadvantage is the fact that a tourniquet deprives the entire extremity of arterial flow, both through collaterals and through the injured artery. In Jahnke's report of the Korean experience (1953), all patients who later underwent amputation following attempts at arterial repair had had a tourniquet applied to the extremity for a long period of time. In Vietnam, tourniquets were seldom found necessary (Rich and Hughes, 1969; Rich, 1970).

RESUSCITATION FROM SHOCK

Most patients with an arterial injury have some degree of shock. In 1957 Morris and colleagues reported that 66 per cent of 136 patients treated for acute arterial injury arrived in hemorrhagic shock and subsequently required an average blood replacement of 2440 ml. By contrast, those not in shock received less than 500 ml of blood. Similarly, in 1961 Ferguson and co-workers found that 44 per cent of 200 patients treated in Atlanta arrived in a state of shock, requiring an average of 2600 ml of blood. The 112 patients not in shock required one-half as much replacement, or an average of only 1300 ml.

In Vietnam, Fisher (1967) reported that in resuscitation of 54 patients, an average of 8.7 units of blood were given per patient, ranging from 2 to 40 units. One-third of the patients required more than 10 units (5000 ml). Similarly, Rich and Hughes

(1969) analyzed blood replacement among 500 patients with arterial injuries in Vietnam, and found that one-half of the group required an average of 4300 ml of blood.

When significant shock is present, it should be corrected promptly by the rapid infusion of appropriate fluids. Until type-specific blood has been located or appropriate cross-matching done, other fluids should be used. Ringer's lactate is readily available and is probably the most useful. There has been considerable interest in the use of unusually large volumes—two to four times the estimated blood loss—of Ringer's lactate. Evidence indicates that these large volumes may cause harm by causing pulmonary congestion, and a policy of giving no more than twice the estimated blood loss would seem prudent. Plasma or dextran is a useful alternative. In urgent instances, unmatched 0-negative blood may be used until type-specified blood is available.

Rapid transfusion is essential to prompt resuscitation, especially if bleeding is continuing. With major abdominal injuries, transfusion through veins in the upper extremities should probably be employed because intra-abdominal bleeding may partly negate the value of fluids infused through veins in the lower extremity.

Broad spectrum antibiotics in large intravenous doses should be started as soon as possible following the arterial injury, continued during the operation and used in the early postoperative period. In Vietnam, the initial use of up to 30 million units of intravenous aqueous penicillin over a 24 hour period, combined with 2.0 gm of intramuscular streptomycin, was fairly routine (Rich and Hughes, 1969) Other broad spectrum antibiotics have been selected by surgeons and used with equal success. In the civilian community, Dillard and associates (1968) reported that they had extensively used antibiotics, in the form of penicillin and chloromycetin; however, they stated that no scientific system had been used to evaluate the results.

MINIMIZING TIME LAG FROM INJURY TO REPAIR

It is well established that the ideal time period for repair of an arterial injury is within six to eight hours after injury. This "golden period" should be the dominant guidepost in planning resuscitation and arterial repair. This time interval is determined chiefly by the tolerance of the muscles of the extremity for ischemia. Recovery is almost certain if arterial flow is re-established within six to eight hours, but beyond this time interval irreversible muscle necrosis is common. The classic experiments of Miller and Welch in 1949 clearly defined the influence of the time interval by restoring blood flow to an extremity after different periods of ischemia. Survival rate was consistently greater than 90 per cent when repair was done within six hours. An additional factor jeopardizing repair after longer periods of time is the development of thrombi in the distal arterial tree; this increases with longer periods of time, especially as muscle necrosis evolves. The haphazard, unpredictable development of distal thrombi is probably the greatest single impediment to successful arterial reconstruction.

It should be emphasized that the time lag is a valuable guideline, but not an absolute criterion. The significance of time lag, of course, depends upon the degree of ischemia present. There are at least four factors which significantly influence the degree of ischemia and similarly influence the significance of time lag. Of the four, the most important is the size of the artery injured. In general, the larger the artery, the more severe the ischemia. Hence, injuries of the iliac artery or the common femoral artery produce more severe is-

chemia than do injuries of the popliteal artery or the superficial brachial artery. The second most significant factor is the degree of impairment of collateral circulation from associated soft tissue injury. This is well illustrated with concomitant fractures, because the hazard of gangrene is greater when an arterial injury is complicated by fracture. This destruction of soft tissue particularly occurs with injuries from high velocity missiles. A third, though less precise, factor is the degree and duration of shock, for this in turn influences the flow of blood through collateral circulation. Finally, ambient temperature, influencing the metabolism of the ischemic extremity, is important because a cold extremity will naturally tolerate ischemia longer than a warm one.

Hence, arbitrary limits cannot be established beyond which repair of an injured artery is futile. The possibility of successful repair may be best evaluated from the musculature in the injured limb. With continuing ischemia, there is a progressive increase in muscle turgor and tone, eventually producing a rigid, hard muscle. The muscular turgor or tone is perhaps the best clinical guide as to whether or not an extremity can be salvaged. This can then be correlated with the overall estimate of the time lag. Occasionally, an extremity may be salvaged 12 to 20 hours after arterial injury because collateral circulation has maintained sufficient flow of blood; however, most extremities will have developed irreversible ischemia by this time. Similarly, in some fortunate instances, collateral circulation is sufficient to maintain viability indefinitely. This is seen in the presence of a pulsating hematoma or an arteriovenous fistula where hemorrhage has stopped but collateral circulation has maintained viability. In such instances, when the viability is no longer in jeopardy, other considerations may be used to choose the proper time for operation. When the time lag has exceeded 10 hours, the hazard of infection from wound contamination is progressively increased and must be carefully evaluated in planning operative repair.

The influence of the average lag time in different wars has been carefully studied. In World War II time lag exceeded 12 hours in most injuries (DeBakey and

Simeone, 1946). They studied a series of 58 vascular injuries in which the time lag between wounding and treatment averaged 15 hours. The dramatic achievements with vascular repairs in the Korean Conflict, in striking contrast to those in World War II, were made possible by the decrease in time lag, a result of helicopter transportation and other logistical factors. Major arterial injuries repaired within nine hours resulted in almost no amputations, while those repaired after nine hours had an amputation rate near 25 per cent.

Time lag was shortened even further in Vietnam. In one study of 225 vascular injuries, most patients reached the hospital within 1.5 hours, and average time from wounding to operation was 2.75 hours (Rich and Hughes, 1969).

To repeat earlier statements, however, when circumstances have resulted in a time lag longer than ideal (greater than eight to 10 hours), arterial repair should be performed in almost all instances, unless the extremity is obviously gangrenous. Whelan and Baugh (1967), encouraging this approach, indicated that the amputation rate with injuries repaired after more than 12 hours was about 50 per cent. They cited a particularly impressive example of a seven year old boy reported by Edwards and Lyons in 1954, where the femoral artery was repaired 24 hours after injury, at which time the toes were black with bullae over the foot and pretibial regions. After resection of a 4 cm contused arterial segment with interposition of a vein graft, only the toes were lost.

In civilian injuries, an average time lag of approximately four hours is usually attainable. In 1957 Morris and co-workers reported an average time of 4.5 hours from injury to definitive treatment in a group of 136 patients. Ferguson and co-authors (1961) described an average time interval between injury and treatment of 3.5 hours in a group of 200 patients treated over a 10 year period in Atlanta. Patman and co-workers (1964) reported a similar experience with a large group of patients, with an average time interval of 3.2 hours; and Dillard and associates (1968) reported similar findings in 85 patients, with an average interval less than six hours (Table 5–1). Drapanas and co-workers (1970)

TABLE 5–1. INITIAL INJURY TO TIME OF ARTERIAL REPAIR* ST. LOUIS, 1958–1966

TIME IN HOURS	NUMBER	PER CENT
Less than 3	62	88.6
3 to 6	4	5.7
6 to 9	2	2.9
12 to 15	1	1.4
18 to 20	1	1.4
Total	70†	100.0

*From Dillard, B. M., Nelson, D. L., and Norman, H. G., Jr., Surgery, *63*:391, 1968.

†This represents 82.4 per cent of 85 arterial injuries. Delay in diagnosis, 15 cases, occurred in 17.6 per cent.

mentioned that the time from injury to operation varied enormously from a few minutes to 30 hours in their series of 226 arterial injuries managed over a 30 year period in New Orleans. However, the average delay for injuries of arteries in the extremities and neck was approximately five hours. In their series the delay was least among survivors of abdominal aortic injuries, with the time lag averaging 36 minutes.

OPERATIVE CONSIDERATIONS

GENERAL CONSIDERATIONS: ANESTHESIA, GENERAL EXPLORATION, AND DÉBRIDEMENT

Anesthesia. The choice of anesthetic agent varies with the ability to control hemorrhage and to restore blood volume before induction of anesthesia. In ideal circumstances, hemorrhage is controlled, blood volume is restored, and anesthesia is then induced. With abdominal and thoracic injuries, however, bleeding may continue during transfusion and even increase as blood pressure is raised. In such instances anesthesia must be induced and operation commenced promptly to control hemorrhage. Under these circumstances, the type of anesthesia must be carefully chosen because the release of vasomotor tone with induction of anesthesia may precipitate severe hypotension. Experiences in Vietnam, however, have shown clearly that modern anesthetic agents can be properly utilized and can effectively enhance resuscitation of patients by permitting prompt exploration and control of intra-abdominal or thoracic bleeding.

Occasionally, local or regional anesthesia may be adequate for injuries limited to an extremity (Patman et al., 1964). The role of regional anesthesia, however, is not great, because wounds are often multiple, and the time needed to effect adequate regional or local anesthesia may unduly delay arterial repair.

General Exploration. The presence of multiple wounds often requires considerable judgment in deciding priorities of treatment. A head injury, abdominal injury, and multiple extremity injuries may be present in the same patient. The obvious priority is to treat those injuries which threaten life most severely and, secondarily, to treat those which threaten loss of the extremity. Such a seemingly obvious point has been overlooked more than once, when prolonged attempts to repair an arterial injury in a patient with multiple injuries resulted in prolonged operating time, massive blood transfusions, and ultimately fatal renal shutdown.

The most frequent concomitant injuries are those involving the head, thorax or abdomen. Immediate thoracic problems can usually be controlled by insertion of an endotracheal tube, rarely a tracheostomy tube, and appropriate intercostal tubes to relieve hemothorax or pneumothorax. Thoracotomy, fortunately, is seldom necessary. With abdominal and intracranial injuries, a decision must be made as to whether surgical exploration should precede, accompany or follow repair of an injured artery. Multiple operating teams are frequently employed to operate upon two or three areas, such as an abdomen, a hand and a leg, simultaneously. In Vietnam as many as four to six surgeons have operated simultaneously upon a single patient.

The most useful monitoring techniques during operation are measurement of central venous pressure, arterial pressure, urine output, and blood gas concentrations. Routine measurement of blood gas concentrations is invaluable in resuscitation of patients with multiple injuries, because acidosis from both respiratory and metabolic causes is frequent and varies unpredictably in severity.

In the preparation of the injured extremity for operation, the entire extremity should be prepared and included in the operative field to permit ready examination of the foot or leg for return of distal pulses and capillary circulation (Fig. 5–3). When possible, an uninflated pneumatic tourniquet may be applied proximally as a reserve mechanism if unexpected hemorrhage is encountered. In such instances, the tourni-

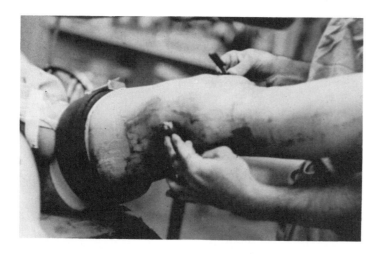

Figure 5–3. To prepare the injury for operation, the entire extremity should be prepared and included in the operative field to permit examination of distal pulses. Control of hemorrhage in this patient was maintained by pressure over the site of the severed superficial femoral artery. In this case a pneumatic tourniquet was applied proximally only for momentary control of hemorrhage. (Rich, N. M., J. Cardiovasc. Surg., *11*:368, 1970.)

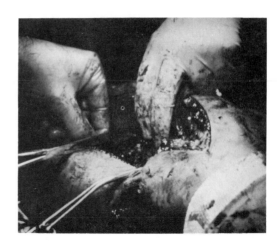

Figure 5-4. Proximal and distal control of the severed ends of the superficial femoral artery controlled the hemorrhage in this patient. An elective incision to provide optimum exposure was utilized to allow prompt application of a nontraumatic vascular clamp to the proximal left superficial femoral artery in this high velocity gunshot wound of the mid-left thigh. (Rich, N. M., J. Cardiovasc. Surg., *11*:368, 1970.)

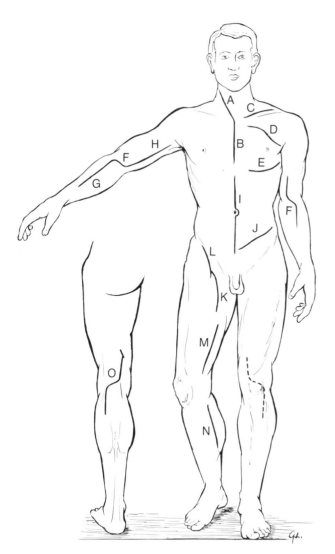

Figure 5-5. Some of the elective incisions that can be utilized in approaching major arteries. Specific details regarding trauma to each major artery are covered in the various chapters throughout this book.

quet may be inflated for a few minutes until the bleeding area is located and controlled.

The surgical incision should be chosen to provide both proximal and distal control of the wounded artery (Figs. 5–4 and 5–5). The original wound should not be used for this purpose unless it corresponds with the proposed elective incision. Normally the incision is directly over and parallel to the course of the underlying artery. Usually proximal control of the artery is obtained, followed by distal control. Once the artery has been identified, it may be temporarily occluded with tapes or vascular clamps. While the artery is kept moistened with saline solution, dissection can be completed to obtain necessary mobilization and exposure of the entire injured area. In the unusual instances where the edges of the lacerated artery are visible in the wound, clamps may be directly applied. However, one should resist the temptation to explore the wound initially and attempt to find the lacerated artery, because dislodgement of a hematoma often results in serious hemorrhage. Hasty or blind application of clamps may irreparably injure adjacent nerves or other structures. In addition to temporary digital control of a bleeding artery and the previously mentioned use of circular tapes and occluding vascular clamps, partial occluding clamps may also occasionally be useful. Small, sharp lacerations of large caliber arteries with minimal trauma to the arterial wall can occasionally be managed by temporarily holding the hemorrhage by use of a partial occluding clamp; this circumvents complete occlusion to a viable structure and decreases the possibility of thrombosis (Fig. 5–6).

Intraluminal control of bleeding may be done with a balloon type of catheter, such as the Fogarty catheter, in unusual instances where direct access to the bleeding artery is difficult. This is an especially useful technique with false aneurysms. The Fogarty catheter technique has been particularly serviceable at Walter Reed General Hospital during operations upon large false aneurysms encased in dense scar tissue. One example is the temporary occlusion of the profunda femoris artery during repair of a false aneurysm of the common femoral

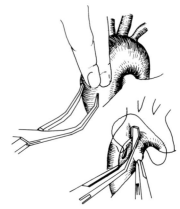

Figure 5–6. Hemorrhage from small lacerations of large arteries can occasionally be controlled temporarily by use of a partial occluding clamp which allows continued distal blood flow.

artery (Fig. 5–7). Once bleeding has been controlled, the wound hematoma can be evacuated and the entire wound irrigated copiously with saline to remove foreign bodies, blood clots and devitalized tissue. In the management of a traumatic wound, copious irrigation is one of the vital principles that will help to prevent infection.

Débridement. During and following irrigation, débridement of injured soft tissues can be done. The degree of débridement varies with the nature of the wound: little débridement is necessary with a sharp puncture wound from a knife, while extensive débridement is required for injury with a high velocity missile and resultant shattering of muscle, bone, and other structures. One of the greatest advances in the treatment of contaminated wounds in the last decades has been the ability to prevent infection in even the most extensively traumatized, contaminated wounds. Probably the three most important principles in prevention of infection are copious irrigation of the wound, adequate débridement, and delayed primary closure of the wound after a few days.

Wound débridement should precede arterial repair because débridement may be erroneously minimized if done after repair has been completed. In more than one instance this has resulted in a disastrous secondary infection, disruption of the arterial repair, and even eventual loss of the extremity.

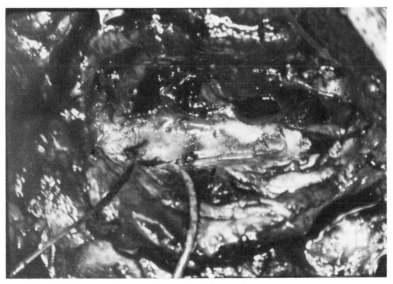

Figure 5–7. Temporary intraluminal occlusion of an artery can be another method of preventing bleeding. Here the Fogarty catheter is used to control temporary back-bleeding from the profunda femoris artery. (W.R.G.H.)

ARTERIAL REPAIR

The repair of an injured artery involves a large number of decisions, some simple and others quite complex. These will be outlined in general terms in this section, and more specific details given in subsequent chapters on specific arterial injuries. Five types of arterial injury are generally recognized: lacerations, transections, contusions, spasm and arteriovenous fistulas. The majority of arterial injuries are either lacerations or transections. Arteriovenous fistulas can often be treated under elective circumstances and are discussed in detail in Chapter 9. The unusual but difficult lesions of *arterial contusion* or *arterial spasm* are considered in detail later in this section.

The basic objectives of arterial repair are débridement of the injured artery, removal of distal thrombi, restoration of continuity without constriction of the lumen or undue tension on the anastomosis, and soft tissue coverage of the site of repair. Depending upon the type of injury, four different techniques may be employed: lateral suture, lateral suture with vein patch, end-to-end anastomosis, and insertion of a vascular graft. The applicability and limitations of these different techniques are analyzed in the following paragraphs.

Débridement. In preparing the injured artery for reconstruction, grossly injured tissue should be excised, but such débridement should be conservative, transecting the vessel where the wall is grossly normal. Although microscopic changes can be found in the adjacent arterial wall of grossly normal-appearing arteries, resection of one or more centimeters of normal appearing artery is unnecessary (see Chap. 2). With high velocity missile wounds, concern has been expressed that an additional margin of normal artery should be excised, but clinically this has been found unnecessary and will often require the insertion of a graft where otherwise a direct anastomosis could have been performed. Rich and associates (1969C) evaluated more than 100 arterial segments from patients in Vietnam and found no correlation between the extent of resection of adjacent normal artery and the ultimate outcome of the arterial repair. Adventitia, one of the greatest sources of tensile strength in an artery, should not be removed to any extent. Removal of a small amount of adventitia may be necessary to prevent strands from protruding into the lumen and constituting a nidus for thrombus formation; otherwise, adventitia should be left intact.

Removal of Distal Thrombi. Removal of thrombi from the distal arterial tree is one of the most crucial aspects of arterial reconstruction, because such thrombi vary to an unpredictable degree in extent and location. Inadequate removal of thrombi is one of the leading causes of failure of arterial reconstruction. Back-bleeding, once considered an index of efficacy of collateral circulation, has been found notoriously unreliable. The degree of such bleeding is influenced by the fortuitous location of a distal tributary. Beyond such a tributary, the lumen may be occluded by a thrombus which will cause gangrene if not removed.

The Fogarty catheter has been a valuable asset in removal of distal thrombi. It probably should be used on a routine basis, advancing the catheter as far as possible into the distal arterial tree, often to the foot or the hand; inflating the balloon; and withdrawing the catheter. This practice was widely employed in Vietnam often with removal of extensive, unsuspected thrombi. Small amounts of heparin, 10 to 25 mg diluted in a saline solution, may be injected into the distal arterial tree at this time to lessen the hazard of subsequent clotting, though the risk of clotting is small if reconstruction is completed within 20 to 30 minutes after the Fogarty catheter has been withdrawn. Systemic heparinization can be employed in unusual circumstances, but it is a distinct hazard in the presence of multiple wounds and is usually unnecessary.

Some experience is necessary to use the Fogarty catheter properly. Undue force in insertion of the catheter has resulted in perforation of the distal artery. The balloon should be tested beforehand, noting the amount of saline required to distend the balloon, as marked on the catheter. Undue distention can produce intensive arterial spasm or even rupture.

Usually the Fogarty catheter is the most effective technique for the removal of distal thrombi. Gentle massage of the distal artery to dislodge thrombus may occasionally be helpful. (See Fig. 5–8). Rarely, incision of an artery at the ankle, such as the posterior tibial, followed by retrograde injection of saline can be useful; but this is cumbersome, not free from risk and far less preferable to effective use of the Fogarty catheter.

A variety of arterial sutures are available, but those generally favored are synthetic sutures (Dacron or Teflon), sizes 5–0 or 6–0. There may be less risk of infection if monofilament sutures are used in the presence of extensive wound contamination. A variety of atraumatic vascular clamps, all modified from the original Pott's principle, are also available. These should be applied gently, using only enough tension to occlude the vessel about 1 cm back from the ends of the transected vessel.

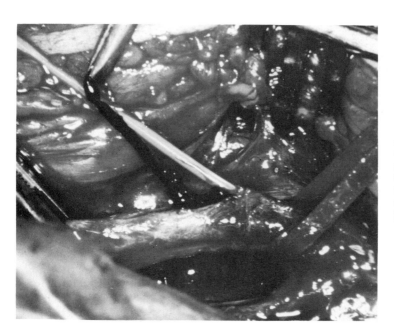

Figure 5–8. A thrombus occasionally may be removed from the artery distal to an area of trauma by gentle massage of the artery; however, the Fogarty catheter is most effective for removing distal thrombi. (W.R.G.H.)

Arterial Reconstruction. LATERAL SUTURE. *Lateral suture* is a technique of repair often overutilized by the inexperienced. It is most commonly applicable to an injury associated with a sharp, penetrating wound, such as a knife, rather than to an injury from a high velocity missile with more arterial destruction. With low velocity missiles, extensive injury to the adjacent arterial wall is unlikely. Best results are usually obtained if the laceration does not involve more than 30 per cent of the circumference of the artery. Also, the technique is safer with larger, rather than small, arteries. In general, lateral repair can be effectively used in no more than 10 to 15 per cent of arterial injuries.

LATERAL SUTURE WITH VEIN PATCH. The use of lateral repair can be enlarged somewhat by the application of an autogenous vein patch to prevent stenosis (Fig. 5–9). However, stenosis can still occur at both the proximal and distal apices of the patch, and care must be taken to incorporate only a minimal amount of arterial wall in the suture line at these points. Otherwise, stenosis can result at the critical angle, even though the vein patch itself is large enough to be somewhat bulbous. Frequently, with a large lateral defect, a better decision is simply to excise the segment and perform a direct anastomosis.

END-TO-END ANASTOMOSIS. *End-to-end anastomosis* or simple anastomosis of the two ends of the injured artery is the technique most effectively employed in over 50 per cent of arterial injuries. Its applicability depends upon the length of artery which has been injured. It is frequently possible to approximate the ends of the injured artery if no more than 2 to 2.5 cm of artery wall have been lost, particularly in the superficial femoral and brachial arteries. Initial inspection of the transected artery may suggest that a larger amount has been destroyed, but the gap is due to elastic recoil of the transected artery. Once vascular clamps have been applied, application of slight tension will readily indicate whether direct anastomosis is feasible (Fig. 5–10). In general, only a slight amount of tension is acceptable in choosing direct anastomosis over the insertion of a vascular graft. Tension can be diminished somewhat by mobilizing the artery proximally and distally for a few centimeters, but important collateral vessels should not be sacrificed (Fig. 5–11). Another maneuver is to flex the joint of the involved extremity to a moderate degree, but when this is employed the joint should be straightened after repair is accomplished to be certain that undue tension is not present. Keeping a joint in flexion for longer than three weeks may lead to serious difficulties from contracture.

In performing the anastomosis, the objective is to approximate the intima of the ends of the vessels without interposing any adventitia. Sutures are normally inserted about 1 mm from the cut end, with 1 mm

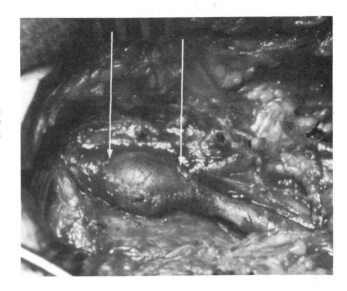

Figure 5–9. An autogenous vein patch graft can be utilized to prevent stenosis of a lateral laceration of a relatively large artery (Rich, N. M., Hobson, R. W., II, Fedde, C. W., and Collins, G. J., Jr.. J. Trauma, *15*:628, 1975. Copyright 1975, The Williams & Wilkins Co., Baltimore.)

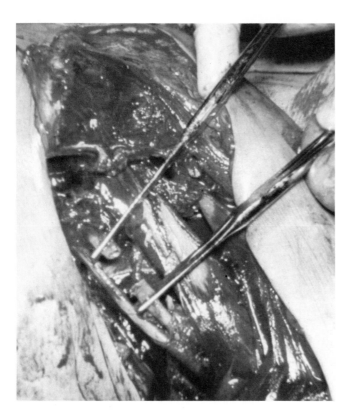

Figure 5–10. Following the application of vascular clamps, a gentle pull to overcome the retraction of the normal artery with its elastic component will usually allow a decision regarding the feasibility of end-to-end anastomosis without tension. (Rich, N. M., Metz, C. W., Jr., Hutton, J. E., Jr., Baugh, J. H., and Hughes, C. W., J. Trauma, *11*:463, 1971. Copyright 1971, The Williams & Wilkins Co., Baltimore.)

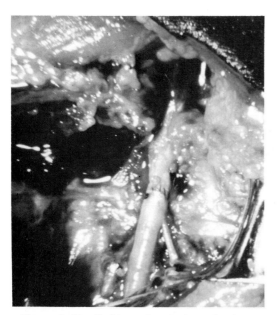

Figure 5–11. End-to-end anastomosis is an ideal method of arterial repair. It is important to avoid tension on the suture line, and the important collateral vessels should be preserved, as shown in this successful end-to-end anastomosis of the popliteal artery. (Rich, N. M., Baugh, J. H., and Hughes, C. W., J. Trauma, *10*:359, 1970.)

between sutures, using a continuous suture for vessels larger than 3 mm internal diameter. Sutures must be gently inserted to avoid laceration of the intima, and the suture line must be carefully observed to avoid constriction or pulling adventitia into the lumen. One technique is to approximate the vessel ends with two sutures 180° apart, complete the anterior one-half of the suture line as a continuous suture, and then rotate the vascular clamps for completion of the posterior one-half of the anastomosis (Fig. 5–12). Another useful technique which obviates the necessity of rotating the clamps is to place one suture directly posterior, 180° away from the surgeon, and then alternately bring each suture line anteriorly as a continuous suture, interrupting it at its midportion anteriorly. If significant resistance is encountered as the suture is drawn through the arterial wall, the thread may be lubricated with sterile petrolatum jelly or mineral oil. Constriction of the suture line can be avoided by cutting the artery on a slight bias and dilating the ends to a slight degree before the sutures are inserted.

After all sutures have been inserted, the

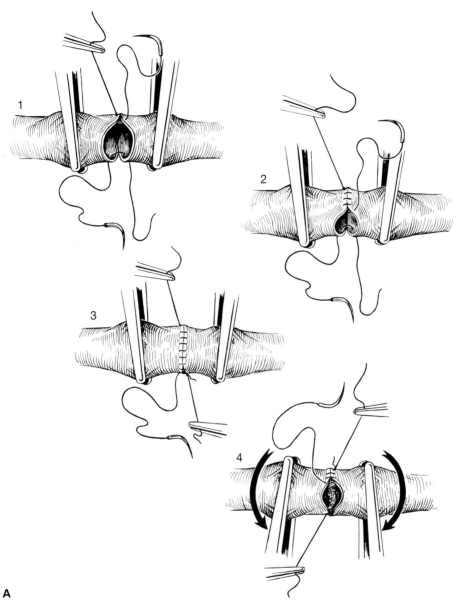

A

Figure 5–12. Various methods that can be used in arterial repair, either end-to-end anastomosis or arterial anastomosis with an arterial substitute. (A) 1, two sutures are used laterally. 2 and 3, an over-and-over stitch is used to complete posterior row. 4, clamps and artery are rotated to complete anterior row.

Illustration continued on following page

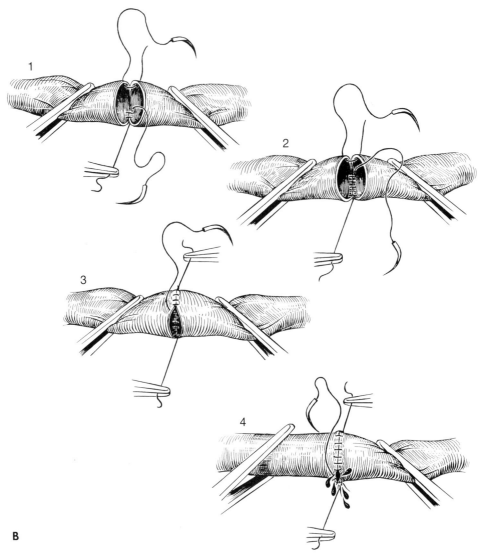

Figure 5–12 *Continued.*   (B) 1 through 4 shows a similar method with two sutures; however, the posterior row is completed from inside and no arterial rotation is required.

Illustration continued on following page

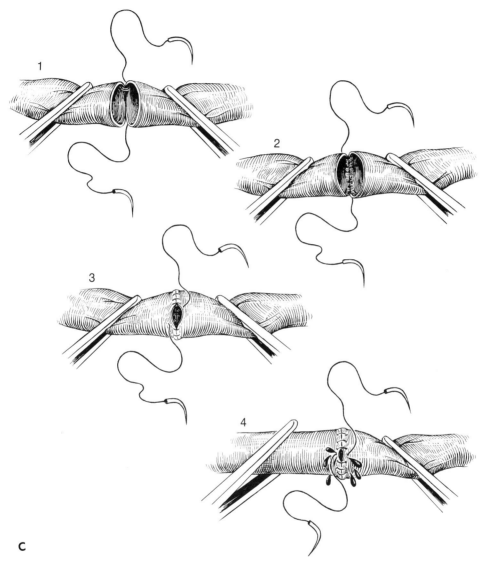

C

Figure 5–12 *Continued.*   (C) 1 through 4 demonstrates the use of one double needle suture starting posteriorly then suturing anteriorly around both sides.

last one or two should be left loose to permit spreading of the edges slightly with a clamp while first the distal arterial clamp and then the proximal clamp are momentarily released to flush blood through the lumen as a safeguard against any thrombi which may have escaped removal beforehand. After the suture line is completed and the clamps released, a vigorous pulse should be palpated immediately beyond the anastomosis, approaching in vigor the pulse that is present proximal to the anastomosis. Significant weakening of the pulse across the site of the anastomosis almost surely indicates constriction or some mechanical defect in the anastomosis which requires revision. A constricted anastomosis readily accumulates platelets, which in turn precipitate thrombosis.

After clamps are released there is normally a slight degree of bleeding from the needle holes. However, this will stop with a few moments of pressure. An area actively spurting blood may require insertion of an additional stitch. This should be done cautiously, however, to avoid laceration. Usually it is best to reapply the clamps for a few moments so sutures are not inserted into an artery under tension. However, when clamps are applied, they cannot be left in place for more than a few minutes. Otherwise a thrombus may form in the lumen and be embolized to the distal arterial tree when the clamps are again released.

Surgicel (reconstituted oxidized cellulose) also may be used occasionally to aid in bringing about a dry suture line.

Arteries smaller than 3 mm internal diameter are probably best repaired with fine 6–0 interrupted sutures, which constrict the lumen to a lesser degree. Optical loupes which magnify two to four times are particularly helpful for performance of these tiny anastomoses (Chase et al., 1963; Kleinert et al., 1963; Gaspar et al., 1968; Spencer, 1971). The possibility of widening the lumen of a small artery with a vein patch, theoretically a useful safeguard to avoid stenosis, has been investigated. Norton and Spencer (1961) evaluated 42 arterial anastomoses upon 2.5 to 4.0 mm arteries in 15 dogs. Six months following operation there was 95 per cent patency of the end-to-end anastomoses, but only 74 per cent patency of the vein patch anastomoses. In the subsequent 16 months, 80 per cent of the end-to-end anastomoses remained patent compared to 75 per cent of the vein patch anastomoses. In most instances a "microsurgical technique" with direct anastomosis gives results better than the insertion of a vein patch with associated creation of turbulent blood flow.

VASCULAR GRAFTS. Vascular grafts are utilized when direct anastomosis is not possible because of excessive tension. Depending upon the type of injury, a graft is needed in about one-third of arterial injuries (Fig. 5–13). In recent experience in Vietnam, grafts were required more frequently because of the large incidence of high velocity wounds. By far the preferable graft is the autogenous reversed greater saphenous vein. This may be taken from the injured extremity if there is not extensive soft tissue injury and loss of major veins. In such instances, it is better to remove the saphenous vein from the opposite extremity. Usually the graft should be taken only after the injured artery has been examined and found unsuitable for direct anastomosis.

The technique for removal of the graft is well defined. Tributaries should be ligated 2 to 3 mm from their origin to avoid constriction of the lumen. During removal of the vein a small amount of adventitia should be left on the vessel, and undue tension, which may disrupt the musculature of the vein, should be avoided. The ends should be carefully marked to be certain that the vein is reversed. If any uncertainty exists, a catheter can be momentarily advanced down the lumen to confirm that obstruction is not present. Gentle dilatation of the vein with heparinized saline should be done after it has been removed, because spasm invariably constricts the lumen to a marked degree (Fig. 5–14). Once dilated with saline, however, the vein does not constrict again. Considerable variation in diameter of the vein exists among different persons, and at different levels in the lower extremity, ranging from as small as 3 mm to as large as 8 mm or more. The ideal graft is one which is only slightly larger than the injured artery. It is preferable to perform the proximal anastomosis first, after which the graft can be distended with blood and the appropriate length more accurately chosen, avoiding either a short graft with tension or a

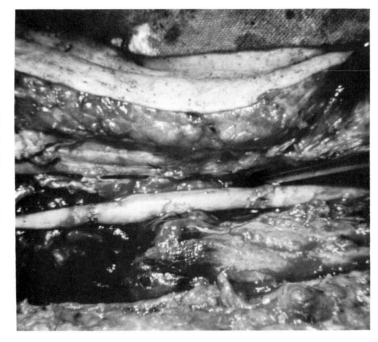

Figure 5-13. If an arterial repair by end-to-end anastomosis is not possible, the use of an autogenous greater saphenous vein graft is most frequently the preferred arterial substitute. (Rich, N. M., Baugh, J. H., and Hughes, C. W., J. Trauma, *10*:359, 1970. Copyright 1970, The Williams & Wilkins Co., Baltimore.)

long, redundant graft. As the distal suture line is completed, as with direct anastomosis, the distal and then the proximal arterial clamps should be momentarily released to flush the anastomotic site with blood.

The saphenous vein is ideal because of its thick wall, which is probably a result of hydrostatic pressure from the normal upright position. However, the cephalic vein can be used when a saphenous vein is not available (Kakkar, 1969). Other veins, however, such as the external jugular, may be too thin walled to withstand arterial pressure without becoming markedly dilated.

There are abundant data published confirming the adequacy of a vein graft as a permanent arterial substitute, principally from bypass operations for occlusive vascular disease. Some periods of follow-up for trauma are now greater than 20 to 30 years. In 1963 Hershey and Spencer reported use of vein grafts in 18 patients during a period in which 139 other arterial injuries were repaired by other techniques. In some instances the brachial vein was used in the arm and the superficial femoral vein in the thigh. Long term evaluation showed uniformly good results. In 1963 Szilagyi similarly stressed that autogenous vein grafts were the graft of choice.

Every effort should be made to use a vein

graft because other types of conduits are much less satisfactory. Plastic prostheses, such as Dacron or Teflon, have the great hazard of infection in the presence of the inevitable contamination. Fortunately, they are necessary only in the unusual instance of extensive injury of a large artery, such as the aorta or common iliac. Fromm and associ-

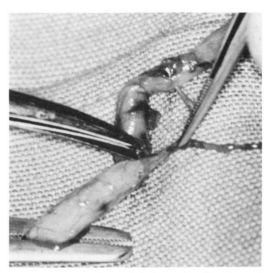

Figure 5-14. General hydrostatic dilatation of the vein with heparinized saline can be performed along with selective removal of excessive and constricting adventitia. (W.R.G.H.)

ates (1970) reported successful insertion of Dacron prostheses in three patients with traumatic injuries of the abdominal aorta. In most arterial injuries in the extremities, however, prostheses have been unsatisfactory. In Vietnam, Dacron prostheses were infrequently used, but over three-fourths of those employed had to be subsequently removed because of different complications (Rich and Hughes, 1972).

Freeze-dried homologous vein grafts have been used in some special instances where an adequate vein was not available, but their long term fate is dubious (Weber et al., 1975). Homologous artery grafts were used in the Korean Conflict (Spencer and Grewe, 1955), but are no longer recommended because of the high frequency of degenerative changes one to three years following insertion.

Rarely, autogenous arterial grafts have been employed, such as the proximal hypogastric artery. In two instances in Vietnam, the profunda femoris artery was used but elective sacrifice of this important collateral vessel is dubious practice. In the unusual instance of traumatic loss of an extremity, an artery may be removed from the amputated extremity and employed as a vascular graft. Although autogenous arteries are the ideal vascular substitute, only in the most unusual situations is this clinically feasible.

Distal pulses after repair, as mentioned earlier, should be immediately palpable in the artery beyond the anastomosis after the vascular clamps are removed. Pedal pulses should soon be palpable also, but in some instances with prolonged spasm these may not be detected for some time, occasionally even for hours. Absence of a palpable pedal pulse, however, is always a cause for serious concern. Several possibilities must be considered. First is the possibility of inadequate anastomosis, producing either constriction or prolapse of a flap of intima. A second consideration is thrombi in the distal arterial tree. A third, less common cause, is the presence of an additional arterial injury in the distal arterial tree. The most favorable possibility is that severe spasm is present and will spontaneously resolve with time. However, this is a dangerous assumption and in such instances operative arteriography should be performed to exclude any of the

first three possibilities. Operative arteriography is of such value that several authors have strongly recommended its routine use after all arterial repairs (DeWeese, 1962; Gaspar et al. 1968; Perdue and Smith, 1968; Engelman et al., 1969). Whether one employs operative angiography or re-exploration of the anastomosis and distal arterial tree depends upon varying circumstances. It should be emphasized, however, that successful repair of an arterial injury should be possible in well over 95 per cent of the patients. Failure of a repair is almost always due to one of several recognized errors in technique.

Soft Tissue Coverage. Soft tissue coverage of the site of arterial repair is mandatory. For unknown biologic reasons, an exposed artery will invariably rupture, even in the absence of arterial injury. This is notably seen following radical neck dissection when necrosis of soft tissue exposes the underlying carotid artery.

Normally, soft tissue coverage is an uncomplicated procedure, and simply involves approximating adjacent soft tissues over the repaired artery and leaving the remaining wound open for delayed primary closure. Problems arise when nonviable tissue is erroneously used to cover the artery; subsequent necrosis of the tissue with resulting exposure of the underlying artery invariably leads to secondary hemorrhage or thrombosis. Problems also arise whenever soft tissue loss is so extensive that simple coverage is not possible. A muscle flap may be rotated in most instances. In the thigh the sartorius muscle is usually available, while in the leg one of the heads of the gastrocnemius can be used. The latissimus dorsi can be used to protect the axillary vessels, and the scalene, levator scapulae, and the trapezius can provide some coverage for the carotid artery. With very extensive soft tissue defects, coverage may be difficult or even impossible. Free grafts of fascia lata or split thickness skin grafts have been employed, but results have been discouraging. Patman and associates (1964) reported that in their management of 256 patients with arterial injuries, coverage was possible in all by either transposition of muscle or by use of relaxing incisions of skin to mobilize a sufficient amount of skin with subcutaneous tissue. Cohen and co-workers (1969) in Vietnam reported more difficulty in war wounds where skin flaps and split thickness skin grafts were used in the absence of available tissue for muscle flaps. They cited that daily inspection and repeated débridement were necessary with much of the wound left open, and that sepsis remained a formidable problem.

A theoretical possibility in unusual instances where adequate soft tissue coverage cannot be obtained would be the insertion of a long vein graft in an extra-anatomic soft tissue position to establish continuity around the area of injury. This unusual approach would be indicated only with an un-usually large soft tissue defect, an extremity clearly threatened with gangrene, and the availability of a vascular surgeon thoroughly experienced with the many pitfalls attending such a complicated procedure.

Arterial Contusion

Arterial contusion in which there is no gross disruption in continuity often poses a difficult problem in management. A frequent error has been to underestimate the severity of the problem and attribute diminution of pulse to associated spasm. The extent of injury often cannot be determined precisely because there is a variable degree

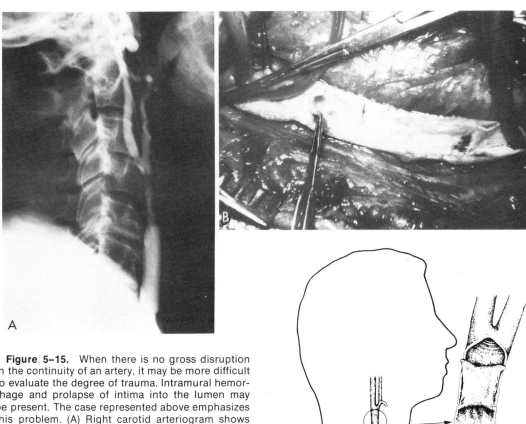

Common Carotid Artery

Figure 5–15. When there is no gross disruption in the continuity of an artery, it may be more difficult to evaluate the degree of trauma. Intramural hemorrhage and prolapse of intima into the lumen may be present. The case represented above emphasizes this problem. (A) Right carotid arteriogram shows abrupt narrowing in the common carotid artery. (B) The operative view of the artery shows the fractured intima to the right and prolapsed intima picked up by forceps to the left. (C) Drawing outlines the transverse fracture of the intima with distal prolapse. (McGough, E. C., Helfrich, C. R., and Hughes, R. K., Am. J. Surg., *123*:724, 1972.)

of disruption of the arterial wall with intramural hemorrhage and prolapse of intima into the lumen (Fig. 5–15). The fracture and prolapse of intimal flaps is the most serious consequence of this lesion because the injured artery may initially be patent. The flow of blood, however, progressively strips the torn intima from the arterial wall to such a degree that within a few hours thrombosis ensues. In some instances the artery can be incised for inspection of the lumen to detect injury to the intima. Useful experiences with such problems were reported by Gryska in 1962, who described excision of areas of damage to the intima followed by end-to-end anastomosis. In some instances the detached intima can be

reapproximated to the arterial wall with multiple fine sutures. In general, realizing the deceptive external appearance of such injuries, it is better to "overtreat" than to "undertreat" such lesions. One example can be given to support this point. A patient injured in Vietnam was noted to have contusion of the brachial artery at the time of surgical exploration. Nothing was done to the artery, but two days later arterial insufficiency developed as the contused segment thrombosed. This was treated by excision of the thrombosed segment and direct anastomosis. However, this delayed repair became infected, and the suture line was disrupted and required ligation. The arm subsequently became necrotic and

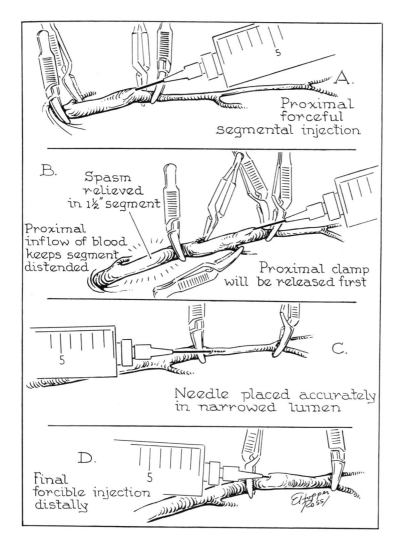

Figure 5–16. If arterial spasm truly exists, mechanical dilatation of the artery by forceful injection of saline into a segment occluded between two vascular clamps may be successful. (Mustard, W. T., and Bull, C., Ann. Surg., *155*:339, 1962.)

an above-the-elbow amputation was required.

Arterial Spasm

Arterial spasm is of particular interest in the management of vascular trauma. Severe spasm of large muscular arteries is an unusual lesion although it can be readily produced experimentally by repeated traction on a segment of artery encircled by a ligature (Kinmonth, 1952). Of fundamental importance is the realization that spasm is myogenic (due to sustained contraction of smooth muscle) and not neurogenic (a result of stimuli through the autonomic nervous system). Accordingly, therapeutic efforts must involve relief of muscle spasm rather than the use of nerve blocks. The typical vasospasm relieved by sympathetic blocks involves only small arteries, which are innervated by the autonomic nervous system. The topical application of papaverine (2.5 per cent concentration) has been the most useful agent (Kinmonth, 1952; Patman et al., 1964). If spasm is not relieved, mechanical dilatation of the artery by forceful injection of saline into a segment occluded between two vascular clamps may be employed (Mustard and Bull, 1962) (Fig. 5–16). If such measures are ineffective, the segment may have to be excised and a vascular graft inserted.

As with arterial contusion, the major clinical hazard is to underestimate the gravity of the arterial obstruction from spasm and assume that it will spontaneously regress. In the past, thrombosis and gangrene have often resulted. One must realize the unpredictability of arterial spasm, and if spasm is not clearly relieved the involved segment should be excised and a graft inserted.

The diagnosis of spasm has too often been used to explain failure of return of pedal pulses after arterial repair. As mentioned earlier, if pulses are not palpable, it is mandatory to demonstrate either by arteriography or by re-exploration that arterial continuity is intact. Separate from the detection of pulses, a particularly useful guideline regarding viability of an extremity is the return of neurological function—the ability to move the toes and the presence of sensation. These findings are valid, of course, only in the absence of peripheral nerve injury. If ischemia is not severe enough to produce loss of neurological function, there is little or no hazard of gangrene. Conversely, ischemia producing loss of neurological function almost always results in gangrene unless circulation is improved.

Ligation of Arterial Injury

Although ligation was the primary method of treatment of arterial injuries during World War II and resulted in gangrene in about one-half of the patients, it is now employed in specific instances where the extremity is not threatened or where prolonged attempts to repair the artery jeopardize life (Fig. 5–17). The frequency of gangrene after ligation can be predicted with

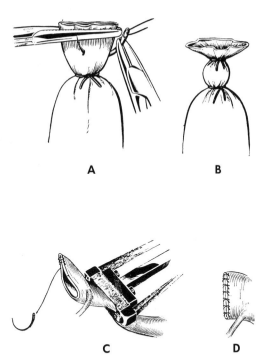

Figure 5–17. Safe methods for obliterating major arteries. (A) A proximal ligature has been applied, and the secondary more distal transfixion ligature is being placed. (B) The artery doubly ligated with sufficient cuff distal to the transfixion ligature to safeguard against having it slip off. (C) Suture closure of a large artery with a running over-and-over type of suture following proximal control with a vascular clamp. (D) The completed closure shows how a collateral vessel in close proximity to the severed end can be preserved by this method of closure. (Linton, R. R., N. Y. J. Med., *49:*2039, 1949.)

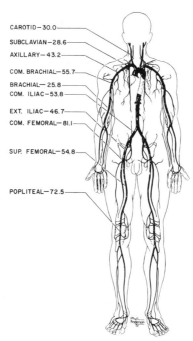

CAROTID—30.0
SUBCLAVIAN—28.6
AXILLARY—43.2
COM. BRACHIAL—55.7
BRACHIAL—25.8
COM. ILIAC—53.8
EXT. ILIAC—46.7
COM. FEMORAL—81.1
SUP. FEMORAL—54.8
POPLITEAL—72.5

Figure 5–18. Variations in frequency of gangrene following ligation of peripheral arteries. (Hughes, C. W., and Bowers, W. F., Traumatic Lesions of Peripheral Vessels. Charles C Thomas, Publisher, Springfield, Illinois, 1961.)

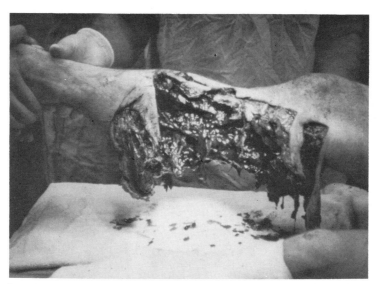

Figure 5–19. Occasionally, primary amputation of an extremity may be indicated because of massive soft tissue destruction and massive trauma to arteries, nerves, bone and veins, despite the fact that some type of vascular reconstruction might be feasible initially. (N.M.R., 2nd Surgical Hospital, 1966.)

reasonable certainty. The risk, of course, is higher with larger arteries: 80 per cent for the common femoral ligation, 40 to 60 per cent for high axillary and high brachial ligation, near 50 per cent for superficial femoral ligation, 20 to 25 per cent for superficial brachial ligation and about 70 per cent for popliteal artery ligation (Fig. 5–18). Ligation of the deep branches of the brachial artery in the arm or of the femoral artery in the thigh usually does not risk viability; however, claudication has been reported following profunda femoris artery ligation (Hughes and Jahnke, 1958). A single artery may usually be safely ligated in the forearm or the leg. In the proximal third, however, repair of the radial, ulnar or tibial arteries is preferable and should be performed if possible. If more than one of these arteries is injured, repair of at least one is urgent because gangrene can exceed 80 per cent when two are ligated.

As mentioned earlier, backflow is a notoriously unreliable guide to the safety of ligation. In the absence of a concomitant peripheral nerve injury, the degree of neurological function permits one to tell within a few hours if an extremity will become gangrenous following ligation. If neurological function is intact, even though signs of ischemia are present, the limb will almost surely survive. Conversely, if the extremity becomes numb and paralyzed following ligation, gangrene is virtually inevitable.

Primary Amputation

In rare instances with massive injury, primary amputation is the treatment of choice. This occurs with massive destruction of soft tissue, including arteries, nerves, bone and veins (Fig. 5–19). Reconstruction of such an extremity, even if viable, simply produces a useless, cumbersome appendage.

Similarly, amputation should be performed when sepsis and disruption of an arterial repair with ensuing complications endanger the life of the patient. Several fatalities resulted in Vietnam from injudicious repeated efforts to preserve an extremity. Some patients were transfused with over 30 liters of blood before amputation was finally performed.

Replantation of a completely severed extremity has been accomplished in a few patients. This can be attempted in unusual circumstances where an extremity has been cleanly severed and primary repair of injured arteries, veins, bone and nerves is feasible. Such techniques are beyond the scope of this text, but the feasibility in unusual instances should be considered. In 1972, Malt and associates reported convincing long term evidence that useful extremities definitely can be obtained by these techniques.

MANAGEMENT OF ASSOCIATED INJURIES

Concomitant Venous Injuries. Major veins accompanying arteries should be preserved whenever possible. Ligation is generally undesirable. Although there has been wide acceptance for repair of arterial injuries in the past 20 years, there has been less interest in repairing venous injuries. A greater emphasis was placed on reconstruction of venous injuries approximately 20 years ago with the repair of large numbers of arteriovenous fistulas in casualties from the Korean Conflict. In addition to the vein damaged in association with an arterial injury, there have also been numerous instances of isolated major venous injuries. The management of venous injuries is discussed in greater detail in Chapter 8.

An example of the problem that might occur is that following the ligation of a concomitant vein, such as the common femoral vein; there is resultant venous stasis of the extremity which is often disabling in either an acute or chronic nature. Careful lateral repair of a laceration of a venous injury can be successful. Also, end-to-end anastomosis is feasible in some wounds. Utilization of autogenous vein grafts in the venous system, particularly in the lower extremities, should be considered. Patency even for only 24 to 72 hours may be sufficient to allow establishment of additional collateral venous return. Recanalization within four to six weeks is a possibility even if there is early thrombosis of the vein graft. The segment of replacement is usually small enough that the remaining uninjured vein will retain functioning valves. When there are concomitant injuries to major arteries and veins, the venous repair should usually be performed prior to completion of the arterial repair. This will eliminate troublesome venous bleeding which might otherwise occur at the time an arterial repair is attempted. This was cited by Murphy in 1897 when he mentioned that venous repair was an accepted procedure. The fears of some that venous repairs are associated with an increase in thrombophlebitis and pulmonary embolization has not been borne out in the follow-up of Vietnam casualties.

Associated Fractures. The presence of an associated fracture may cause additional problems in managing the patient with vascular trauma (see Chap. 7). Whatever the technique of the fracture treatment, reduction should be accomplished prior to the vascular operation to be certain that arterial length is sufficient and that the artery is not unduly stretched or later disturbed. Occasionally, the extremity may be shortened by fracture and anastomosis of the artery can be more easily carried out. If the fracture is managed by traction, careful consideration must be given to the fate of the arterial anastomosis. Careful observation to detect the development of symptoms and signs of arterial insufficiency, evidence of undue stretching of the repair or evidence of compression by the fracture must be instituted. If readjustment of the traction does not improve the situation, evaluation of the arterial repair by angiography or operation is often indicated. If the limb is placed in a cast after operation, the cast must be split or bivalved to the skin for its full length to allow for the possibility of postoperative swelling and to permit immediate access to the site of the repair in case secondary hemorrhage occurs. External fixation is usually sufficient to manage the fracture. Although unstable fractures can compromise the vascular repair, internal fixation of the fracture is rarely indicated and should be avoided in acute care of contaminated fractures because of the increased risk of infection.

Interposition of viable muscle between an arterial repair and the fracture is indicated in an attempt to obviate secondary injury or compression of the artery from bone fragments or developing callous. In managing Vietnam casualties, there have been several instances where spicules of bone have caused additional arterial injuries and unstable fractures have disrupted arterial repairs. A large civilian series reported by Perry and associates (1971) revealed that they also followed specific priorities of repair when there were fractures associated with arterial injuries. In their experience this included stabilization of long bone fractures prior to vascular repair.

Associated Nerve Injuries. There is rarely any indication for repair of concomitant nerve injuries (see Chap. 7). The success of nerve repair with long term follow-up is just as good when the nerve repairs are delayed for a period of approximately several weeks. Of the small number of primary repairs performed in Vietnam, there has been a known disruption of three upper extremity nerve repairs in patients seen at Walter Reed General Hospital.

At the time of the initial débridement, the ends of the nerves can be tagged with a fine wire suture to facilitate identification at a second operation. It is also extremely important to have a diagram of the wound delineating the extent and location of the nerve injury.

ADJUNCTIVE MEASURES

Although somewhat controversial, anticoagulation may help in preventing distal thrombus formation. Murry (1940) presented an early review of the merits of using heparin in vascular repairs. Systemic heparinization is rarely indicated. "Distal heparinization" utilizing a fairly small amount of heparin, between 15 and 30 mg of dilute heparin solution, will be of value. Although this heparin is obviously disseminated fairly rapidly, an initial return of heparin, rather than blood, is frequently seen with release of the clamp 30 minutes after placing the heparin in an ischemic limb. Heparin can easily be instilled directly into the distal arterial tree by needle or catheter. There is rarely any need to consider countering the effect with protamine. Anticoagulation should not be continued in the postoperative period because of the danger of continued bleeding from open wounds or hematoma formation in the area of injury. It must be remembered that heparin will not salvage a poorly performed repair and it will not alter an artery filled with clot which might have been removed by proper use of the Fogarty catheter.

Perry and associates (1971) have advocated irrigating the distal arterial tree with copious amounts of cool, balanced salt solution containing a one to ten dilution of heparin in combined arterial and venous injuries. They believe that this technique retards intravascular thrombosis by removal of the foreign elements of the blood and by the anticoagulation effect of the heparin.

The operative and postoperative use of dextran has been advocated by some in managing vascular injuries. This must be kept in the surgeon's armamentarium and may be of value if anticoagulation cannot be used. Low molecular weight dextran (1.5 to 3.0 gm per kg per day) has aided in the prevention of the propagation of thrombus, according to some authors, and it might be of particular value when venous grafts are placed in the venous system.

A properly performed fasciotomy can be an extremely important adjunctive procedure, particularly in lower extremity vascular injuries. The problem of "too little, too late" should be avoided. On the other hand, there is no need for routine fasciotomy or for the routine use of four-compartment fasciotomy, combined with fibulectomy. Individual case selection and proper surgical judgment are of paramount importance. With ischemia of an extremity, pain followed by hypesthesia, anesthesia and paralysis occur. Muscle fasciculation may be noted, followed by fixation of the muscles. All degrees of muscle necrosis may occur depending on the severity and period of ischemia. In prolonged ischemia the entire compartment may become necrotic and be lost. With spotting necrosis and replacement by fibrous tissue, Volkmann's contracture occurs. Although the anterior compartment of the leg is one of the most vulnerable compartments for such changes, the flexor compartment of the forearm is also quite vulnerable. The primary ischemia from the vascular injury may not be the only contributing factor to

complications in the vascular injury patient. After the blood supply is returned to such areas, the previously ischemic capillaries extravasate fluid to the surrounding tissues. This in turn may obstruct venous return in a closed compartment and a vicious cycle is generated.

An adequate fasciotomy can frequently be performed without extending the skin incision the entire length of the extremity (Fig. 5–20). Although limited skin incisions are used, the vertical plane allows extension of the fascial incision by dissecting scissors beneath the intact skin both proximally and distally to relax the fascia completely. There is little danger of additional injury in this method, although care must be taken to avoid the peroneal nerve and to avoid disturbing bleeding. In addition, great care must be taken to insure that the fasciotomy is adequate. If the edema is initially severe or progressively becomes severe, the skin may be constrictive and should also be opened the full length of the fasciotomy incision.

A fasciotomy through the subperiosteal fibulectomy technique may have merit in that it decompresses all four major compartments of the leg (Fig. 5–21). This procedure may have no more morbidity than three long incisions and is the ideal method if the fibula is already fractured. The four-compartment decompression also insures that the deep fascia enclosing the soleus muscle is incised.

Although there are a few surgeons who feel that fasciotomy should be avoided and although there are hundreds of vascular repairs performed which have been successful without the use of fasciotomy, experience in Vietnam and the civilian communities has led us to believe that fasciotomy should be seriously considered under the following circumstances:

1. A delay of more than six hours between injury and primary repair.

2. Combined arterial and venous injuries, particularly at the popliteal level.

3. Severe shock with a prolonged period of hypotension.

4. Associated massive soft tissue trauma.

5. Massive edema, either preoperatively or postoperatively.

It is recognized that there is some morbidity associated with fasciotomy. In a few

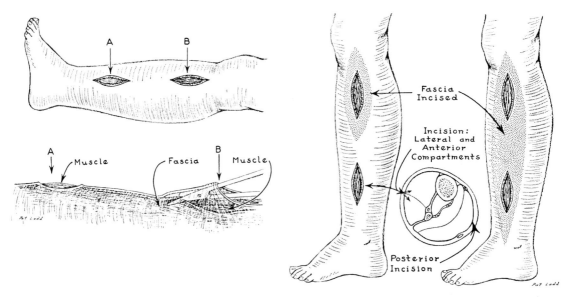

Figure 5-20. The technique of fasciotomy through limited skin incisions can be adequate and effective if performed early. The enveloping fascia can be incised for the full length of the leg through one or two small skin incisions. This method, however, is applicable only if fascia and not skin is the constricting factor. (Patman, R. D., Poulos, E., and Shires, G. T., Surg. Gynec. Obstet., *118*:725, 1964.)

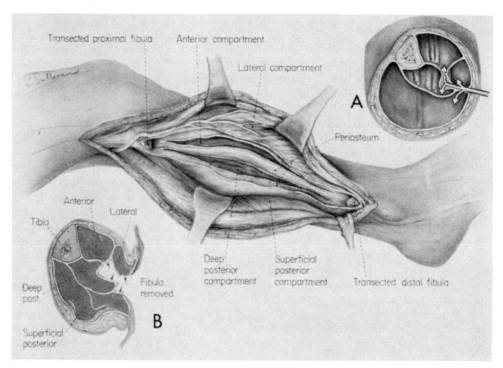

Figure 5-21. In selected patients, a fasciotomy by means of the subperiosteal fibulectomy technique may have merit in obtaining adequate decompression of all four major compartments of the leg. The completed fibulectomy-fasciotomy is shown. Insert (A) is a cross-section at the mid-calf level. The arrows indicate the direction to be followed for four-compartment decompression. Insert (B) shows the area decompressed. (Ernst, C. B., and Kaufer, H., J. Trauma, *11*:365, 1971. Copyright 1971, The Williams & Wilkins Co., Baltimore.)

isolated instances, fasciotomy incisions have become infected and led to subsequent amputation in the Vietnam casualties. Although most fasciotomy incisions can be reapproximated primarily, it may be necessary to cover the fasciotomy site with split thickness skin grafts to obtain local wound healing several weeks after the initial injury. Fasciotomy is no substitute for restoring arterial continuity. If performed late in the course of the injury, fasciotomy should not be expected to reverse changes of irreversible ischemia in the muscles. On the other hand, if a fasciotomy is not performed when the arterial· repair is performed several hours following injury, recognition of the muscle necrosis may be delayed. The phenomenon of intact skin, a live foot, but a dead leg may occur. The gastrocnemius-soleus muscle group may become necrotic. This may not be recognized because of the intact overlying skin and the fact that pedal pulses are restored by arterial reconstruction. The result may be renal shutdown and a fatal outcome.

As with other adjunctive measures, sympathetic block and sympathectomy are not substitutes for adequate arterial repair. They have been utilized infrequently. It is of interest to note that Williams and co-workers (1969) demonstrated an increased blood flow beyond the repair site following a sympathetic block. The use of vasodilating drugs has also been limited and appears to offer very little assistance in managing patients with acute arterial injuries.

POSTOPERATIVE CONSIDERATIONS

During the postoperative period, particular attention must be given to the patient with an arterial repair. Frequent observation is mandatory because the rather sudden onset of complications can be catastrophic. In the immediate postoperative period, the blood volume and pressure must be maintained. Sudden and prolonged hypotension predisposes to thrombosis of the sites of arterial repair, as well as of the distal small vessels. There is very little use for vasoconstrictors, except as a temporary expedient, because hypo-tension during the postoperative period is usually manifested by deficient blood volume and the treatment is blood replacement.

General comments can be made regarding at least 90 per cent of the arterial wounds involving major arteries to the extremities. The distal involved extremity must be examined frequently in the first 24 hours. The fingers and toes should be exposed for assessment of capillary filling, skin temperature and color. Distal pulses should be checked hourly by the nurse and frequently by the surgeon. Marking the patient's skin with a pen, such as a small "X" over the dorsalis pedis pulse, can be helpful, in addition to giving verbal instructions to nurses or house staff, who can then readily feel in the correct place for the pulse with some knowledge of the prior quality of the pulse. Circular bandages should not be used on extremities because they almost invariably result in constriction, especially if there is increasing edema. The development of edema in the subfascial closed compartments must be watched for, particularly in the lower extremities. If a tightness develops in the closed compartments or if the patient starts to develop a neuropathy, fasciotomy over the length of the space should be performed without delay as previously outlined in this chapter. Capillary filling is not a particularly good sign of arterial patency except when it is unequivocally rapid and of excellent quality. Superficial venous distention and venous filling may be helpful in determining the adequacy of distal blood flow.

If pulses disappear any time during the postoperative period, serious consideration must be given to returning the patient to the operating room for re-exploration of the wound. An arteriogram may be helpful if there is some doubt about the occlusion of the artery. In both civilian and military situations, returning the patient to the operating room can be a difficult decision if the patient is particularly ill or if there is infection present. This is where it is particularly important to be able to assess the status of the collateral circulation in determining the viability of the extremity. In the combat zone, additional operations have frequently been associated with a higher rate of complications, especially those secondary to infection. In Vietnam, because the majority of wounds were grossly contaminated, there was a high incidence of infection with repeated operations. The only time that reoperation should be indicated following an early failure of a vascular repair is to prevent loss of limb. A viable extremity can be treated with supportive measures and an additional reconstructive vascular procedure performed at a later date under more stable conditions. By providing additional information regarding the status of the collateral circulation, the Doppler (ultrasonic sounding device) has been particularly helpful in determining extremity viability following failure of a vascular repair. (see Chap. 4).

After arterial surgery the injured limb should be kept level with the body or in slight flexion; it usually should not be elevated. If the extremity has been flexed, gradual extension is encouraged to avoid contracture. Active ·muscle exercises are begun in the early postoperative period while immobilization in bed is necessary. As soon as other injuries permit, ambulation should be allowed and increased rapidly, particularly after delayed primary closure of soft tissues has been successfully accomplished.

Delayed primary closure of the contaminated wound in four to six days is important in the early identification of wound infections. If there is no infection evident at this time, good wound healing can usually be anticipated. Antibiotics should be used routinely in the postoperative period. Wounds should be cultured, and specific organisms present after the first few days can be treated with the appropriate antibiotic.

Anticoagulation should not be employed in the immediate postoperative period following vascular reconstruction because of the danger of hemorrhage and hematoma formation. Dextran might be of some value in the early postoperative period if there is small vessel thrombosis or if a venous repair has been performed. Sympathetic blocks have limited value in the postoperative period. Sympathectomy is rarely indicated.

When arterial continuity has been restored in an extremity in which the muscle tissue is of questionable viability, the patient must be closely observed for the following:

1. Decreased urinary output: evidence of acute renal insufficiency.

2. Increased fever and pulse rate: evidence of wound infection.

3. Increased pain, toxicity, confusion, fever and pulse rate: evidence of clostridial myosites.

Evidence of any of these clinical states may be indications for excision of necrotic muscle tissue or even for amputation of a nonviable limb. Otherwise, it is safe to defer amputation and observe the patient for four or five days until a line of demarcation is established.

RESULTS

In the military experience of the last 20 years, the overall amputation rate of approximately 50 per cent following the practice of ligation of major arteries has been lowered to about 13 per cent following the practice of routine arterial repair. Improved results should be expected and obtained in more stable civilian situations. It must also be remembered that amputation, although a final measure, is only one method of determining the success of managing vascular trauma.

The theoretical value of suturing vascular injuries was recognized during World War I; but it was also realized that the number of cases in which it would be possible to perform vascular repair as extremely limited. Makins (1919) was able to collect only 19 cases where immediate suture of acute arterial wounds had been carried out in the British experience in World War I. Sencert (1918) felt that ligature should be used to arrest hemorrhage from vascular wounds and that indications for suture were exceptional. DeBakey and Simeone (1946) pointed out that although débridement, practiced in World War II, supplemented by chemotherapeutic measures diminished the fear of infection (which presumably discouraged a wide variety of vascular suture in World War I), the instances of suture repair of vascular injury continued to be very limited. Lateral wounds sufficiently localized to allow suture repair were seldom seen, and the majority of the wounds were accompanied by wide spread destruction of tissue with such loss of arterial substance that end-to-end anastomosis was rarely feasible. Suture was used in only 81 cases in the series of 2471 arterial wounds in American troops. There were only three end-to-end anastomoses: the common femoral, the superficial femoral and the popliteal arteries. The majority of the cases had small lateral lacerations involving one-third or less of the circumference of the vessel. It is of interest that only one wound was a sharp, clean laceration which has been caused by a bayonet following an accidental injury (Fig. 5–22). Of the 81 repairs in the World War II collective study, the amputation rate was reduced to 36 per cent compared to the overall amputation rate of 49 per cent when ligation was used as the primary management of the arterial injury.

With the growing interest in vascular surgery after the end of World War II, the Korean Conflict was timely in that it provided large numbers of patients and an opportunity to prove the practicability of the repair of acute vascular injuries under battlefield conditions. During the early Korean experience there were only isolated attempts to perform arterial repairs, and the majority of the injured arteries were ligated. Ligation of major arteries in Korea

resulted in an amputation rate of 51.4 per cent (Hughes, 1958), which was essentially the same as the experience in World War II. Later, investigators of surgical research teams reported a total of 130 vascular repairs, with amputation rates varying from 8.8 per cent to 12.5 per cent—an average of 11 per cent (Jahnke and Howard, 1953; Jahnke and Seeley, 1953; Hughes, 1954). The collective review of 304 arterial injuries from the Korean Conflict, which included the Navy experience reported by Spencer and Grewe (1955) as well as the previously mentioned Army experience, revealed an overall amputation rate of 13 per cent.

The earliest published series of vascular injuries from Vietnam was a collective study of 108 patients with 116 arterial injuries, which included the personal experience of one of us (NMR), with an amputation rate of 8.3 per cent (Fisher, 1967). Considerable variation has existed in the reports from both individual hospitals or groups of hospitals in Vietnam. Chandler and Knapp (1967) reported 118 patients with 126 vascular repairs, with an amputation rate of 19.8 per cent. Their follow-up extended to an average of 23 days after injury. Levitsky and co-authors (1968) reported a series of 55 patients who underwent vascular repairs with an amputation rate of 3.8 per cent.

The establishment of the Vietnam Vascular Registry at Walter Reed General Hospital in 1966 initiated the attempt to

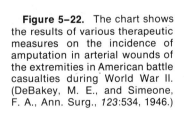

Figure 5–22. The chart shows the results of various therapeutic measures on the incidence of amputation in arterial wounds of the extremities in American battle casualties during World War II. (DeBakey, M. E., and Simeone, F. A., Ann. Surg., *123*:534, 1946.)

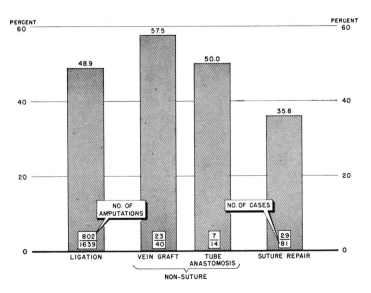

record and follow all who sustained vascular injuries in Vietnam. At the time of the first report from the Registry, 500 soldiers who had received vascular injuries in Vietnam had their medical cases documented with follow-up to the time that they were returned to duty or discharged from the military (Rich and Hughes, 1969). Of the 500 patients, 344 had 365 major arterial injuries. The amputation rate after repair of these vascular injuries was 12.7 per cent, almost identical to the amputation rate reported from the Korean Conflict. In an interim report from the Registry, the method of management of 1000 acute major arterial injuries included the use of autogenous vein grafts in approximately 46 per cent of the cases, and end-to-end anastomosis in approximately 38 per cent of the cases (Table 5–2). Surprisingly, lateral suture was utilized in approximately 9 per cent of the injuries. Prostheses were used in only four patients, and autogenous artery grafts were used in three patients; ligation of the injured artery was necessary in 15 patients. Fifty-five repairs were listed as questionable because there was some confusion as to the exact type of repair. A description stating "the artery was repaired" is inadequate and should not be used by responsible surgeons. Although there was a complication rate of approximately 30 per cent, many of the complications were corrected successfully, some of them even at the time of the initial procedure. It is important also to emphasize that other patients with complications remained asymptomatic. The mortality rate

TABLE 5–2. ARTERIAL REPAIRS NEW ORLEANS, 1942–1969* RECONSTRUCTION POSSIBLE IN 83.2 PER CENT OF 226 PATIENTS

METHOD	NUMBER	PER CENT
Suture	82	43.2
Resection and suture	53	28.4
Vein graft	30	16.0
Prosthetic graft	14	7.6
Patch angioplasty	9	4.8
Total	188	100.0

*Modified from Drapanas, T., Hewitt, R. L., Weichert, R. F., and Smith, A. D., Ann. Surg., *172*:351, 1970.

was slightly less than 2 per cent in this most recent war experience. In contrast to the small group of surgeons in special research teams who performed the repairs during the Korean Conflict, in Vietnam hundreds of surgeons trained in essentially all of the major training programs in the United States, both civilian and military, successfully performed vascular repairs.

In the past 20 years, varying results in civilian experience have been reported. In the early experience in Houston in treating 136 acute civilian arterial injuries, Morris and associates (1957) reported that it was possible to do a primary arterial repair in 93 patients: 68.4 per cent of the 136 injuries. End-to-end anastomosis was possible in approximately 85 per cent of those injuries that were repaired, and the remaining 14 injuries were treated with a homograft. Lord and associates (1958) gave an early follow-up of the use of 12 autogenous vein grafts which were followed as long as seven years, with maintenance of patency and no development of aneurysmal dilatation. In their overall experience, Ferguson and co-authors (1961) reported 88 patients with acute arterial injury repairs: 44 per cent of their total of 200 patients. Arterial replacement was necessary in only seven patients. Patman and associates (1964) found that ligation was necessary in slightly more than one-fourth of their 271 arterial injuries. However, they emphasized that it was only in the early years of their series that ligations of major arteries were performed as a life-saving measure under extreme circumstances. Otherwise, ligation was usually limited to arteries the size of

TABLE 5–2. METHOD OF MANAGEMENT OF ACUTE MAJOR ARTERIAL INJURIES IN VIETNAM*

METHOD	NUMBER	PER CENT
Autogenous vein graft	459	45.9
End-to-end anastomosis	377	37.7
Lateral suture	87	8.7
Prosthesis	4	0.4
Autogenous artery	3	0.3
Questionable	55	5.5
Ligation	15	1.5
Total	1000	100.0

*From Rich, N. M., Baugh, J. H., and Hughes, C. W., J. Trauma, *10*:359, 1970.

TABLE 5–4. METHOD OF MANAGING
ARTERIAL INJURIES
DALLAS, 1962–1968*

PROCEDURE	NUMBER	PER CENT
Lateral	66	26.5
Anastomosis	107	43.0
Autograft	27	10.8
Prosthetic graft	7	2.8
Ligation	42	16.9
Total	249	100.0

*Modified from Perry, M. O., Thal, E. R., and Shires, G. T., Ann. Surg., *173*:403, 1971.

the distal radial, ulnar and tibial arteries. Dillard and co-authors (1968) reported that an end-to-end anastomosis with lateral suture technique was possible in repairing arterial grafts in 34 of 35 penetrating injuries caused by knives or glass. Drapanas and co-workers (1970) found that arterial reconstruction was possible in 83.2 per cent of their 226 patients with arterial trauma. They found that direct suture or resection and primary anastomosis was possible in

70 per cent of the reconstructions (Table 5–3). Perry and associates (1971) stated that lateral repair and end-to-end anastomosis were possible in the majority of 249 patients with arterial injuries (Table 5–4).

MASS CASUALTY SITUATION

In the event of mass casualties, either in the combat zone or in a civilian disaster, there may be a shortage of trained personnel, available medical supplies may be limited and time may be at a premium. Treatment of victims with vascular wounds should be one of the highest priorities, second only to maintaining a patent airway, controlling hemorrhage and salvaging an extremity. Under the mass casualty situation, however, major vascular injuries may have to be treated by little more than arresting hemorrhage, and a certain portion of damaged limbs will have to be sacrificed following the more expedient method of ligation.

CHAPTER 6

SEQUELAE OF ACUTE ARTERIAL TRAUMA

Complications following unsuccessful arterial repair will be emphasized in this chapter. These complications can also result from acute arterial trauma without attempted arterial repair. The following are the three most important complications:

    I. Thrombosis
    II. Infection
    III. Stenosis

Brief comment will also be given to the following miscellaneous complications:

    IV. Miscellaneous
        A. Acute
            1. Errors in diagnosis
            2. Edema
            3. Embolization
            4. Disseminated intravascular coagulopathies
        B. Delayed
            1. Chronic pain
            2. Decreased function
            3. Ischemic changes
            4. Systemic complications
            5. Arteriovenous fistulas and false aneurysms
            6. Arteriosclerotic changes
            7. Aneurysmal graft changes
    V. Morbidity and Mortality Rates

There are numerous problems associated with attempts to obtain accurate statistics associated with the management of acute arterial trauma. Makins' World War I study in 1919 was an excellent example of the confusion that results from inclusion of both acute and nonacute lesions (false aneurysms and arteriovenous fistulas with delayed recognition) in a single series. DeBakey and Simeone (1946) pointed out that it was important to know all circumstances about a series of cases of arterial injuries before drawing conclusions from comparative studies. They emphasized this by showing that the association of concomitant fractures with arterial injuries could increase the amputation rate to about 60 per cent, compared to approximately 43 per cent when arterial injuries existed alone. Despite all limitations of comparing various reports of experiences with acute arterial trauma, it is important to analyze results and formulate conclusions. Results can only be improved by continually evaluating all related material.

There is confusion in attempting to interpret actual complication rates associated with attempted arterial repair. In many reports there is no mention of an overall complication rate. In other reports there is no separation of numerous systemic complications associated with generalized trauma from those complications specifically related to unsuccessful arterial reconstruction. In the preliminary report from the Vietnam Vascular Registry (Rich and Hughes, 1969), there was a complication rate of approximately 28 per cent with major arterial repairs (Table 6–1). The majority of these initial complications, however, were successfully treated by an additional procedure, often during the initial anesthetic. In this report, revisions during one operation were counted separately in an attempt to determine the etiology of repair failure. An example would be thrombosis at the suture line requiring further arterial resection and an additional

TABLE 6–1. INITIAL COMPLICATIONS OF MAJOR ARTERIAL REPAIRS IN VIETNAM*

ARTERIES	DISRUPTION	STENOSIS	THROMBOSIS	AMPUTATION RATE No.	Per Cent
Common carotid		(1†)	4 (1†)		
Axilliary	1	2 (1†)	8 (4†)	1	4.5
Brachial	5 (6†)	2 (1†)	16 (6†)	3	2.9
Iliac	(1†)		1 (1†)	0	0.0
Common femoral	2 (5†)	(1†)	4	2	8.3
Superficial femoral	8 (14†)	2	14 (3†)	12	10.3
Popliteal	2 (4†)	1	20 (10†)	25	32.5
Total:	18 (30†)	7 (4†)	67 (25†)		

*From Rich, N.M., and Hughes, C.W., Surgery, *65*:218, 1969.
†These figures represent complications in addition to the complication of initial repair of acute arterial injuries in Vietnam. Many of these initial complications were successfully repaired at the time of the initial operation or during the very early postoperative period.

reconstruction. Multiple procedures were not unusual in individual patients, ultimately including as many as five or six separate procedures. This explains part of the additional number of complications. Also, many patients with a residual complication, such as a thrombosed axillary or brachial arterial repair, remained asymptomatic and did not require additional operations. In the interim report from the Vietnam Vascular Registry (Rich et al., 1970A) which evaluated the results of 1000 acute major arterial injuries, the overall complication rate was approximately 30 per cent (Table 6–2). Again, many of these complications were successfully managed at the time of the initial operation—for example, a very stenotic lateral suture repair changed to excision of the injured artery, or a successful

TABLE 6–2. COMPLICATIONS ASSOCIATED WITH ARTERIAL REPAIR: MANAGEMENT OF 1000 ACUTE MAJOR ARTERIAL INJURIES*

	PATIENTS	PER CENT
COMPLICATIONS	301	30.1
Thrombosis	193	
Hemorrhage with or without infection	46	
Massive tissue necrosis, sepsis, venous insufficiency, etc., resulting in amputation	62	
DEATHS	17	1.7

*Modified from Rich, N.M., Baugh, J.H., and Hughes, C.W., J. Trauma, *10*:359, 1970. Copyright 1970, The Williams & Wilkins Company, Baltimore.

end-to-end anastomosis done under tension changed to additional debridement with an autogenous saphenous vein graft replacement. In the civilian community, Moore and associates (1971), in reporting 250 arterial injuries, described a comparable complication rate of 21 per cent.

THROMBOSIS

Acute arterial thrombosis is the most important complication because it is relatively common compared to other complications, and successful correction is usually possible. As stated earlier, it is difficult to compare complication rates regarding various types of arterial repair. Lateral suture repair and end-to-end anastomosis are usually best achieved when there is minimal destruction; in more extensive wounds an autogenous saphenous vein graft is necessary to restore arterial continuity. On the other hand, it is important to determine the complication rate for each specific type of arterial repair. In small lacerated lesions, the results of lateral repair have been excellent in the short term follow-up. Hughes (1955) was able to perform lateral arteriorrhaphy in approximately 10 per cent (20) of 211 arterial repairs. Spencer and Grewe (1955) reported a higher incidence in performing 13 lateral repairs, nearly 15 per cent of 89 arterial repairs. In these lateral repairs there was only one instance of thrombosis and only one amputation necessary. Lateral repair was utilized when 20 to

TABLE 6–3. TREATMENT AND RESULTS IN SIX PATIENTS WHO LOST PULSES: EARLY POSTOPERATIVE PERIOD*

ARTERY REPAIRED	TIME P.O. PULSE LOST	TREATMENT	TREATMENT RESULT	FINAL RESULT
Subclavian	6 hr	Observation	Extremity remained viable	Exsanguinating hemorrhage into chest
Femoral	1 hr	Sympathectomy	Extremity remained viable	Cool, pulseless but viable extremity
Femoral	24 hr	Fasciotomy of leg	Pulse returned third day	Normal function
Femoral	1 hr	Thrombectomy	Pulses restored	Normal extremity
Femoral	4 hr	Thrombectomy	Pulse restored	Normal extremity
Femoral	12 hr	Sympathectomy	Gangrene	Supracondylar amputation

*Modified from Ferguson, I.A., Sr., Byrd, W.M., and McAfee, D.K., Ann. Surg., *153*:980, 1961.

30 per cent or less of the vessel circumference was lacerated, and this probably contributed to the success. In contrast, however, Jahnke (1958) reported a late thrombosis rate of 47 per cent in those cases repaired by lateral suture during the Korean Conflict. It is possible that lateral repair was used in lesions in which more than 30 per cent of the circumference of the artery was traumatized in many of the patients in this latter series. If there was inadequate arterial debridement and inaccurate intimal approximation at the time of repair, leaving an inadequate lumen, thrombosis of the compromised lumen was likely.

Ferguson and co-workers (1961) in an early civilian report outlined the relatively early loss of pulses in six of their patients following arterial repair, the type of treatment instituted and the final results obtained (Table 6–3). In two patients in whom thrombectomy of the repair site was performed in the early postoperative period, pulses were restored, and the final result was a normal extremity. In one large civilian series of arterial trauma, Perry and associates (1971) found an early occlusion rate of 9.1 per cent, with 19 early occlusions following 207 arterial repairs (Table 6–4). Eight of these occlusions were successfully re-operated upon, resulting in a corrected 5.2 per cent failure rate. The failures were essentially equally divided between major arteries of the upper and lower extremities. They found that failures in their series of arterial repairs were equally distributed among the various types of repairs employed. They did not find that the specific technique of arterial repair

TABLE 6–4. COMPLICATIONS ASSOCIATED WITH 207 ARTERIAL REPAIRS: CIVILIAN SERIES FROM DALLAS*

ARTERY	OCCLUSION	RE-OP SUCCESSFUL	INFECTION
Axillary	2		1
Brachial	4	2	3
Radial-ulnar	4	1	
Renal	1		
Iliac			1
Femoral	5	4	3
Carotid	1		
Popliteal	2	1	
Total:	19	8	8

Initial failure of repair = 9.1%
Failure of repair after reoperation = 5.2%

*Modified from Perry, M.O., Thal, E.R., and Shires, G.T., Ann. Surg., *173*:403, 1971.

TABLE 6–5. COMPLICATIONS OF ARTERIAL REPAIRS FROM VIETNAM EVALUATED AT WALTER REED GENERAL HOSPITAL*

ARTERY	INFECTION AND/OR HEMORRHAGE	THROMBOSIS OF THE REPAIR	STENOSIS OF THE REPAIR	TOTAL
Carotid	1	4	2	7
Axillary	0	7	3	10
Brachial	1	16	1	18
Femoral	7	2	4	13
Popliteal	2	5	2	9
Total:	11 (19%)	34 (60%)	12 (21%)	57

*Modified from Rich, N.M., Baugh, J.H., and Hughes, C.W., Arch. Surg., *100*:646, 1970. Copyright 1970, The American Medical Association.

could be implicated as a factor in the ultimate failure. Failure was due to an anastomosis under tension or stenosis at the anastomotic site, with either end-to-end arterial anastomosis or arterial tube graft anastomosis. In the Vietnam experience thrombosis was the most frequent complication following attempted arterial repair (Tables 6–1 and 6–2). In the evaluation of 57 patients at Walter Reed General Hospital with complications of arterial repair initially performed in Vietnam, approximately 60 per cent of the complications involved thrombosis (Table 6–5). In this series thrombosis of the brachial arterial repairs comprised nearly one-half of all thromboses. Only 10 of the 34 patients required additional arterial reconstruction because of symptoms of arterial insufficiency (Table 6–6).

Various technical errors or difficulties can contribute to thrombosis of an attempted arterial repair (Fig. 6–1). This may or may not result in distal ischemia leading to nonviability of an extremity, depending on the availability of collateral circulation. The following technical problems are

some of the factors that can contribute to thrombosis: (1) inadequate arterial debridement; (2) a second adjacent arterial injury; (3) residual distal arterial thrombus; (4) severe stenosis at the suture line caused by the suture line being pulled too tight; (5) severe stenosis at the suture line because there was not sufficient arterial wall remaining for an attempted lateral suture repair; (6) undue tension on the suture line associated with a significant missing arterial segment; (7) if used, various problems associated with a graft, such as twisting, making the graft too long to cause a kink and external compression of the graft; (8) inability to perform venous repair when no effective venous return exists.

Inadequate arterial debridement can leave residual ischemic arterial wall where platelets and thrombin can be deposited to result in thrombosis, or the area can become aneurysmal and rupture. Also, inadequate debridement can leave residual intimal flaps which can cause thrombosis. In the early days of the Korean Conflict, there was a thrombosis rate of over 70 per cent following primary arterial repair (Jahnke,

TABLE 6–6. COMPLICATIONS OF ARTERIAL REPAIRS: 57 VIETNAM CASUALTIES TREATED AT WALTER REED GENERAL HOSPITAL*

COMPLICATION	ADDITIONAL OPERATIONS	NO OPERATIONS
Infection and/or Hemorrhage	9	2
Thrombosis	10	24
Stenosis	5	7
Total:	24 (42%)	33 (58%)

*Modified from Rich, N.M., Baugh, J.H., and Hughes, C.W., Arch. Surg., *100*:646, 1970. Copyright 1970, The American Medical Association.

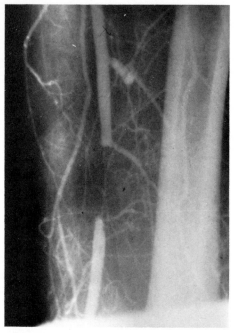

Figure 6–1. An arteriotomy performed in Vietnam in the mid-brachial artery resulted in a short segmental thrombosis as demonstrated in this left brachial arteriogram. Although there were no palpable distal pulses, the patient had a viable hand through excellent collaterals and was limited only by neurologic deficits. (Rich, N.M., Baugh, J.H., and Hughes, C.W., Arch. Surg., *100*:646, 1970. Copyright 1970, American Medical Association.)

operatively, as well as close postoperative monitoring, are important.

Residual distal thrombus can result in thrombosis of an otherwise technically successful arterial repair. Use of heparinization during the arterial repair and checking for the quantity and quality of arterial "back-bleeding" can be useful. However, it must be remembered that there can be what is interpreted as adequate back-bleeding with significant distal thrombus still being present. Careful passage of a Fogarty balloon catheter into the major distal arterial vessels can be useful in retrieving distal thrombus (Fig. 6–3). Also, an intraoperative angiogram can be useful in determining whether residual thrombus persists or not (Fig. 6–4). Cohen and co-workers (1969) mentioned that occasionally an apparent simple arterial reconstruction in Vietnam did not function. At re-operation, or during postamputation dissection, extensive thrombosis of the run-off vessels was evident. Multiple factors can contribute

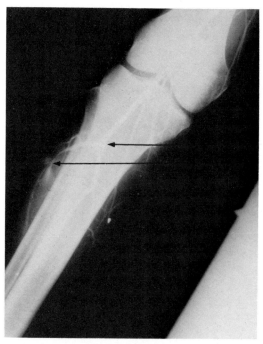

Figure 6–2. The possibility of multiple arterial injuries must be considered in the injured patient. This angiogram demonstrates an unsuspected false aneurysm of the distal popliteal artery (upper arrow), as well as a clinically obvious false aneurysm of the anterior tibial artery (lower arrow). (Vietnam Vascular Registry No. 5189, N.M.R.)

1958). It was felt that this was due to the anastomosis of arterial ends or edges of the wounded artery after the loose, fragmented adventitia was merely trimmed. This problem is discussed in more detail in Chapter 4. Williams (1968) and Brisbin and associates (1969) reported that inadequate debridement of the damaged artery and surrounding tissues was a limiting factor in continued patency of arterial repairs in their Vietnam experience. Perry and associates (1971) felt that although there was no persuasive evidence, these factors contributed to failures in their studies.

Multiple arterial lesions may exist (Fig. 6–2). A second adjacent lesion may cause a persistent failure despite the technically successful primary arterial repair. Intraoperative angiography including the repair site and run-off vessels will help eliminate this problem. Also, repeated evaluations in the operating room and immediately post-

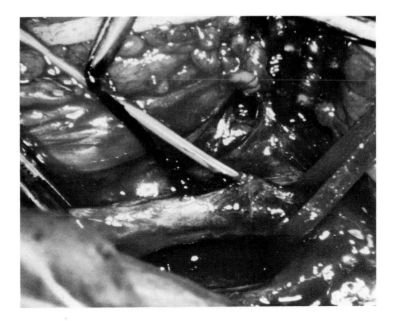

Figure 6–3. Careful passage of the Fogarty balloon catheter into distal vessels can be helpful in retrieving residual thrombus. (N.M.R., W.R.G.H., 1969.)

to the failure and compound the difficulty in determining the most significant complicating factor. This is demonstrated by the case of one Vietnam casualty who had distal arterial thrombus, massive soft tissue destruction and acute venous hypertension (Fig. 6–5).

Meticulous surgical technique must be utilized in performing arterial repairs. A "purse string" effect must not be created by excessive pulling on the suture if a continuous suture line is being performed. Interrupted sutures may help prevent this complication in small vessels. Also, lateral suture repair must not be performed in small vessels or in larger vessels where a large portion of the artery is missing. This problem can be eliminated by using an au-

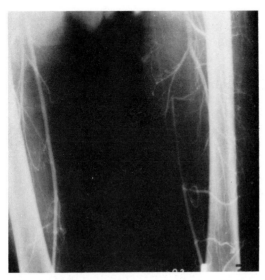

Figure 6–4. Angiogram performed in a Vietnam casualty demonstrates residual thrombus in the left superficial femoral artery contrasted by normal flow on the right. (N.M.R., W.R.G.H., 1970.)

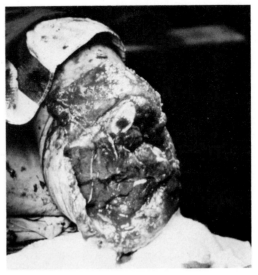

Figure 6–5. When amputation is required, inspection for distal arterial and venous thrombosis should be performed in determining multiple factors which contribute to failure of vascular repairs. (N.M.R., 2nd Surgical Hospital, Vietnam, 1966.)

togenous saphenous vein patch graft or by
utilizing excision of the damaged artery
followed by end-to-end anastomosis.
Thrombosis of the repair site can also
occur if there is undue tension on the suture line. Important collateral branches
should not be sacrificed, and joints should
not be immobilized in severe flexion in an
attempt to perform an end-to-end anastomosis when a significant segment of the artery has been removed. On the other hand,
the elastic nature of the artery will cause retraction of the ends. Sound surgical judgment must be exercised in determining
whether an end-to-end anastomosis can be
performed safely or whether an arterial replacement conduit will be necessary to accomplish a successful repair.

If a replacement conduit is needed to effect successful arterial reconstruction, the
graft must not be twisted when put into
place. Also, leaving the graft too long can
result in a kink that can lead to thrombosis.
External compression can add to the possibility of thrombosis. Moore and associates
(1971) mentioned a patient shot in the
popliteal artery in whom a lateral repair
of the injured popliteal vein was possible.
When pulses disappeared eight hours
postoperatively, immediate reexploration
revealed a redundant and kinked vein
graft. This was revised following thrombectomy, and the patient's subsequent
course was uneventful. Figure 6–6 demonstrates a vein graft of excessive length
in one of the Vietnam casualties. Turbulence in the blood flow caused by grafts
that are either too wide or too narrow in
diameter can also lead to thrombosis.
Figure 6–7 shows the thrombosed segment of a piece of Dacron 10 mm in diameter which was used in an attempt to
reconstruct a much smaller axillary to a
proximal brachial arterial defect.

One fairly accurate method of determining whether or not the arterial repair has
been initially successful and whether the
distal arterial tree is patent is to palpate for
distal pulses. However, this is not always
possible in such injuries as those to the internal carotid artery. Even the establishment of a palpable distal pulse does not insure long term success. In an early civilian
series of 136 acute arterial injuries, Morris

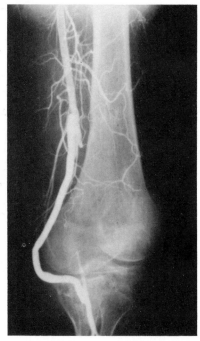

Figure 6–6. An autogenous saphenous vein graft
used to reconstruct the popliteal artery in a Vietnam
casualty is demonstrated angiographically to be excessive in length with some kinking. (Vietnam Vascular Registry No. 612, N.M.R.)

and associates (1957) found that pulses
were restored immediately in 73 patients
and that there was a delayed return of
pulses in other patients (Table 6–7). Their
experience emphasized what has been generally accepted; distal pulses should readily
be palpable following arterial repair. Drapanas and co-workers (1970) reported that
pulses were palpable immediately postoperatively in 80 per cent of patients with
repair of arterial injuries in extremities.
Diffculties arise if there are no palpable distal pulses. The majority of these early complications can be corrected (see Chap. 5). It
may be necessary to perform a second
operation in the immediate postoperative
period if early thrombosis occurs and there
is a question of viability of the extremity.
However, if viability is maintained despite
thrombotic occlusion of the repair, additional operation can be avoided. This
would be particularly imperative in a combat zone or in a civilian situation when the
patient's general condition would not tolerate an additional procedure. Repeated

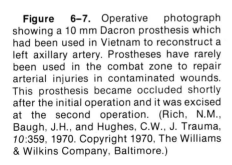

Figure 6–7. Operative photograph showing a 10 mm Dacron prosthesis which had been used in Vietnam to reconstruct a left axillary artery. Prostheses have rarely been used in the combat zone to repair arterial injuries in contaminated wounds. This prosthesis became occluded shortly after the initial operation and it was excised at the second operation. (Rich, N.M., Baugh, J.H., and Hughes, C.W., J. Trauma, *10*:359, 1970. Copyright 1970, The Williams & Wilkins Company, Baltimore.)

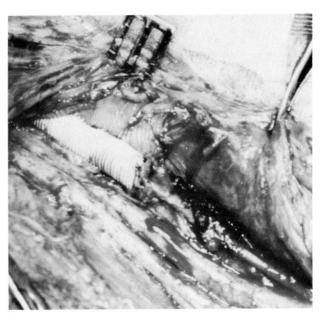

operations are also followed by a higher incidence of infection that may jeopardize life as well as limb. Additional operations can be performed at an elective time if symptoms of arterial insufficiency persist. Collateral circulation, however, may develop to the point where the patient is essentially asymptomatic despite the presence of thrombosis of a major artery and may not require an additional operation (Fig. 6–8). The ultrasonic sounding device (Doppler) can be used in the early postoperative period to determine the extent of collateral flow distal to the arterial occlusion. Lavenson and co-authors (1971), from their Vietnam experience, demonstrated that additional operations in the high risk group could be successfully delayed.

Confusion followed by disastrous results may occur if the diagnosis of arterial spasm is entertained rather than accepting the probability that thrombosis has occurred in the artery. In Vietnam a widely accepted belief was that if one thought of spasm, the spelling should be "C-L-O-T." Numerous methods have evolved to attempt to relieve spasm. Sympathetic blocks, when employed to differentiate spasm from arterial trauma, have confused the problem and caused unwarranted delay in management of arte-

TABLE 6–7. RESULTS OF TREATMENT IN 136 CASES OF ACUTE ARTERIAL INJURY: HOUSTON EXPERIENCE PRIOR TO JULY 31, 1956*

TREATMENT	TOTAL CASES	PULSES RESTORED IMMEDIATELY	PULSES RESTORED BUT DELAYED	NO PULSES VIABLE	AMPUTATION	DEAD
Repair	93	70	11	2	7	3
Suture	79	62	9	1	6	1
Graft	14	8	2	1	1	2
Ligation	32	0	1	24	5	2
Exploration	4	3	0	1	0	0
None	7	0	0	0	0	7
Total:	136	73	12	27	12 (8.8%)	12 (8.8%)

*Modified from Morris, G.C., Jr., Creech, O., Jr., and DeBakey, M.E., Am. J. Surg., *93*:565, 1957.

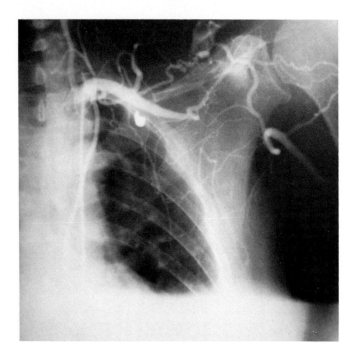

Figure 6–8. The importance of collateral circulation is emphasized by this angiogram, which shows occlusion of the mid-axillary artery with reconstitution of the brachial artery by thoracoacromial and circumflex humeral arteries. (Levin, P.M., Rich, N.M., and Hutton, J.E., Jr., Arch. Surg., *102*:392, 1971. Copyright 1971, American Medical Association.)

rial injuries. Even under direct vision, diagnosis of arterial spasm has been erroneously made when there was actually an intimal rupture or a subintimal hematoma which was not evident from external arterial inspection. Nevertheless, true segmental arterial spasm may occur associated with arterial injury. This may occur adjacent to the recognized trauma and be diagnosed at the time of arterial repair. Papaverine hydrochloride, 1 per cent procaine hydrochloride, warm packs applied locally and hydrostatic dilatation of the involved segment have been successfully employed.

INFECTION

Infection causing disruption of an arterial repair can lead to sudden and dramatic hemorrhage, with exsanguination as a potential fatal outcome. As in other areas of surgery, prevention is far better than treatment. Prompt diagnosis of arterial injury, use of appropriate antibiotics, adequate wound debridement, restoration of vascular continuity as soon as possible and adequate systemic nutrition should all help prevent vascular infection. Close observation in the postoperative period of the patient's general status, as well as the charac-

ter of the local wound, is mandatory. Prompt and aggressive regional treatment of an adjacent infection may prevent a vascular infection. Elimination of as much foreign material as possible in any type of reconstruction is important in contaminated wounds (Fig. 6–9).

Additional vascular repair should not be attempted in an infected area. Not only is additional repair usually subjected to an early failure from infection, but also the patient's life is endangered by exsanguination or septicemia. Ligation of the proximal and distal arteries in the area of the infected arterial repair is mandatory as a minimal procedure. Records in the Vietnam Vascular Registry are replete with numerous instances in which attempts to perform additional vascular repairs in the presence of infection were followed by subsequent disruption of arterial repairs with various degrees of resulting complications. For example, in a patient with trauma to the popliteal vessels, a greater saphenous vein graft was utilized to reconstruct the popliteal artery. Approximately two weeks later there was massive arterial bleeding from the wound. An attempt was made to repair a hole in the vein graft; however, three days later there was recurrent massive arterial hemorrhage, and it was neces-

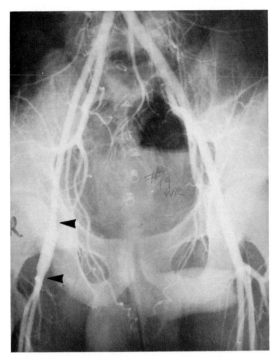

Figure 6–9. Although patency of this 5 cm piece of Dacron (between arrows) used to repair the right common femoral artery in Vietnam was maintained, surrounding infection finally necessitated removal of the prosthesis approximately six weeks later at Walter Reed General Hospital. (Rich, N.M., Baugh, J.H., and Hughes, C.W., J. Trauma, *10*:359, 1970. Copyright 1970, The Williams & Wilkins Co., Baltimore.)

sary to ligate the distal superficial femoral artery. Occasionally, it may be necessary to reconstruct the arterial supply using an extra-anatomical location to maintain extremity viability. Arterial ligation together with an extra-anatomical bypass through an uninvolved anatomical region, however, is no panacea for success. This was established by one patient at Walter Reed General Hospital who had a disrupted common femoral arterial repair. Because of obvious nonviability of the patient's lower extremity without restoration of arterial continuity, a greater saphenous vein graft was utilized in an extra-anatomical position through the obturator canal. Unfortunately, despite meticulous technique and utilization of all known precautions, this bypass also became infected, and removal was necessary. Interestingly, the extremity remained viable after this additional period of time. There are a number

of procedures that can be used in an aggressive approach to the infected wound which might be successful. This is particularly true if the infection is recognized early and treatment instituted immediately. Redebridement, muscle flap transposition, instillation of antibiotics in the wound through catheters in a continuous manner, or at scheduled intervals, and massive systemic antibiotic therapy have all been successful adjuvant measures in difficult cases.

There are few statistics regarding the incidence of management of infected arterial repairs following trauma in the civilian community. Drapanas and co-workers (1970) reported an infection rate of approximately 5 per cent. They noted that infection occurred at the site of injury in extremity wounds, and the majority of these patients subsequently required amputations. Perry and associates (1971) found a 3.5 per cent wound infection rate (Table 6–4). They did not believe that there was any constant correlation between the presence of infection and ultimate failure of repair in their series. In only two cases, one brachial arterial repair and one femoral arterial repair, did the infection appear to be significantly involved in delayed postoperative thrombosis.

In the Vietnam experience, infection was the second most common complication following attempted arterial repair (Tables 6–1 and 6–2; Fig. 6–10). Among 57 patients with complications of arterial repair initially performed in Vietnam who were later seen at Walter Reed General Hospital, approximately 19 per cent had infection (Table 6–5). Brisbin and co-authors (1969) reviewed the cases of six patients with secondary disruption of arterial repairs performed in Vietnam (Table 6–8). The following violations of vascular surgical precepts were outlined by Brisbin and co-workers as contributing to secondary disruption of vascular repairs:

1. Primary skin closure in a war wound.
2. Placement of a vascular graft in an area of established infection.
3. Inadequate soft tissue debridement in an attempt to conserve tissue for coverage of a vascular repair.
4. Attempted direct repair of a disrupted anastomosis in the presence of infection.

TABLE 6–8. SIX CASES OF DELAYED RUPTURE OF VASCULAR REPAIR IN VIETNAM*

Case No.	Missile	Type Repair	Days of Repair to Rupture	Vessel Involved	Site of Rupture	Reason for Rupture	Comments
1	MFW	Vein graft	7	Popliteal	Artery distal to graft	Infection, inadequate debridement	AK amputation due to massive muscle necrosis
2	MFW	Vein graft	17	Superficial femoral	Proximal anastomosis	Primary wound closure, inadequate debridement	AK amputation due to sciatic nerve palsy
3	AK–47 bullet	Vein graft	13	Superficial femoral	Body of graft	Primary wound closure, infection	Limb survival with bypass graft
4	MFW	Direct anastomosis	7	Superficial femoral	Artery distal to anastomosis	Inadequate debridement, artery and muscle	Limb survived with ligation
5	M–14 bullet	Vein graft	25	Superficial femoral	Body of graft	Infection, inadequate debridement, exposed graft	Limb survived with ligation
6	AK–47 bullet	Vein graft	6	Superficial femoral	Both anastomoses	Erosion of artery by bone	Limb survived with ligation

*Modified from Brisbin, R.L., Geib, P.O., and Eiseman, B., Arch. Surg., *99*:787, 1969. Copyright 1969, The American Medical Association.

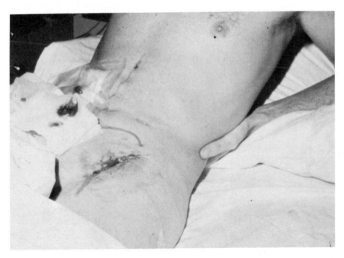

Figure 6–10. Numerous procedures, including local antibiotic application, through a catheter, were attempted to preserve the arterial repair in this patient. However, continued infection required removal of the Dacron prosthesis in the left external iliac artery. Following subsequent wound healing, an autogenous greater saphenous vein bypass graft was possible to restore arterial continuity. (Rich, N.M., Baugh, J.H., and Hughes, C.W., J. Trauma, *10*:359, 1970. Copyright 1970, The Williams & Wilkins Company, Baltimore.)

5. Inadequate debridement of a damaged vessel.

6. Suture repair of a lateral arterial laceration in a war wound.

7. Failure to perform fasciotomy.

8. Permitting a vascular graft to remain uncovered with soft tissue.

9. Proximal detachment of the sartorius muscle to cover a vascular graft when the muscle has been deprived of its blood supply by necessary debridement.

STENOSIS

Two major types of stenosis can develop as a complication of attempted arterial repair. The first is a purely technical complication caused by pulling too tightly on the suture during the repair, attempting to perform a lateral repair without sufficient remaining arterial wall, suturing arterial wall where residual damage remains, placing too much tension on the suture line or some other problem related to the suture line itself (Fig. 6–11). This should be readily apparent if an intraoperative arteriogram is obtained, and corrective measures can be performed, usually another repair using more meticulous technique, as outlined in Chapter 5.

The second major type of stenosis usually develops from intimal hyperplasia at the suture line which manifests itself over a matter of weeks or months. A representative example would be one young soldier returning from Vietnam with what appeared clinically to be a successful autogenous interposition vein graft repair of the right distal axillary artery to proximal right brachial artery. At the time of his first examination at Walter Reed General Hospital approximately one month after wounding, he had bounding radial and ulnar pulses in the right upper extremity, and there was no bruit audible along the repair site. Two months later, however, a bruit was heard over the repair site in his right arm, and it was thought that his right radial pulse was somewhat weaker. At three months following the initial repair, the patient complained of easy fatigability in his right upper extremity with moderate exercise; he had a loud bruit over the repair site, and his radial pulse was very weak with no palpable ulnar pulse. Angiography was performed and revealed a marked stenosis at the proximal suture line (Fig. 6–12). When this area of the repair was surgically exposed, there was a marked thrill over the stenotic anastomosis; however, the external appearance of the anastomosis did not allow a full appreciation of the degree of stenosis (Fig. 6–13). It was

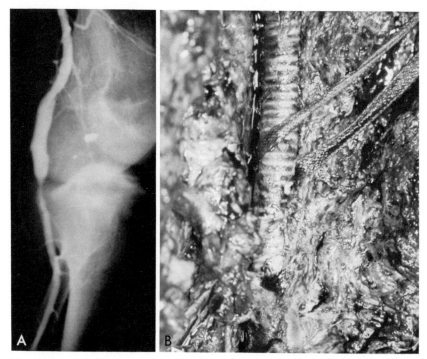

Figure 6–11. *(A)* Arteriogram demonstrating severe stenosis of the distal anastomosis of an autogenous saphenous vein graft to the left popliteal artery. Clinically, there was a high-pitched bruit over the repair site. A small segmental resection with reanastomosis at Walter Reed General Hospital corrected the problem and the patient then became asymptomatic. (Rich, N.M., Baugh, J.H., and Hughes, C.W., Arch. Surg., *100*:646, 1970. Copyright 1970, American Medical Association.)

(B) Dense scar tissue surrounds this 5 cm piece of Dacron used to repair the right superficial femoral artery. Early thrombosis and subsequent intermittent claudication necessitated replacement of this prosthesis with a saphenous vein graft, which was successfully performed at Walter Reed General Hospital. (Rich, N.M., Baugh, J.H., and Hughes, C.W., J. Trauma, *10*:359, 1970. Copyright 1970, The Williams & Wilkins Company, Baltimore.)

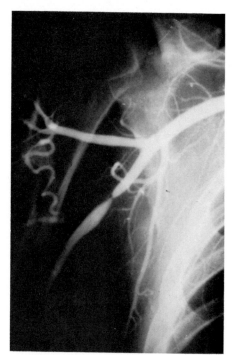

Figure 6–12. Arteriogram demonstrating severe stenosis of the proximal anastomosis of an autogenous saphenous vein graft at the right brachial-axillary artery junction which was performed in Vietnam. Although prominent collateral circulation developed between the humeral circumflex and deep brachial arteries, the patient developed discomfort with repetitive motion of his right hand. (See Figs. 6–13 and 6–14.) (Rich, N.M., Baugh, J.H., and Hughes, C.W., Arch. Surg., *100*:646, 1970. Copyright 1970, American Medical Association.)

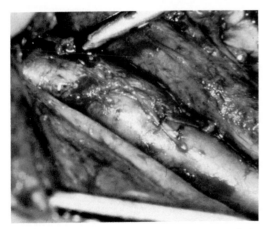

Figure 6–13. The external appearance of the proximal suture line, shown angiographically to be very stenotic (see Fig. 6–12), did not reveal the extent of the pathology. (N.M.R., W.R.G.H., 1968.)

possible to excise the short segment of marked stenosis (Fig. 6–14) and to reconstruct continuity successfully by a new end-to-end anastomosis. Within a five-year follow-up period, there was no clinical evidence of re-stenosis.

Whether or not all stenoses will progress to ultimate occlusion is debatable. We have seen patients in the Vietnam Vascular Registry who have an audible bruit over the repair site. In the past, if there were no associated symptoms, angiography was not performed. However, we are reaching a more aggressive point in the follow-up and we are attempting to provide further definition of this problem.

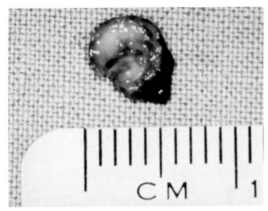

Figure 6–14. The resected segment at the stenotic proximal suture line, described in Figures 6–12 and 6–13, shows nearly total occlusion caused by intimal hyperplasia. (N.M.R., W.R.G.H., 1968.)

MISCELLANEOUS COMPLICATIONS

There are numerous other potential or actual complications which can be associated with attempted arterial reconstruction. As with any major operation, injury to other structures can occur. Particular care should be taken to preserve major venous return and to identify and preserve adjacent nerves.

ACUTE COMPLICATIONS

Errors in Diagnosis. Failure to recognize a second associated or adjacent arterial injury can result in thrombosis and ultimate arterial repair failure. There may also be improper identification of arteries. A thorough knowledge of anatomy is mandatory. Confusion can exist at times, however, particularly when massive tissue destruction has occurred. An example of this problem occurred in Vietnam when surgeons reported ligation of a "large" profunda femoris artery. It was not until several days later, when it was noted that there were no palpable distal pulses in the injured extremity, that an arteriogram was obtained to confirm that the proximal right superficial femoral artery rather than the profunda femoris artery had been ligated (Fig. 6–15). There also may be a failure to recognize arterial trauma associated with fractures.

Edema. Persistent swelling with or without associated venous trauma which is obvious has been associated with some arterial trauma. Drapanas and co-workers (1970) particularly emphasized development of marked edema as a distressing complication that occurred within a few hours after restoration of arterial flow to a previously ischemic limb. Despite apparent successful arterial repair with fasciotomies performed to decompress the muscles, progressive edema following restoration of arterial flow in an injured extremity was seen in 41 patients in their series (Table 6–9).

Embolization. Thrombus from either the site of arterial injury or the site of arterial repair can embolize into distal arterial branches. This is discussed in more detail

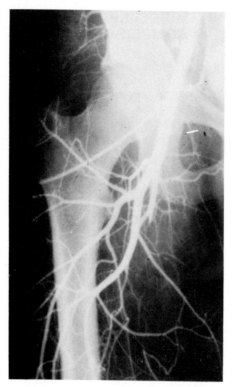

Figure 6–15. A knowledge of anatomy is mandatory to prevent complications as noted above. It was documented in Vietnam that a "large" profunda femoris artery was ligated. This angiogram later confirmed the clinical suspicion that the superficial femoral was the artery that was ligated. (Vietnam Vascular Registry No. 1129, N.M.R.)

TABLE 6–9. EDEMA FOLLOWING REPAIR OF MAJOR ARTERIAL INJURIES OF EXTREMITIES*

ARTERIES REPAIRED	NUMBER	NUMBER WITH EDEMA
Subclavian	16	3
Axillary	12	2
Brachial	39	10
Iliac and common femoral	16	9
Superficial femoral	31	11
Popliteal	14	6
Total:	128	41

Factors Possibly Contributing to the Edema:

Shock	17
Ischemia, severe	16
Vein injured	21

*Modified from Drapanas, T., Hewitt, R.L., Weichert, R.F., and Smith, A.D., Ann. Surg., *172*:351, 1970.

in Chapter 9 as one of the potential complications associated with false aneurysms. In some unusual situations such as axillary or brachial arterial trauma caused by prolonged use of crutches, some lesions have presented as mural thrombus with distal embolization or aneurysm formation with distal embolism (see Chap. 14).

Disseminated Intravascular Coagulopathies. Although some details are not completely understood, numerous clotting defects can be induced by multiple blood transfusions. It can become an appreciable problem manifested by diffuse uncontrollable oozing after approximately 500 ml of blood replacement. The hazard increases with each successive unit of blood. The oozing may continue despite all measures, and death can result. Patman and co-workers (1964) mentioned that this occurred in 2 of their 21 patients who died, an incidence of approximately 10 per cent of the total deaths.

DELAYED COMPLICATIONS

Chronic Pain. Drapanas and co-workers (1970) found chronic pain was a complaint in 10.2 per cent of patients in their series with salvaged extremities who had major extremity arterial trauma.

Decreased Function. White and associates (1968) documented some specific problems in infants and children associated with thrombosis of a major artery. They presented the case of a 3 year old boy who had cardiac catheterization via the left femoral artery. One year later the circumference of his left thigh was 2 cm less than that of the right, and the left calf was 1 cm less than the opposite. The left leg was also 1 cm shorter when measured by radiographic scanogram. Reduced limb growth can occur following major lower extremity arterial occlusions in growing children.

Ischemic Changes. The limb which is ischemic after vascular injury often exhibits a contracture resembling Volkmann's ischemic contracture. This condition may be reversible if the blood supply is restored within a reasonably short period of time. When circulation returns, however, muscles tend to swell. If fasciotomies with adequate incisions in the skin and long inci-

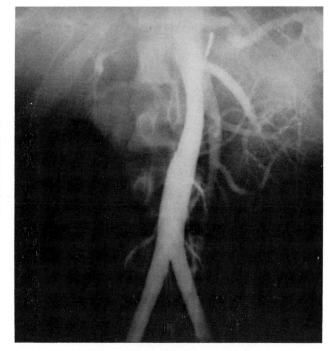

Figure 6-16. Anteroposterior view of this aortogram shows extrinsic pressure against the right infrarenal aorta. This false aneurysm of the abdominal aorta was caused by an M-26 grenade fragment in Vietnam. Identification was delayed three months, when the patient was evaluated for hypertension. (Rich, N.M., Clarke, J.S., and Baugh, J.H., Surgery, *66*:492, 1969.)

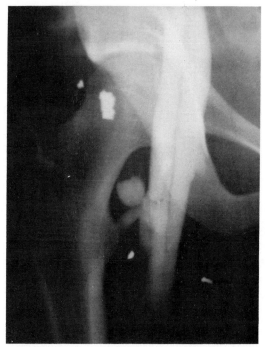

Figure 6-17. Angiogram demonstrating an arteriovenous fistula at the level of the right common femoral arterial bifurcation. As frequently found with arteriovenous fistulas, there is a false aneurysm adjacent to the fistula. (Rich, N. M., Hobson, R. W., II, and Collins, G. J., Jr., Surgery, *78*:817, 1975.)

sions in the fascia are not performed promptly, continued edema of the muscle within the closed fascial compartment terminates in ischemia and necrosis. Delay in performing adequate fasciotomy in the presence of increasing muscular swelling may result in compression of vessels with resultant muscle necrosis and nerve damage. These changes are more prone to occur in the anterior compartment in the lower extremity and the flexor compartment of the forearm. All degrees of muscle necrosis may occur, depending on the severity and period of ischemia. In prolonged ischemia an entire compartment may become necrotic and lost. With spotty necrosis and replacement of fibrous tissue, Volkmann's contracture occurs.

Systemic Complications. The development of an aortoenteric fistula following repair of a traumatic wound of the aorta or iliac arteries is rare. One patient in Vietnam developed an aortoenteric fistula within a short period of time following a common iliac arterial repair. Approximately two weeks after wounding, infection and hemorrhage developed. The distal aorta was ligated, and an opening in the small bowel was sutured. One week subsequent to the second operation, the patient developed a small bowel fistula and pelvic abscess, with death ensuing within several days.

Arteriovenous Fistulas and False Aneurysms. If acute arterial injury is initially overlooked, false aneurysms (Fig. 6–16) and arteriovenous fistulas (Fig. 6–17) can develop. Successful reconstruction at a later date has usually been possible, as was noted in Chapters 9 and 10.

Arteriosclerotic Changes. There is an increased potential for complications in the diseased artery compared to the normal artery. Arteriosclerotic material can be dislodged to form a nidus for thrombosis, or it can embolize to cause distal obstruction and thrombosis.

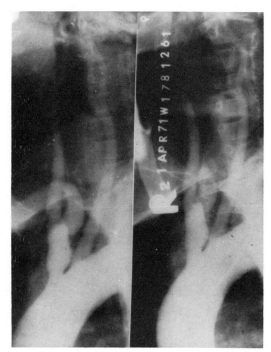

Figure 6–19. Fusiform dilatation of this autogenous saphenous vein graft is noted on this arch angiogram about five years after an aorto-innominate bypass. (N.M.R., Vietnam Vascular Registry No. 4591.)

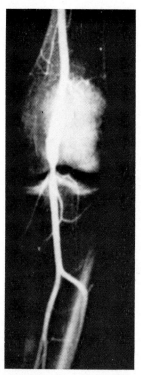

Figure 6–18. Arteriogram demonstrating a somewhat dilated autogenous popliteal vein graft six months after it was used at Walter Reed General Hospital to replace the missing segment of the accompanying popliteal artery caused by injury. Actually the dilatation had occurred at implantation when the popliteal vein was used rather than a preferred greater saphenous vein. In this case, both the popliteal artery and vein had been transected by a seat spring loosened in an automobile accident. (Whelan, T.J., Jr., and Baugh, J.H., Year Book Medical Publishers, Inc., Chicago, February 1967).

Aneurysmal Graft Changes. This complication is infrequent as related to diagnosis and documentation (Fig. 6–18). It probably occurs more frequently than has been previously recognized. Nevertheless, the true significance of generalized fusiform aneurysmal dilatation in an autogenous vein graft used as an interposition replacement to restore arterial continuity is not completely understood at this point. In the Vietnam experience, it has generally been recognized that the autogenous greater saphenous vein is the best conduit for segmental arterial replacement. Nevertheless, similar to recent reports regarding diffuse fusiform aneurysmal dilatation in autogenous greater saphenous vein grafts used in aortorenal bypass, a disturbing finding has occurred in several individual Vietnam casualties. One patient had an autogenous greater saphenous vein graft used as a bypass of his occluded innominate artery from the ascending portion of the arch of the aorta to the innominate bifurcation. Approximately five years later fusiform aneurysmal dilatation was noted in this vein graft, which has

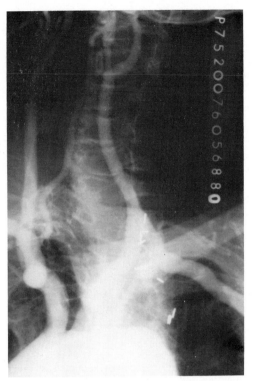

Figure 6–20. There is some fusiform aneurysmal dilatation of the greater saphenous vein seen on angiographic follow-up in 1974. A left carotid–axillary bypass was performed in 1970. (Vietnam Vascular Registry No. 5422, N.M.R.)

remained patent (Fig. 6–19). Another patient had a left carotid-axillary arterial bypass utilizing an autogenous greater saphenous vein graft in 1970. A follow-up arteriogram in 1974 revealed some fusiform aneurysmal dilatation in this bypass (Fig. 6–20).

MORBIDITY AND MORTALITY RATE

Although amputation is only one method of determining the ultimate success of an attempted repair of a major extremity artery, it is a final result. The amputation rate remained at approximately 13 per cent in the Vietnam experience, similar to the Korean experience; however, many factors were involved in these statistics. Attempts were made at limb salvage in Vietnam which had not previously been made in other wars. Also, the Vietnam statistics include longer term follow-up. This is reflected by the statistics of both Fisher (1967) and Cohen and associates (1969), who reported approximately an 8 per cent amputation rate in Vietnam. Rich and Hughes (1969) recorded that nearly one-third of the amputations were performed in the relatively early follow-up period after patients were evacuated from Vietnam. Amputation rates have generally been lower in civilian experience (Tables 6–7, 6–10 and 6–11). Additional details can be found in chapters discussing specific arterial injuries.

The incidence of death following acute arterial trauma is an unknown entity. Many injured patients who die of their injuries have an associated exsanguinating hemorrhage which may or may not be recognized. Associated injuries contribute to the mortality rate. There is a considerable range in the mortality rate from approximately 2 per cent to approximately 20 per cent

TABLE 6–10. MORBIDITY AND MORTALITY ASSOCIATED WITH ARTERIAL INJURIES: 181 PATIENTS TREATED IN NEW ORLEANS*

	AMPUTATIONS		DEATHS	
ARTERIES REPAIRED	No.	Per Cent	No.	Per Cent
Subclavian	1	6.2	4	25.0
Axillary	1	8.3	0	0.0
Brachial	1	2.5	0	0.0
Radial and ulnar	0	0.0	0	0.0
Iliac and common femoral	0	0.0	4	25.0
Superficial femoral	3	9.6	2	6.4
Popliteal	6	42.8	0	0.0
Anterior, posterior tibial	1	14.3	0	0.0
Total:	13	7.1	10	5.5

*Modified from Drapanas, T., Hewitt, R.L., Weichert, R.F., and Smith, A.D., Ann. Surg., *172*:351, 1970.

TABLE 6–11. COMPLICATIONS IN SURVIVING PATIENTS WITH MAJOR EXTREMITY ARTERIAL INJURY*

VESSEL		BLEEDING	AMPUTATIONS
Subclavian	11		
Axillary	12		1
Brachial	32	1	
Radial and ulnar combined	8		1
Aorta	12		
Iliac	15		
Femoral	63	3	
Popliteal	12		1
Total:	165	4	3 (1.8%)

*Modified from Perry, M.O., Thal, E.R., and Shires, G.T., Ann. Surg., *173*:403, 1971.

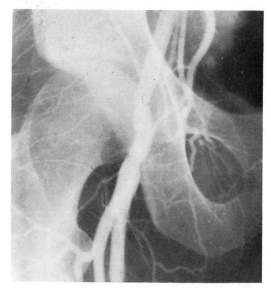

Figure 6–21. Five years after insertion of this 5 cm piece of Teflon into the right common femoral artery in 1964 in Saigon, this patient complained of increasingly severe intermittent claudication in the right lower extremity. Note particularly the marked degree of stenosis at the proximal anastomosis. Successful replacement with an autogenous greater saphenous vein graft was performed at Walter Reed General Hospital. (Rich, N.M., Baugh, J.H., and Hughes, C.W. J. Trauma, *10*:359, 1970. Copyright 1970, The Williams and Wilkins Company, Baltimore.)

among large civilian series. Representative examples are found in Tables 6–7 and 6–10. Further reference can be found in other chapters regarding specific arterial injuries. The interim report from the Vietnam Vascular Registry documented a mortality rate of 1.7 per cent among 1000 major acute arterial injuries (Rich et al., 1970A).

FOLLOW-UP

To any scholar interested in vascular trauma, it is readily apparent that there are very few centers that can obtain long term follow-up of their patients who sustained major vascular trauma (Fig. 6–21). Many inherent problems occur from the beginning. Some patients injured are not the most reliable, having suffered gunshot wounds in street brawls and similar affairs. Other patients may not reside in the locale of the hospital where they are treated. Maintaining current addresses for patients in our changing society, which sees numerous moves for most families, is difficult at best.

The Vietnam Vascular Registry material has provided a somewhat unique opportunity to obtain long term follow-up on the majority of nearly 7500 patients in a young, healthy age group who sustained arterial trauma. This allows a more comprehensive review of the true incidence and significance of various complications associated with attempted repair of arterial injuries.

CHAPTER 7

CONCOMITANT FRACTURES AND NERVE TRAUMA

There is universal agreement among surgeons that immobilization of concomitant fractures associated with major arterial trauma is important in obtaining optimum healing. However, there is considerable controversy regarding how this immobilization should be secured. Many surgeons have advocated routine use of internal fixation of some long bone fractures in their civilian practice, particularly when a concomitant arterial injury exists. On the other hand, during recent military experience, especially in Vietnam, surgeons have generally felt that internal fixation of fractures should be avoided because of the increased potential for infection in contaminated wounds. Major combat experience in the past 30 years has substantiated the widely accepted belief that external immobilization of fractures, including those with concomitant arterial injuries, can be successfully utilized in the majority of combat casualties.

Less controversy has existed regarding the management of injured nerves. Delayed repair of nerves for three to six weeks, as was advocated in World War II, has been accepted except for an unusual situation. Recent civilian experience, however, has demonstrated that good results can be obtained with primary nerve repair in civilian wounds.

First, this chapter will review the asso-

ciation of concomitant fractures with arterial trauma. This will be followed by a review of trauma to adjacent nerves associated with arterial injuries.

The interested reader is also referred to specific chapters for additional information. For example, Chapter 13 should be referred to for further details of subclavian arterial trauma associated with fracture of the clavicle and Chapter 24 for information on popliteal arterial trauma associated with fractures about or dislocation of the knee.

FRACTURES AND DISLOCATIONS

Incidence

The true incidence of the association between fractures and vascular trauma is difficult to establish because of wide variation in individual reports. It has been stated repeatedly that 10 to 50 per cent of arterial injuries are associated with fractures of adjacent bones. Another way to evaluate the incidence of concomitant injuries is to determine how many patients with fractures also have associated vascular injuries. In studies of fractures of long bones, the incidence of associated arterial injuries has been documented to be as high as 3 per cent. Rosental and colleagues (1975) found a 2 per cent incidence of arterial trauma in about 1000 femoral fractures treated at Los Angeles County Hospital between 1968 and 1973. Sher (1975) reported an incidence of arterial trauma of 0.28 per cent (10 patients) among 355 patients with long bone fractures or with associated dislocation of the respective joint.

The incidence of dislocations or subluxations causing arterial trauma is even more difficult to determine than the incidence of associated fractures. Although dislocations occur more rarely than fractures, numerous case reports underscore the diagnostic dilemma that often exists with a dislocation and questionable vascular injury.

Among 1000 acute major arterial injuries in Vietnam, concomitant fractures were noted in 28.5 per cent of the patients (Rich et al., 1970A) (Table 7–1). The percentage of fractures associated with certain specific arterial injuries was higher than the overall fracture percentage (Table 7–2). In one Registry report which reviewed 150 popliteal arterial injuries, concomitant fractures existed in 49.3 per cent (Rich et al., 1969A). However, individual reports from Vietnam demonstrated that this rate was not constant. Hewitt and associates (1969) reported that approximately 50 per cent of their 62 patients with arterial injuries had concomitant fractures. This included fractures with 8 out of the 10 popliteal arterial injuries, 10 out of the 24 superficial femoral arterial injuries and 9 out of the 21 brachial arterial injuries. These percentages are somewhat higher than those in an earlier report by Fisher (1967), who found fractures to be associated with about 32 per cent of the vascular injuries treated in Army

TABLE 7–1. CONCOMITANT INJURIES ASSOCIATED WITH 1000 ACUTE MAJOR ARTERIAL INJURIES: VIETNAM VASCULAR REGISTRY*

INJURIES	NO.	PER CENT
Bone	285	28.5
Vein	377	37.7
Nerve	424	42.4

*Modified from Rich, N. M., Baugh, J. H., and Hughes, C. W., J. Trauma, *10*:359, 1970.

TABLE 7–2. FREQUENCY OF BONE INJURIES ASSOCIATED WITH ACUTE ARTERIAL TRAUMA: COMBAT EXPERIENCE*

ARTERY	NO.	FRACTURE	PER CENT
Axillary	59	16	27.1
Brachial	283	96	33.9
Iliac	26	2	7.6
Common femoral	46	9	19.5
Superficial femoral	305	72	23.6
Popliteal	217	87	40.0
Total:	936	282	30.1

*Unpublished data from the Vietnam Vascular Registry based on the vast majority of patients whose records were included in the Interim Registry Report (Rich, N. M., Baugh, J. H., and Hughes, C. W., J. Trauma, *10*:359, 1970).

hospitals during the initial Vietnam experience of 1965 and 1966.

Although there are no specific data correlating fractures with arterial injuries during World War II, Elkin and Shumacker (1955) reported about a 31 per cent incidence of fractures with false aneurysms and arteriovenous fistulas: 38 fractures with 159 aneurysms, and 99 fractures with 288 arteriovenous fistulas. In Korea, individual investigators found varying percentages. Spencer and Grewe (1955) found 20 fractures accompanying 54 popliteal and femoral arterial injuries: an incidence of about 37 per cent. Hughes (1954) noted only 15 per cent in a series of 79 acute vascular injuries.

In civilian experience, the incidence of concomitant fractures associated with arterial trauma has ranged widely. Smith and co-workers (1963) reported that fractures were associated with 10 per cent of the arterial injuries in their series. Dillard and associates (1968) stated that 7 of their 85 arterial injuries were associated with fractures, and an additional injury was associated with a dislocation. The arterial injuries in this series consisted of three brachial, two subclavian, two superficial femoral and one popliteal arterial injury, again an incidence of approximately 10 per cent. Drapanas and associates (1970) reported an 8.3 per cent incidence of long bone fractures in patients with extremity arterial injuries. Hardy and co-workers

TABLE 7-3. CIVILIAN ARTERIAL TRAUMA DUE TO BLUNT TRAUMA ASSOCIATED WITH FRACTURE OF LONG BONES: HENRY FORD HOSPITAL*

CASE NO.	AGE SEX	TYPE OF BLUNT TRAUMA	SITE AND TYPE OF FRACTURE	ARTERIAL INJURY Location	ARTERIAL INJURY Type	DURATION ARTERIAL OCCLUSION (HR)
1	16 M	Thrown from speeding car; landed on abducted hyper-extended right knee	Tibial plateau	Popliteal bifurcation	Disruption; thrombosis	72
2	63 M	Obese (240 lb); stumbled into ditch, falling on right thigh	Spiral comminuted fracture distal femur	Distal superficial femoral	Contusion; thrombosis	72
3	63 M	300 lb casing struck anterior right thigh	Compound comminuted fracture distal femur	Distal superficial femoral	Contusion; thrombosis	5
4	55 M	Right thigh caught between bumpers by backing car	Compound comminuted fracture distal femur	Proximal popliteal	Disruption; thrombosis	4
5	18 M	Car struck motorcycle rider, pinning left ankle to ground	Compound comminuted fracture distal tibia and fibula	Anterior and posterior tibial	Disruption anterior tibial; thrombosis posterior tibial	7
6	11 M	Right anterior leg struck by car bumper	Transverse fracture proximal tibia and fibula	Popliteal bifurcation	Avulsion anterior tibial; thrombosis popliteal	75
7	35 M	Grinding wheel broke, striking medial aspect right arm	Compound comminuted fracture distal humerus	Brachial	Disruption	3
8	32 M	Roll of steel plate fell, striking anterior right knee	Compound comminuted fracture proximal tibia and fibula	Popliteal bifurcation	Avulsion anterior tibial; disruption popliteal	4
9	58 M	Right leg struck from side by car bumper	Comminuted fracture proximal tibia and fibula	Popliteal	Compression by hematoma and plaster cast	6
10	26 M	Driver's left elbow wedged between seat and frame in car accident	Compound comminuted fracture distal humerus	Brachial	Contusion and intimal tear; thrombosis	26

*Modified from Smith, R. F., Szilagyi, D. E., and Elliott, J. P., Jr., Arch. Surg., 99:315, 1969.

(1975) reported a 17 per cent incidence of osseous injury among 360 cases of arterial trauma in their extensive experience in Jackson. Bole and colleagues (1976) found a 14.7 per cent incidence of fractures: 18 associated with 126 arterial injuries.

Recent individual reports emphasize specific associated injuries and note a larger number of injuries than previously reported. An example is the report by Natali and co-authors (1975), which documented 10 cases of subclavian arterial trauma in association with fracture of the clavicle.

Smith and associates (1969) found the association of long bone fractures with concomitant blunt arterial trauma to be relatively uncommon. They were able to tabulate the results of 10 patients treated for arterial injuries associated with fractures of bones of the extremities at Henry Ford Hospital in Detroit between January 1, 1964, and December 31, 1968 (Table 7–3). All 10 patients were males ranging in age from 11 to 63 years. The most common site of trauma was the lower extremity, particularly the region of the knee. In a subsequent report, which was limited to their experience with penetrating arterial injuries of the neck and limbs, Smith and colleagues (1974) found a 19 per cent incidence of associated fractures: 22 of 127.

White and associates (1968) emphasized an increasing awareness of peripheral arterial injuries in infants and children with the development of pediatric referral centers and the use of more refined diagnostic methods. One of the three major categories that they described in their experience from Johns Hopkins Hospital involved arterial injuries associated with trauma to an extremity.

Etiology

The types of wounds producing an association between fractures and major arterial injuries differ in military and civilian experience. The combat wounds are generally larger in extent, with more massive tissue destruction caused by high velocity missiles. In the course of determining the nature of the wounding agent in various Vietnam vascular injuries, a significant factor emerged when fractures were associated with major arterial trauma. Although in previous reports from the Registry fragments constituted the wounding agent in the majority of patients with vascular injuries (Rich and Hughes, 1969; Rich et al., 1970A), in this small series of concomitant fractures and arterial injuries, 20 patients, or nearly 69 per cent of the total, sustained high velocity gunshot wounds (Table 7–4). The wounding power of missiles, especially those of high velocity, was noted to be of particular importance. (Experimental details are given in Chapter 3.) In Figure 7–1 the wounding power of a high velocity 7.62 mm bullet fired from an AK–47 assult rifle is shown. This bullet produced a comminuted fracture of the femur.

Not only do the etiologic factors vary between military and civilian experience; they vary within civilian experience as well. Included among the civilian data are missile wounds, blunt trauma, and falls. Sher (1975) reported that all injuries in his series were the result of vehicular accidents. If blunt trauma is severe enough to cause a fracture of one of the long bones of an extremity, adjacent arteries can be damaged either by direct force against the artery associated with the initial trauma or by indirect force from stretching during displacement of the fracture. An early report is that of Bergan (1963), who postulated the following as causes of arterial occlusion in supracondylar fractures of either the femur or the humerus: (1) pressure on the artery from the dislocated fracture; (2) spastic

TABLE 7–4. ETIOLOGY OF THE WOUNDING AGENT: CONCOMITANT FRACTURES ASSOCIATED WITH MAJOR ARTERIAL INJURIES TREATED BY INTERNAL FIXATION IN VIETNAM*

Etiology	No.	Per Cent
Gunshot wound	20	69
Fragment wound	6	21
Blunt trauma	2	7
Electric saw	1	3
Total:	29	100

*Modified from Rich, N. M., Metz, C. W., Hutton, J. E., Baugh, J. H., and Hughes, C. W., J. Trauma, *11*:463, 1971.

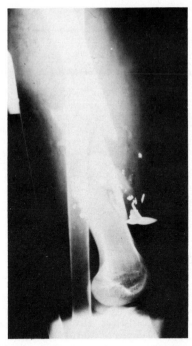

Figure 7-1. This roentgenogram demonstrates the wounding power of a high velocity 7.62 mm bullet fired from an AK–47 assault rifle. Most of the jacket and some of the fragments may be seen lying adjacent to the comminuted fracture of the femur in a soldier treated at the 2nd Surgical Hospital in 1966 in Vietnam. (Rich. N.M., Metz, C.W., Hutton, J.E., Baugh, J.H., and Hughes, C.W., J. Trauma, *11*:463, 1971. Copyright 1971, The Williams & Wilkins Company, Baltimore.)

a passenger forced by the collision against the dashboard and front windshield.

Arterial and venous injuries can also result from treatment of fractures and dislocations. This avoidable complication should be uncommon. However, vascular injuries have occurred with orthopedic procedures other than the management of fractures. Ferguson (1914) described an infant who developed an arteriovenous fistula following an osteotomy of the femur for genu valgum. Indeed, vascular injuries can occur during a variety of elective orthopedic operative procedures (Hughes, 1958B; DeBakey et al., 1965). General appreciation of these potential injuries, particularly in the lower extremities, is probably insufficient. Operations on the lumbar intervertebral discs carry the risk of potential vascular trauma because the abdominal aorta, inferior vena cava, and iliac vessels lie along the ventral border of the lumbar vertebra and are separated from the intervertebral disc spaces only by the anterior longitudinal ligament. Instruments can inadvertently pass too far ventrally through the anterior longitudinal ligament and injure either major arteries or veins (see Chap. 21). (Jarstfer and Rich, 1976).

Clinical Pathology

The close association between the neurovascular bundle and the long bones of the extremities helps to explain the frequent correlation between a fracture and vascular trauma, particularly with penetrating injuries such as high velocity gunshot wounds (Fig. 7–2). The fracture may vary from a linear fracture with minimal displacement in a closed wound to an open comminuted fracture. In reviewing the Vietnam experience, Rich and co-workers (1970A) found that all fractures were comminuted and all but one were of the open type (Fig. 7–3). Only one patient had blunt trauma with a closed comminuted fracture (Fig. 7–4). Blunt trauma causing a displaced linear fracture in a closed wound is more frequent in civilian injuries. A dislocation may have had a spontaneous reduction, or it may be obvious because of the deformity.

A variety of pathologic lesions can occur with fractures of long bones of the extrem-

contraction of the arterial wall; (3) rupture and rolling up of the intimal layer with thrombosis and occlusion of the artery; and (4) total rupture of the artery. Table 7–3 shows the various causes of blunt trauma associated with fracture of long bones in civilian experience in Detroit.

There are many anecdotal reports of vascular compromise accompanying fractures at unusual sites. The following is a representative example. Stein and associates (1971) reported a rare instance of arterial injury associated with fracture of the scapula. The axillary artery was actually ruptured. In a review covering 20 years, they could find only one other similar reported case in the world's literature. In this other case, the axillary artery was thrombosed without rupture. The patient was a 19 year old male involved in an automobile accident with an oncoming vehicle. He was

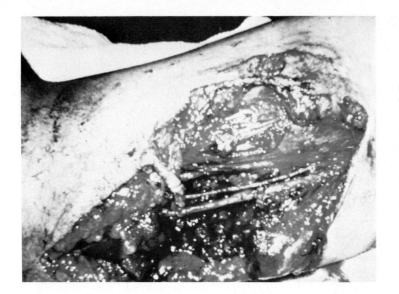

Figure 7–2. Massive soft tissue destruction in the right arm of this helicopter door gunner was caused by a high velocity .50 caliber bullet. In addition to the brachial arterial trauma, there were also concomitant osseous, venous and nerve injuries. (Rich, N.M., Baugh, J.H., and Hughes, C.W., J. Trauma, *10*:359, 1970. Copyright 1970, The Williams & Wilkins Company, Baltimore.)

ities. These range from total disruption of the artery to contusion and subsequent thrombosis at the site of an intimal tear or subintimal hematoma (Fig. 7–5). De Nayer

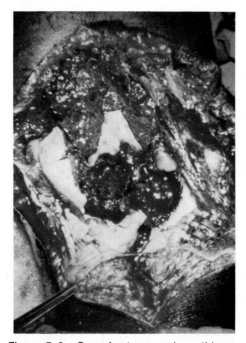

Figure 7–3. Open fractures such as this comminuted fracture of the distal femur caused by an artillery fragment, in the center of the wound, were often associated with vascular injuries in Vietnam because of the close proximity of the neurovascular bundle. (Rich, N.M., Milit. Med., *133*:9, 1968.)

and associates (1973) reviewed 17 patients with arterial trauma combined with major fractures. Contusions and thrombosis occurred in eight arterial injuries, the artery was disrupted in seven, and the remaining two patients had arterial compression (Table 7–5). Bergan (1963) demonstrated experimentally that stretching of a femoral artery was followed by rupture of the intima and the media before the more elastic outer part of the arterial wall was torn. This would allow the flow of the blood stream to roll up the ruptured intimal layer with resultant thrombosis which would occlude the artery. Venous injury usually is manifested by a laceration, disruption or thrombosis (see Chap. 8).

A variety of arterial injuries can accompany closed fractures. The artery may be lacerated, or even transected, by sharp bone fragments from the fracture. Similar trauma can also occur to veins. Contusion of the vessel wall may be noted. In the arteries this may be associated with a subintimal hematoma or with an intimal flap and medial dissection, with ultimate thrombosis of the artery. Hematoma formation, or even edema, may be severe enough to cause arterial occlusion within a closed fascial compartment. Arterial spasm can occasionally occur in close proximity to a fracture, significantly compromising the distal circulation. However, it is unwise to assume that obvious arterial insufficiency is caused by arterial spasm. Only by explora-

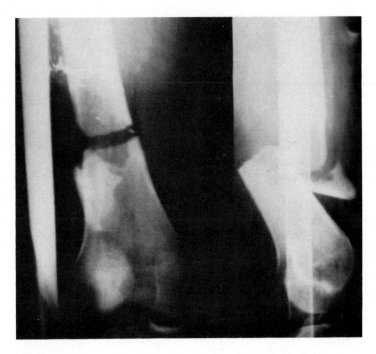

Figure 7–4. Closed fractures of the distal femur or dislocation of the knee occasionally occurred in Vietnam, particularly in crews involved in helicopter crashes. Posterior displacement of a fracture of the distal femur caused blunt trauma to the popliteal artery. Thrombosis of the artery was not initially recognized. An above-the-knee amputation was ultimately required. (Rich, N.M., *in* Dale, W.A. (Ed.), Management of Arterial Occlusive Disease. Year Book Medical Publishers, Chicago, 1971.)

tion can the exact type and extent of arterial trauma be determined.

Because neurovascular bundles are in close proximity to joint capsules, the possibility of vascular trauma must be considered in the management of dislocations. A common example is found with posterior dislocations of the knee. These injuries and resultant problems were recently discussed by Hardy and colleagues (1975). The tibial plateau can directly traumatize the popliteal artery, which is stretched under tension (Fig. 7–6). Complete dislocation is not a prerequisite for arterial damage. Injuries of the knee are occasionally complicated by popliteal arterial thrombosis. Clinically, the arterial lesions can be either a rupture or a segmental thrombosis. In eight patients described by Kennedy (1959), rupture of the popliteal artery was present in only

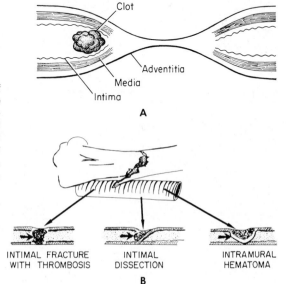

Figure 7–5. (A) This diagram shows one form of injury involving laceration and retraction of both the intima and media with an intact adventitia and no external hemorrhage. (Makin, G.S., Howard, J.M., and Green, R.L., Surgery, *59*:203, 1966.) (B) This diagram shows additional causes of occlusion of the artery with only part of the arterial wall involved. (Saletta, J.D., and Freeark, R.J., Ortho. Clinics in Am., *1*:93, 1970.)

TABLE 7–5. VASCULAR LESIONS: 17 CASES*

LOCATION	CONTUSIONS-THROMBOSES	RUPTURE	COMPRESSION
Upper extremity　(3)	None	1 Dislocation	1 Dislocation 1 Humeral fracture
Lower extremity　(14)	4 Femoral fractures 4 Tibial fractures	1 Dislocation 2 Femoral fractures 3 Tibial fractures	None
Total:	8	7	2

*Modified from De Nayer, P., Jaumin, P., and Linard, D., Acta Chir. Belg., 72:427, 1973.

one. Kennedy also demonstrated rupture of the popliteal artery in cadavers by using a stress machine.

Schwartz and Haller (1974) documented the challenging case of a 5 year old child with an open anterior hip dislocation with femoral vessel transection (Fig. 7–7).

Anatomical location plays a significant role in the clinical pathology. This is emphasized by the vulnerability of the popliteal artery to injury during adjacent fracture or dislocation, due in part to its relatively fixed position at entry and exit points in the popliteal fossa (Fig. 7–8). The adductor magnus tendon proximally and the fibrous arch over the soleus muscle distally establish relatively fixed points, as do some fascial attachments to the posterior capsule of the joint where there is also a mid-genicular artery. Other arteries vulnerable to injury include the subclavian artery beneath the clavicle, the brachial artery adjacent to the humeral shaft and supracondylar portion of the humerus and the superficial femoral artery near the femoral shaft. Lord and Irani (1974), in describing the mechanisms of injury of arterial trauma, noted that in their Australian civilian practice open and closed injuries occurred in about equal frequency with gunshort wounds and other types of penetrating injuries. They emphasized that

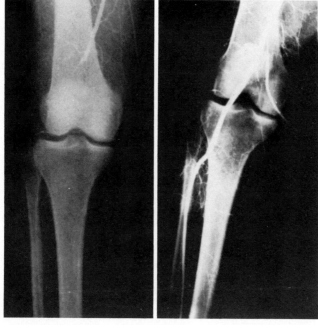

Figure 7–6. (A) Arteriogram demonstrating occlusion of the popliteal artery in a 21 year old man who sustained a posterior dislocation of the knee in a motorcycle accident. (B) Patency of popliteal artery following resection and repair. (Doty, D.B., Treiman, R.L., Rothschild, P.D., and Gaspar, M.R., Surg. Gynecol. Obstet., 125:284, 1967.)

A　　　　　　　　B

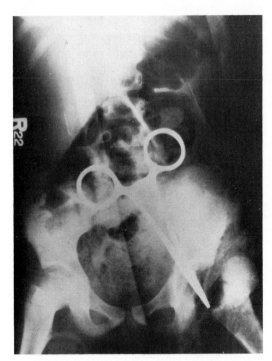

Figure 7-7. This admission x-ray, with a clamp pointing to the left hip dislocation, provided additional information in the case of a 5 year old girl who sustained an open anterior hip dislocation with transection of the femoral vessels after being struck by an automobile. (Schwartz, D.L., and Haller, A.J., Jr., J. Trauma, *14*:1054, 1974. Copyright 1974, The Williams & Wilkins Company, Baltimore.)

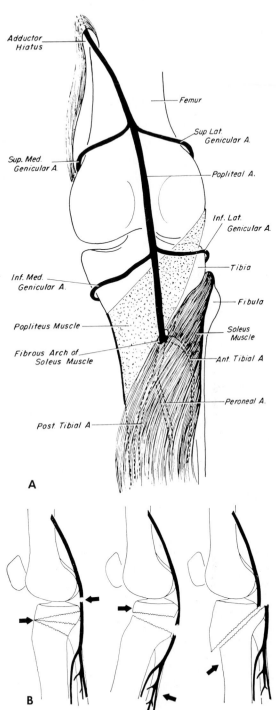

Figure 7-8. (A) This diagrammatic representation outlines the relationship of the popliteal artery to the structures about the knee. (B) The mechanism of arterial injury in proximal tibial fractures includes direct trauma to the popliteal space, hyperextension with stretching or tearing of the popliteal artery and bone injury to the popliteal artery by a displaced fragment. (Haas, L. M., and Staple, T. W., South. Med. J., *62*:1439, 1969.)

in their experience closed arterial injuries were often related to fractures and dislocations. Figure 7–9 documents the statistics compiled from the Australian experience. In reviewing the literature of vascular complications following dislocation of the shoulder, Archambault and co-workers (1959) noted that these injuries are relatively infrequent. They cited the review by Cranley and Krause of the literature from 1918 to 1956, which identified only eight cases in addition to the two added by the authors themselves. Two new cases of damage to the axillary artery were subsequently reported by McKenzie and Sinclair (1958). Guibe's 1911 article in French was cited as reporting 57 cases collected from 10 different authors. Guibe noted that one of the prevalent mechanisms of injury was for a horse to rear up suddenly and pull on the driver's extended shoulder. Another mechanism limited to the "horse and buggy days" occurred when a person fell out of a

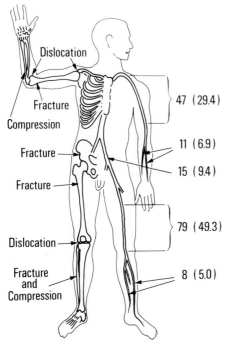

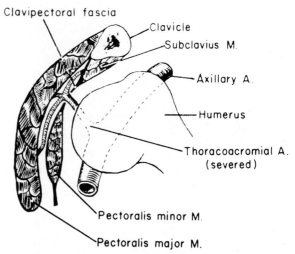

Figure 7–9. This composite diagram shows the type of orthopedic trauma most likely to cause closed arterial injuries (left) and the number, with percentage in brackets, of injuries affecting individual arteries as compiled from the Australian experience (right) (Annetts et al. [1970] and Little and May [1972]: cases from St. Vincent's Hospital, Sydney, Australia). Note that injuries were more common in the lower limb than in the upper limb and proximal arteries were affected more frequently than distal vessels. (Lord, R. S. A., and Irana, C. N., J. Trauma, *14*:1042, 1974. Copyright 1974, the Williams & Wilkins Company, Baltimore.)

Figure 7–10. The above drawing demonstrates how the dislocated head of the humerus displaces the axillary artery and subsequently tears the acromioclavicular artery at its origin. The anchoring effect of the clavipectoral fascia on the acromioclavicular artery facilitates such a process. (Archambault, R., Archambault, H. A., and Mizeres, N. J., Am. J. Surg., *97*:782, 1959.)

buggy and was dragged by an extended arm. Archambault and associates (1959) stated that the most common cause of dislocation of the shoulder at the present time is a fall on the extended arm. They described a 47 year old schoolteacher who fell down basement stairs and dislocated her left shoulder. Frequently, collaterals are torn. In order of incidence, these are the subscapular, circumflex and long thoracic arteries. Ecchymosis in the axilla by tamponade of the head of the humerus against the axillary artery may be a delayed complication. With reduction of the dislocation, the tamponade is removed and active hemorrhage from the axillary artery can then take place. Figure 7–10 illustrates the anatomical considerations involved in

trauma of the thoracoacromial artery in anterior dislocation of the shoulder.

Injuries to the musculoskeletal component of the thorax can be associated with unusually severe myocardial injuries. Actual disruption can occur (see Chap. 17).

If there is unrecognized vascular trauma associated with either an open or closed fracture, false aneurysms and arteriovenous fistulas may develop (see Chaps. 9 and 10). The former would occur with arterial trauma and the latter if a venous injury is in continuity with the arterial injury. Cameron and co-workers (1972) reviewed the problem of false aneurysms complicating closed fractures (Table 7–6). They added 4 cases from their hospital in London, Ontario, to 10 cases from the literature.

Clinical Features

There may be an obvious open wound with protruding bone from a comminuted fracture. The fracture may be less apparent if it is nondisplaced and caused by blunt trauma without disruption of the integument. A dislocation may be obvious because of marked joint deformity or obscure because of spontaneous reduction.

TABLE 7–6. REPORTED CASES OF FALSE ANEURYSMS COMPLICATING CLOSED FRACTURES*

AUTHOR	YEAR	ARTERY INVOLVED	FRACTURE
Robson	1957	4th lumbar artery	Fractured spinous processes and traumatic spondylolisthesis
Crellin	1963	Anterior tibial artery	Fracture upper third tibia
Meyer	1964	Profunda femoral artery	Subtrochanteric osteotomy
Dameron	1964	Profunda femoral artery	Screw in blade plate
Staheli	1967	Popliteal artery	Fracture distal femoral shaft
Smith	1963	One false aneurysm with closed fracture in 61 arterial injuries; site not stated	
Stein	1958	Anterior tibial artery	Fracture of tibial plateau
Bassett	1964	Profunda femoral artery	Blade plate for subtrochanteric osteotomy
Bassett	1966	Thoracic aorta	11th dorsal vertebra
Harrow	1970	Right internal iliac	Pelvis

*Modified from Cameron, H. S., Laird, J. J., and Carroll, S. E., J. Trauma, *12*:67, 1972.

Massive extremity swelling may make diagnosis of a fracture or dislocation more difficult. Bleeding may or may not be present. This may be arterial (see Chap. 4) or venous (see Chap. 8) bleeding. Arterial insufficiency may be noted (see Chap. 4). There may be an associated thrill or bruit over the area of injury (see Chaps. 9 and 10).

Diagnostic Considerations

A high index of suspicion and a thorough, and often repeated, evaluation are mandatory to reduce diagnostic errors. The possibility of vascular trauma should be considered with any fracture or dislocation. However, there are certain fractures which are more frequently associated with vascular injuries than others. This is emphasized by the remaining enigma of recognizing and successfully treating injuries of the popliteal area. Only instability of the knee may be found in a swollen extremity following spontaneous reduction of a dislocation.

Roentgenograms should be obtained in two views: anterior-posterior and lateral. The extent of fracture or dislocation can often be delineated better than by physical examination alone. There may be scattered osseous fragments or missile fragments adjacent to a neurovascular bundle.

Angiography can be particularly helpful in determining the type and location of a vascular injury associated with a fracture. This is especially true with a closed fracture (Fig. 7–11). Distal pulses might be palpable even if there is an associated arterial injury from either blunt trauma or external com-

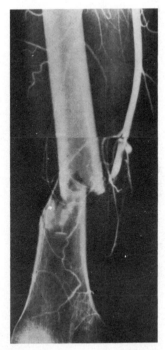

Figure 7–11. This arteriogram shows obstruction of the superficial femoral artery at the level of the fracture. The femoral shaft fracture is located at the junction of the middle and lower thirds of the shaft. (Kootstra, G., Schipper, J. J., Boontje, A. H., Klasen, H. J., and Binnendijk, B., Surg. Gynecol. Obstet., *142*:399, 1976.)

pression from an associated fracture. Intimal disruption and subintimal hematoma may not cause thrombosis of the artery for a number of hours. Also, multiple vascular injuries may exist, or the site may be at a level different from that suspected. An example of the latter is a patient admitted to Walter Reed Army Medical Center who had been struck from behind by a bumper of an automobile. The patient presented with an obvious supracondylar fracture of the femur and distal arteriovenous fistula of the involved extremity. An angiogram was performed, and the actual site of occlusion was identified in the mid-popliteal region (Fig. 7–12). The arterial injury had been caused by a dislocation of the knee rather than by the ends of the femoral fracture (Fig. 7–13). Angiography has not been as useful in the combat zone (Rich et al., 1971A). With the typically open contaminated wounds in which debridement was indicated, it was usually felt to be most expeditious to move the patient directly to the operating room.

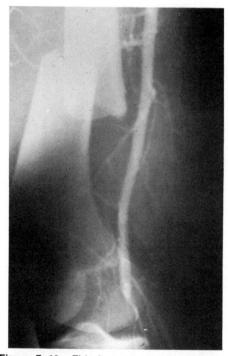

Figure 7–12. This femoral arteriogram failed to demonstrate anticipated arterial trauma adjacent to the obvious femoral fracture. However, there was total occlusion of the mid-popliteal artery caused by an unsuspected subluxation of the knee, which had subsequently reduced. (W.R.G.H., 1973.)

Venography can also be of value in identifying major venous injuries. This is emphasized by a case report from Walter Reed General Hospital (Yosowitz et al., 1972) (Fig. 7–14).

Whether or not fractures are evident, blunt trauma to the chest wall, such as occurs from the steering wheel during automobile accidents, should alert one to the possibility of myocardial damage. Serial electrocardiograms should be obtained. Abnormal changes in the tracings may signify myocardial trauma ranging from mild contusion to myocardial rupture. If rupture of the myocardium has occurred and the patient has survived the initial trauma, signs and symptoms of pericardial tamponade may be significant, and heart sounds may be distant. Repeated physical examination (particularly auscultation over the heart) should be performed, because myocardial damage may be manifest by the early development of a cardiac murmur (DeBakey et al., 1965). Cardiac catheterization will probably be indicated to identify the exact anatomical myocardial damage.

Surgical Treatment

Reports from the literature indicate that in the management of this combination of injuries [i.e., fracture of long bones with arterial injury due to blunt trauma], diagnosis is frequently delayed until the opportunity to salvage the extremity is lost or temporizing measures are utilized in the false hope that the vascular impairment does not represent arterial damage requiring prompt treatment.

Smith, R. F., Szilagyi, D. E.,
and Elliot, J. P., Jr., 1969

The above quotation epitomizes the problem of delay in recognizing arterial and venous injuries with concomitant fractures. Additional details regarding management of arterial and venous trauma, respectively, may be found in Chapters 5 and 8. Because vascular injuries frequently occur with fractures and can occasionally occur with various orthopedic procedures, orthopedic surgeons should have a thorough understanding of these injuries and a knowledge of the methods that are available to correct them.

Recognition of an arterial injury associated with fractures is imperative. This has

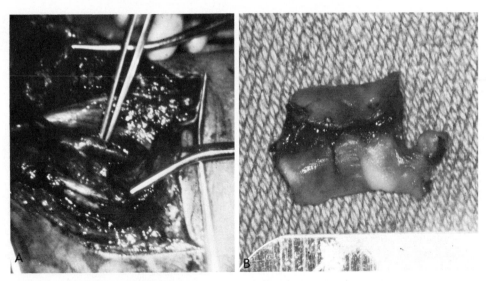

Figure 7–13. The external appearance of the popliteal artery injured by a knee dislocation, which was described in Figure 7–12, showed a contusion (A). A longitudinal resection was made through the resected segment of popliteal artery, and this demonstrated an impressive laceration of the intima where a thrombus had formed to occlude the popliteal artery (B). (N.M.R., W.R.G.H., 1973.)

been emphasized repeatedly. Exploration of the artery may be necessary to rule out arterial trauma associated with a fracture. This may be the only way that a subintimal hematoma or intimal tear with medial dissection can be differentiated from arterial spasm. Frequently, arteriotomy may be necessary to determine whether or not the intima remains intact. If there is a short segment of arterial injury, resection may be carried out, followed by either an end-to-end anastomosis or an interposition autogenous vein graft repair. On the other hand, it may also be possible to reattach the

intima above and below the area of obvious trauma with interrupted, double-armed, 6–0 synthetic vascular sutures, both needles being passed from within the arterial lumen to secure the knot outside the arterial lumen. A patch graft (again autogenous venous tissue is preferred) may be used to insure that there is no compromise of the diameter of the lumen. If there is a long segment of injury, either a direct replacement or a bypass procedure — usually with the autogenous greater saphenous vein — may be the method of choice.

Occasionally with open comminuted frac-

Figure 7–14. This drawing represents bilateral fractures of the superior and inferior pubic rami with resultant iliac vein laceration caused by blunt trauma to the pelvis of a 27 year old female struck on the left side in a hit and run automobile accident. (Yosowitz, P., Hobson, R. W., II, and Rich, N. M., Am. J. Surg., *124*:91, 1972.)

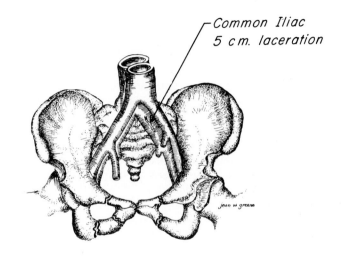

Common Iliac
5 c m. laceration

tures involving either the ulna and radius or the tibia and fibula, associated vascular and soft tissue trauma may be so extensive that direct repair is impossible. In extremely severe injuries involving massive tissue destruction, primary amputation may be indicated. Sympathectomy may be helpful in extremities in which viability is marginal.

Controversy continues regarding the best method of immobilizing a fracture associated with an arterial injury. Many civilian surgeons have been satisfied with internal fixation. In the military experience, external immobilization has been the method of choice. There is general agreement that adequate fracture immobilization should be achieved. It is becoming more obvious that in unusual circumstances, neither internal nor external fixation of fractures will provide ideal immobilization. The following quotation from one civilian study is representative:

[These data] add further support to the military contention that the success of the arterial anastomosis in combined fracture-arterial injuries is unrelated to the method of fracture management, provided a reasonable amount of fracture immobilization is achieved.

Connolly, J., et al., 1969

It is a principle accepted by many, particularly in civilian practice, that internal fixation of an associated fracture should be performed prior to arterial repair to prevent disruption of the arterial anastomosis by fracture motion. Many civilian orthopedic and vascular surgeons believe that internal fixation is the most satisfactory method of stabilizing the fracture and of safeguarding the vascular repair. However, Connolly and associates (1969) emphasized that it remains unproved whether fracture stabilization in this manner contributes more to the vascular repair than the trauma accompanying it detracts. Ideal stabilization of the fracture is usually not possible anyway, even with internal fixation. In addition, external immobilization properly performed is usually sufficient for managing these fractures, particularly in combat experience (Fig. 7–15).

Of paramount importance is the general agreement that immobilization of a frac-

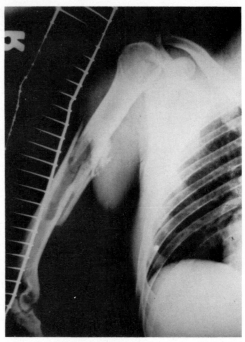

Figure 7–15. Immobilization of fractures associated with vascular injuries is imperative. The wire splint seen on this roentgenogram provided temporary external immobilization for the fracture of the right midhumerus caused by a missile from a Claymore mine (seen in the low chest wall). More definitive external immobilization was performed with a plaster cast at the definitive treatment center. (Rich, N. M., Milit. Med., *133*:9, 1968.)

ture is desired. Also, an attempt should be made to prevent wound infection and to insure early wound healing. With the massive tissue destruction caused by high velocity missiles (such as the wounds recently seen in Vietnam), internal fixation is less ideal than it might be in civilian practice. It has seemed unwarranted to accept the additional risk of infection by placing foreign material, such as an intramedullary rod, into a contaminated wound if it can be avoided.

Although no attempt is made to review the general management of the traumatized patient, several features should be emphasized. Fractures should be reduced and aligned as accurately as possible with salvage of as much as possible, discarding only the small, detached, avascular fragments. Sharp, projecting spicules of bone fragments, which might jeopardize a vascular repair, can be rongeured. If internal fixation of a fracture is considered necessary, it is important to expedite that portion of the operation to avoid prolonged ischemia. Gaspar and associates (1968) described a patient in whom meticulous bone repair lasting several hours jeopardized the viability of the extremity. They believed, as have others in civilian practice, that it is best to stabilize the bone prior to repairing the artery to prevent disruption of the arterial repair during osseous manipulation and to avoid additional injury, even possible disruption, during immobilization of the fracture. If an extremity is shortened due to an osseous defect, arterial repair may actually be facilitated, allowing an end-to-end anastomosis. If end-to-end anastomosis of the concomitant arterial injury is not possible, autogenous venous substitutes, usually from the greater saphenous vein, are the material of choice. Arterial prostheses should be avoided in contaminated wounds. Repair of concomitant venous injuries should be facilitated, as well as repair of the arterial injury. Fasciotomies should be performed when indicated.

Plaster slab splints have generally been inadequate for external immobilization of fractures. A circular plaster cast which can immobilize the joints above and below the fracture has been utilized in an attempt to provide stabilization of the majority of fractures. The cast should be bivalved all the way to the skin. It was demonstrated in Vietnam that there is essentially no place for monovalved casts. Bivalving of the cast for transportation and evacuation from Vietnam was considered mandatory. Additional stabilization of the fracture by external means has included utilization of the Steinmann pin through the tibial tubercle, which can be incorporated in the plaster cast for associated femoral fractures (Fig. 7–16). Balanced suspension methods have also been utilized even in the Vietnam combat situation (Fig. 7–17).

In addition to bivalving, windowing of the cast should be performed when appropriate. This will allow a check of the patency of the vascular repair by palpating distal pulses.

Primary amputation of a severely involved extremity may be indicated (Fig. 7–18). This Vietnam casualty was wounded in the posterior thigh by three high velocity bullets from a .30 caliber (7.62 mm) machine gun. The massive destruction of soft tissue, the complete disruption of the neurovascular bundles and the large defect in the distal femur all resulted from the high velocity effect of these bullets. Although technically it would have been possible to restore vascular continuity, it was elected to perform an amputation in this patient.

Figure 7–16. Utilizing external immobilization in the combat zone, a Steinmann pin was inserted into the tibial tubercle in this patient to assist in obtaining fracture immobilization. The Steinmann pin was then incorporated into the bivalved plaster cast (N.M.R., 2nd Surgical Hospital, 1966). (Rich, N. M., Metz, C. W., Hutton, J. E., Baugh, J. H., and Hughes, C. W., J. Trauma, 11:463, 1971. Copyright 1971, The Williams & Wilkins Company, Baltimore.)

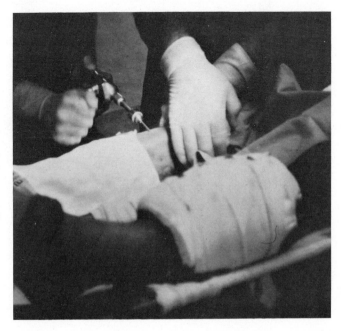

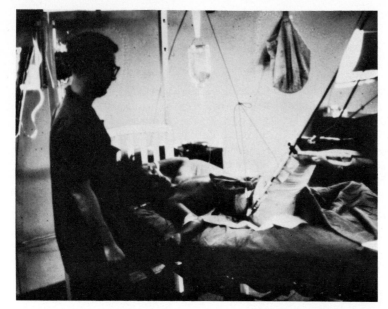

Figure 7–17. In the hospitals in Vietnam it was possible to utilize balanced suspension as part of the method of external immobilization of fractures. This enemy soldier received treatment identical to that of American military casualties (J.E.H., 91st Evacuation Hospital, 1968). (Rich, N. M., Metz, C. W., Hutton, J. E., Baugh, J. H., and Hughes, C. W., J. Trauma, *11*: 463, 1971. Copyright 1971, The Williams & Wilkins Company, Baltimore.)

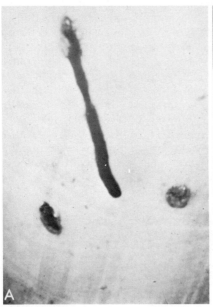

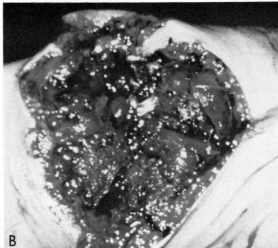

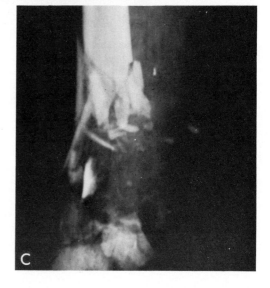

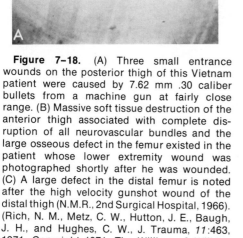

Figure 7–18. (A) Three small entrance wounds on the posterior thigh of this Vietnam patient were caused by 7.62 mm .30 caliber bullets from a machine gun at fairly close range. (B) Massive soft tissue destruction of the anterior thigh associated with complete disruption of all neurovascular bundles and the large osseous defect in the femur existed in the patient whose lower extremity wound was photographed shortly after he was wounded. (C) A large defect in the distal femur is noted after the high velocity gunshot wound of the distal thigh (N.M.R., 2nd Surgical Hospital, 1966). (Rich, N. M., Metz, C. W., Hutton, J. E., Baugh, J. H., and Hughes, C. W., J. Trauma, *11*:463, 1971. Copyright 1971, The Williams & Wilkins Company, Baltimore.)

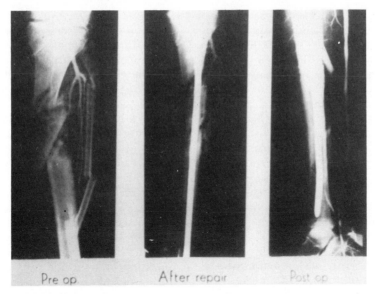

Figure 7–19. The preoperative angiogram shows destruction of the tibial and peroneal arteries. No filling occurred on repeat films following stabilization and reduction. The distal bypass is shown in the postoperative angiogram. Extended vein bypass grafts to the posterior tibial artery, in a manner similar to those used to the distal tibial and peroneal arteries in patients with arteriosclerotic occlusive disease, were useful in preventing gangrene in four patients with ischemia resulting from long bone fractures and significant arterial disruption in the lower extremities. (Evans, W. E., and Bernhard, V. M., J. Trauma, *11*:999, 1971. Copyright 1971, The Williams & Wilkins Company, Baltimore.)

There are situations in which there is even more massive destruction of a limb, and the decision for primary amputation may be even less difficult to make. On the other hand, particularly in civilian vascular injuries, arterial bypass can now salvage limbs that might have been amputated 10 years ago. Evans and Bernhard (1971) stated that some massive injuries in and around the popliteal area might have associated long bone fracture with loss of the popliteal artery and its proximal branches. They suggested using distal tibial bypass procedures similar to those used in patients with arteriosclerotic obliterative disease, where vein grafts were extended to the distal tibial and peroneal arteries (Fig. 17–19). They had four patients between 1967 and 1969 in whom conventional bypass procedures were precluded because of the extent of popliteal artery and proximal tibial and peroneal arterial trauma.

Postoperative Care

In the postoperative period, fractures associated with acute arterial injuries must remain immobilized. On occasion, it is difficult to obtain ideal immobilization by either external or internal means. Usually, however, external fixation will provide adequate immobilization as previously outlined. The method of immobilization may have to be changed for transportation of the patient.

Close observation with repeated examinations is mandatory to insure continued patency of vascular repair.

For specific management of various fractures and of complications such as unstable fractures and osteomyelitis, the reader is referred to standard orthopedic textbooks.

Results

Because of the continuing controversy surrounding immobilization of fractures, an evaluation of the fate of internally fixed fractures in the Vietnam combat zone was carried out (Rich et al., 1971A). Although the majority of these concomitant fractures were treated by external immobilization, internal fixation was occasionally used. At the time the two techniques were compared, the fighting in Southeast Asia had provided the largest number of casualties who had repairs of acute vascular injuries in any war. Given the many variables encountered in the combat zone, it is difficult to compare military experience with civilian experience. Nevertheless, it is important to point out that 10 patients, or 36 per cent, required amputation after internal fixation of fractures associated with major arterial injuries (Rich et al., 1971A). This amputation rate is considerably higher than the 13.5 per cent overall amputation rate reported from the Registry (Rich et al., 1970A). The amputation rate for those whose concomitant fractures were treated by external immobilization was approximately 20 per cent, emphasizing that the presence of a fracture with a major arterial injury increases the complication rate.

In determining the fate of the internal fixation devices, more than one-half (16) had been removed at the time of the study (Table 7–7). Of those patients having their internal fixation devices removed, nine had developed infection in the intramedullary canal, requiring removal of the device. Five of these patients subsequently underwent amputation. Of the nine patients under discussion, two had their primary intramedullary rods replaced, one at three days and one at nine days. Subsequently, both patients developed infection with resulting amputation in one and nonunion in the other. Of the 12 patients (43 per cent) with internal fixation devices that remained in place at the time of this study, only five remained entirely asymptomatic. Three patients who had internal fixation of their

fractures utilizing plates or screws still retained the devices without any known complications. One patient had chronic osteomyelitis of the fracture site, and an additional four patients had local infections in the region of the device at the time of the last available follow-up. Two additional patients had remaining intramedullary rod fixation of femoral fractures above an amputation which was required after arterial repair failure and subsequent distal arterial thrombosis.

Despite an attempt to discourage use of internal fixation of fractures in Vietnam, a few surgeons used their individual judgment in selecting internal fixation as the best method for providing fracture immobilization in a specific situation. One of the authors (NMR) was involved in such a decision, which was influenced by recent experience of disruption of a brachial arterial repair on the fourteenth postoperative day, caused by motion of a comminuted humeral fracture. Figures 7–20 through 7–22 demonstrate the case of a patient who had a large fragment wound of the left humerus with an associated distal axillary arterial injury. After an intramedullary rod had been inserted to provide stabilization of the open comminuted humeral fracture, it was possible to perform an end-to-end anastomosis of the axillary artery. Fortunately, the long term follow-up of this patient revealed no complications associated with the procedure. Hewitt and co-authors (1969) stated that internal fixation of femoral fractures was used whenever possible. Hirsch (1971) stated that, in the experience of his group in Vietnam, it was more common to see massive bone destruction in the upper extremity than in the lower extremity. Their major problem with these upper extremity wounds was immobilization of fractures. Finding that it was difficult to use plaster for external immobilization, they resorted to internal fixation.

Some surgeons are adamant advocates of internal fixation of fractures associated with concomitant arterial trauma. Hull and Hyde (1967) reported the case of a 13 year old boy with a fracture of the left femur and an ischemic leg. They described repair of the femoral artery by end-to-end anastomosis, with the fracture treated by skeletal traction. On the seventh postoperative day,

TABLE 7–7. FATE OF INTERNAL FIXATION DEVICES IN THE TREATMENT OF CONCOMITANT FRACTURES: VASCULAR INJURIES IN VIETNAM*

REMOVED............ 57%		REMAINING 43%	
Infection and amputation	5	Asymptomatic	5
Infection	4	Above amputation	2
Amputation	3	Chronic infection	1
Elective	3	Local infection	2
Displacement	1	Uncertain	2
Total:	16		12

*Rich, N. M., Metz, C. W., Hutton, J. E., Baugh, J. H., and Hughes, C. W., J. Trauma, *11*:463, 1971. Copyright 1971, The Williams & Wilkins Company, Baltimore.

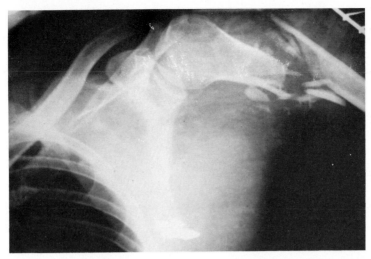

Figure 7–20. An open comminuted fracture of the left humerus is demonstrated in this roentgenogram of a patient who sustained a large fragment wound from an exploding artillery round. There was an associated left axillary arterial injury (N.M.R., 2nd Surgical Hospital, 1966). (Rich, N. M., Metz, C. W., Hutton, J. E., Baugh, J. H., and Hughes, C. W., J. Trauma, *11*:463, 1971. Copyright 1971, The Williams & Wilkins Company, Baltimore.)

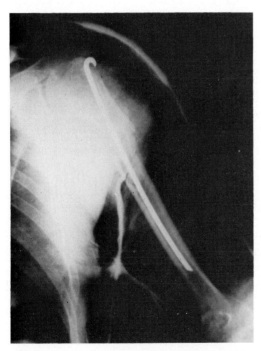

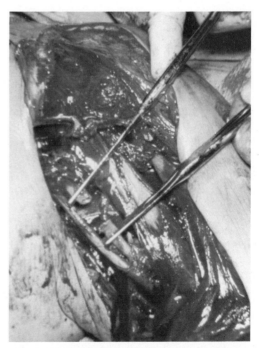

Figure 7–21. Internal fixation utilizing an intramedullary rod was obtained in this left humeral fracture. An associated left axillary arterial injury was repaired by end-to-end anastomosis (Fig. 7–22) (N.M.R., 2nd Surgical Hospital, 1966). (Rich, N. M., Metz, C. W., Hutton, J. E., Baugh, J. H., and Hughes, C. W., J. Trauma, *11*:463, 1971. Copyright 1971, The Williams & Wilkins Company, Baltimore.)

Figure 7–22. After adequate debridement and internal fixation of the humeral fracture shown in Figure 7–21, it was possible to restore arterial continuity without undue tension by end-to-end anastomosis of the left axillary artery (N.M.R., 2nd Surgical Hospital, 1966). (Rich, N. M., Metz, C. W., Hutton, J. E., Baugh, J. H., and Hughes, C. W., J. Trauma, *11*:463, 1971. Copyright 1971, The Williams & Wilkins Company, Baltimore.)

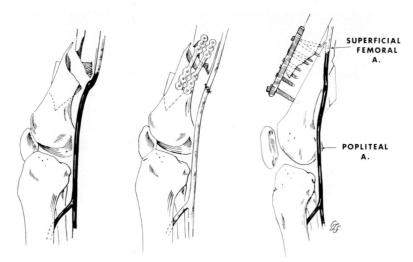

SUPERFICIAL
FEMORAL
A.

POPLITEAL
A.

Figure 7–23.   (Left) Displaced fracture of distal femur with contusion and thrombosis of superficial femoral artery. (Center) Fracture reduced and immobilized with two 6-hole plates. Injured arterial segment excised and reconstructed by end-to-end anastomôsis. (Right) Rethrombosis of femoral artery (A) by pressure of displaced bone fragment resulting from inadequate internal fixation. (Smith, R. F., Szilagyi, D. E., and Elliott, J. P., Jr., Arch. Surg., 99:315, 1969.)

when the patient was taken back to the operating room for the application of a cast, his arterial anastomosis thrombosed during transportation and the manipulation necessary for casting. The thrombus was not recognized, presumably because of the cast, until the following day, and it became necessary to perform an above-the-knee amputation. The authors offer the following conclusion:

Despite the presence of contamination and opinions to the contrary, internal fixation in patients with associated fractures and vascular anastomosis is mandatory.

An equal number of studies may be cited to support the opposing view. One example reported by Smith and co-workers (1969) involved internal fixation of a spinal comminuted fracture of the femur with two 6-hole plates. By the fifth postoperative day, it was clinically obvious that the fracture was unstable, and a roentgenogram revealed that the plate fixation had separated (Fig. 7–23). Skeletal traction and a custom-made splint were then utilized unsuccessfully in an attempt to achieve stabilization of the fracture. Because progressive signs of ischemia occurred, on the 20th postoperative day an above-the-knee amputation had to be performed.

A good summary of the success and failure rates with internal and external fixation techniques is provided by Smith and associates (1969) (Table 7–8).

In the final analysis, the mere presence of a concomitant fracture severely compromises the chances for successful repair. DeBakey and Simeone (1946), in recording World War II injuries, found that the incidence of subsequent amputation was 60 per cent when a fracture was associated with an arterial injury, compared with only 43 per cent when there was no fracture complicating the injury (Table 7–9). McNamara and colleagues (1973) reported the experience at the 24th Evacuation Hospital in Vietnam (Table 7–10). Both the failure and amputation rates increased when concomitant fractures accompanied brachial, superficial femoral and popliteal arterial injuries. A dramatic example is the increase in arterial repair failure rate from 6.3 per cent without associated fractures to 58.8 per cent when fractures accompanied popliteal arterial trauma.

In civilian experience, poor results also plague fractures and dislocations associated with arterial injuries. Procrastination and a failure to appreciate the signs and symptoms of arterial insufficiency magnify the problem. Failure to explore the artery early

TABLE 7–8. PRINCIPLES OF MANAGEMENT OF CIVILIAN ARTERIAL INJURY DUE TO BLUNT TRAUMA ASSOCIATED WITH FRACTURE OF LONG BONES: HENRY FORD HOSPITAL*

CASE No.	TREATMENT OF FRACTURE	TREATMENT OF ARTERIAL INJURY	FOL-LOW-UP (MO)	RESULT		
				Orthopedic	Vascular	Functional
1†	Internal fixation knee joint with intramedullary rod	Debridement; catheter thrombectomy; posterior tibial to anterior tibial end-to-end repair	54	Fracture healed	Arterial repair patent by x-ray; residual trophic changes foot	Syme's amputation 3 yr postop; no major limitations
2	Open reduction; onlay plate fixation	Excision contused segment; catheter thrombectomy; end-to-end repair	2	Fracture displaced	Rethrombosis due to unstable fracture	Above-the-knee amputation; died pulmonary embolus
3	Open reduction; crossed rod fixation	Excision contused segment; catheter thrombectomy; end-to-end repair	48	Fracture healed	Arterial repair patent by pulse and x-ray	Slight limitation knee flexion
4	Skeletal traction	Catheter thrombectomy; end-to-end repair	42	Fracture healed	Arterial repair patent by pulse and x-ray	Slight limitation knee flexion
5	Open reduction; onlay plate fixation	End-to-end repair anterior tibial; catheter thrombectomy posterior	41	Fracture reduction stable	Thrombosis; gangrene foot	Below-the-knee amputation; active in sports
6	Posterior plaster mold	Ligation anterior tibial; catheter thrombectomy; excision segment popliteal; end-to-end repair	38	Fracture healed	Arterial repair patent by pulse and x-ray	Mild intermittent claudication
7	Open reduction; intramedullary rod and onlay plate fixation	Debridement; end-to-end repair	37	Nonunion; bone graft 14 mo postoperatively; fracture healed	Arterial repair patent by pulse	Moderate limitation elbow motion; residual nerve deficit; working
8	Bivalved long leg plaster cast	Ligation anterior tibial; catheter thrombectomy; debridement popliteal; end-to-end repair	31	Fracture healed	Arterial repair patent by pulse and x-ray	Mild traumatic arthritis; working
9	Internal fixation tibia with intramedullary rod and bolt	Removal plaster cast; evacuation popliteal space hematoma	10	Fracture healed	Arterial repair patent by pulse and x-ray	Mild traumatic arthritis; full activity
10	Open reduction; intramedullary rod fixation	Excision contused segment; catheter thrombectomy; end-to-end repair	5	Fracture healed	Arterial repair patent by pulse	Slight limitation elbow extension

*Modified from Smith, R.F., Szilagyi, D.E., and Elliot, J.P., Jr., Arch. Surg., 99:315, 1969.
†Refer to Table 7–3.

TABLE 7–9. THE COMPLICATING INFLUENCE OF CONCOMITANT FRACTURES WITH ARTERIAL WOUNDS, INCREASING THE INCIDENCE OF AMPUTATION OF EXTREMITIES AMONG AMERICAN BATTLE CASUALTIES IN WORLD WAR II*

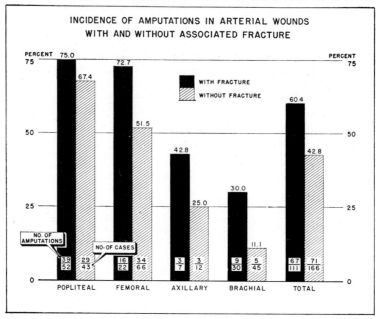

*DeBakey, M. E., and Simeone, F. A., Ann. Surg., *123*:534, 1946.

and to correct the arterial obstruction in arterial trauma associated with concomitant fractures and dislocations produces nearly a 100 per cent amputation rate in the lower extremities (Gardner, 1952); (Miller, 1957). According to Hoover (1961), dislocations of the knee nearly always result in injury to the popliteal artery and subsequent amputation unless the popliteal artery is repaired soon after the injury. Doty and colleagues (1967) summarized a 15 year experience in Los Angeles County Hospital, which started in 1948. They found that 18 of 23 patients with fractures and associated arterial injuries required major amputations: an amputation rate of about 78 per cent. Makin and co-workers (1966) found that 9 of their 16 patients with combined arterial trauma and fractures ultimately required an amputation. They advocated a more aggressive approach to the management of arterial injuries complicated by fractures and dislocations.

In contrast to the experience in Vietnam, where patients reached a definitive surgical center in only a few hours in the majority of cases, Makin and colleagues (1964) found that 10 of 16 patients in their study received treatment after a 12 hour period.

Rosental and associates (1975) reported 21 vascular injuries associated with femoral

fracture (Table 7–11). There were 19 vascular repairs at the time of acute injury; however, an average interval of 15 hours occurred between the time of injury and repair (Table 7–12). Two major amputations were required, and there were three cases of anterior tibial compartment necrosis. Of 11 patients who had external immobilization, two eventually required amputation because of massive soft tissue injury. Kootstra and colleagues (1976) reported limb salvage in six of eight patients with femoral shaft fracture and associated superficial femoral arterial trauma.

In addition to method of repair, failure to appreciate presenting signs and symptoms and inordinate delay in performing operative repair, certain exceptional circumstances may influence the outcome of the injuries. Major extremity arteries can become entrapped between the ends of a fractured long bone (Fig. 7–24). Reduction of a closed fracture may not release the artery. Also, whether or not the artery is released from the entrapment by direct surgical intervention, the possibility of intimal fracture with thrombosis of the artery must be considered.

White and associates (1968) presented the case of a 4 year old girl who sustained a comminuted supracondylar fracture of

TABLE 7-10. INCIDENCE OF USE OF VEIN GRAFT TO REPAIR ARTERIAL INJURY WITH CONCOMITANT FRACTURE: VIETNAM EXPERIENCE*

	TOTAL CASES	TOTAL FRACTURES	AMPUTATION						FAILURE†					
			Without Fracture		With Fracture		Total		Without Fracture		With Fracture		Total	
			No.	%	No.	%	No.	%	No.	%	No.	%	No.	%
Brachial	64	20 (humerus)	0	0	2	10	2	3.1	1	2.3	2	10	3	4.7
Superficial femoral	65	23 (femur)	2	4.7	7	30	9	13.8	3	7.1	8	34.8	11	16.9
Popliteal	49	17 (tibia)	1	3.1	5	29.4	6	12.2	2	6.3	10	58.8	12	24.5
Totals:	178	60	3	2.5	14	23.3	17	9.6	6	5.1	20	33.3	26	14.6

*Modified from McNamara, J. J., Brief, D. K., Stremple, J. F., and Wright, J. K., J. Trauma, *13*:17, 1973.
†Amputation, ligation, or loss of pulse.

TABLE 7–11. VASCULAR INJURIES ASSOCIATED WITH FRACTURES OF THE FEMUR: INJURY, TREATMENT AND RESULTS*

CASE NO./ AGE, YR/ SEX	TRAUMA	SITE AND TYPE OF FRACTURE	TREATMENT OF FRACTURE	ARTERIAL INJURY	ARTERIAL REPAIR TIME TO REPAIR	RESULT
1/16/M	Gunshot wound (.38 caliber)	Distal third, compound comminuted	H & P suspension	Through and through, proximal one-third of superficial femoral artery	End-to-end repair (10½ hr)	Minor amputation, tips of toes
2/44/M	Blunt	Middle third, closed	Intramedullary rod	False aneurysm, profunda femoris artery	Ligation of profunda femoris artery (5 mo)	Good
3/42/F	Blunt	Middle third, comminuted	Compression plate, fasciotomy	Intimal flap, superficial femoral artery	Resection and end-to-end anastomosis (17½ hr)	Below-knee amputation
4/23/M	Gunshot wound (.30-06 caliber)	Middle third, comminuted	Kirschner wire traction	Popliteal blast injury	Autogenous vein graft (12 hr)	Below-knee amputation
5/21/M	Blunt	Distal third, compound comminuted	Jewett nail, fasciotomy	Popliteal thrombosis	Resection and end-to-end anastomosis (15½ hr)	Above-knee amputation
6/13/M	Blunt	Middle third, comminuted	Tibial pins, traction	Intimal flap, superficial femoral artery	Autogenous vein graft (25½ hr)	"Hammer toe" due to nerve injury
7/33/M	Blunt	Middle third, comminuted massive degloving injury	Steinmann pins	Transected superficial femoral	Autogenous vein graft (10 hr)	Above-knee amputation
8/24/M	Gunshot wound	Distal third	Tibial pin suspension	False aneurysm, popliteal artery	Autogenous vein graft (8 weeks)	Peroneal nerve palsy due to false aneurysm
9/28/M	Blunt	Proximal third, open	Tibial pin traction	Transected superficial femoral	End-to-end anastomosis (6½ hr)	Good
10/15/M	Blunt	Distal third, comminuted open	Steinmann pins	Transected superficial femoral artery	End-to-end anastomosis (17½ hr)	Anterior compartment syndrome
11/30/M	Blunt	Middle third, compound comminuted	Compression plate	Intimal flap, popliteal artery	Autogenous vein graft (12½ hr)	Good
12/39/M	Blunt	Middle third	Intramedullary rod	Laceration, superficial femoral artery	Resection and end-to-end anastomosis (27 hr)	Good
13/29/M	Blunt	Middle third, comminuted	Traction	Laceration, popliteal artery	End-to-end anastomosis (8 hr)	Died fourth postoperative day of fat embolus

TABLE 7–11. VASCULAR INJURIES ASSOCIATED WITH FRACTURES OF THE FEMUR: INJURY, TREATMENT AND RESULTS (*Continued*)*

CASE NO./ AGE, YR/ SEX	TRAUMA	SITE AND TYPE OF FRACTURE	TREATMENT OF FRACTURE	ARTERIAL INJURY	ARTERIAL REPAIR TIME TO REPAIR	RESULT
14/12/M	Blunt	Middle third	Pin and suspension, fasciotomy	Contusion and thrombosis, superficial femoral artery	Resection and end-end-to-end anastomosis (7½ hr)	Good
15/26/M	Blunt	Distal third	Intramedullary rod, fasciotomy	Transected popliteal artery	End-to-end anastomosis (38 hr)	Necrosis of anterior compartment muscles
16/20/M	Blunt	Middle third	Compression plate fasciotomy	Laceration, superficial femoral artery	End-to-end anastomosis (18 hr)	Necrosis of anterior compartment muscles
17/51/M	Gunshot wound	Distal third, comminuted	Tibial pin traction, fasciotomy	Transected popliteal artery	Autogenous vein graft (14 hr)	Good
18/42/M	Shotgun blast	Distal third, compound comminuted	Tibial pin traction	Transected superficial femoral artery	Autogenous vein graft (9 hr)	Sciatic nerve deficit
19/24/M	Blunt	Distal third, compound comminuted	Compression plate, fasciotomy	Popliteal artery avulsion	Autogenous vein graft (11 hr)	Good
20/19/F	Blunt	Distal third	Compression plate, fasciotomy	Transected superficial femoral artery	Autogenous vein graft (21 hr)	Anterior compartment syndrome
21/29/M	Shotgun	Middle third	Femoral pins and cast	Superficial femoral artery penetration	End-to-end anastomosis (7 hr)	Good

*Rosental, J. J., Gaspar, M. R., Gjerdrum, T. C., and Newman, J., Arch. Surg., *110*:494, 1975.

TABLE 7–12. VASCULAR INJURIES ASSOCIATED WITH FRACTURES OF THE FEMUR: RESULTS OF INTERNAL AND EXTERNAL FIXATION*

RESULTS (19 ACUTE CASES)	BONE FIXATION	
	Internal	External
Good or fair (causalgia, nerve injury, minor amputation)	3	8
Anterior compartment necrosis	3	0
Major amputation	2	2
Death	0	1 (fat embolus)
Total	8	11

*Rosental, J. J., Gaspar, M. R., Gjerdrum, T. C., and Newman, J., Arch. Surg., *110*:494, 1975. Refer also to Table 7–11.

the humerus. Despite reduction of the fracture within one hour, circulation in the hand remained poor. The brachial artery was explored 24 hours later and released from its trapped position between the ends of the fracture. A thrombectomy of the artery was also carried out.

Movement of the fracture can lacerate the repaired artery or areas of the artery adjacent to the repair. Movement may also place excessive tension on the suture line and may destroy important collateral vessels. Cohen and associates (1969) documented the case of a patient with an unstable fracture. He had sustained multiple fragment wounds in Vietnam which fractured the right humerus. An associated brachial artery injury was repaired with a short segment of saphenous vein graft, and the bone ends were aligned with application of a cast. Bleeding occurred eight days following the initial operation, and at

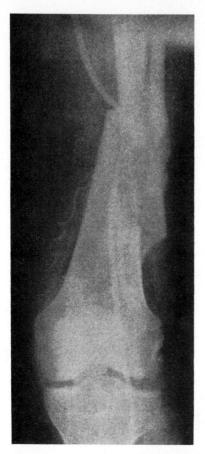

Figure 7–24. Entrapment of the distal superficial femoral artery in this femoral fracture is demonstrated angiographically. (Stokes, J. M., and McAfee, C. A., J. Trauma, 5:162, 1965. Copyright 1965, The Williams & Wilkins Company, Baltimore.)

reoperation the proximal bone fragment was found to have lacerated the artery. An additional repair was performed, followed by the application of skeletal traction. However, bleeding recurred within 48 hours, infection became evident, and it was necessary to perform an above-the-elbow amputation.

Among specific fractures associated with vascular trauma, pelvic fractures can produce some of the most disastrous results. This is emphasized by the report of Patterson and Morton (1973), who surveyed 633 patients with pelvic fracture and dislocation treated at Vancouver General Hospital between 1960 and 1966. There were 88 deaths, with a gross mortality rate of 13.9 per cent. Nine deaths were considered to

be coincidental to the injury, and fractures of the pelvis were considered the terminal event in 17 deaths. However, in 62 patients death was directly due to a complication of the injury. Among this third group, hemorrhagic shock was the major cause of death in 37 patients; these were considered by the authors to be salvageable.

Follow-Up

Continued long term follow-up of the special study group of Vietnam casualties will provide additional information from recent combat experience.

Civilian series contain few long term results for patients with combined fractures and arterial trauma. The following case (Bergan, 1963) represents one of a limited number of reports available. A 10 year old female sustained a supracondylar fracture and a fracture of the shaft of the femur in an automobile accident. Arterial insufficiency of the extremity below the popliteal artery was obvious, and reposition of the fracture had no influence on improving the arterial flow. At the time of open reduction of the fracture, occlusion of the popliteal artery corresponding to the site of the supracondylar fracture was demonstrated. There was no rupture in the outer arterial wall. An arteriotomy showed thrombus within the artery, and removal of the clot revealed an intimal rupture with a circular rolling up of the intima. After endarterectomy was performed and the arteriotomy was sutured, the arterial circulation was restored and a good distal peripheral pulse was noted. Six months later, arteriography revealed a patent popliteal artery. The patient remained free from symptoms for five years after the accident.

Final functional results are an important measure of success. Many months, or several years, may pass before this can be established (Table 7–8). Sher (1975) documented good final functional results in 8 of 10 patients (Table 7–13).

NERVE INJURIES

Problems of vascular trauma are markedly increased when there are associated

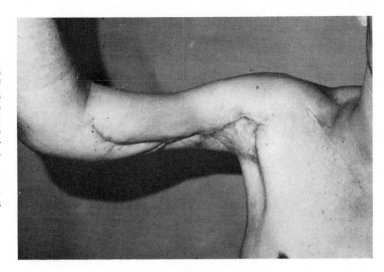

Figure 7–29. Long term follow-up of patients such as this young officer with thrombosis of his right axillary arterial repair is important. Concomitant nerve deficits, venous insufficiency and massive soft tissue loss were actually his limiting factors as far as functional use of his extremity was concerned. (Rich, N. M., Baugh, J. H., and Hughes, C. W., J. Trauma, *10*:359, 1970. Copyright 1970, The Williams & Wilkins Company, Baltimore.)

(1976) recently emphasized the value of identifying the ends of major nerves that had been severed. In their "Plea to Emergency Room Physicians" they noted that it would be helpful to the neurologic, orthopedic or other surgeon performing secondary repair of peripheral nerves for the primary surgeon to mark the severed ends with colored, nonabsorbable sutures or metal clips or to bring the ends together, not for primary repair but to prevent the ends from retracting. Details of nerve repair are outlined in numerous texts of neurosurgery and orthopedics.

As emphasized earlier, prompt splinting and control of edema are of paramount importance in preventing deformity until nerve regeneration is complete.

Results

Elkin and Woodhall (1944) reported their World War II experience with combined vascular and nerve injuries. They emphasized that there was a higher incidence of these injuries than was seen in World War I. Shumacker and Stokes (1950) augmented the clinical experience with an experimental study of combined vascular and neurologic injuries, in which the effect of somatic and sympathetic denervation was examined. Learmonth (1952–53) outlined his approach to combined neurovascular lesions. Woodhall and Nulsen (1953) outlined their management of nerve injuries. They emphasized that the best nerve regeneration

occurs when the nerve has been severed and repair has been properly performed within three months. The regeneration potential for nerves varies considerably and is beyond the scope of this review. Optimum mechanical function depends on prevention of muscular contracture and joint stiffening. Physiotherapy is extremely important in obtaining optimum function and habitual use.

In civilian experience, Smith and associates (1974) reported primary nerve repair in 28 per cent of patients who had combined arterial trauma: 16 of 56 injuries. Delayed repair was used in three cases. No repair was performed in 37 patients who had only various degrees of contusion. The disability rate was 79 per cent following repair and 51 per cent when injuries were more limited.

Bole and co-workers (1976) reported only one initial repair of 10 nerve injuries. This was a repair of a transected median nerve. Again, to emphasize a difference between civilian and military injuries, Kline and Hackett (1975) reported their operative and recording experience with 200 major nerve injuries.

Follow-Up

Detailed follow-up is required to determine the functional extremity ability following repair of associated nerve injuries.

Figure 7–29 emphasizes the type of combined injury that can result in a residual limiting deficit.

CHAPTER 8

VENOUS INJURIES

It could be recorded in history that outstanding contributions based on experience of managing Vietnam casualties by American military surgeons did as much to stimulate and direct interest and success in repair of venous injuries as was established during the Korean Conflict with repair of arterial injuries.

Vietnam Vascular Registry, NMR, 1976

Although repair rather than ligation of arterial injuries has been widely and enthusiastically accepted for the past 20 years, the same approach has not developed for venous injuries (Fig. 8–1). In most instances these are simply treated by ligation. There are several reasons for this paucity of interest in repair: First, many veins can be ligated and little or no disability follows. Even when very large veins are ligated, the extremity may not be threatened, although months or years later venous insufficiency may appear. Second, the effectiveness of repair of many venous injuries is yet uncertain. With the low pressure in the venous

system, thrombosis is much more common than it is after repair of arterial injuries. Acquisition of data to show the effectiveness of repair is particularly difficult because there is no simple method for determining patency of a venous reconstruction; with arterial repair, simple palpation of a peripheral pulse is usually adequate.

The degree of disability from chronic venous insufficiency is not recognized by many, for it may become evident only months or years after injury. A clinical example of disability from venous stasis, edema, skin pigmentation and ulceration following ligation of the superficial femoral

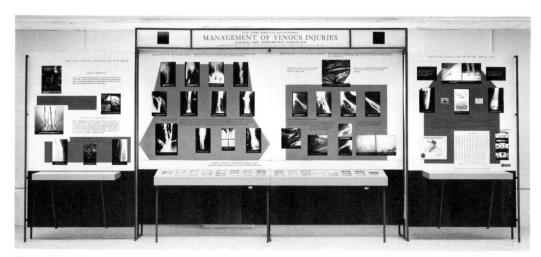

Figure 8–1. This exhibit, entitled "Management of Venous Injuries: Clinical and Experimental Evaluation," has been used to stimulate an increased interest in the repair of venous injuries. Although repair of arterial injuries has been accepted during the past 20 years, all too often the repair of venous injuries has been treated with minimal interest and even disdain. (A.F.I.P. Photograph.)

and greater saphenous veins is shown in Figure 8–2. Because of the uncertainty of the importance and the effectiveness of repair of venous injuries, an analysis and a preliminary report from the Vietnam Vascular Registry were prepared in 1970; this report encouraged the repair of major veins in the lower extremities (Rich et al., 1970 B). Although data thus far are meager and the effectiveness of some types of venous reconstruction is yet unproved, certain clinical guidelines are now well established.

Venous repair may be important in at least three circumstances. First, with popliteal injuries, repair of the vein may be

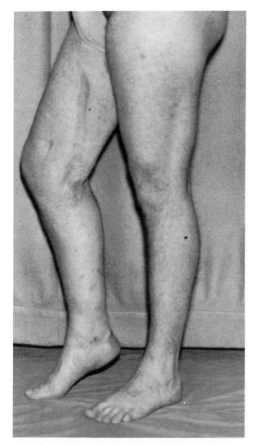

Figure 8–2. Chronic venous insufficiency has been seen in the Registry with increasing frequency in patients who had lower extremity venous ligation in Vietnam. In addition to edema, other changes similar to the post-phlebitic syndrome have been evident, including venous stasis changes in the skin and even some superficial ulcerations. Some of these changes are present in the right lower extremity of this patient, who had ligation of his superficial femoral vein. (W.R.G.H., 1969.) (Vietnam Vascular Registry #225, N.M.R.)

necessary to prevent loss of the leg despite successful arterial reconstruction. This observation was first made during the Korean Conflict and has been confirmed repeatedly since that time. A major factor in this decision is the anatomy of the popliteal space, where an injury often critically impedes venous return from the lower extremity. Second, venous repair may be necessary in the presence of massive soft tissue injury in the lower extremities, where the widespread loss of soft tissue interrupts venous return to a crucial degree. Thirdly, repair should be routinely considered with large veins, especially when the damage is proximal to the profunda femoris, to prevent chronic venous insufficiency. This includes the common femoral, the external and the common iliac veins.

For a long time a natural concern with repair of venous injuries was the fear of producing venous thrombosis and pulmonary embolization. Although an apparently likely hazard, this dangerous sequence has been surprisingly absent. Conceivably, small emboli may not be recognized clinically, but the absence of clinically detectable pulmonary emboli has been uniformly documented in both the Vietnam Vascular Registry and in previous reports by others.

HISTORICAL REVIEW

Several excellent reviews of the development of vascular surgery have been published in recent years (Rob, 1972; Shumacker, 1969; Haimovici, 1963). Two earlier outstanding references are Guthrie (1912) and Murphy (1897). As early as 1816, Travers supposedly closed a small wound in a femoral vein. In 1830, G. J. Guthrie reported more precisely that he closed a laceration of the internal jugular vein by placing a tenaculum through the cut edges, after which he tied a suture around the tenaculum to constitute a lateral ligature. In 1878, Agnew used lateral sutures to close venous wounds. Only a year earlier, Eck had performed the first vascular anastomosis by suturing the portal vein to the inferior vena cava. Schede in 1882 in Germany is generally given credit for performing the first successful lateral suture repair of a laceration in a vein in clinical practice, and he advocated repair of wounds of the femoral veins in man.

In the late 19th century other surgeons who, with apparent success, sutured wounds of veins include Billroth, Braun of Koenigsberg and Schmidt. In his experimental laboratory, Hirsch in 1881 successfully repaired divided veins in dogs. When Dörfler in 1889 outlined his method of arterial repair, he recommended the same technique for repairing veins. Haimovici (1963) described Dörfler's method:

The essential features of this method consisted of the use of fine, round needles and fine silk and his suture was continuous, embracing all of the coats of the vessel. From his experience, although limited to 16 cases, he concluded that aseptic silk thread in the lumen of the vessel does not necessarily lead to thrombosis, and therefore, the penetration of the intima was not contraindicated.

In 1889 Kümmel performed the first clinical end-to-end anastomosis of a femoral vein. In 1901 Clermont successfully reunited the ends of a divided vena cava with a continuous fine silk suture. A month later the lumen of the vena cava was found to be smooth and unobstructed at the site of the anastomosis. Jensen in 1903 was successful in four of seven operations in anastomosing transected veins, using a continuous suture technique.

In World War I the clinical use of lateral suture repair of venous lacerations was reported by Goodman (1918). He reported experiences with five patients with vascular injuries in whom a lateral suture repair of venous lacerations was done in four, involving two popliteal and two superficial femoral veins. The defects ranged from 5 mm to 20 mm in length. The results are unknown as there was no follow-up evaluation.

The importance of venous repair was surely minimized by the proposal of Makins in 1917 that the concomitant vein should be ligated when an arterial injury was treated by ligation. The results reported by Makins to support this hypothesis were later found to have no statistical significance (Table 8–1). The influence persisted even until World War II. Data from World War II showed no benefit from ligation of the concomitant vein, however (DeBakey and Simeone, 1946). During the Korean Conflict repair of injuries of major veins was again undertaken in selected patients (Hughes, 1959).

One of the most bizarre recommendations in the history of vascular surgery is the mid-19th century recommendation that ligation of the concomitant uninjured artery should be done when a venous injury was treated by ligation. Apparently this astonishing recommendation was first made by Gensoul in 1833, who feared the hazards of venous engorgement if the vein alone was ligated. Other surgeons (Dupuytren, 1839; Chassaignac, 1855; Langenbeck, 1861; Pilcher, 1886) made similar recommendations, although these were intended primarily to minimize hemorrhage with venous injuries (Simeone et al., 1951).

TABLE 8–1. A COMPARISON OF THE RESULTS OF LIGATIONS OF THE ARTERY ALONE WITH THOSE OF SIMULTANEOUS LIGATIONS OF ARTERY AND VEIN*

	ARTERY ALONE				ARTERY AND VEIN			
ARTERY	Number of Cases	Good Result	Gangrene	Per Cent Gangrene	Number of Cases	Good Result	Gangrene	Per Cent Gangrene†
Subclavian	4	3	1	25.0	1	1	...	0.0
Axillary	6	5	1	16.6	4	4	...	0.0
Brachial	13	10	3	23.0	1	1	...	0.0
Femoral	32	24	8	25.0	32	25	7	21.0
Popliteal	24	14	10	41.6	28	22	6	21.4
Tibial	4	4	...	0.0	1	1	...	0.0
Carotid	18	12	6	33.3	4	3	1	25.0
Total	101	72	29	28.0	71	57	14	19.7

*Modified from Montgomery, M. L., Arch. Surg., *24*:1016, 1932. Copyright 1932, American Medical Association.
†All the percentages were added to the table by me, except the total percentages, which appear in Makins' original table.

Moreover, during the Korean Conflict, there was a renewal of interest in repair of the involved vein during the elective repair of arteriovenous fistulas that usually was performed several months after the initial injury. Traditionally such fistulas were treated by ligation of both the artery and the vein. The technique of repair gradually evolved to include repair of the artery and often repair of the concomitant vein. Successful results in such patients generated some enthusiasm for repair of acute venous injuries (Hughes, 1958):

. . . noted 63 per cent major vein injuries accompanying major artery injuries. A number of other vein injuries were treated in which there was no arterial involvement. Most of these vein injuries were treated by ligation, but in some, ligations resulted in various degrees of venous stasis. On rare occasion, massive venous stasis resulted in amputation of the extremity. To eliminate this complication, two investigators . . . sic Hughes and Spencer independently . . . began the repair of major veins. They reported 20 major veins repaired, all by lateral suture except one which was repaired by direct anastomosis. Some of these are known to have thrombosed later without complications. No embolic complications resulted.

A review concerned primarily with the management of venous injuries in civilian practice was published by Gaspar and Treiman in 1960; it described injuries of 52 major veins in 51 patients. Venous reconstruction when performed was usually by lateral suture.

During the Vietnam Conflict, with the interest and experience resulting from the necessity of treating thousands of vascular injuries, there was a significant effort to perform venous repairs in the last five years of the conflict (1968–1972). In a recent symposium on venous surgery in the lower extremities at Walter Reed Army Institute of Research, the combined experiences of both civilian and military surgeons were summarized (Swan et al., 1975).

SURGICAL ANATOMY

Unlike the arterial system, there is considerable variation in the configuration of the venous system. It frequently has been stated that the only consistency in the venous system is its inconsistency. Anomalous pathways and additional veins running parallel to the main vein are found frequently.

This presentation will concentrate on the major veins of the venous system that may be of particular importance to the vascular surgeon (Fig. 8–3). The regions covered include the neck, the upper extremities and the thorax, the lower extremities and the abdomen.

The internal jugular vein is the major vein in the neck that returns the blood from the brain and the superficial parts of the face and the neck. It begins in the jugular foramen at the base of the skull as a continuation of the transverse sinus. There is an internal jugular vein on either side of the neck that passes in a vertical direction to the level of the sternoclavicular articulation, where it joins the subclavian vein and forms the innominate vein at the base of the neck. It lies lateral to the internal carotid artery near its origin and then lateral to the common carotid artery lower in the neck. It is one of three structures in the carotid sheath along with the carotid artery and the vagus nerve. The latter descends between and behind the vein and artery. The left internal jugular vein is generally smaller than the right, and each contains a pair of valves which are placed approximately 2.5 cm above the termination of the vessel. There are numerous other veins in the neck which have less significance: external jugular, facial, anterior jugular and vertebral veins.

VEINS OF THE ARM

The superficial veins of the upper extremity and thorax are generally of minimal significance. Deep veins accompany major arteries and constitute venae comitantes of the arteries. Valves are found in most of the deep veins. The cephalic vein begins in the radial part of the dorsal venous network. It is one superficial vein that is important because of its frequent use for intravenous infusions and as a possible donor site. It has numerous communications, including one with the basilic vein at the elbow level. As it ascends, it passes between the pectoralis major and the deltoideus muscles. It terminates in the axillary vein just below the clavicle. The

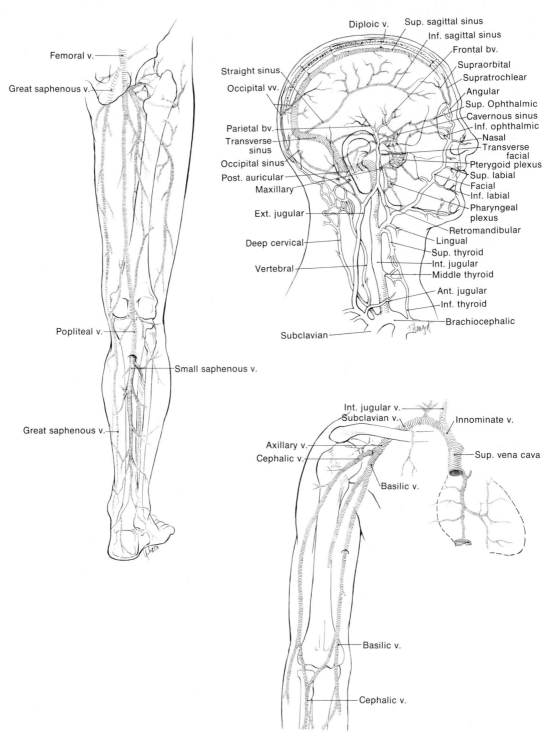

Figure 8–3. Artist's conception of the major venous anatomy that is particularly important to the surgeon. Repair of major venous injuries is advocated for large caliber veins under most conditions. See also Figure 8–4.

basilic vein begins in the ulnar part of the dorsal venous network and descends on the ulnar side of the forearm before passing obliquely in the groove between the biceps brachii and pronator teres muscles. It passes upward along the medial border of the biceps brachii and the brachial artery to the lower border of the teres major muscle, where it joins the brachial veins to form the axillary vein. The brachial veins are placed on either side of the brachial artery and have numerous tributaries. The axillary vein begins at the junction of the basilic and brachial veins near the lower border of the teres major and terminates as the subclavian vein at the outer border of the first rib. It lies on the medial side of the axillary artery. The medial cord of the brachial plexus is in close proximity. There are a pair of valves opposite the lower border of the subscapularis muscle. The subclavian vein is a continuation of the axillary vein, and it extends from the outer border of the first rib to the sternal end of the clavicle, where it unites with the internal jugular vein to form the innominate vein. A very important anatomic feature finds the subclavian vein behind the clavicle and separated from the subclavian artery medially by the scalenus anticus muscle. There are usually a pair of valves in the subclavian vein.

The innominate veins, which have no valves, are formed by the internal jugular and subclavian veins on either side at the base of the neck. The right innominate vein is about 2.5 cm in length, compared to the left innominate vein which is about 6 cm in length. Each begins behind the sternal end of the clavicle, and they unite behind the upper half of the manubrium to the right side to form the superior vena cava. The superior vena cava, approximately 7 cm in length, returns blood from the upper half of the body. Formed by the union of the two innominate veins near the cartilage of the right first rib close to the sternum, it descends vertically to end in the upper part of the right atrium. The azygos system will not be included in this review.

VEINS OF THE LEG

In the lower extremities there are superficial and deep venous systems similar to those found in the upper extremities. Of the superficial veins, the greater saphenous vein deserves mention because of its value in collateral venous return and as an autogenous donor graft. It begins on the medial margin of the dorsum of the foot and ascends in front of the medial malleolus. It passes upward on the medial aspect of the calf and thigh and ends about 3 cm below the inguinal ligament after passing through the fossa ovalis to end in the femoral vein. The deep veins of the lower extremity accompany the arteries. The popliteal vein is formed by anastomosis of the anterior and posterior tibial veins at the lower border of the popliteus muscle. It ascends through the popliteal fossa to pass under the adductor magnus tendon, where it becomes the femoral vein. Although it is deep in location, it is usually called the superficial femoral vein at that point because it accompanies the superficial femoral artery. The superficial femoral vein is lateral to the artery in the lower portion of the thigh. As it passes upward, it lies on the medial side of the artery. About 4 cm below the inguinal ligament it is joined by the profunda femoris vein. Near its termination it is joined by the greater saphenous vein. There are usually four valves in the popliteal vein and three valves in the superficial femoral vein. The common femoral vein is a short segment of the femoral vein above the termination of the greater saphenous vein and below the inguinal ligament. The external iliac vein is the continuation of the femoral vein, which begins behind the inguinal ligament. It passes upward along the brim of the pelvis. It ends opposite the sacroiliac articulation, where it joins the hypogastric vein to form the common iliac vein. It lies medial to the artery on the right side and gradually passes behind the artery near its termination. On the left side it lies medial to the artery throughout its length. The external iliac vein frequently has one valve, and occasionally it has two valves. The common iliac veins, after being formed by the union of the external iliac and hypogastric veins, pass obliquely upward toward the right side, where they end near the fifth lumbar vertebra by joining to form the inferior vena cava. The right common iliac vein is shorter than the left and is nearly vertical

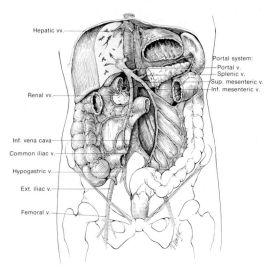

Figure 8-4. The portal venous system also has surgical importance. Repair of the portal vein or superior mesenteric vein may be necessary to maintain intestinal viability.

in its direction. The left common iliac vein passes upward in an oblique path. It is initially situated on the medial side of the common iliac artery, and then passes behind the artery. There are no valves in the common iliac veins. The inferior vena cava returns blood to the heart from the body below the diaphragm. It is formed by the common iliac veins on the right side of the fifth lumbar vertebra. It ascends on the right side of the aorta and terminates in the lower and posterior part of the right atrium. Important tributaries include the two renal veins and the hepatic veins.

OTHER VEINS

The portal system deserves mention because it returns the blood from the greatest part of the digestive tract (Fig. 8-4). The portal vein is approximately 8 cm in length and is formed at the level of the second lumbar vertebra by the superior mesenteric and splenic veins. It divides into a right and left branch to enter the respective lobes of the liver.

INCIDENCE

The true frequency of venous injuries is undetermined, for many surgeons consider them unimportant and often do not report them. This is particularly true in the case of combined arterial and venous injuries. Analysis of the Vietnam experience found numerous cases in which venous trauma was not documented in the records.

The first major interest in the frequency of venous injuries in military trauma was during the Korean Conflict. In analysis of 180 acute vascular injuries (Table 8-2), Hughes (1954) found nearly as many injuries in major veins (71) as there were in major arteries (79).

Similarly, in civilian practice the frequency of venous trauma has been documented only occasionally, most reports describing only arterial trauma. There are numerous large series of arterial injuries reported that give no details regarding venous trauma. The report by Gaspar and Treiman (1960) is one of the first to have a detailed analysis of venous injuries alone. In a group of 228 patients with vascular injuries at the Los Angeles County General Hospital over a period of 10 years, about 22 per cent (51 patients) had venous injuries. The superficial femoral vein was most frequently injured (nine times). The inferior vena cava and the internal jugular vein were each injured eight times, and the brachial veins seven. In 1966 an additional 40 patients were added to the original series in a supplementary report by Trei-

TABLE 8-2 INCIDENCE OF ACUTE VASCULAR TRAUMA IN KOREAN CASUALTIES*

VESSEL	NUMBER	PER CENT
Major arteries	79	43.9
Major veins	71	39.4
Minor arteries	30	16.7
Total	180	100.0

*Modified from Hughes, C. W., Surg. Gynecol. Obstet., 99:1, 1954. By permission of Surgery, Gynecology & Obstetrics.

TABLE 8-3. INCIDENCE OF VENOUS INJURIES*

Vein	Number 1948– 1958	Number 1958– 1963	Total 1948– 1963	Per Cent
Axillary-brachial	8	5	13	14.1
Innominate-subclavian	3	5	8	8.7
Superior vena cava	1	0	1	1.1
Inferior vena cava	8	4	12	13.0
Iliac	7	4	11	12.0
Femoral	11	6	17	18.5
Other	14	16	30	32.6
Total	52	40	92	100.0

*Modified from Treiman, R. L., Doty, D., and Gaspar, M. R., Am. J. Surg., *111*:469, 1966.

man and associates. The frequency of venous injury in the different locations is shown in Table 8–3.

In the preliminary Vietnam Vascular Registry report, approximately one-fourth of the patients had venous trauma (Table 8–4) (Rich and Hughes, 1969). There were only 28 injuries of isolated veins, and the majority of the venous injuries were combined with arterial trauma. The increased incidence of venous trauma when associated with arterial trauma was emphasized in an interim Registry report, which documented concomitant venous injuries in 37.7 per cent of cases with acute major arterial trauma (Table 8–5) (Rich et al., 1970 A).

ETIOLOGY

The variety of wounding agents producing venous trauma is virtually endless. The paucity of reports specifically devoted to venous injury, however, precludes complete documentation.

As might be expected, fragments and

TABLE 8-4. INCIDENCE OF VENOUS TRAUMA– PRELIMINARY VIETNAM VASCULAR REGISTRY REPORT (500 PATIENTS)*

Total vascular injuries	718	
Venous injuries	194	(27.0%)
Isolated	28	(14.4%)
Combined	166	(85.6%)

*Modified from Rich, N. M., and Hughes, C. W., Surgery, *65*:218, 1969.

TABLE 8-5. CONCOMITANT VENOUS TRAUMA ASSOCIATED WITH ACUTE ARTERIAL TRAUMA*

Cases	1000	
Venous injuries	377	(37.7%)

*Modified from Rich, N. M., Baugh, J. H., and Hughes, C. W., J. Trauma, *10*:359, 1970. Copyright 1970, The Williams & Wilkins Co., Baltimore.

high velocity missiles cause most venous injuries in military casualties. In an analysis of 1000 acute major arterial injuries in Vietnam, which included 377 concomitant venous injuries, 60 per cent were produced by fragment wounds and 35 per cent by bullets (Rich et al., 1970 A). Some venous injuries resulted from wounds with the primitive punji stick, a unique variety of trauma in Southeast Asia.

In the civilian report by Gaspar and Treiman (1960), most injuries (52) were produced by sharp instruments (Table 8–6). An almost equal number were caused by missiles, and only nine were produced by blunt instruments. One injury was an iatrogenic laceration of the inferior vena cava that occurred during an abdomino-perineal resection.

With the great strides in vascular and cardiac angiography and catheterization, there has been an increasing frequency of iatrogenic trauma to the venous system in the past 20 years. The reported cases of lost catheters in veins are too numerous for this review. Mathur and associates (1971) summarized previous reports and included removal of a catheter fragment from a subclavian vein with a Fogarty balloon catheter (Fig. 8–5). Thrombosis, sepsis and phlebitis have also complicated the use of

TABLE 8-6. ETIOLOGY OF MAJOR VENOUS TRAUMA–LOS ANGELES*

Wounding Agent	Number	Per Cent
Sharp instruments	23	44.2
Missiles	20	38.5
Blunt instruments	9	17.3
Total	52	100.0

*From Gaspar, M. R., and Treiman, R. I., Am. J. Surg., *100*:171, 1960.

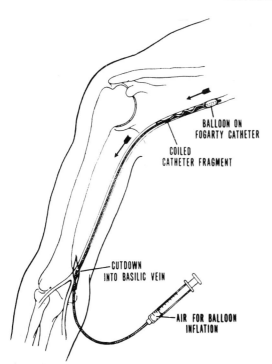

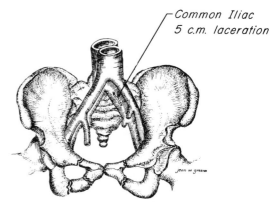

Figure 8–6. Artist's illustration of a 5 cm laceration of the left common iliac vein caused by blunt trauma. There were associated bilateral fractures of the superior and inferior pubic rami. (Yosowitz, P., Hobson, R. W., II, and Rich, N. M., Am. J. Surg., *124*:91, 1972.)

Figure 8–5. Numerous techniques have been utilized to retrieve catheter fragments. This drawing shows a Fogarty balloon catheter used to remove a piece of a catheter that was accidentally sheared off by the needle. (Mathur, A. P., Pochaczevsky, R., Levowitz, B. S., and Feraru, F., J.A.M.A., *217*:481, 1971.)

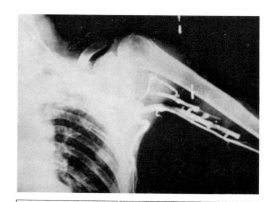

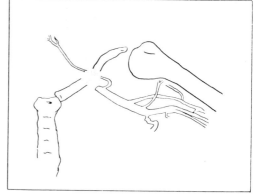

indwelling catheters; this was well reviewed by McDonough and Altemeier (1971). Iatrogenic venous trauma has been associated with the majority of major operations at one time or another. A not uncommon surgical error has been the inadvertent injury of the common femoral vein during stripping of the greater saphenous system, usually from lack of recognition of the common femoral vein. An unusual example is the report by Zabin in 1950 of an accidental tear of the inferior vena cava, complicating cholecystectomy.

Venous injuries also have resulted frequently from fractures. With pelvic fracture, hemorrhage from such injury may be lethal. Motsay and associates (1969) emphasized the problems of injury of the iliac vein with fractures of the pelvis, describing experiences with three cases and emphasizing the threat of exsanguination unless hemorrhage was promptly controlled. Yosowitz and coworkers (1970) described the fatal case of

Figure 8–7. The venogram above and the outlined sketch below demonstrate total left subclavian vein obstruction three months after the patient sustained a fracture of the left clavicle (see also Figs. 28–25 and 28–26). (Witte, C. L., and Smith, C. A., Arch. Surg., *93*:664, 1966. Copyright 1966, American Medical Association.)

laceration of an iliac vein by blunt trauma (Fig. 8–6). An unusual experience described by Witte and Smith (1966) was the case of a 45 year old laborer with a displaced fracture of the left clavicle that had developed a prominent callus. Four weeks after injury, pain and swelling abruptly appeared in the left arm, with subsequent edema and pain after minimal exercise. Venography and subsequent surgical exploration confirmed obstruction of the subclavian vein from the newly formed callus (Fig. 8–7). When the left supraclavicular fossa was explored, the obstructed subclavian vein was found enmeshed in callus near the original fracture site.

CLINICAL PATHOLOGY AND PATHOPHYSIOLOGY

Although statistics are incomplete, most venous injuries that have been repaired have been lacerations that occur from stab wounds. But with injuries from high velocity missiles, as in military casualties, transection is more common. Because of the anatomic proximity of arteries and veins in many areas of the body, the possibility of concomitant arterial injury should always be suspected when a venous injury is found. In a series of 90 patients with 126 intra-abdominal vascular injuries reported by Perdue and Smith (1968), 12 of 27 patients with iliac vein injuries also had injuries of the iliac artery (44 per cent). Certainly the converse is equally true, for injury of the concomitant vein is frequent with arterial injury. This is especially the case with injury of the popliteal artery; in one series it occurred in 116 of a total of 217 injuries (53 per cent) (Rich et al., 1970 A).

Pertinent experimental research warrants special mention. An evaluation of the hemodynamics of venous occlusion in an experimental model found an immediate decrease in femoral artery blood flow, reported by Barcia and associates in 1972 and Wright and Swan in 1973. These authors demonstrated that femoral venous ligation in the canine hindlimb resulted in a 50 per cent to 75 per cent reduction in femoral arterial blood flow, with a marked increase in femoral venous pressure as well as an increase in peripheral resistance. Hobson and associates (1973) extended the investigation over a 72-hour period and emphasized the critical aspects of these physiological changes in the early hours (Figs. 8–8 and 8–9). These studies, as well as numerous other problems, are included in the recent

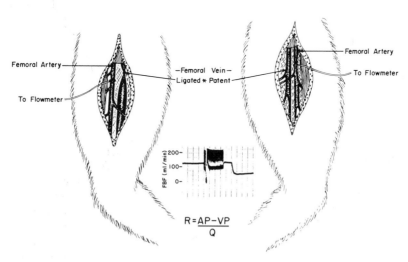

Figure 8–8. Stimulated by the work of Barcia and associates (1972) and Wright and Swan (1973), Hobson and co-workers (1973) used an experimental model as diagrammed above to determine femoral arterial blood flow, femoral venous pressure and peripheral resistance related to femoral venous ligation over a 72-hour period. (Hobson, R. W., II, Howard E. W., Wright C. B., Collins, G. J., and Rich, N. M. Surgery, 74:824, 1973.)

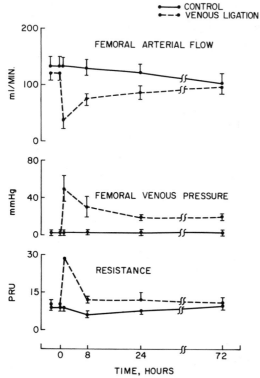

Figure 8–9. Femoral arterial blood flow, femoral venous pressure and peripheral resistance in the canine hindlimb are compared immediately and at 8, 24 and 72 hours after femoral venous ligation (dashed line) with control values from the opposite hindlimb (solid line). Data are presented as a mean ± standard and show an initial marked reduction in femoral arterial flow with a gradual return to normal within 72 hours, as well as changes in femoral venous pressure and resistance. (Hobson, R. W., II, Howard, E. W., Wright, C. B., Collins, G. J., and Rich, N. M., Surgery, 74:824, 1973.)

symposium on venous trauma (Swan et al., 1975).

CLINICAL FEATURES

Most venous injuries occur in the extremities, principally because the relatively superficial location of many veins makes them more vulnerable to injury (Table 8–7). Usually there is dark, steady bleeding from the wound instead of the bright red spurting blood of an arterial injury. In a closed wound, a massive hematoma may develop. Such a hematoma, of course, also

TABLE 8–7. FREQUENCY OF CONCOMITANT VENOUS INJURIES ASSOCIATED WITH ACUTE ARTERIAL TRAUMA*

ARTERY	NUMBER	VENOUS INJURIES	PER CENT
Axillary	59	20	33.8
Brachial	283	54	19.0
Iliac	26	11	42.3
Common femoral	46	17	36.9
Superficial femoral	305	139	45.5
Popliteal	217	116	53.5
Total	936	357	37.9

*Modified from Rich, N. M., Hughes, C. W., and Baugh, J. H., Ann. Surg., 171:724, 1970.

results from trauma to multiple small vessels or from arterial trauma. Consequently, many venous injuries often are first recognized at surgical exploration.

Acute venous insufficiency following arterial trauma may evolve in the first 12 to 24 hours. Massive edema and a cool, bluish extremity are the principal clinical findings. The clinical pattern of chronic venous insufficiency, a familiar one because of the frequency of thrombophlebitis in surgical patients, includes edema, varices, brown pigmentation of the skin and stasis ulcers.

DIAGNOSTIC CONSIDERATIONS

Roentgenograms may be of help in identifying a missile or the path of a missile near a major vein. Fractures also may be disclosed, which may be associated with venous injuries. Venography has seldom been used for diagnosis but may be useful in certain instances. Reynolds and Balsano (1971) used pelvic venography with simultaneous injections in the femoral vein to demonstrate integrity of the iliac vein in 25 patients with pelvic fractures. Gerlock and associates (1976) evaluated penetrating injuries of the extremities.

The Doppler ultrasound unit may become a useful diagnostic tool in the management of venous disease. Experiences with 210 patients were reported by Siegel and co-workers in 1968, who compared findings using the Doppler unit with observations from venography, operation or autopsy. The clinical diagnosis of thrombosis was accurate in only 5 per cent of the cases,

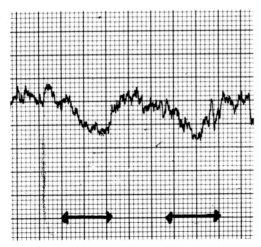

Figure 8-10. This recording from the ultrasonic sounding device (Doppler) demonstrates normal flow through the left femoral vein during deep respiration in a patient who had a lateral repair of a laceration of the femoral vein. (Rich, N. M., Hughes, C. W., and Baugh, J. H., Ann. Surg., *171*:724, 1970.)

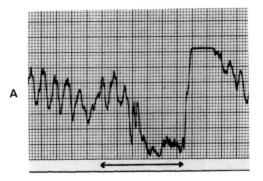

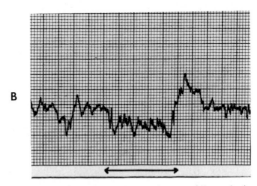

Figure 8-12. The ultrasonic sounding device (Doppler) records normal depression with rapid elevation (A) of the right common femoral vein after the Valsalva maneuver. In contrast, this characteristic flow pattern was absent (B) when the Doppler was placed over the left common femoral vein above the occluded femoropopliteal veins (see Fig. 8-13). (Rich, N. M., Hughes, C. W., and Baugh, J. H., Ann. Surg., *171*:724, 1970.)

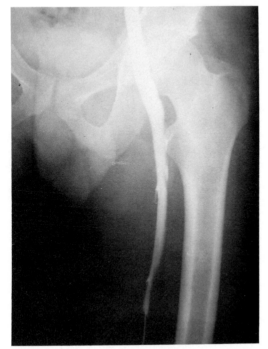

Figure 8-11. To substantiate the Doppler impression of patency of the left femoral vein (see Fig. 8-10), this venogram was performed, and it demonstrated wide patency. (Rich, N. M., Hughes, C. W., and Baugh, J. H., Ann. Surg., *171*:724, 1970.)

whereas the Doppler examination was accurate in 86 per cent. A diagnosis of deep vein valvular incompetence was only 15 per cent accurate on clinical examination and 97 per cent by Doppler examination. The device has also been of value in determining patency of venous repairs, especially in the lower extremities (Rich et al., 1970 B). An ultrasound tracing is shown in Figure 8-10 that demonstrates normal flow through a femoral vein during deep inspiration. Patency of the vein was confirmed with a venogram (Fig. 8-11). The contrast in flow pattern over patent and occluded veins during a Valsalva maneuver is shown in Figures 8-12 and 8-13. At present the Doppler unit is frequently used at Walter Reed Army Medical Center.

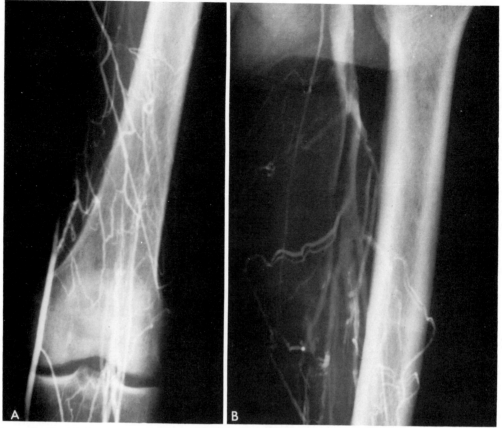

Figure 8–13. (A) Occlusion of the left greater saphenous vein and the superficial femoral vein is demonstrated by phlebography. Some small venous channels have appeared. (B) Venous collaterals can carry flow from the lower extremity and re-establish flow in the left common femoral and iliac veins (see Doppler tracings in Fig. 8–12). (Rich, N. M., Hughes, C. W., and Baugh, J. H., Ann. Surg., *171*:724, 1970.)

SURGICAL TREATMENT

I recently closed an opening three-eighths of an inch long in the common jugular with five continuous silk sutures. Small openings in veins have frequently been closed with lateral suture.

Despite the above quote recorded over 70 years ago (Murphy, 1897), there have been few reports devoted exclusively to the management of major venous injuries (Gaspar and Treiman, 1960; Rich et al., 1970 B). A collective review of experimental and clinical evaluation of grafts in the venous system was published by Haimovici and coworkers in 1970. A 1973 symposium on experiences with lower extremity venous trauma was reported by Swan and colleagues (1975).

As this is the only chapter in this monograph specifically concerned with venous injuries, some principles of resuscitation are emphasized here which are also presented in other chapters concerned with arterial injuries. This repetition is done for the convenience of the reader, concentrating all material on venous injuries in one chapter.

GENERAL CONSIDERATIONS AND RESUSCITATION

Shock is common, especially if active hemorrhage is still present. As with arterial injuries, multiple injuries are frequent, so complete examination should be done promptly. Hemorrhage can usually be controlled by judicious pressure or packing, except with penetrating injuries of the body cavities. In such instances immediate operation may be necessary before profound shock can be controlled. Shock should be treated by rapid infusion of whole blood and appropriate electrolyte solutions. Antibiotics should be given routinely. At operation adequate wound débridement is essential, just as with any violent trauma. Often arterial and venous injuries are both present, raising the question of which should be repaired first. Normally the injured artery should be required first to minimize anoxia in the distal extremity. In some instances, though, it may be more expeditious to repair the venous injury first, either for hemostasis or for better exposure of the arterial injury.

At least five different methods of repair may be considered for venous injuries (Rich et al., 1975 F). These are listed in order of popularity of use:

1. Ligation
2. Lateral suture repair
3. End-to-end anastomosis
4. Venous patch graft
5. Venous replacement graft

Ligation, of course, has been used for most injuries. Most clinical data at present are concerned with techniques of lateral suture repair. It should be emphasized that there is a great lack of data concerning other techniques, such as end-to-end anastomoses, patch grafts or venous replacement grafts. Though theoretically satisfactory, there are not enough data presently available to estimate the likelihood of success of a venous replacement graft inserted for injuries in different parts of the body.

The surgical incision should be adequate to expose the vein proximal and distal to the point of injury. If the entrance and exit wounds cannot be extended for exposure, an elective incision should be made over the course of the injured vein and the vein isolated proximal and distal to the point of injury. Copious irrigation with saline is useful for both visualization and removal of foreign material. Bleeding can usually be controlled temporarily with digital pressure until clot and debris have been irrigated away. The combination of encircling tapes and a tourniquet is a simple, atraumatic form of control which may be preferable to vascular clamps if exposure is limited. With tangential injuries of large veins, a partial occluding vascular clamp, such as a Satinsky or a Cooley clamp, may be used.

This avoids the necessity of wider mobilization of the vein and also permits the flow of blood to continue.

Before repair is started, the vein should be explored both proximally and distally for thrombi. The Fogarty balloon catheter is most useful, though occasional difficulty is encountered during retrograde insertion because of competent valves. Gentle manipulation is necessary to avoid perforation. If venous occlusion is necessary for a long time, heparin should be administered locally or systemically.

During reconstruction meticulous technique is crucial. This is more critical than with arterial injuries because of the greater tendency for venous repairs to thrombose. A fine synthetic vascular suture on a small needle will minimize bleeding from needle holes. As the suture is drawn through the lumen, care should be taken to prevent drawing strands of adventitia into the lumen, which may become a nidus for a thrombus. When a continuous suture is used, less tension is applied than that employed in an arterial anastomosis so as to avoid circular construction. Leaving the loops of a continuous suture somewhat loose may create a few leaks, but bleeding will usually stop with mild pressure. The apparent simplicity of venous repair often deceives the inexperienced operator, who may feel the problem to be simpler than the more frightening arterial repair with violent hemorrhage and threatened loss of the extremity. Actually, the necessity for a more meticulous technique is one reason why thrombosis is more common with the inexperienced operator. As opportunity for clinical experience is limited, practice with experimental models is of considerable value.

With lateral suture repair, as with arterial repairs, the principal consideration is to avoid undue constriction of the lumen. A typical experience is shown in Figure 8–14 with lateral repair of an injury of the popliteal vein. Occasionally, autogenous venous patches may be useful.

When repair cannot be done by lateral suture, reconstruction by either end-to-end anastomosis or insertion of a vascular graft can be considered. As mentioned earlier, data are yet inadequate to be certain of the

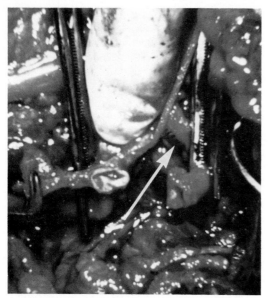

Figure 8-14. This operative photograph demonstrates a lateral suture repair of the popliteal vein (arrow) that was carried out prior to repair of the artery at the 2nd Surgical Hospital in Vietnam in 1966. (N.M.R.)

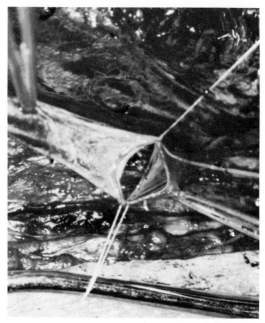

Figure 8-15. This photograph demonstrates the use of two sutures in performing a venous end-to-end anastomosis, which is carried out in a continuous fashion. Surgeons who are successful with this technique in the experimental model will have an improved success rate in the clinical situation (Rich, N. M., Hobson, R. W., II, Wright, C. B. and Swan, K. G., *in* Swan, et al. (Eds.), Venous Surgery in the Lower Extremity. Warren H. Green Publishers, Inc., St. Louis, 1975.)

effectiveness of either type of reconstruction in different areas of the body, although isolated experiences thus far are encouraging.

VENOUS GRAFTS

The only truly satisfactory venous graft is an autogenous one. A great deal of experimental work has been done to investigate other materials, including Teflon, Dacron, bovine heterografts, pericardium, peritoneum, intestine, homografts and various newer synthetics (Haimovici et al., 1970; Swan et al., 1975). Synthetic grafts are usually considered in the repair of large veins, usually the inferior or superior vena cava.

When a graft is used, tension must be scrupulously avoided because of the susceptibility of the low pressure venous system to constriction and thrombosis (Fig. 8-15). Hence, a graft should be chosen that appears a bit longer than necessary. Various maneuvers can be used if there is a disparity in the size of the graft and the recipient vein. Several of these are shown in Figure 8-16, including "fishmouthing" the end.

Cutting the graft and vein diagonally or cutting through a major tributary are other methods of increasing the diameter. One of the clinical problems associated with the use of autogenous venous grafts is shown in Figure 8-17. Even using the technique of "fishmouthing" on the small autogenous vein graft placed into a larger recipient vein, a smaller diameter still existed in the graft. Turbulence and eddying result and are factors that contribute to the thrombosis of this type of graft.

REPAIR OF VENA CAVA INJURIES

As mentioned earlier, most interest in grafts has been in their use for reconstruction of the venae cavae; there is no acceptable autogenous vein graft for these large vessels. Good long-term results have been obtained, however, by making composite

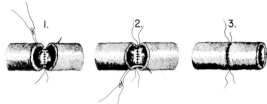

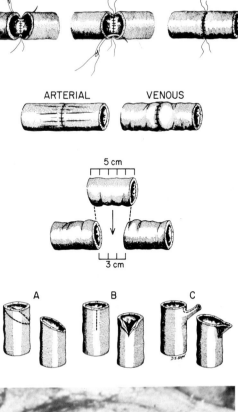

Figure 8–16. These drawings outline principles that have been useful in performing venous anastomoses. The loops of a continuous suture line should be left somewhat more loose than those used in an arterial suture line to prevent constriction. Venous replacements should be longer than the area lost and approximately the same diameter. Diagonal cuts, "fishmouthing" and use of a branch can help prevent stenosis at a suture line, particularly when the graft is smaller than the recipient vein. (Rich, N. M., Hobson, R. W., II, Wright, C. B., and Swan, K. G., *in* Swan, K. G., et al. (Eds.), Venous Surgery in the Lower Extremity. Warren H. Green Publishers, Inc., St. Louis, 1975.)

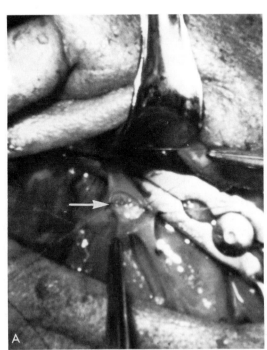

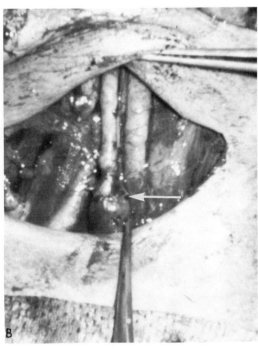

Figure 8–17. This operative photograph demonstrates some of the clinical problems involved in attempting to place a much smaller autogenous vein graft in a large recipient vein. Even when techniques such as "fish mouthing" are used (A), the ends of the graft and the smaller diameter of the graft (B) contribute to turbulence and eddying of flow with subsequent thrombosis. (Rich, N. M., Hobson, R. W., II, Wright, C. B., and Swan, K. G., *in* Swan, K. G., et al. (Eds.), Venous Surgery in the Lower Extremity. Warren H. Green Publishers, Inc., St. Louis, 1975.)

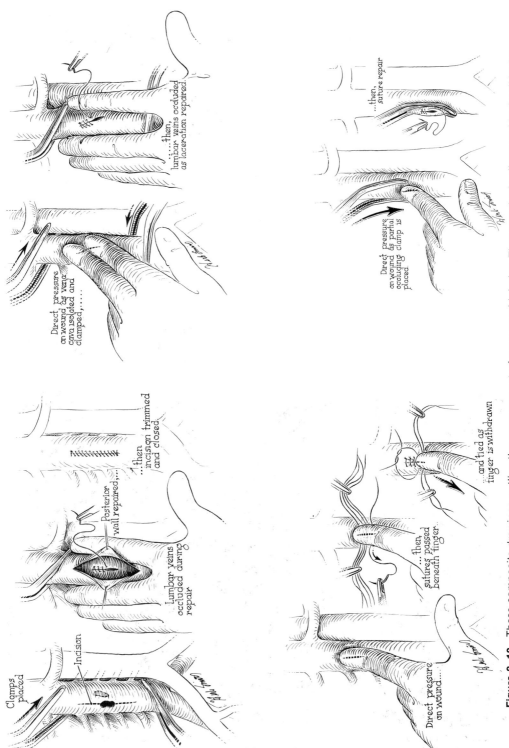

Figure 8–18 These composite drawings outline the management of vena caval injuries. These methods, discussed in detail in the text, can be utilized in injuries to the large vein. (Quast, D. C., Shirkey, A. L., Fitzgerald, J. B., Beall, A. C., Jr., and DeBakey, M. E., J. Trauma, 5:3, 1965, The Williams & Wilkins Co., Baltimore.)

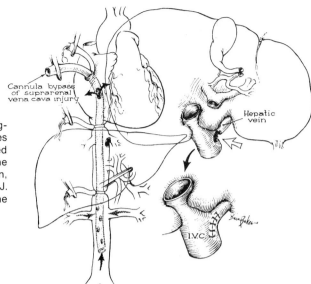

Figure 8–19. Similar to the method originally described by Schrock and associates (1968), an internal vena caval shunt is used during repair of the hepatic portion of the inferior vena cava. (Bricker, D. L., Morton, J. R., Okies, J. E., and Beall, A. C., Jr., J. Trauma, *11*:725, 1971. Copyright 1971, the Williams & Wilkins Co., Baltimore.)

grafts from two or three segments of saphenous vein opened longitudinally and then sewn together to make a single graft of larger diameter.

Haimovici and colleagues in 1970 emphasized that the patency of grafts in the venous system was considerably higher in the superior vena cava and its tributaries than in the inferior vena cava. This may be because higher pressure is developed in the more dependent venous system.

With injury of the vena cava, the mortality rates remain high. Quast and co-workers (1965) reported an overall mortality rate of 49 per cent among 69 patients with such injuries. These authors outlined a number of techniques that can be considered with lacerations of the inferior vena cava as illustrated in Figure 8–18. Schrock and co-authors in 1968 and Bricker and colleagues in 1971 both described an internal vena cava shunt to maintain venous return during repair. This is needed for injury of the cava proximal to the point of entry of the renal veins. This shunt, introduced through the right atrium, is illustrated in Figure 8–19.

PERTINENT EXPERIMENTAL STUDIES

Since experience with the repair of venous injuries is still evolving, pertinent experimental studies over the past 25 years are briefly summarized here. In 1947 Johns helped to stimulate a renewed interest in venous grafts when he reported an experimental study of suture and nonsuture methods for venous anastomoses. Collins and Douglass (1964) utilized operative microscopic methods in an attempt to improve the technique of small venous anastomoses. Waddell and associates (1964), using the National Research Council–Vogelfanger vascular stapler, cross-exchanged short segments of valve-bearing autogenous and homologous vein segments in dogs. McLachlin and colleagues (1965) also used the stapling apparatus with vein grafts containing competent valves to replace an incompetent valve segment. Cerino and co-workers (1964) showed that small caliber femoral autogenous vein grafts remained patent in most experiments, and patency progressively improved with experience. Earle and co-workers (1960) described the technique of obtaining a graft with a wider lumen by suturing short segments together (Fig. 8–20). Benvenuto and colleagues (1962) recommended a slight variation in composite venous autografts by using multiple segments in a similar procedure. Unfortunately, there is a distressing lack of follow-up data with many of these techniques of forming compilation vein grafts, so they remain simply experimental concepts.

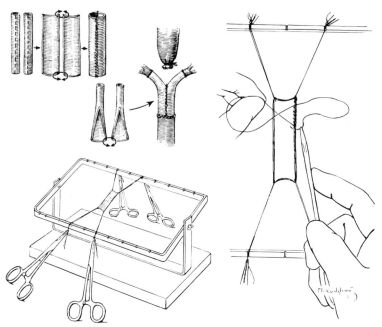

Figure 8–20. The compilation graft is a method of obtaining a wider lumen from autogenous vein grafts by suturing short segments together. There is, however, minimal clinical experience reported with the compilation graft. (Earle, A. S., Horshey, J. S., Villavicencio, J. L., and Warren, R., Arch. Surg., *80*:119, 1960. Copyright 1960, American Medical Association.)

An important concept was introduced by Hardin in 1962 when he used a graft of saphenous vein to relieve chronic venous obstruction (Fig. 8–21). This method was further developed by Dale in 1966 in his technique of cross-over saphenofemoral bypass to relieve iliofemoral occlusion (Fig. 8–22). The technique included dissection of the greater saphenous vein on the contralateral side, with division of the vein in the distal thigh. It was then irrigated with heparinized saline, brought upward, passed through a suprapubic tunnel, and connected to the common femoral vein with an end-to-side anastomosis.

In 1967 Turney showed remarkable ingenuity in the application of this technique in an unusual injury in Vietnam:

. . . gunshot wound of the left groin, completely transecting the femoral artery at the bifurcation associated with complete transection of the common femoral vein. There was a fracture of the femur which was débrided. We then used a segment of the left saphenous vein to connect the common femoral to the superficial femoral artery. After the blood was turned back into the leg it became grossly enlarged on the operating

table because there was no venous drainage. Since the left common femoral vein had been ligated above the inguinal ligament, it was my feeling that a cross-over vein graft would give better drainage. Therefore the right greater saphenous vein was dissected and tunneled subcutaneously over the pubis and anastomosed end-to-end into the left femoral vein. Following this the leg returned to normal size with a pink color. In three days delayed primary closure of the wound was done and I personally saw the venous anastomosis which was obviously patent at that time.

A number of adjuvant measures have been employed to improve the patency of grafts in the venous system, including the administration of anticoagulants, Dextran, or fibrinolytic agents, and the use of sympathectomy and distal arteriovenous fistulas (Figs. 8–23 and 8–24). The practicality of these methods remains questionable (Swan et al., 1975). Johnson and Eiseman (1969) and Rabinowitz and Goldfarb (1971) have employed a temporary arteriovenous fistula during venous reconstruction. It was Johnson and Eiseman who presented the first clinical use of an arterio-

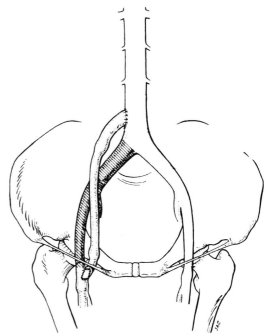

Figure 8–21. This diagrammatic illustration of the operative technique of bypass saphenous grafts for the relief of venous obstruction of the lower extremity was outlined for patients who had venous occlusion secondary to both disease and injury. Patent follow-up venograms demonstrated successful results. (Hardin, C. A., Surg. Gynecol. Obstet., *115*: 709, 1962.)

venous fistula to maintain patency of a graft in the venous system. Their patient was a 51 year old woman who had bilateral varicose vein strippings during which the left common femoral vein was ligated to control bleeding. Because the patient had severe swelling and pain in the left leg and thigh, an 8 cm segment of thrombosed common femoral vein was excised four months later, and a segment of internal jugular vein was inserted as a vein graft. Blood flow appeared to be sluggish in the autograft; there-

Figure 8–22. The technique of crossover vein grafting (the Palma operation). Used for chronic venous occlusion, it can also be applied to some acute venous injuries. (Dale, W. A., Surgery, *59*:117, 1966.)

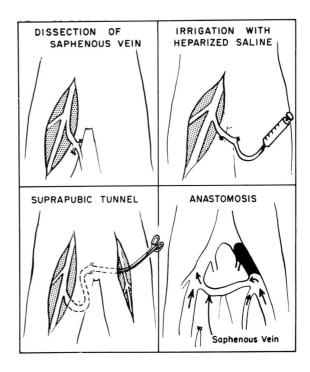

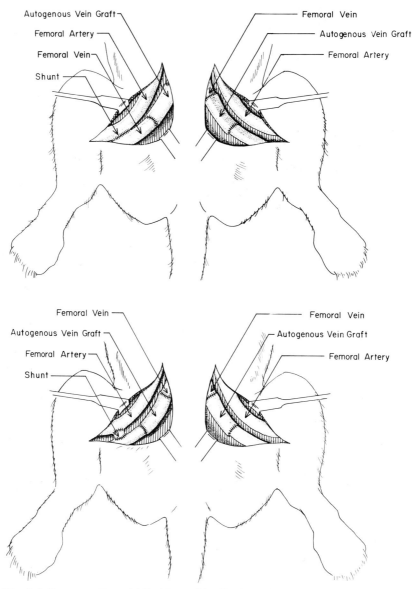

Figure 8–23. Artist's conception of (A) side-to-side distal arteriovenous shunt in the canine right lower extremity with the left side acting as the control, and (B) H-type distal arteriovenous shunt in the canine right lower extremity with a control vein graft on the left side. These models were used in experimental work at Walter Reed Army Institute of Research in an attempt to determine the value of distal arteriovenous fistulas in improving the patency rate in venous reconstruction. (Levin, P. M., Rich, N. M., Hutton, J. E., Jr., Barker, W. F., and Zeller, J. A., Am. J. Surg., *122*:183, 1971.)

fore it was decided to use a Dacron graft measuring 2 cm in length and 8 mm in diameter to create an H-type arteriovenous fistula between the superficial femoral artery and vein 4 cm distal to the venograft. The venograft immediately swelled and remained turgid with the increased blood flow. The leg was temporarily swollen until the arteriovenous shunt was removed after three weeks. Thereafter, pain and swelling subsided rapidly, and a venogram performed seven months later revealed patency of the venous graft. Rabinowitz and Goldfarb (1971) reported a case of a pa-

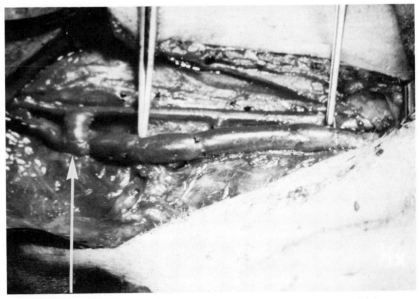

Figure 8–24. Operative photograph showing the H-type arteriovenous fistula, which measures approximately 1 cm in length and 8 mm in diameter (arrow), constructed approximately 2 to 3 cm distal to the suture line of the vein graft (between two vascular forceps) in the femoral vein of the canine model. Patency of the autogenous vein graft in the venous system was enhanced by the adjuvant distal arteriovenous fistula. (Rich, N. M., Levin, P. M., and Hutton, J. E., Jr., *in* Swan, K. E., et al. (Eds.), Venous Surgery in the Lower Extremity. Warren H. Green Publishers, Inc., St. Louis, 1975.)

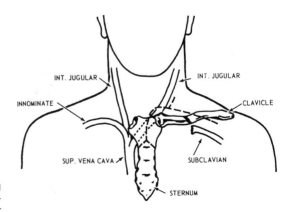

Figure 8–25. Schematic diagram demonstrating the operative procedure utilized to relieve obstruction of a left subclavian vein. The left internal jugular vein was mobilized and anastomosed in an end-to-end fashion to the distal left subclavian vein. (Witte, C. L., and Smith, C. A., Arch. Surg., *93*:664, 1966. Copyright 1966, American Medical Association.)

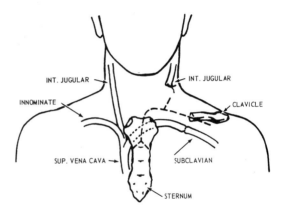

tient with an axillosubclavian venous thrombosis. An autogenous saphenous vein graft was interposed between the distal axillary vein and the proximal internal jugular vein. In addition, an arteriovenous fistula was constructed between the distal right radial artery and the basilic vein. Three weeks after the operation, the arteriovenous fistula was closed because of the decrease in swelling and pain. A venogram performed four months after the original procedure was interpreted to show a patent graft slightly larger than the majority of veins in the basilic venous system. There may be some theoretic disadvantages to the use of the distal arteriovenous fistula (Levin et al., 1971; Hobson et al., 1973).

Ingenuity of some of the venous repairs has been emphasized in case reports. The report by Witte and Smith (1966) represents a successful example. Their patient had a fractured clavicle with resultant obstruction of the left subclavian vein (Fig. 8–25). When they explored the left supraclavicular fossa, the subclavian vein was found enmeshed in callus near the original fracture site. The left internal jugular vein was mobilized and divided high in the neck, after which it was anastomosed in an end-to-end fashion to the distal subclavian vein. Over a nine-month follow-up, during which the patient was engaged in heavy lifting, he had no arm pain or swelling. Follow-up venography demonstrated patency of the anastomosis (Fig. 8–26).

Operative venography is an adjunct that may be of value during reconstruction because palpation is less valuable in venous reconstructions than it is in arterial recon-

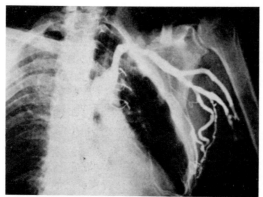
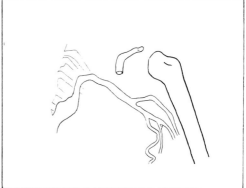
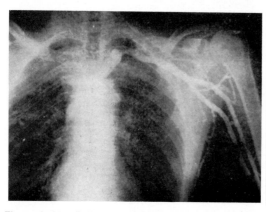
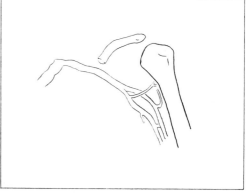

Figure 8–26. Follow-up venograms at three weeks and nine months demonstrate patency of an end-to-end internal jugulosubclavian vein shunt. Note the absence of collateral venous channels that were present on the preoperative studies when the left subclavian vein was occluded. (Witte, C. L., and Smith, C. A., Arch. Surg., 93:664, 1966. Copyright 1966, American Medical Association.)

TABLE 8–8. THE REPAIR OF SEVEN VEIN INJURIES IN KOREA*

Vein Injured	Number	Method of Repair	Result
Common femoral	2	1 Lateral suture	Viable extremity
		1 Venous homograft	Gangrene
Superficial femoral	1	Lateral suture	Gangrene
Popliteal	4	Lateral suture	Viable extremities

*Modified from Spencer, F. C., and Grewe, R. V., Ann. Surg., *141*:304, 1955.

structions. With a venogram, either a stenotic area or a residual thrombus within the lumen may be found.

POSTOPERATIVE CARE

In addition to general supportive care of associated injuries, specific attempts should be made after operation to minimize or eliminate edema of the involved extremity. This is particularly true when large veins, especially the inferior vena cava, have been ligated. Early and vigorous postoperative care to prevent massive edema should be started promptly, employing both elevation of the legs and careful wrapping with elastic support. Subsequently, as the patient ambulates, continued elastic support is not often needed above the knee. Disability from chronic venous insufficiency can be greatly minimized by early effective use of elastic support. This requires frequent inspection and periodic adjustment of both the type and degree of support. This simple factor is probably mismanaged more often than any other form of supportive care in patients with chronic venous insufficiency.

RESULTS

The data of one of the first reports regarding the method of venous repair and immediate results were derived from experiences during the Korean Conflict (Table 8–8) (Spencer and Grewe, 1955). These observations were noted:

Massive venous occlusion appeared to be the chief cause of gangrene in three cases. Extensive soft tissue injuries had destroyed most of the large veins, including the long and short saphenous veins and popliteal vein. Massive edema

appearing after arterial repair progressed to gangrene within 48 to 72 hours. The arterial tree was demonstrated to be patent in the amputated extremity. There was widespread dilatation and congestion of the distal venous bed.

All of the four extremities survived in which the popliteal artery and vein were repaired, but the number of cases is too small to permit any conclusions regarding value of the venous repair. Postoperative venograms were not made. There were no instances of pulmonary embolism.

In a summation of the Korean conflict experience, Hughes (1958) reported a total of 20 venous repairs (Table 8–9). All were done by lateral suture except for one end-to-end anastomosis.

In the report of civilian experience by Gaspar and Treiman in 1960, 10 lacerations were repaired by lateral suture; these represented only one-fifth of the 52 injuries encountered. Six of these ten were for injuries of the inferior vena cava. All but one of the patients recovered, apparently with a good result from the venous reconstruction. In the remaining cases, 27 ligations were performed, with a good result in 21. Six could not be evaluated because of three deaths from associated injuries and three amputations due to concomitant arterial injury. For various reasons the venous injury was not treated in 15 patients, eight of whom

TABLE 8–9. VENOUS REPAIR: KOREAN CONFLICT EXPERIENCE*

Type of Repair	Number	Per Cent
Lateral suture	19	95
End-to-end anastomosis	1	5
Total	20	100

*Modified from Hughes, C. W., Ann. Surg., *147*:555, 1958.

TABLE 8–10. MANAGEMENT OF 92 VENOUS WOUNDS*

OPERATION	(1948-1958) NUMBER	(1948-1958) PER CENT	(1958-1963) NUMBER	(1958-1963) PER CENT
Simple ligation	27	52	14	35
Repair	10	19	19	48
Direct anastomosis	0		2	
Lateral suture repair	10		16	
Other	0		1	
No exploration	15	29	7	17
Total	52	100	40	100

*Modified from Treiman, R. L., Doty, D., and Gaspar, M., Am. J. Surg., *111*:469, 1966.

subsequently developed arteriovenous fistulas, which probably could have been avoided if exploration had been done. A supplemental report was published by Treiman and associates in 1966, by which time repair was being utilized in nearly 50 per cent of venous injuries encountered. Experiences with the total series of 92 injuries are shown in Table 8–10.

In Vietnam, approximately one-third of the venous injuries were repaired (Table 8–11) (Rich et al., 1970 B). This was confirmed by both the initial and interim Registry reports. Interest was concentrated particularly on major veins in the lower extremities (Table 8–12). Eighty-five per cent of the repairs were by lateral suture (Table 8–13). As experience increased, end-to-end anastomoses and autogenous vein grafts were used more frequently. Unfortunately, the effectiveness of these methods of reconstruction cannot be precisely measured without late venograms. Though of no statistical significance, important information has been obtained through the Registry at Walter Reed Army Medical Center about specific cases. Several are illustrated as follows: (1) patency of superficial femoral vein one month following lateral repair (Fig. 8–27); (2) patency of common femoral

vein repaired by lateral suture both anteriorly and posteriorly with resulting constriction (Fig. 8–28); and patency of superficial femoral vein repaired with autogenous saphenous vein patch graft (Fig. 8–29). Not all repairs were successful, as shown in the following illustrations: (1) thrombosis of end-to-end popliteal venous repair (Fig. 8–30); (2) thrombosis of an end-to-end anastomosis between greater saphenous vein and superficial femoral vein (Fig. 8–31); and (3) thrombosis of a saphenous vein graft inserted in the superficial femoral vein (Fig. 8–32). Figure 8–33 demonstrates the problem of chronic venous insufficiency following ligation of the right popliteal vein. There is inadequate development of venous collateral circulation, and the patient has signs of severe, chronic venous insufficiency.

Sullivan and co-workers (1971), working at the 12th Evacuation Hospital in Vietnam, performed perhaps the most significant study on the management of injuries of the popliteal vein. In a group of 35 popliteal vascular injuries, there were 27 injuries of the popliteal vein, 21 of which were repaired. Venograms were performed on 11 patients within the first 72 hours after operation which showed a patent repair in eight. Figure 8–34 shows patency of an end-to-end anastomosis, while Figures 8–35 and 8–36 show patency of an autogenous vein graft. Perhaps of even greater importance was the finding that massive edema did not occur in any of the 21 patients who had primary repair of the venous injury, compared with severe venous insufficiency and morbidity in four patients in whom the vein was ligated.

Fitchett and co-workers in 1969 described experiences with 10 patients who had incurred trauma to the internal jugular vein.

TABLE 8–11. REPAIR OF VENOUS INJURIES—VIETNAM VASCULAR REGISTRY*

REGISTRY	INJURIES	REPAIRS	PER CENT
Initial report	194	64	32.9
Interim report	377	124	32.9

*Modified from Rich, N. M., Hughes, C. W., and Baugh, J. H., Ann. Surg., *171*:724, 1970.

TABLE 8–12. METHODS OF MANAGING VENOUS TRAUMA: LOCATION OF VASCULAR INJURIES—INTERIM VIETNAM VASCULAR REGISTRY REPORT*

LOCATION		ARTERIES	CONCOMITANT VEINS	LIGATION	REPAIR
Neck	Carotid	50	14	10	4
Chest	Innominate	3	1	0	1
	Subclavian	8	4	1	3
Upper extremity	Axillary	59	20	18	2
	Brachial	283	54	42	12
Abdomen and pelvis	Abdominal aorta	3	1	0	1
	Common iliac	9	6	6	0
	External iliac	17	5	3	2
Lower extremity	Common femoral	46	17	8	9
	Superficial femoral	305	139	83	56
	Popliteal	217	116	82	34
Total		1000	377	253	124

*Modified from Rich, N. M., Hughes, C. W., and Baugh, J. H., Ann. Surg., *171*:724, 1970.

Nine of the 10 were treated by ligation, while lateral repair was done in one. There were no significant sequelae. As ligation of the internal jugular vein is well tolerated, it would seem pointless to attempt repair if anything more complicated than lateral suture is necessary.

It is remarkable that there were no known cases of pulmonary embolization recognized after venous repair in the initial Vietnam series, which included 124 reconstructions (Rich et al., 1970 B). In a later follow-up evaluation, nonfatal pulmonary emboli have been seen infrequently. One patient had repair by lateral suture of a lacteration of the common and superficial femoral veins. Ten days later, after his evacuation to Japan, a venogram showed thrombosis at the site of repair. He had clinical signs of a small pulmonary embolus, later substantiated by a lung scan.

Text continued on page 186

TABLE 8–13. REPAIR OF VENOUS INJURIES—INTERIM VIETNAM VASCULAR REGISTRY REPORT*

TYPE OF REPAIR	NUMBER	PER CENT
Lateral suture	106	85.5
End-to-end anastomosis	10	8.1
Vein interposition graft	5	4.0
Vein patch graft	3	2.4
Total	124	100.0

*Modified from Rich, N. M., Hughes, C. W., and Baugh, J. H., Ann. Surg., *171*:724, 1970.

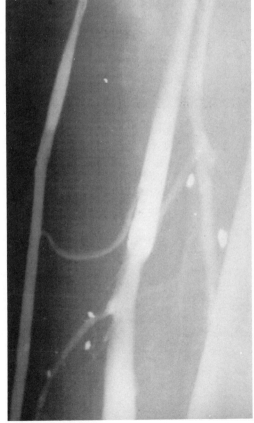

Figure 8–27. Patency of the superficial femoral vein is demonstrated by phlebography approximately one month after repair in a 20 year old Vietnam casualty who developed a superficial femoral arteriovenous fistula from multiple fragment wounds. (Rich, N. M., Hughes, C. W., and Baugh, J. H., Ann. Surg., *171*:724, 1970.)

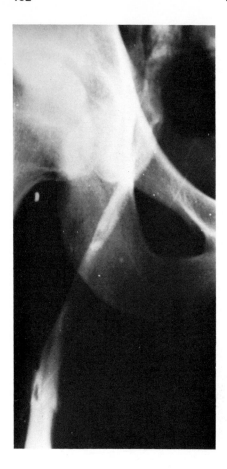

Figure 8-28. Although there is a constriction at the common femoral vein repair site, adequate flow is demonstrated by phlebography. Note the absence of any venous collaterals. Suture of an anterior and posterior laceration caused by a small, low velocity fragment was successful in this patient. (Rich, N. M., Hughes, C. W., and Baugh, J. H., Ann. Surg., *171*: 724, 1970.)

Figure 8-29. The distal superficial femoral vein in this patient was repaired with an autogenous greater saphenous vein patch graft. This venogram shows successful repair and the patency of the vein at the junction with the popliteal vein. (Rich, N. M., Hughes, C. W., and Baugh, J. H., Ann. Surg., *171*:724, 1970.)

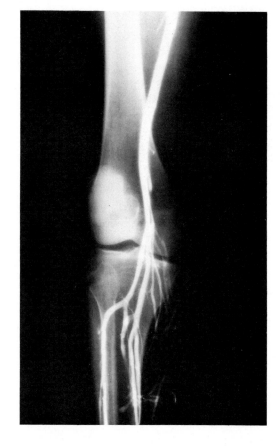

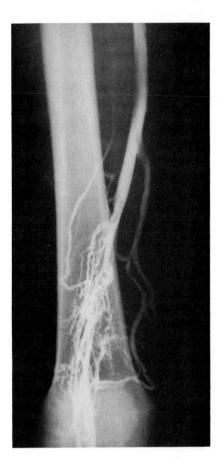

Figure 8–30. Thrombosis of an end-to-end vein repair of the popliteal vein is demonstrated in this venogram. Although there appears to be adequate venous collateral flow, this patient initially had significant pedal edema. (Rich, N. M., Hughes, C. W., and Baugh, J. H., Ann. Surg., *171*:724, 1970.)

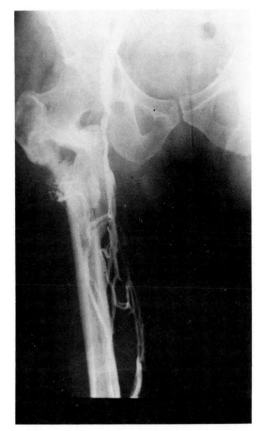

Figure 8–31. By use of the subtraction technique, good venous collateral circulation is seen one year after an attempt was made to restore venous return by end-to-end anastomosis of the greater saphenous vein to the superficial femoral vein. This repair was performed in Vietnam in 1967 by Dr. Paul M. James. (Rich, N. M., Hughes, C. W., and Baugh, J. H., Ann. Surg., *171*:724, 1970.)

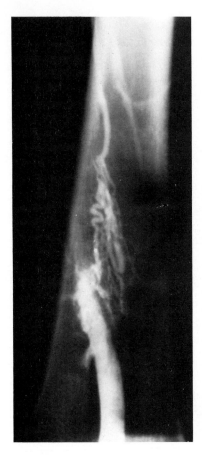

Figure 8–32. The autogenous greater saphenous vein graft to the superficial femoral vein was occluded, as demonstrated in this venogram obtained 3½ months after repair. Deep collateral veins, as well as a patent superficial venous system, were adequate, and the patient had no significant edema clinically. (Rich, N. M., Hughes, C. W., and Baugh, J. H., Ann. Surg., *171*:724, 1970.)

Figure 8–33. After ligation of the right popliteal vein, this venogram demonstrated poor venous collateral return. The patient had persistent pedal edema and will have additional difficulties in the future from chronic venous insufficiency. (Rich, N. M., Hughes, C. W., and Baugh, J. H., Ann. Surg., *171*:724, 1970.)

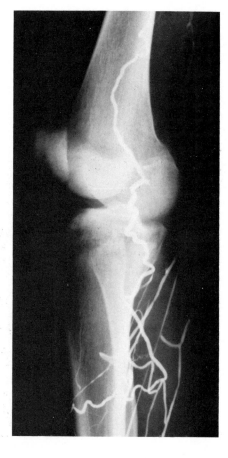

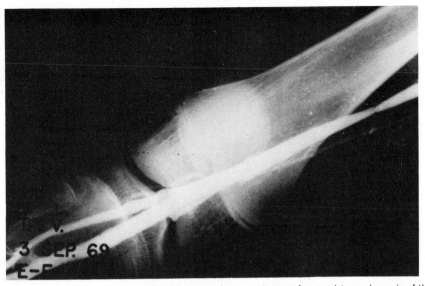

Figure 8–34. This venogram performed in Vietnam shows patency of an end-to-end repair of the popliteal vein four days later. (Sullivan, W. G., Thornton, F. H., Baker, L. H., LaPlante, E. S., and Cohen, A., Am. J. Surg., *122*:528, 1971.)

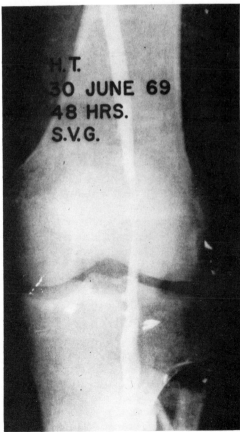

Figure 8–35. The above venogram was obtained 48 hours after an autogenous vein graft repair of the popliteal vein. The artery had been repaired by end-to-end anastomosis. (Sullivan, W. G., Thornton, F. H., Baker, L. H., LaPlante, E. S., and Cohen, A., Am. J. Surg., *122*: 528, 1971.)

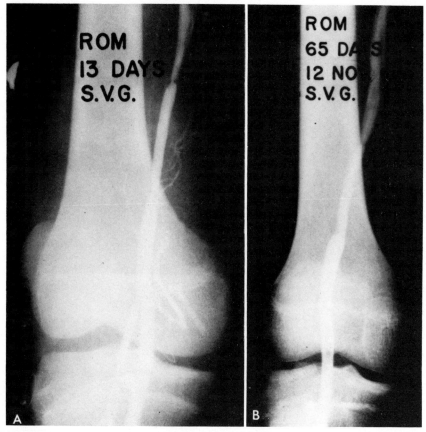

Figure 8–36. These two venograms were performed at the 12th Evacuation Hospital in Vietnam in 1969. Patency of the autogenous saphenous vein grafts in the popliteal vein was demonstrated at 13 days (A) and 65 days (B). The popliteal artery had also been repaired with a vein graft. There had been extensive soft tissue trauma in the popliteal area, and the saphenous vein had also been destroyed. (Sullivan, W. G., Thornton, F. H., Baker, L. H., LaPlante, E. S., and Cohen, A., Am. J. Surg., *122*:528, 1971.)

In this regard it should be remembered that the sequelae following ligation, principally stasis and phlebitis, can also result in pulmonary embolism. In the series reported by Gaspar and Treiman (1960), thrombophlebitis developed in three of 21 patients after ligation, a frequency of about 15 per cent.

FOLLOW-UP

As mentioned earlier in this chapter, valid statistical data are still badly needed to determine the best method of venous repair, especially when end-to-end venous anastomoses of vein grafts are required. Only by such long term evaluation can the

reliability of different types of venous reconstruction be determined. Figure 8–37 demonstrates patency of a compilation graft of autogenous greater saphenous vein used successfully to repair a defect in the left common femoral vein. Although it is important to know that this repair was successful in the immediate postoperative period, it is also important to know whether long term patency can be anticipated.

The second important area in which long term data are needed is frequency of significant venous insufficiency following ligation. As venous insufficiency may not develop for several years, often after repeated episodes of phlebitis induced by stasis from the original vein ligation, long periods of observation are necessary. Another consideration is the possibility of

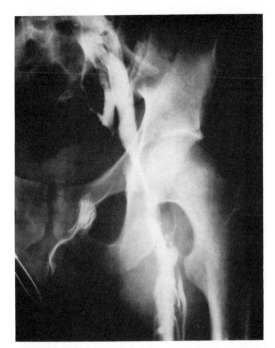

Figure 8–37. Clinical success is demonstrated angiographically by the patent compilation vein graft used to repair an injured common femoral vein. (Courtesy of Dr. William G. Sullivan.)

delayed venous reconstruction in some patients with chronic venous insufficiency following ligation. In such patients serial venography may be useful. This is shown in a report by Rich and Sullivan (1972) of a patient with recanalization of an autogenous vein graft in the popliteal vein (Fig. 8–38 and Fig. 8–39). Early recanalization can be seen in Figure 8–40. Additional phlebograms are needed in the extended follow-up period, and some findings have been encouraging, such as the long term patency 3½ years after lateral suture repair (Fig. 8–41). The importance of repair of the popliteal vein when associated with injuries of the popliteal artery is discussed in further detail in Chapter 25.

Recently, additional experience has been accumulated regarding the use of adjunctive measures. Schramek and co-authors (1974, 1975) in Israel have used a branch of the profunda femoris artery to reconstruct a distal arteriovenous fistula with an autogenous vein graft for repair of the femoral vein in three patients (Fig. 8–42).

Text continued on page 190

Figure 8–38. This venogram was performed 72 hours postoperatively at the 12th Evacuation Hospital in the Republic of Vietnam. It revealed thrombosis of the autogenous cephalic vein graft placed in the right popliteal vein. (Rich, N. M., and Sullivan, W. G., J. Trauma, *12*:919, 1972. Copyright 1972, The Williams & Wilkins Co., Baltimore.)

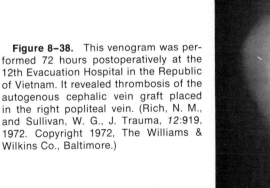
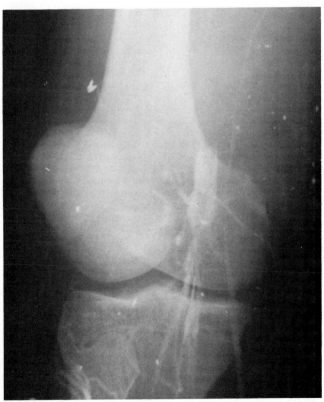

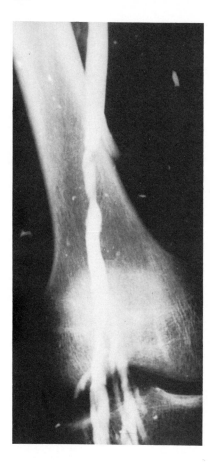

Figure 8-39. An additional venogram was performed at Walter Reed General Hospital approximately 4½ months following a venogram performed in Vietnam (see Fig. 8–38). Note recanalization of the 3-cm cephalic vein graft in the right popliteal vein. (Rich, N. M., and Sullivan, W. G., J. Trauma, *12*:919, 1972. Copyright 1972, The Williams & Wilkins Co., Baltimore.)

Figure 8-40. This venogram shows minimal recanalization of a segment of the left greater saphenous vein which was used to repair the right popliteal vein 2½ months earlier in Vietnam. Also note some of the remaining collateral venous development. Interestingly, the patient had no distal edema. (Rich, N. M., and Hobson, R. W., *in* Swan, K. E., et al. (Eds.), Venous Surgery in the Lower Extremity. Warren H. Green Publishers, Inc., St. Louis, 1975.)

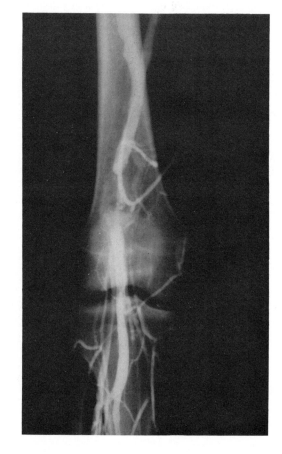

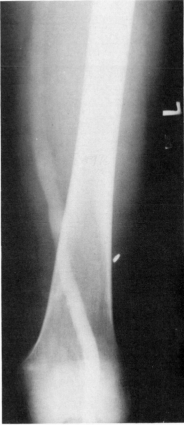

Figure 8–41. Venogram demonstrating patency of the popliteal vein at its junction with the superficial femoral vein. Note the metallic fragments that caused the injury. The vein was repaired by lateral suture 3½ years earlier in Vietnam. Repair of concomitant venous injuries is advocated as one of the methods that will help lower the relatively high amputation rate associated with popliteal artery trauma. (Rich, N. M., Jarstfer, B. S., and Geer, T. M., J. Cardiovasc. Surg., *15*:340, 1974.)

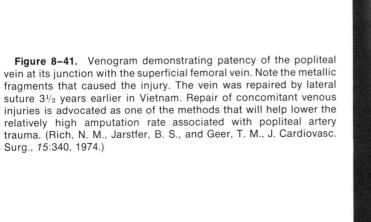

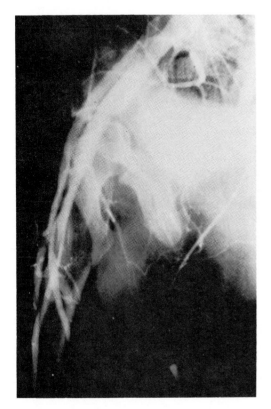

Figure 8–42. This arteriogram reveals patency of an autogenous vein graft in the common femoral vein, with a functioning distal arteriovenous fistula using a branch of the profunda femoris artery. (Schramek, A., Hashmonai, M., Farbstein, J., and Adler, O., J. Trauma, *15*:816, 1975. Copyright 1975, The Williams & Wilkins Co., Baltimore.)

TABLE 8–14. INCIDENCE OF EDEMA
FOLLOWING LIGATION AND REPAIR OF
INJURED POPLITEAL VEINS*

MANAGEMENT	NUMBER	WITH EDEMA	PER CENT
Ligation	57	29	50.9
Repair	53	7	13.2

*Modified from Rich, N. M., Hobson, R. W., II, Collins, G. J., Jr., and Andersen, C. A., Ann. Surg., *183*:365, 1976.

A recent study from the Vietnam Vascular Registry (Rich et al., 1976) evaluates the management and long-term follow-up of 110 patients with isolated popliteal venous trauma. Nearly an equal number were repaired and ligated. Thrombophlebitis and pulmonary embolism were not significant complications in this series. The only pulmonary embolus occurred after ligation of an injured popliteal vein. However, there was a significant increase in edema in the involved extremity following ligation of the popliteal vein (Table 8–14).

Rich and associates (1977D) also provided a 10-year follow-up of 51 former Vietnam casualties who had lower extremity venous injuries repaired using autogenous interposition venous grafts. Only one patient, or 2 per cent, developed thrombophlebitis in the post-operative period and this was transitory in nature (Table 8–15).

TABLE 8–15. COMPLICATIONS OF
VENOUS REPAIR USING
AUTOGENOUS VENOUS GRAFTS*

COMPLICATION	NUMBER	PER CENT
Thrombophlebitis	1	2.0
Pulmonary embolism	0	0.0
Amputation	0	0.0
Death	0	0.0

EDEMA	NUMBER	PER CENT
None	34	66.6
Early	11	21.6
Residual	6	11.8
Totals	51	100.0

*Fifty-one patients. From Rich, N. M., Collins, G. J., Jr., Andersen, C. A., and McDonald, P. T., J. Trauma, *17*:512, 1977. Copyright 1977, The Williams & Wilkins Co., Baltimore.

CHAPTER 9

ARTERIOVENOUS FISTULAS

If it should be found by experience, that a large artery, when wounded, may be healed up by this kind of suture, without becoming impervious, it would be an important discovery in surgery. It would make the operation for the Aneurysm still more successful in the arm, when the main trunk is wounded; and by this method, perhaps, we might be able to cure the wounds of some arteries that would otherwise require amputation, or be altogether incurable.

Mr. Lambert, 1762, Newcastle-upon-Tyne (Letter to Dr. Hunter)

It is generally accepted that the first successful arterial repair was performed by Hallowell in 1759. His comments emphasize his realization that repair of false aneurysms and arteriovenous fistulas could be valuable. The diagnosis, pathophysiology and surgical management of arteriovenous fistulas and false aneurysms have stimulated the intellectual curiosity and challenged the technical abilities of surgeons for more than 200 years. These lesions are often found in association, and they are frequently discussed together, despite the variable aspects that exist. Appropriate emphasis will be given where indicated.

Because of the outstanding contributions of Matas, Halsted, Reid, Holman, Elkin, Shumacker, Hughes and others and a plethora of reports from three major armed conflicts in this century, considerable documentation exists regarding princi-

ples of diagnosis and management of arteriovenous fistulas and false aneurysms. During the Korean Conflict, Hughes, Jahnke, Spencer and co-workers documented that arterial repair could be successful, even in a combat zone. Consequently, more vascular repairs were done at the time of initial wounding, with a resultant decrease in the number of arteriovenous fistulas and false aneurysms which required later repair. With the rapid progress which was made in vascular surgery in the 10 years preceding the increased American military involvement in Southeast Asia in 1965, hundreds of well-trained young surgeons from both military and civilian training programs were available and eager to perform vascular repairs during the fighting in the Republic of South Vietnam.

With the establishment of the Vietnam

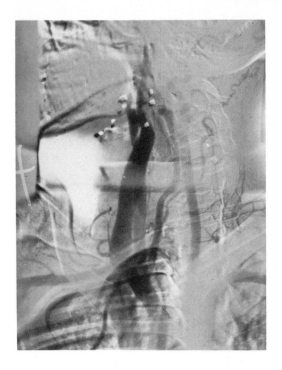

Figure 9-1. Multiple fragments from various exploding devices were responsible for the majority (87.3 per cent) of arteriovenous fistulas and false aneurysms in this study. The subtraction study of an arch angiogram helped to confirm the clinical impression of an arteriovenous communication in the patient's right neck at the level of the common carotid bifurcation. Excision of the fistula with ligation of the external carotid artery and venorrhaphy of the internal jugular vein were performed at Walter Reed Army Medical Center in 1971. (Rich, N. M., Hobson, R. W., II, and Collins, G. J., Jr., Surgery, 78:817, 1975.)

Vascular Registry at Walter Reed Army Medical Center in 1966, an effort was made to document as accurately as possible all vascular injuries that occurred among American casualties in Southeast Asia and to provide long term follow-up of these casualties. The initial analysis was important in providing guidelines for determining the ultimate success or failure following various types of repairs. It was believed that there would be relatively few arteriovenous fistulas and false aneurysms, compared to other recent wars. Nevertheless, it was recognized that a number of factors, such as multiple wounds and other more serious problems, might lead to delayed recognition of both arteriovenous fistulas and false aneurysms. In later follow-up from the Registry, it was shown that there were more arteriovenous fistulas and false aneurysms than initially anticipated. The Registry report provided an analysis of information gathered over a nine year period from nearly 7500 records of American casualties showing that there were 558 arteriovenous fistulas and false aneurysms among 509 combat casualties (Rich et al., 1975D) (Fig. 9-1).

HISTORY

William Hunter (1757, 1762) provided documention more than 200 years ago that the heart enlarged in a patient with an arteriovenous fistula and that arterial dilatation occurred proximal to an arteriovenous communication (Table 9-1). Norris (1843) noted the recurrence of physical findings associated with an arteriovenous aneurysm 10 days after ligation of the artery above and below the fistula. Nicoladoni (1875) and Branham (1890) described slowing of the heart with pressure occlusion of an arteriovenous communication, and their names are often associated with this physical finding (the Nicoladoni-Branham sign). Annadale (1875) described the successful management of a popliteal arteriovenous fistula by ligature of the popliteal artery and vein. Eisenbrey (1913) described pathologic changes associated with arteriovenous aneurysms of the superficial femoral vessels (Fig. 9-2). Holman (1937), in his classic monograph, described the pathophysiology associated with abnormal communications between arterial and venous circulations. Holman (1940, 1962) has also

TABLE 9–1. ACHIEVEMENTS AND UNDERSTANDING IN TREATING ARTERIOVENOUS FISTULAS: REPRESENTATIVE HISTORICAL NOTES

AUTHOR	YEAR	CONTRIBUTION
Hunter	1757	Recognized an abnormal communication between an artery and vein. Described the associated thrill and bruit. Eliminated the thrill and bruit by pressure over the proximal artery or site of communication. Noted tortuosity and dilatation of the artery proximal to the fistula.
Norris	1843	Cured an arteriovenous fistula by double arterial ligation.
Breshet	1833	Described two patients in whom ligation of the artery proximal to the arteriovenous communication was followed by gangrene.
Nicoladoni	1875	The first to demonstrate the remarkable slowing of the pulse rate by compression of the artery proximal to the arteriovenous fistula.
Branham	1890	Emphasized the slowing of the pulse rate by obliterating a large acquired arteriovenous fistula (Branham-Nicoladoni sign).
Stewart	1913	Noted that the heart diminished in size within 10 days after elimination of the arteriovenous fistula.
Gunderman	1915	The first to mention an increase in blood pressure on obliteration of an acquired arteriovenous fistula.
Reid	1920	Presented experimental evidence of cardiac enlargement in the presence of an arteriovenous fistula.
Nanu et al.	1922	Accurately described the effect on the blood pressure of closure of the arteriovenous fistula.
Franz		Observed an increase in skin temperature and an increase in extremity growth in the presence of a femoral fistula of 18 months duration in a 12 year old boy.
Holman	1937	Clarified many of the anatomical and hemodynamic variations seen with arteriovenous fistulas.

provided more recent reviews of the pathophysiology of arteriovenous fistulas. Osler (1893, 1905) made a number of early observations on arteriovenous fistulas. His respect for these lesions is exemplified by a quotation from an article written in 1905: "The great danger of operating is in the gangrene which is apt to follow."

Halsted made numerous contributions in the field of vascular surgery, including the management of arteriovenous fistulas. His remarks regarding the case presentation by Bernheim in 1916, when the latter utilized an interposition autogenous saphenous vein graft as a replacement for a popliteal aneurysm, emphasize his interest in arterial repair (Halsted, 1916). He noted the important contributions of Carrel and specifically stated that the operation of Lexer, which Bernheim also was advocating, was "the ideal operation." Reid, in two important contributions (1920, 1925), described abnormal arteriovenous communications.

Using the vast World War II experience, Elkin (1945, 1955) and Shumacker (1946, 1950) and their co-workers documented a number of important findings. Shumacker (1946) outlined the surgical approach to various arteriovenous fistulas and false aneurysms. He recognized the important work of Matas (1901, 1903), who made significant contributions to the present management of both arteriovenous fistulas and false aneurysms.

The management of 215 arteriovenous fistulas and false aneurysms during the Korean Conflict was reported by Hughes and Jahnke (1958).

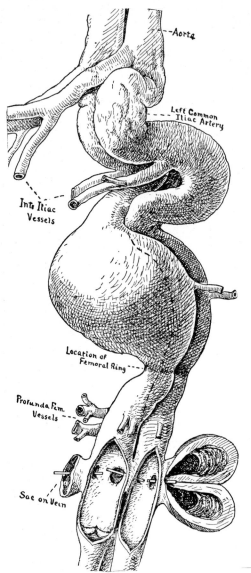

Aorta

Left Common Iliac Artery

Int. Iliac Vessels

Location of Femoral Ring

Profunda Fem. Vessels

Sac on Vein

Figure 9–2. An arteriovenous communication with extensive vascular alterations. (Eisenbrey, A. B., J.A.M.A., *61*:2155, 1913.)

INCIDENCE

It is difficult to determine the true incidence of arteriovenous fistulas. Some series combine congenital with traumatic lesions. False aneurysms may or may not be included. Some reports of arterial lesions include arteriovenous fistulas and others do not. Often the diagnosis is not made until years later. As an example, arteriovenous fistulas are still diagnosed at this time among World War II veterans, more than 30 years after their original injury.

Encouraged by Halsted, Callander (1920) made a literature review of 447 arteriovenous fistulas to 1914, including some from World War I. In one of the earliest reports of management of combat-incurred arteriovenous fistulas, Soubbotitch (1913) reported an insignificant percentage of vascular injuries: 77 injuries to large blood vessels among 20,000 wounded. The numerous separate reports by Elkin, Shumacker, Freeman and others from their vast experience during World War II are included in a final bound report (Elkin and DeBakey, 1955). A total of 593 arteriovenous fistulas were treated; however, there was no incidence given for this lesion among World War II combat casualties. In the Korean Conflict 202 patients were treated for 215 arteriovenous fistulas and false aneurysms, with notation made for an incidence among all combat casualties (Hughes and Jahnke, 1958).

The only statistic from the Vietnam experience of any value was an incidence of approximately 7 per cent of arteriovenous fistulas and false aneurysms among nearly 7500 American casualties in Southeast Asia who suffered some type of vascular trauma. When Heaton and co-authors (1966) evaluated the initial military surgical practices of the United States Army in Vietnam, they recorded the following: "The lessons learned in Korea, the advances made in the technics of vascular surgery, the increased numbers of surgeons trained in vascular technics, plus rapid evacuation, new instruments and antibiotics have resulted in practically all arterial injuries occurring in Vietnam being repaired primarily with a high degree of success, so that only rarely do patients develop an arteriovenous fistula or false aneurysm." The factors mentioned certainly played a significant role in limiting the number of arteriovenous fistulas and false aneurysms. With time, however, an increasing number of arteriovenous fistulas and false aneurysms were recorded. In many cases these occurred in patients sustaining multiple small fragment wounds over a large portion of the body which made it impractical to explore every artery in which a vascular injury might be present.

Hewitt and Collins (1969) reported a 10 per cent incidence of arteriovenous fistulas among 60 patients with arterial injuries treated between December, 1966, and October, 1967, at the 18th Surgical Hospital (MA) and during November, 1967, at the 71st Evacuation Hospital in Vietnam. Five of the six lesions were acute arteriovenous fistulas which were noted upon admission of the patients to the hospital within one to six hours following injury.

Civilian reports of vascular trauma have increased in the past 20 years, and some include reviews of experience in managing arteriovenous fistulas. Patman and associates (1964) included 6 patients with arteriovenous fistulas among their 256 patients with civilian arterial injuries: an incidence of 2.3 per cent. Drapanas and co-authors (1970) stated that because the immediate repair of all acute arterial injuries is advocated, the development of serious delayed complications, including arteriovenous fistulas and false aneurysms, should largely be prevented. They found that chronic arteriovenous fistulas and false aneurysms declined noticeably during the last period of their study—between 1958 and 1969—at Charity Hospital in New Orleans (Fig. 9–3). Hewitt and co-workers (1973) reported a 6.8 per cent incidence—14 cases—of acute arteriovenous fistulas among 206 patients with acute arterial inju-

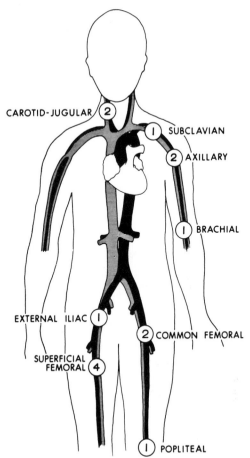

Figure 9–4. Distribution of acute arteriovenous fistulas in 14 out of 206 patients with acute civilian arterial injuries in New Orleans: an incidence of 6.8 per cent. (Hewitt, R. L., Smith, A. D., and Drapanas, T. J. Trauma, *13*:901, 1973. Copyright 1973, The Williams & Wilkins Company, Baltimore.)

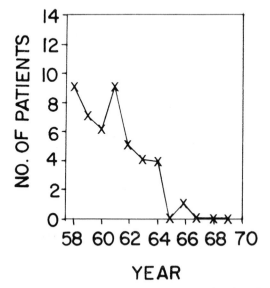

Figure 9–3. The number of patients with chronic arteriovenous fistulas and false aneurysms admitted to Charity Hospital in New Orleans on the Tulane Service between 1958 and 1969. There has been a notable decline in the incidence of these vascular injuries with delayed recognition. (Drapanas, T., Hewitt, R. L., Weichert, R. F., and Smith, A. D., Ann. Surg., *172*:351, 1970.)

ries treated on the Tulane University Surgical Service (Fig. 9–4).

The incidence of arteriovenous fistulas compared to that of false aneurysms has varied from one series to another. Shumacker and Carter (1946) studied 364 arteriovenous fistulas and false aneurysms in 351 individuals. There were 245 arteriovenous fistulas and 119 aneurysms, with 206 and 82, respectively, operated upon at one of the three Vascular Centers, Mayo General Hospital, established by the Army Surgeon General during World War II (Fig. 9–5; Table 9–2). In the 1964 series of Patman and associates from Dallas, there were 17 patients who developed late complications, but only 5 arteriovenous fistulas were reported, compared with 12 false aneurysms. Thus in their series the false an-

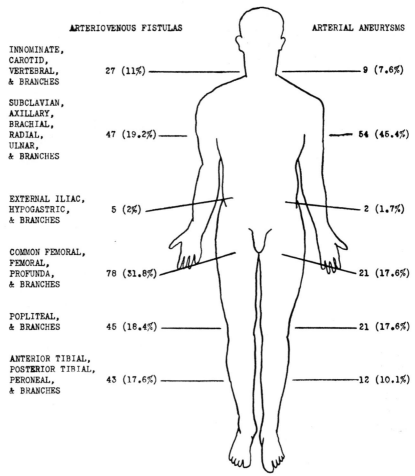

Figure 9-5. General distribution of arteriovenous fistulas and false aneurysms in a study from the Mayo General Hospital during World War II. (Shumacker, H. B., Jr., and Carter, K. L., Surgery, *20*:9, 1946.)

TABLE 9-2. COMPARISON OF INCIDENCE OF ARTERIAL ANEURYSMS AND ARTERIOVENOUS FISTULAS IN THE MAIN PERIPHERAL ARTERIES: MAYO GENERAL HOSPITAL, WORLD WAR II*

| | ARTERIOVENOUS FISTULAS | | ARTERIAL ANEURYSM | |
ARTERY INVOLVED	No.	Per Cent	No.	Per Cent
Subclavian	10	4.1	5	4.2
Axillary	12	4.9	15	12.6
Brachial	13	5.3	28	23.5
Common femoral and femoral	66	26.9	17	14.3
Popliteal	42	17.1	21	17.6

*Shumacker, H. B., Jr., and Carter, K. L., Surgery, *20*:9, 1946.

eurysms outnumbered the arteriovenous fistulas two to one, a ratio opposite to that reported by Hughes and Jahnke (1958) from the Korean experience.

Seeley and associates (1952) reported that arteriovenous fistulas occurred at least twice as often as false aneurysms in 106 cases seen at Walter Reed General Hospital. The majority of the patients sustained their injury in the earlier part of the Korean Conflict. The incidence was nearly equal in the Vietnam experience (Rich et al., 1975D), although there were fewer arteriovenous fistulas than false aneurysms (Table 9–3). Arteriovenous fistulas and false aneurysms are frequently found together in various anatomical configurations (Figs. 9–6 and 9–7). Shumacker and Wayson (1950) outlined the development

TABLE 9–3. ARTERIOVENOUS FISTULAS AND FALSE ANEURYSMS VIETNAM VASCULAR REGISTRY*

LESIONS	NO.	PER CENT
False aneurysms	296	53.1
Arteriovenous fistulas	262	46.9
Total:	558	100.0

*Rich, N. M., Hobson, R. W., II, and Collins, G. J., Jr., Surgery, *78*:817, 1975.

of arteriovenous fistulas, showing that pulsating hematomas may present initially, with well-formed saccular aneurysms developing subsequently. Notes made at the time of operation and upon examination of the excised specimen permitted an analysis of

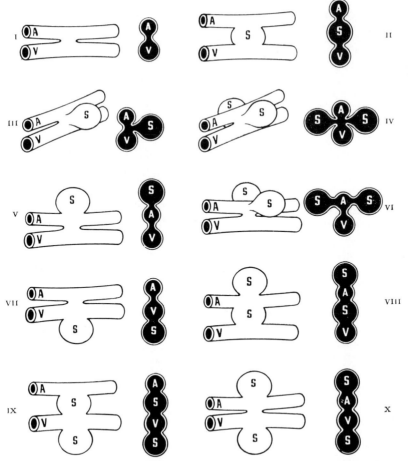

Figure 9–6. This diagrammatic representation of various types of arteriovenous fistulas and associated aneurysms evolved from a study of 195 cases of arteriovenous fistulas. There was an associated aneurysm in 60 per cent of the arteriovenous fistulas. Symbols: A, artery; V, vein; S, sac. (Shumacker, H. B., Jr., and Wayson, E. E., Am. J. Surg., 79:532, 1950.)

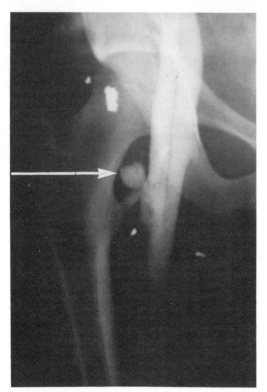

Figure 9–7. Femoral angiogram demonstrating an arteriovenous fistula at the level of the right common femoral arterial bifurcation. There is an associated false aneurysm (arrow). Arteriorrhaphy of the origin of the profunda femoris artery and venorrhaphy of the common femoral vein were successfully accomplished at Walter Reed Army Medical Center in 1970. (Rich, N. M., Hobson, R. W., II, and Collins, G. J., Jr., Surgery, 78:817, 1975.)

the presence or absence of an aneurysm in 195 cases of arteriovenous fistula. There was no associated aneurysm in 78 cases, or 40 per cent. The 60 per cent majority had one or more aneurysms. Multiple lesions may also exist in various anatomical sites (Table 9–4).

There is a wide variation in the regional distribution of arteriovenous fistulas. This may include specific arteries, as well as regional areas. During a 15 year period from 1947 through 1962, 50 patients with arteriovenous fistulas were admitted to the Baylor University College of Medicine affiliated hospitals in Houston. The greatest number of these lesions were found in the extremities, the lower extremities being more frequently involved than the upper (Table 9–5). Vollmar and Krumhaar (1968) found that nearly 50 per cent of the arteriovenous fistulas in their series were lo-

TABLE 9–4. ARTERIOVENOUS FISTULAS AND FALSE ANEURYSMS— MULTIPLE LESIONS AT VARIOUS ANATOMICAL SITES: VIETNAM VASCULAR REGISTRY*

PATIENTS	LESIONS	TOTAL
468	1	468
35	2	70
4	3	12
2	4	8
509		558

*Rich, N. M., Hobson, R. W., II, and Collins, G. J., Jr., Surgery, 78:817, 1975.

calized in the lower extremities (Fig. 9–8). Next in frequency were fistulas of the upper extremities and shoulders (27 per cent), head and neck (22.5 per cent) and trunk (2 per cent).

Table 9–6 outlines representative World War II statistics concerning predominantly lower extremity injuries, specifically those involving the femoral and popliteal vessels. Involvement of major (Table 9–7) and minor (Table 9–8) vessels was outlined for the Korean experience by Hughes and *Text continued on page 202*

TABLE 9–5. LOCATION OF ARTERIOVENOUS ANEURYSMS: BAYLOR UNIVERSITY COLLEGE OF MEDICINE AFFILIATED HOSPITALS*

LOCATION	No.
Popliteal	9
Femoral	9
Brachial	6
Common carotid	5
Radial	2
Subclavian	2
External carotid	2
Internal carotid	2
Posterior tibial	2
Temporal	2
Aortic arch	1
Internal iliac	1
External iliac	1
Occipital	1
Internal maxillary	1
Thyrocervical	1
Uterine	1
Peroneal	1
Medial circumflex femoral	1
Total:	50

*Beall, A. C., Jr., Harrington, O. B., Crawford, E. S., and DeBakey, M. E., Am. J. Surg., 106:610, 1963.

LOCALIZATION OF 200 TRAUMATIC ARTERIOVENOUS FISTULAE

(Surg. Clin of the Univ. of Heidelberg, 1939 - 1967).

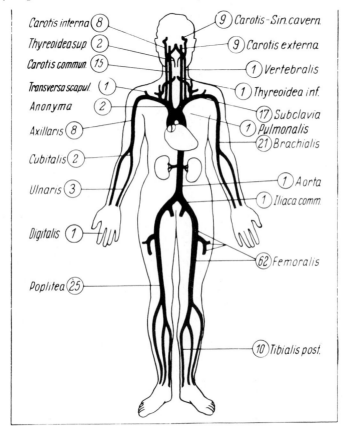

Figure 9–8. In the cases seen at Heidelberg University, nearly 50 per cent of the arteriovenous fistulas were found in the lower extremities. (Vollmar, J., and Krumhaar, D., *in* Hiertonn, T., and Rybeck, B. (Eds.), Traumatic Arterial Lesions. Research Institute of National Defense, Stockholm, Sweden, 1968.)

TABLE 9–6. DISTRIBUTION OF FALSE ANEURYSMS AND ARTERIOVENOUS FISTULAS: MAYO GENERAL HOSPITAL*

ARTERY INVOLVED	ARTERIOVENOUS FISTULAS: No. of Cases			ARTERIAL ANEURYSMS: No. of Cases		
	Operation at M.G.H.	Operation Elsewhere	"Spontaneous Cure"	Operation at M.G.H.	Operation Elsewhere	"Spontaneous Cure"
Aorta	1					
Innominate				1		
Internal carotid	3			2		
External carotid	3					
Common carotid	6		1	1	1	2
Vertebral	4					
Lingual	1					
Occipital	1					
Cirsoid, nose, ear	2					
Superior temporal	2			1		
Transverse cervical	1	1				
Deep cervical				1		
Internal mammary	1					
Subclavian	6	3	1	5		
Axillary	12			13	2	
Branch axillary	4			2		
Brachial	11	1	1	22	5	1
Radial	1	1		2		
Ulnar	4	2		2		
External iliac		1		1		
Hypogastric	1					
Superior gluteal	2			1		
Obturator	1					
Common femoral	3	2				1
Femoral	47	13	1	6	9	1
Profunda femoris	6			2		
Branch profunda	2	2	1	2		
Popliteal	41	1		14	6	1
Geniculate	4					
Posterior tibial	21	5		1	4	2
Anterior tibial	5	1		2	1	
Peroneal	5	1			1	
Branches in calf	5			1		
Total	206	34	5	82	29	8

*Shumacker, H. B., Jr., and Carter, K. L., Surgery, *20*:9, 1946.

TABLE 9–7. LOCATION OF TOTAL MAJOR VESSEL LESIONS: ARTERIOVENOUS FISTULAS— KOREAN EXPERIENCE*

Vessel	Arterio-venous Fistulas	False Aneurysms	Total
Common carotid	7	2	9
Internal carotid	3	–	3
Subclavian	6	2	8
Axillary	9	11	20
Brachial	10	9	19
Iliac	3	1	4
Common femoral	7	1	8
Superior femoral	24	7	31
Popliteal	22	10	32
Total:	91	43	134

*Hughes, C. W., and Jahnke, E. J., Jr., Ann. Surg., *148*:790, 1958.

TABLE 9–8. LOCATION OF ARTERIOVENOUS FISTULAS—TOTAL MINOR VESSEL LESIONS TREATED: KOREAN EXPERIENCE*

Vessel	Lesions		Treatment			Total
	Arterio-venous Fistulas	False Aneurysms	Ligation	Sponta-neous Closure	Anasto-mosis	
Occipital	1	1	2	–	–	2
Supraorbital	–	1	1	–	–	1
Superior temporal	2	1	3	–	–	3
Vertebral	3	–	3	–	–	3
Superior thyroid	–	1	–	1	–	1
Inferior thyroid	2	–	2	–	–	2
Thoracoacromial	2	–	2	–	–	2
Thoracodorsal	2	1	3	–	–	3
Posterior humeral circumflex	1	1	2	–	–	2
Subscapular	1	–	–	–	1	1
Profunda brachii	–	1	1	–	–	1
Radial	2	4	5	–	1	6
Ulnar	2	2	4	–	–	4
Posterior interosseous	1	–	1	–	–	1
Anterior interosseous	2	–	2	–	–	2
Digital	–	1	1	–	–	1
Profunda femoris	10	–	10	–	–	10
Muscular branch femoral	–	1	1	–	–	1
Circumflex femoral, lateral	1	1	2	–	–	2
Inferior Genu	2	1	3	–	–	3
Posterior tibial	11	2	12	1	–	13
Peroneal	8	1	9	–	–	9
Anterior tibial	3	3	6	–	–	6
Dorsalis pedis	–	1	1	–	–	1
Deep Mantar	1	–	1	–	–	1
Total:	57	24	77	2	2	81

*Hughes, C. W., and Jahnke, E. J., Jr., Ann. Surg., *148*:790, 1958.

TABLE 9–9. ARTERIOVENOUS FISTULAS AND FALSE ANEURYSMS—ANATOMICAL LOCATION: VIETNAM VASCULAR REGISTRY*

LOCATION	NO.	PER CENT
Head/neck	42	7.5
Upper extremity	134	24.0
Thorax	17	3.1
Abdomen	22	3.9
Lower extremity	343	61.5
Total:	558	100.0

*Rich, N. M., Hobson, R. W., II, and Collins, G. J., Jr., Surgery, 78:817, 1975.

Jahnke (1958). The Vietnam data centered around lower extremity involvement (Table 9–9), the superficial femoral and popliteal arteries being most frequently injured (Table 9–10).

There are hundreds of reports of specific or unusual arteriovenous fistulas. Complete analysis is beyond the scope of this review. Creech and associates (1965) presented a series of traumatic arteriovenous fistulas at unusual sites, including the superior gluteal, hepatic-portal, coronary and vertebral vessels. Conn and associates (1971) reported challenging arterial injuries, including an aortocaval fistula, an iliac arteriovenous fistula and a mesenteric arteriovenous fistula, in eight patients.

Other representative reports include the following (additional information can be found in specific chapters): Hunt and associates (1971) reported their experience in managing five arteriovenous fistulas of major vessels in the abdomen. One of the cases was unique in that the authors could find no previous report of a successful repair of a fistula between the aorta, the renal vein and the portal vein (Fig. 9–9). They also described immediate repair of a mesenteric arteriovenous fistula and other fistulas involving the portal and renal veins. Dillard and associates (1968) reported one case in which a 29 year old female was stabbed in the right flank and three years later was found to have severe hypertension. After correction of the renal arteriovenous fistula, the patient's blood pressure returned to normal.

TABLE 9–10. ARTERIOVENOUS FISTULAS AND FALSE ANEURYSMS—ARTERIAL INJURIES: VIETNAM VASCULAR REGISTRY*

ARTERY	ARTERIOVENOUS FISTULAS	FALSE ANEURYSMS	TOTAL	PER CENT
Common carotid	6	5	11	2.0
Internal carotid	2	4	6	1.1
External carotid	2	3	5	0.7
Vertebral	6	2	8	1.4
Subclavian	1	7	8	1.4
Axillary	10	8	18	3.2
Brachial	22	33	55	9.9
Radial	2	25	27	4.8
Ulnar	8	15	23	4.1
Innominate	1	1	2	0.4
Thoracic aorta	0	2	2	0.4
Abdominal aorta	0	1	1	0.2
Common iliac	1	1	2	0.4
External iliac	0	6	6	1.1
Internal iliac	0	1	1	0.2
Common femoral	4	7	11	2.0
Superficial femoral	57	31	88	15.8
Deep femoral	17	20	37	6.6
Popliteal	41	28	69	12.4
Posterior tibial	30	33	63	11.3
Anterior tibial	20	18	38	6.8
Peroneal	12	12	24	4.3
Miscellaneous	20	33	53	9.5
Total:	262	296	558	100.0

*Rich, N. M., Hobson, R. W., II, and Collins, G. J., Jr., Surgery, 78:817, 1975.

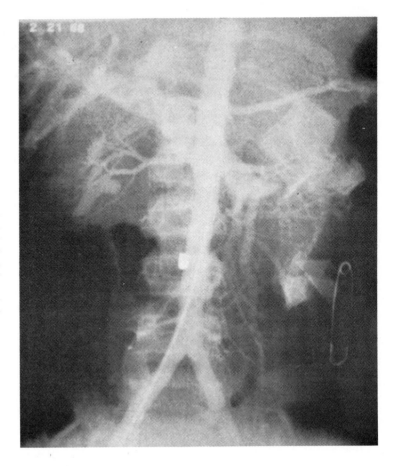

Figure 9–9. Abdominal aorta injured by small caliber bullet. This angiogram reveals the tip of the catheter in the area of injury; the portal vein fills selectively. The additional injury to the renal vein could not be shown simultaneously in this unique lesion involving the aorta, the renal vein and the portal vein. (Hunt, T. K., Leeds, F. H., Wanebo, H. J., and Blaisdell, F. W., J. Trauma, *11*:483, 1971. Copyright 1971, The Williams & Wilkins Company, Baltimore.)

ETIOLOGY

Although arteriovenous fistulas may be either acquired or congenital, we are essentially concerned with those that are acquired by trauma. On the other hand, one cannot be knowledgeable about acquired arteriovenous fistulas without also understanding the anatomical and pathophysiologic aspects of congenital arteriovenous fistulas (Table 9–11). Long standing acquired arteriovenous fistulas must be differentiated from congenital arteriovenous fistulas, because there is a considerable difference in their surgical management, as well as the final results. An acquired arteriovenous fistula can have one, or possibly two, communications, whereas the communications between the arteries and veins

TABLE 9–11. ARTERIOVENOUS FISTULAS: 10 YEAR EXPERIENCE AT THE MAYO CLINIC*

	CONGENITAL	ACQUIRED
AV fistulas of the extremities	80	17
Aorta–inferior vena cava fistulas	0	7
Pulmonary AV fistulas	47	0
Renal AV fistulas	0	6
AV fistulas of the portal system	0	1
AV fistulas of the neck and face	11	4
Pelvic AV fistulas	1	5
AV fistulas of the chest wall	0	2
Total:	139	42

*Modified from Gomes, M. M. R., and Bernatz, P. E., Mayo Clin. Proc., *45*:81, 1970.

TABLE 9–12. ARTERIOVENOUS FISTULAS AND FALSE ANEURYSMS—ETIOLOGY OF INJURY: VIETNAM VASCULAR REGISTRY*

WOUNDING AGENT	No.	PER CENT
Fragment	487	87.3
Bullet	59	10.6
Blunt	7	1.2
Punji stick	5	0.9
Total:	558	100.0

*Rich, N. M., Hobson, R. W., II, and Collins, G. J., Jr., Surgery, 78:817, 1975.

TABLE 9–13. ETIOLOGY OF 200 TRAUMATIC ARTERIOVENOUS FISTULAS: SURGICAL CLINIC OF THE UNIVERSITY OF HEIDELBERG, 1939–1967*

WOUNDING AGENT	No.	PER CENT
War projectiles	177	88.5
Fractures	10	5.0
Stab wounds	7	3.5
Iatrogenic trauma	4	2.0
Gunshot wounds (civil)	2	1.0
Total:	200	100.0

*Vollmar, J., and Krumhaar, D., in Hiertonn, T., and Rybeck, B. (Eds.), Traumatic Arterial Lesions. Research Institute of National Defense, Stockholm, Sweden, 1968.

in the congenital type of arteriovenous fistula may be myriad.

Usually an arteriovenous fistula results from a simultaneous injury of an artery and adjacent vein which permits blood to flow directly from the injured artery into the vein. Penetrating injuries are usually responsible for these lesions. In military injuries penetrating missiles are the major cause, and in civilian injuries stab wounds, as well as missile wounds, are associated with these lesions. The largest series of arteriovenous fistulas have been associated with recent combat wounds which have occurred during wars in the past century (Table 9–12). Both gunshot and fragment wounds have created arteriovenous fistulas which have been recognized either in the immediate or acute state, or after a delayed period of several weeks or months. One of the ironies of the combat situation in Vietnam, where modern weapons have been employed, is that the primitive punji stick has also caused arteriovenous fistulas. One of the authors (NMR) saw such an injury of the anterior tibial artery and vein at the 2nd Surgical Hospital in 1966.

Vollmar and Krumhaar (1968), based on their experience with 200 traumatic arteriovenous fistulas treated at the Surgical Clinic at the University of Heidelberg between 1939 and 1967 (Table 9–13), reported that two World Wars greatly increased the incidence of traumatic arteriovenous fistulas.

In civilian experience many arteriovenous fistulas result from stab wounds, although they can also be caused by bullets. However, these are usually low velocity gunshot wounds. Beall and associates (1963) reported that the majority—36 of 50—of ar-

teriovenous fistulas in their 15 year study of civilian vascular injuries resulted from gunshot wounds (Table 9–14).

Sako and Varco (1970) reported their experience in managing 57 patients with congenital and acquired arteriovenous fistulas of the extremities, abdomen and chest wall during a 20 year period (1949–1969). Less than 50 per cent, or 25 patients, had acquired arteriovenous fistulas. The etiology of these injuries included small arms fire in nine, penetration with a knife or glass in six, a shell fragment or land mine explosion in three, multiple puncture for cardiac catheterization in two, blunt injury of the hand in one, pelvic fracture in one, renal needle biopsy in one, rupture of an aneurysm in one, and following gastrectomy in one.

Although it is infrequent, traumatic arteriovenous fistulas have been reported after both major and minor surgical proce-

TABLE 9–14. TYPES OF INJURIES RESULTING IN ARTERIOVENOUS ANEURYSMS: BAYLOR UNIVERSITY COLLEGE OF MEDICINE AFFILIATED HOSPITALS*

TYPE OF INJURY	No.
Gunshot wounds	36
Stab wounds and lacerations	10
Shrapnel injuries	3
Blunt trauma	1
Total:	50

*Beall, A. C., Jr., Harrington, O. B., Crawford, E. S., and DeBakey, M. E., Am. J. Surg., 106:610, 1963.

dures (Fig. 9–10). The vessels which have been involved include the superior thyroid (Ransohoff, 1935), renal (Muller and Goodwin, 1956), intercostal (Reid and McGuire, 1938), uterine (Elkin and Banner, 1946) and aortocaval (DeBakey et al., 1958). Pridgen and Jacobs (1962) reviewed three postoperative arteriovenous fistulas treated in a three year period at Vanderbilt University. They emphasized the necessity for exercising extreme care to avoid accidental injury to vessels during any surgical procedure. In one of their cases they also emphasized that "en masse" ligation must be carefully avoided. They felt that the suture ligature had passed through the right superior epigastric artery and vein in one of their patients to result in an arteriovenous communication. Arteriovenous fis-

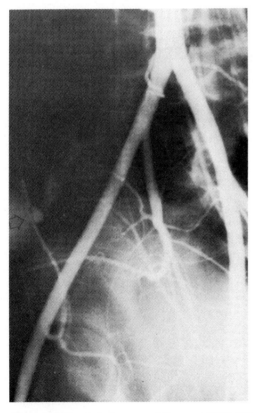

Figure 9–10. Arteriogram of the aortoiliac vessels demonstrating an inferior epigastric artery false aneurysm which occurred as a complication of abdominal retention sutures. (Loello, F. V., and Nunn, D. B., Surgery, 74:460, 1973.)

tulas have occurred following mass ligature of the renal vessels during nephrectomy and of the blood supply to the thyroid gland during thyroid lobectomy. One case report from Walter Reed General Hospital documented the development of an arteriovenous fistula following subtotal gastric resection (Blackwell and Whelan, 1965) (Fig. 9–11).

Beattie and associates (1961) presented the case of a 25 year old man with an arteriovenous fistula of the superior thyroid vessels. Approximately 18 months earlier he had had a partial thyroidectomy for primary thyrotoxicosis. The superior thyroid pedicles were each ligatured with one ligature of No. 40 linen thread. Approximately five months after his partial thyroidectomy, the patient noted swelling in his neck and was aware of a "humming" in the region of the swelling. After angiographic demonstration of the superior thyroid arteriovenous fistula between the superior thyroid artery and vein, excision of the remnant of the left lobe of the thyroid gland was accomplished.

There have been unusual forms of arteriovenous fistulas reported following essentially every type of surgical operation and every type of diagnostic or therapeutic procedure; for example, an arteriovenous fistula was reported following removal of an intervertebral disk with injury to the iliac artery and vein (see Chap. 21). Another such fistula occurred following a percutaneous transaxillary angiogram performed at Walter Reed General Hospital. Lester (1966) described arteriovenous fistulas as a complication of selective vertebral angiography. One of these lesions has also been treated at Walter Reed General Hospital.

White and associates (1968) stated that there was an increasing awareness of peripheral arterial injuries in infants and children. One of their patients, a three month old female, had a right femoral vein, right heart catheterization, to investigate a small ventricular septal defect and mild pulmonic stenosis. Over the following three years, she developed borderline heart failure, with a pulse rate of 120 and an increase in her heart size. At the age of 4½ years, a thrill was noted over the left groin, and the

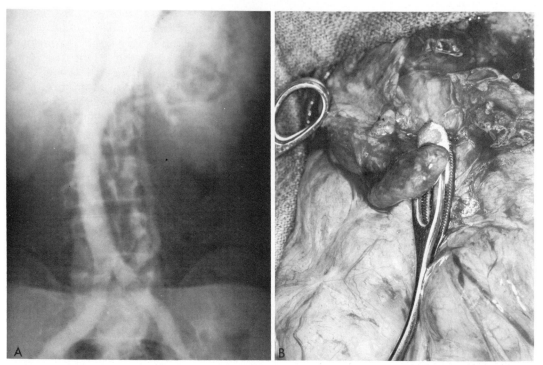

Figure 9–11. (A) Antegrade aortogram showing large anomalous artery to the left of the aorta communicating with veins in the lower part of the abdomen. (B) The specimen in situ showing the artery ending in a cul-de-sac communicating with dilated veins. The Kütner dissector has been placed beneath the arteriovenous fistula. The transverse colon and mesocolon lie inferior to the fistula. (Blackwell, T. L., and Whelan, T. J., Jr., Am. J. Surg., *109*:197, 1965.)

left leg was 2 cm longer than the right. The proximal fibula epiphysis was present on the left and not on the right. A large arteriovenous fistula (Fig. 9–12) was demonstrated between the profunda femoris ar-

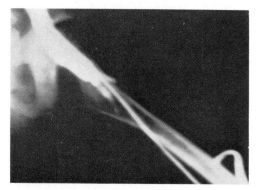

Figure 9–12. Angiogram demonstrating an arteriovenous communication between the right profunda femoris artery and the deep femoral vein following arterial puncture for blood gas analysis. Over the subsequent three years, the patient was in borderline heart failure, with an increased heart rate and an increased growth in her lower extremity. (White, J. J., Talbert, J. L., and Haller, J. A., Jr., Ann. Surg., *167*:757, 1968.)

tery and profunda femoris vein. Arterial blood gases had been measured and samples obtained from arterial punctures of the right femoral artery. The needle must have been inserted in a lateral and downward direction, penetrating the femoral vein before puncturing the femoral artery for the blood samples. A direct arteriovenous fistula was created by the needle. After ligation of this fistula and without sacrifice of either artery or vein, over the next several months her pulse rate gradually returned to normal and her cardiac failure cleared.

Lord and associates (1968) presented the case of a profunda femoris arteriovenous fistula caused by passage of a Fogarty arterial catheter. At the time of their report, they stated that there were two other similar incidences in the literature. Subsequent reports include those of Rob and Battle (1971) and Gaspard and Gaspar (1972) (Fig. 9–11).

Arteriovenous fistulas occasionally occur with fractures (additional details are given in Chapter 7). Harris (1963) reported an arteriovenous fistula following closed frac-

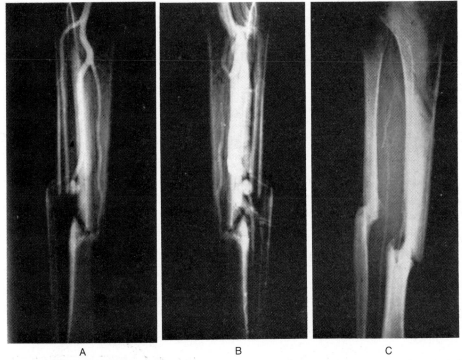

A   B   C

Figure 9–13. (A) Closed fracture of the tibia and fibula; the arteriogram shows an arteriovenous fistula of the peroneal artery and the arterial phase of filling. (B) The arteriogram shows the venous phase of filling of the peroneal arteriovenous fistula. (C) A postoperative arteriogram following excision of the fistula. Note the rapid advance and union of the fracture of the tibia and fibula following excision of the fistula. (Harris, J. D., Br. J. Surg., *50*:774, 1963.)

ture of the tibia and fibula in a 35 year old male (Fig. 9–13). Vascular injuries have occurred with orthopedic procedures other than those involved in the management of fractures. Ferguson (1914) presented an infant who developed an arteriovenous fistula following an osteotomy of the femur for genu valgum.

Anthopoulos and associates (1965) reported the unusual case of a 23 year old female, who at age nine had sustained a human bite at the base of the finger. The authors believed that the arteriovenous fistula of the fifth finger developed as a complication of the human bite. There was spontaneous, periodic, subungual spurting of arterial blood, as well as increased growth, venous distention, increased local temperature and more rapid growth of the nail. Surgical excision of the aneurysmal sacs and ligation of visible communications on two separate occasions resulted in relief of symptoms and enabled the patient to resume her occupation as a typist.

PATHOPHYSIOLOGY

As a student at The Johns Hopkins Medical School in 1917, my curiosity about arteriovenous fistulas was aroused and repeatedly whetted by Dr. Halsted's recurring expressions of great puzzlement at the occasional massive enlargement of the heart to the point of cardiac failure and at the marked dilatation of the proximal artery that could accompany an arteriovenous fistula, usually one of long duration. Equally puzzling was the fact that this heart enlargement and arterial dilatation occurred with some but not all fistulas.

Emile Holman, 1971

There is a series of anatomical and pathologic changes which evolves when an arteriovenous fistula is produced (Fig. 9–14). An arteriovenous fistula is an abnormal communication between the arterial and venous systems which creates a shorter circuit in relation to the heart by allowing blood to pass from the higher peripheral resistance of the arterial system to the lower peripheral resistance of the venous

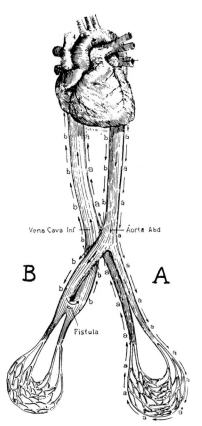

Figure 9–14. This schema shows the circulation in the presence of a right femoral arteriovenous fistula establishing a second circuit of blood. A progressively increasing volume of blood is sequestered in circuit B as long as resistance in the fistula circuit is less than resistance in the capillary bed in circuit A. (Holman, E., Arteriovenous Aneurysm: Abnormal Communications Between the Arterial and Venous Circulations. The Macmillan Company, New York, 1937.)

fistula. If the rim of the arteriovenous fistula is rigid from fibrosis, there is more tendency to limit the volume of shunt of blood. On the other hand, a distensible

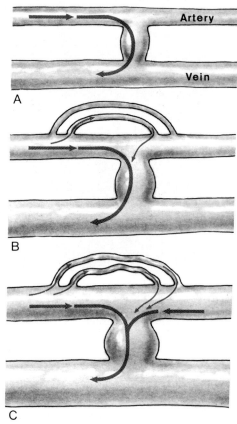

Figure 9–15. (A) Immediately following the development of an arteriovenous fistula there is shunting of blood from the artery through the fistula into the vein, from which it returns to the heart. This results in a decrease in peripheral vascular resistance, a fall in diastolic blood pressure and an increase in heart rate. The venous pressure rises in the involved vein. Peripheral blood flow is decreased in the involved artery. (B) After several weeks, collateral circulation enlarges around the fistula because of the decreased vascular resistance at the site of the fistula. As the collateral circulation develops, the involved artery and vein also dilate, increasing the amount of blood flowing through the fistula. (C) After several years, extensive dilatation may develop about a fistula with marked enlargement of collateral circulation. In addition, there is enlargement of the artery immediately distal to the fistula, through which blood flows in a retrograde fashion through the fistula toward the heart. The vein may enlarge to marked proportions, creating varicosities in the extremity. Ultimately such progressive dilatation after a period of years may result in congestive heart failure from the increased cardiac output. (Spencer, F. C., *in* Schwartz, S. I., et al. (Eds.), Principles of Surgery. McGraw-Hill Book Company, New York, 1974.)

system (Fig. 9–15). This secondary circuit, which has a constant tendency to divert the arterial blood into the lower resistance venous system through the fistula, causes a number of hemodynamic disturbances. The effective systemic blood flow is reduced, and there is a decreased mean systemic arterial pressure. However, there is an increase in the blood volume, total cardiac output, stroke volume, heart rate, left atrial pressure and pulmonary arterial pressure, as has been described by Holman (1937, 1968).

Holman also emphasized that the size of the arteriovenous fistula, the location of the communication in the vascular tree and the distensibility of the vascular rim are the factors that determine the volume of blood that is diverted through the arteriovenous fistula's border permits progressive increase of the blood shunted through the secondary circuit of the fistula, with additional increase in the blood volume and dilatation of the heart. Lewis (1940) demonstrated that the entire circuit gradually dilates to accommodate the increased volume of blood flow; this includes dilatation of the cardiac chambers, the arterial tree proximal to the fistula, the proximal vein and vena cava and even the arteriovenous fistula itself. Nakano and De Schryver (1964) studied the effects of arteriovenous fistulas on systemic and pulmonary circulation and stated that the increase in cardiac output was essentially a result of the increase in stroke volume, noting that the heart rate may change very little.

Holman (1965) reviewed abnormal arteriovenous communications with particular reference to the delayed development of cardiac failure. He emphasized that <u>low resistance in the venous system to the shunt of blood at the site of the fistula and the decrease in peripheral perfusion distal to the arteriovenous fistula were strong stimuli for the development of collateral circulation.</u> Holman (1940) documented significant structural changes in both the arteries and veins associated with the hemodynamic disturbances of an arteriovenous fistula. With a small communication, the vein gradually assumes the appearance of an artery, and it may not be easily distinguished from the artery at the end of six to nine months. In contrast, with larger fistulas, the vein may become so distended that it appears to be a false aneurysmal sac. As has been known since the first description by Hunter in 1757, the artery proximal to the arteriovenous fistula can become dilated; however, Holman (1940) stated that dilatation of the artery can also occur distal to the fistula. It is not only the initial injury that creates the arteriovenous fistula; the arterial walls at the fistula or proximal to it may become rigid as a result of deposition of fibrous tissue, or the lumen may even become stenotic by contraction of surrounding fibrous tissues.

Some arteriovenous fistulas may be associated with a decreased resistance in the peripheral arterial tree. The consequent enlargement of superficial venous collaterals can be mistaken for changes associated with chronic venous insufficiency. We saw one Vietnam casualty at Walter Reed General Hospital who had been treated for varicose veins of his left lower extremity for five years, when in actuality the increase in his left thigh and associated superficial varicosities were associated with an acquired femoral arteriovenous fistula.

According to Petrovsky and Milonov (1967), the structural changes that occur in the walls of both the arteries and the veins associated with an arteriovenous fistula are called "venization" of arteries and "arterialization" of veins. The alterations in the venous walls are easier to understand because they can be caused by an abrupt increase in the venous pressure and can be considered a consequence of adaptation to new conditions. There is more difficulty in explaining or understanding the changes in the artery. Petrovsky and Milonov (1967) performed experiments which showed thickening of the media of the venous wall due to an increase in the amount of muscular and connective tissue elements, marked elastosis of all layers of the vessel wall, intimal thickening and an increase in the vasa vasorum, which made it resemble the wall of an artery. They saw an increase in muscular fibers and fibrosis in the arterial wall, with a corresponding increase of mucopolysaccharides and extracellular fibers, elastosis and later dystrophy of the elastic fibers, focal necrosis of connective tissue elements in the adventitia and diminution of the vasa vasorum. It was felt that a decrease in the oxidative process accounted for the accumulation of mucopolysaccharides, the extra cellular fibrosis and the elastolysis (decrease in oxidative processes and tissue hypoxia which result from a decreased blood supply in the arterial wall).

Holman (1940) stated that hemodynamic changes caused by arteriovenous fistulas were reversible. However, some structural changes may not be reversible, e.g., dilatation of the proximal artery associated with an arteriovenous fistula of long standing which may not regress if aneurysmal deterioration of the wall has occurred. Also, cardiac enlargement associated with long standing arteriovenous fistulas and dilatation may not revert to normal.

Eisenbrey emphasized the extensive alterations in both the artery and vein up to the bifurcation of the aorta and vena cava in a patient with a superficial femoral arteriovenous fistula (see Fig. 9–2). The patient complained of shortness of breath and presented symptoms of cardiac insufficiency. Eighteen years earlier, the patient had been shot in the thigh with a small caliber (probably .22 caliber) rifle bullet. Terminal illness allowed necropsy examination of the aneurysmal dilatation and tortuosity of the artery and vein.

Recent studies have augmented the original and monumental contributions of Holman. Schenk and associates (1957) evaluated the regional hemodynamics of experimental acute arteriovenous fistulas. Their objective was to use the newer electronic methods for pressure and flow measurements to investigate the pressure-flow changes which occurred immediately upon opening an experimental fistula. Figure 9–16 summarizes the pressure-flow data in a representative model.

Johnson and co-workers (1967) studied the cardiad vein negative pressure in arteriovenous fistulas with a plastic model. They demonstrated creation of a negative pressure in the cardiad vein, the result of transformation of energy, and explained this by the use of the principles of flow through a conduit (Fig. 9–17).

Johnson and Blythe (1970) evaluated eight patients with arteriovenous fistulas

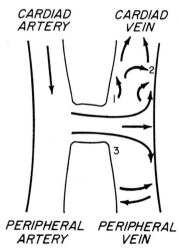

Figure 9–17. Flow pattern through fistula. In model, pressure at *1* was −20 millimeters of mercury, at *2* it was −5 millimeters of mercury, and at *3* it was −4 millimeters of mercury, emphasizing the negative pressure in the cardiad vein and arteriovenous fistula. (Johnson, G., Jr., Peters, R. M., and Dart, C. H., Jr., Surg. Gynecol. Obstet. *124*:82, 1967.)

created for hemodialysis over a period of three years. Their study demonstrated that peripheral arteriovenous fistulas created for hemodialysis in patients with chronic renal failure result in a slight increase in cardiac output and pulse rate and a decrease in the total peripheral resistance. Although these alterations in hemodynamics did not lead to perceptible cardiac strain, a warning was made that physicians managing these patients should be cognizant of this possibility, especially in patients on long term hemodialysis.

CLINICAL PATHOLOGY

The capillary circulation is bypassed in an arteriovenous fistula when there is a direct communication between an artery and a vein. Although this type of communication can be a normal function of the microcirculation, the arteriovenous fistula becomes pathologic when its size or location causes significant hemodynamic alterations. An arteriovenous fistula may be established immediately after a penetrating injury in which blood flows directly from the injured artery into the vein. On the other hand, thrombus may surround the

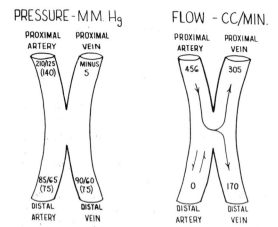

Figure 9–16. Schematic summary of pressure-flow data in a representative animal after a large femoral arteriovenous fistula was opened. (Schenk, W. G., Bahn, R., Cordell, A. R., and Stephens, J. G., Surg. Gynecol. Obstet., *105*:733, 1957.)

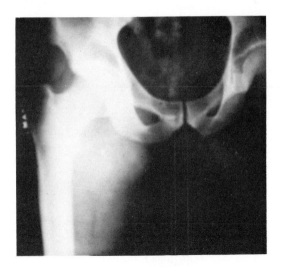

Figure 9-18. This small fragment wound of the upper right thigh created an arteriovenous fistula that was not diagnosed initially. The surrounding increased density on the roentgenogram was caused by an associated pulsating hematoma. (Rich, N. M., J. Cardiovasc. Surg., *11*:3, 1970.)

arteriovenous fistula, and the communication may not be obvious until days or weeks later when the surrounding clot becomes liquefied (Fig. 9–18).

Once a traumatic arteriovenous fistula has been established, there is usually little difficulty in its recognition. The previous history of trauma, the finding of a prominent pulsation and palpable thrill and the presence of an audible machinery-like murmur or any combination of these findings should alert one to the presence of an arteriovenous fistula. A bruit often appears over the site of an arteriovenous communication within a matter of hours after the establishment of the lesion. Other signs and symptoms which can develop distal to an arteriovenous fistula include intermittent claudication, edema (Fig. 9–19) and prominent veins (Fig. 9–20) which are often accompanied by bluish discoloration of the skin and venous stasis. The last two findings result from shunting of the arterial blood into the venous system.

More than 200 years ago, in 1757, William Hunter recognized an abnormal communication between an artery and a vein and accurately described the thrill and bruit associated with the communication. He noted that he could eliminate both the thrill and the bruit by pressure over either the proximal artery or the site of the com-

Figure 9-19. Edema can be associated with arteriovenous fistulas. The massive swelling of the left lower extremity in this Vietnam casualty is obvious. He had a femoral arteriovenous fistula of five years' duration; however, he had been treated as a patient with varicose veins. (Vietnam Vascular Registry #630, NMR, 1972.)

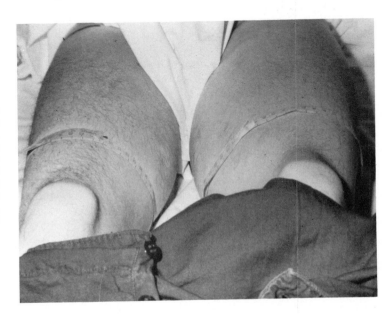

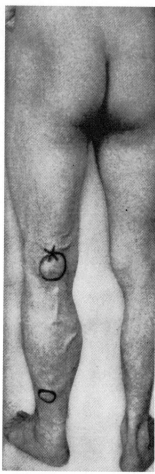

Figure 9–20. The position of an arteriovenous fistula and pulsating venous lakes (circled); note the difference in size of the two lakes. The site of the fistula is indicated by a cross. (Holman, E., Arch. Surg., 7:64, 1923.)

munication. He also documentated his observation of tortuosity and dilatation of the artery proximal to the fistula.

Nicoladoni in 1875 is generally given credit for being the first to demonstrate the remarkable fact that the pulse rate could be lowered by compression of the artery proximal to the arteriovenous fistula. Fifteen years later, in 1890, Branham again called attention to the reduction of the pulse rate by obliteration of a large acquired arteriovenous fistula. This phenomenon is frequently referred to as the Branham-Nicoladoni sign.

The most mysterious phenomenon connected with the case, one which I have not been able to explain myself, or to obtain a satisfactory reason for from others, was slowing of the heart's beat, when compression of the common femoral was employed. This began to be noticeable after the wound had entirely healed. The patient was apparently well, with exception of the injured vessel, which necessitated his confinement to bed. This symptom became more marked until pressure of the artery above the wound caused the heart's beat to fall from 80 to 35 or 40 per minute, and so to remain until the pressure was relieved.

Harris H. Branham, 1890

While working as a student of Halsted, Reid established that there was enlargement of the heart in the presence of an arteriovenous fistula. In 1913, Stewart noted that the heart diminished in size within 10 days after elimination of the fistula.

CLINICAL FEATURES

If the patient has had a penetrating injury, the possibility of an arteriovenous fistula must be recognized; however, this may not be immediately obvious. As previously noted, if the arteriovenous communication has surrounding thrombus, the classic findings of a thrill and bruit may not exist until several days or weeks later. There may be little evidence of vascular trauma in the way of blood loss or loss of peripheral pulses (Fig. 9–21). The patient may or may not be aware of a buzzing sensation when his fingers are placed over the area of the arteriovenous communication. One patient in the Registry had originally been wounded in Korea; however, it was nearly 15 years later, when he was piloting a helicopter in Vietnam, that he noticed a buzzing sensation in his popliteal fossa. It may be more unusual for the patient to present with one of the complications of arteriovenous fistula, such as infection within the vascular system, peripheral embolization or congestive heart failure.

Errors in diagnosis can exist. Patients with arteriovenous fistulas have been treated for years for varicose veins (see Fig. 9–19). Venous hypertension with resultant varices, peripheral pigmentation and ulceration from venous insufficiency can confuse the diagnosis; however, the classic findings

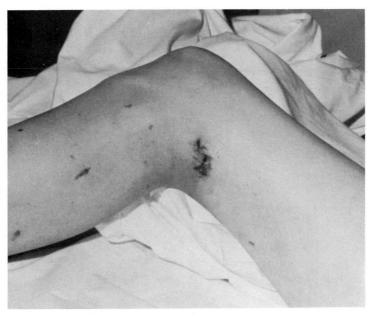

Figure 9–21. A small wound may deceive the casual observer as to the extent of underlying vascular pathology. This patient later developed an expanding mass associated with a popliteal arteriovenous fistula and false aneurysm. (Vietnam Vascular Registry #2513, NMR, 1971.)

of a thrill and bruit should be carefully sought.

There may or may not be a soft, diffuse mass on physical examination. Depending on the period of time that the arteriovenous fistula has existed, dilated veins may surround the area. A thrill, with its maximal component during systole, is usually felt very easily on palpation. A "machinery murmur" is usually heard easily on auscultation, the loudest part of the continuous murmur occurring during systole. Detection of this classic finding differentiates an arteriovenous fistula from an arterial false aneurysm. The Nicoladoni-Branham sign, which has been previously described, is another significant finding if a slowing pulse can be demonstrated when the fistula is obliterated by digital compression. Ironically, this test was not positive in many of the Vietnam casualties with arteriovenous fistulas. The peripheral resistance increases when the fistula is digitally occluded, causing the blood pressure to rise, with reflex slowing of the heart rate and consequent slowing of the pulse. The temporary bradycardia results from a neurogenic reflex mediated through pressure-sensitive receptors in the carotid sinuses and great vessels.

With large arteriovenous fistulas and a large shunting of blood, cardiac enlargement and, more rarely, cardiac failure may occur (Fig. 9–22). Smith and co-authors (1963) found the most serious complication of arteriovenous fistulization—left ventricular myocardial failure—in two of their patients. One of these was a 16 year old male who had been shot in the right thigh with a .22 caliber rifle bullet. Nine days after the accident the patient developed a gallop rhythm and severe dyspnea. A chest roentgenogram revealed a marked enlargement of the cardiac shadow. An emergency operation was performed to correct a common femoral arteriovenous communication. The signs of congestive cardiac failure regressed in three weeks. These authors pointed out that there was a regrettable error of omission in the immediate exploration of the wound. They felt that the rapid development of cardiac decompensation, which made surgical intervention most urgent, was an unusual aspect of the case.

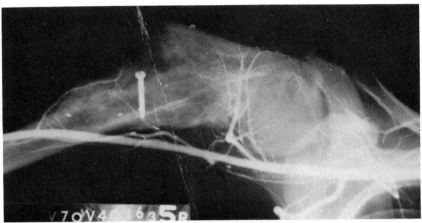

Figure 9–30. A repeat arteriogram, performed six weeks later, demonstrating that the arteriovenous communication in the axillary vessels (see Fig. 9–29) is no longer present. Elective operative closure had not been performed because of a wound infection. The site of "thrombosis" is visible as a small, contrast-filled saccule on the inferior surface of the axillary artery. (Billings, K. J., Nasca, R. J., and Griffin, H. A., J. Trauma, *13*:741, 1973. Copyright 1973, The Williams & Wilkins Company, Baltimore.)

ing mass was noted in the right axilla, and there was a continuous bruit and thrill over the mass. An axillary arteriovenous fistula was demonstrated by angiography (Fig. 9–29). Treatment of other multiple wounds was carried out, and during the first week in November the axillary mass was no longer palpable. A repeat arteriogram demonstrated that there had been spontaneous closure of the arteriovenous fistula (Fig. 9–30). Two similar patients — Vietnam casualties — were seen at Walter Reed General Hospital.

RESULTS

Annandale (1875) reported the successful ligature of a popliteal artery and vein in the treatment of a traumatic popliteal arteriovenous fistula. Pick (1883) reported the case of a 28 year old male who sustained a gunshot wound of the thigh with a resultant arteriovenous fistula of the femoral vessels. He stated that the only operative procedure which appeared to hold any hope for success was ligature of the artery above and below the point of communication. According to Murphy (1897), Von Zoege-Manteuffel successfully repaired a femoral arteriovenous aneurysm by lateral suture of the wall in 1895. When the first end-to-end arterial anastomosis in man

was reported by Murphy (1897), he described his successful treatment in 1896 of a common femoral arteriovenous fistula. In addition to the end-to-end arterial anastomosis following resection of the damaged portion of the artery he also closed the wound in the vein by lateral venorrhaphy. Bickham (1904) suggested that the Matas endoaneurysmorrhaphy could be employed for the intravascular repair of arteriovenous fistulas. He also recommended transverse closure of the defects in the vascular walls as a practical method of preserving the continuity of both the injured artery and vein. Matas emphasized the reason for failure when partial ligation was used in the treatment of arteriovenous fistulas was the remaining patency in other vessels not ligated (Fig. 9–31).

Soubbotitch (1913) reported on the military experience in the Serbo-Turkish and Serbo-Bulgarian Wars. There were 16 different surgeons who performed ligation of large vessels on 41 arteries and 4 veins and partial suture on 17 vessels — 8 arteries and 9 veins. Circular suture was employed on 15 vessels — 11 arteries and 4 veins — to bring the total number of vessels sutured to 32 (19 arteriorrhaphies and 13 venorrhaphies). The 60 arteries and 17 veins made a total of 77 injuries to the larger blood vessels among 20,000 wounded. Osler (1915) stated that there was agreement with a

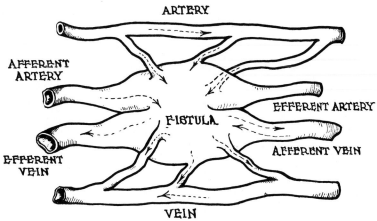

Figure 9–31. Schematic drawing showing the communications of an arteriovenous fistula and the necessity of not only quadruple ligation but also complete excision including all branches. (Matas, R., *in* Keen's Surgery. Vol. VII. W. B. Saunders Company, Philadelphia, 1921.)

conclusion arrived at by Soubbotitch, senior surgeon at the Belgrade State Hospital, from his experience in the Balkan War, "that arteriovenous aneurysms should be operated upon, as they offer small prospect of spontaneous cure, although they often remain stationary for a long time and cause relatively little trouble."

World War I contributed little significant data compared to World War II. Because competent vascular surgeons were chosen to head three centers for vascular surgery during World War II, a large number of arteriovenous fistulas and arterial aneurysms were managed. Elkin and Shumacker (1955) outlined the techniques of operative treatment of 585 arteriovenous fistulas (Table 9–15). Arterial repair was used in only 34 lesions.

The representative material that follows covers a small portion of the World War II experience. Freeman and Shumacker (1955) outlined various approaches in the management of arteriovenous fistulas. Figure 9–32 shows one of the approaches, which involved:

1. Mass ligation of the fistula.
2. Quadruple ligation and division of the main vessels with excision of the fistula.
3. Transvenous closure of the arterial opening.
4. Repair of the opening in both the artery and the vein.

Shumacker (1948A) stressed the impor-

tance of maintaining arterial continuity in the repair of aneurysms and arteriovenous fistulas. In his early experience he performed only four reparative procedures—2.9 per cent of 138 cases involving the innominate, common carotid, extracranial internal carotid, subclavian, axillary, brachial, iliac, common femoral, femoral and popliteal arteries. In later experience, he repaired 52.6 per cent of the arteries: 30 of 57 cases. This included lateral arteriorrhaphy, end-to-end anastomosis and vein graft repair (Table 9–16). The types of autogenous interposition venous grafts used range from the saphenous to a branch of the femoral. Figures 9–33 and 9–34 reveal patency of the venous grafts and no dilatation of the grafts in the early follow-up period of 7 to 10 weeks.

Shumacker (1948A) also used oscillometric studies to evaluate the patency of arterial repair (Table 9–17). The results of oscillometry were good in those cases in which arterial repairs remained patent and poor in those in which arterial repair failed due to thrombosis.

Hughes and Jahnke (1958) performed an end-to-end anastomosis in the majority of arteriovenous fistulas (61 of 134) from the Korean Conflict (Table 9–18). As a result of the Korean Conflict, over 200 patients with false aneurysms and arteriovenous fistulas, 133 of the injuries involving major vessels, were seen at Walter Reed

Text continued on page 225

TABLE 9–15. TECHNIQUES OF OPERATIVE TREATMENT IN 585 ARTERIOVENOUS FISTULAS: WORLD WAR II EXPERIENCE*

Location	Arterial Repair	Quadruple Ligation and Excision	Ligation Alone (Mass Proximal, Distal, or Proximal and Distal)	Total Cases
Upper extremity:				
Axillary		32		32
Brachial		29		29[1]
Cervical, transverse		1		1[2]
Humeral, posterior circumflex		1		1
Interosseous, common		1		1
Radial		2		2
Scapular, transverse		2		2
Subclavian	1	16	1	18[3]
Ulnar		9		9
Lower extremity:				
Calf, to muscles of		4		4
Circumflex, lateral		1		1
Femoral	16	124	1	141[4]
Geniculate		5		5
Gluteal, inferior		1		1
superior		3		3
Peroneal		24	1	25
Plantar		6		6
Popliteal	11	91		102
Profunda femoris		19		19
branch		2		2
Tibial		87		87
Head and neck:				
Carotid	5	29	14	48[3]
Cirsoid		9		9
Lingual		1		1
Occipital		1		1
Temporal, superficial		3	2	5
Vertebral		8	5	13
Trunk:				
Aorta–vena cava	1			1
Hypogastric		1		1
Iliac		9		9
Innominate			1	1
Mammary, internal		1		1
Obturator–iliac vein		1		1
Subscapular		2		2
Thoracoacromial		1		1
Total:	34	526	25	585

This total does not include:

[1] 2 fistulas, 1 in which method of management not stated, and 1 in which spontaneous cure occurred.

[2] 1 fistula in which method of management not stated.

[3] fistula in which spontaneous cure occurred.

[4] 3 fistulas, 1 in which methods of management not stated, and 2 in which spontaneous cure occurred.

*Elkin, D. C., Shumacker, H. B., Jr., *in* Elkin, D. C., and DeBakey, M. E., (Eds.), Vascular Surgery in World War II. Government Printing Office, Washington, D. C., 1955.

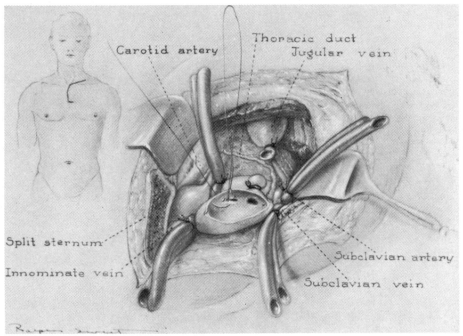

Figure 9–32. Transvenous repair of an arteriovenous fistula involving the left subclavian artery and innominate vein. Insert shows the surgical approach to the lesion which was used to manage a World War II combat casualty at DeWitt General Hospital in 1945. (Freeman, N. E., and Shumacker, H. B., Jr., *in* Elkin, D. C., and DeBakey, M. E. (Eds.), Vascular Surgery in World War II. Government Printing Office, Washington, D.C., 1955.)

TABLE 9–16. CASES IN WHICH CONTINUITY OF ARTERY WAS RESTORED BY VEIN TRANSPLANT*

Case No.	Age of Patient	Duration of Lesion in Months	Type of Lesion	Location of Lesion	Preoperative Sympathectomy	Length of Vein Graft in CM	Source of Vein Graft	Period of Follow-up in Months	Result
1	26	4.2	AV and saccular aneurysms	Femoral, distal 3rd	0	2	Saphenous	3	Excellent
2	19	5	AV	Femoral, middle 3rd	0	2	Branch of femoral	3	Excellent
3	26	4	AV	Femoral, distal 3rd	+	5	Saphenous	3	Excellent
4	35	?	Saccular aneurysm	Popliteal, middle 3rd	+	2	Small saphenous	4	Excellent
5	36	6 yr	Saccular aneurysm	Femoral, proximal 3rd	0	2.5	Femoral	1.5	Excellent
6	24	5.3	Saccular aneurysm	Brachial, middle 3rd	0	2.5	Saphenous	1.2	Thrombosis; good circulation maintained

*Shumacker, H. B., Jr., Ann. Surg., *127:*207, 1948.

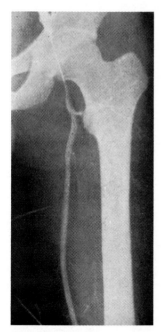

Figure 9–33. This arteriogram taken 10 weeks after repair of a fistula between the femoral and profunda femoral arteries and the femoral vein, with resection and end-to-end anastomosis of the profunda femoral artery proximally to the superficial femoral artery distally, shows no narrowing at the suture line after 70 per cent Diodrast was injected into the common femoral artery. (Shumacker, H. B., Jr., Ann. Surg., *127*:207, 1948.)

large number of similar wounds in 1967 and 1969. The time from injury to recognition of the lesion was arbitrarily divided into four cagegories — immediate, early, delayed and remote. The largest number of lesions was recognized in the early period of 1 to 30 days: 273 or 48.9 per cent (Table 9–20). Nearly an equal number were diagnosed in the delayed period between one and six months. In the remote group, all but 7 of the 35 patients had recognition and treatment of their lesions in less than two years. Only two had recognition and treatment of their lesions after more than five years following the initial injury, and both were treated in less than six years. Nearly an equal number of lesions were treated in the intermediate hospitals in

Text continued on page 228

General Hospital. The lesions were excised, with reparative or reconstructive surgery of the major vessel, without loss of a single limb. Treatment of minor vessel lesions has previously been outlined in Table 9–9. Repair of major veins was performed whenever possible to prevent venous insufficiency (see Chap. 8). This venous repair was possible in about 30 per cent of major veins involved in fistula formation. Cardiac dilatation was common with large fistulas; however, only two patients showed cardiac failure.

Rich and associates (1975D) reported the experience from Vietnam. Of 558 lesions identified in 509 patients, there were almost an equal number of arteriovenous fistulas (262) and false aneurysms (296). As might be anticipated by the number of American troops committed to Southeast Asia in that year, the largest number of lesions resulted from wounds in 1968 (Table 9–19). There were also a relatively

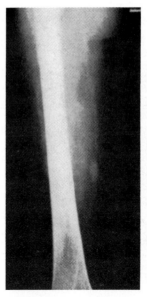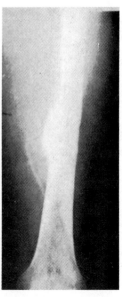

Figure 9–34. The arteriogram on the left, taken seven weeks after repair of an arteriovenous fistula between the superficial femoral artery and vein, with interposition of a segment of a large branch of the femoral vein 2 cm in length, reveals that the venous insert and the artery have relative diameters about equal to those observed at completion of the operation (Case 2). The arteriogram on the right shows that there is no dilatation of the venous segment of a 2 cm piece of saphenous vein used to reconstruct the superficial femoral artery after resection of an arteriovenous fistula and saccular aneurysm involving the femoral vessels (Case 1). There was no dilatation at the completion of the anastomosis, and no dilatation was seen on this arteriogram performed 10 weeks later. (Shumacker, H. B., Jr., Ann. Surg., *127*:207, 1948.)

TABLE 9–17. OSCILLOMETRIC STUDIES AFTER ARTERIAL REPAIR*

TYPE OF REPAIR	ARTERY REPAIRED	NO. OF CASES	OSCILLOMETRY AT ANKLE OR WRIST		OSCILLOMETRY AT CALF OR FOREARM		OSCILLOMETRY AT THIGH OR ARM	
			Reading Average	Per Cent of Reading in Contralateral Limb	Reading Average	Per Cent of Reading in Contralateral Limb	Reading Average	Per Cent of Reading in Contralateral Limb
Ligation of fistula	Femoral	5	2.3	96	5.1	96	3.5	95
	Popliteal	4	5.1	75	7.6	95	...	...
Lateral arteriorrhaphy	Subclavian	2	2.5	83	3.8	70	4.5	88
End-to-end suture	Axillary	2	1.0	37	1.5	41	2.2	44
	Brachial	4	2.5	83	2.8	51	...	...
	Femoral	1	3.0	60	4.5	50	7	100
Vein transplantation	Femoral	4	3.1	67	4	50	4	67
	Popliteal	1	2.0	67	3	43	...	...
Successful repairs	Total:	24	2.9	79	4.3	68	4.0	68
Unsuccessful repairs	Total:	5	1.0	17	0.9	16	0.5	18

*Shumacker, H. B., Jr., Ann. Surg., *127*:207, 1948.

TABLE 9–18. TOTAL OPERATIONS FOR MAJOR VESSEL LESIONS: MILITARY SERIES FROM THE KOREAN CONFLICT*

VESSEL	LIGATION AND EXCISION	ANASTO-MOSIS	VEIN GRAFT	ARTERY GRAFT	LATERAL REPAIR	DIVISION OF FISTULA	SRONTA-NEOUS CLOSURE	TOTAL
Common carotid	—	6	—	—	—	1	2	9
Internal carotid	2	—	—	—	—	1	—	3
Subclavian	3	2	2	1	1	1	3	8
Axillary	4	8	2	1	2	—	—	20
Brachial	6	9	1	1	1	1	—	19
Iliac	—	3	—	1	—	—	—	4
Common femoral	—	3	2	1	—	2	—	8
Superficial femoral	6	14	9	—	—	2	—	31
Popliteal	9	16	3	1	—	2	1	32
Total:	30	61	17	6	4	10	6	134

*Hughes, C. W., and Jahnke, E. J., Jr., Ann. Surg., *148:*790, 1958.

TABLE 9–19. ARTERIOVENOUS FISTULAS AND FALSE ANEURYSMS—YEAR OF INJURY: VIETNAM VASCULAR REGISTRY*

Year	No.	Per Cent
1963	1	0.2
1964	0	0.0
1965	11	2.0
1966	44	7.9
1967	116	20.8
1968	249	44.6
1969	124	22.2
1970	5	0.9
1971	7	1.2
1972	1	0.2
Total:	558	100.0

*Rich, N. M., Hobson, R. W., II, and Collins, G. J., Jr., Surgery, *78*:817, 1975.

TABLE 9–21. ARTERIOVENOUS FISTULAS AND FALSE ANEURYSMS—HOSPITAL LOCATION FOR REPAIR: VIETNAM VASCULAR REGISTRY*

Location	No. of Repairs	Per Cent
Vietnam	57	10.2
Japan, etc.	238	42.7
CONUS	251	45.0
No repair	12	2.1
Total:	558	100.0

*Rich, N. M., Hobson, R. W., II, and Collins, G. J., Jr., Surgery, *78*:817, 1975.

Japan and similar Far West locations as were treated in the continental United States (Table 9–21). Several hundred different surgeons were involved in these repairs. Approximately one-fifth of these operations were performed at Walter Reed Army Medical Center.

Table 9–22 outlines the method of treatment utilized for the various arterial and venous injuries. Arterial ligation was utilized in 290 lesions: 52.0 per cent. Compelling problems often caused this method to be used over the favored and desired arterial repair. Infection, associated injuries, poor general condition of the patient and involvement of smaller caliber arteries were considered. The over-all mortality rate for the 509 patients was 1.8 per cent: seven deaths (Table 9–23). Even considering this low mortality rate, only two deaths could be

directly attributed to the vascular problem. The morbidity rate of 6.3 per cent included 35 complications: hemorrhage in 14, thromboses in 12, stenosis in 2 and persistent, immediately adjacent or recurrent arteriovenous fistulas requiring additional operations in 7.

Experience in the civilian hospitals is increasing. Hershey (1961) encountered a technical complication. The artery proximal to the arteriovenous fistula had dilated and become fragile; it was crushed by a clamp, and a hematoma developed (Fig. 9–35).

Beall and associates (1963) repaired 8 of 50 arteriovenous fistulas within 24 hours of

TABLE 9–20. ARTERIOVENOUS FISTULAS AND FALSE ANEURYSMS—TIME OF DIAGNOSIS: VIETNAM VASCULAR REGISTRY*

Time	No.	Per Cent
Immediate (24 hr)	22	3.9
Early (1 to 30 days)	273	48.9
Delayed (1 to 6 mo)	228	40.9
Remote (>6 mo)	35	6.3
Total:	558	100.0

*Rich, N. M., Hobson, R. W., II, and Collins, G. J., Jr., Surgery, *78*:817, 1975.

TABLE 9–22. ARTERIOVENOUS FISTULAS AND FALSE ANEURYSMS—METHOD OF MANAGEMENT: VIETNAM VASCULAR REGISTRY*

Type	No.	Per Cent
Arterial:		
Ligation	290	52.0
End-to-end anastomosis	143	25.6
Vein graft	57	10.2
Lateral suture	40	7.2
Prosthesis	2	0.3
Miscellaneous	26	4.7
Total:	558	100.0
Venous:		
Ligation	138	52.7
Suture	79	30.1
Miscellaneous	45	17.2
Total:	262	100.0

*Rich, N. M., Hobson, R. W., II, and Collins, G. J., Jr., Surgery, *78*:817, 1975.

TABLE 9–23. ARTERIOVENOUS FISTULAS AND FALSE ANEURYSMS— MORTALITY AND MORBIDITY RATES: VIETNAM VASCULAR REGISTRY*

	No.	Per Cent
Deaths	7	1.8
Morbidity		
Amputations	8	1.7
Complications	35	6.3

*Rich, N. M., Hobson, R. W., II, and Collins, G. J., Jr., Surgery, *78*:817, 1975.

injury; an additional 17 were repaired within 24 hours to 3 months following injury. However, there was a delayed repair of more than three months following injury for 23, or nearly 50 per cent, of the lesions. No repair was performed for two of the arteriovenous fistulas. Excision and repair was utilized for 27 lesions and ligation and excision for 17 lesions. No deaths were reported. There were no amputations required. Not counting two patients lost in follow-up who had no treatment, 42 were asymptomatic. Six patients were symptomatic following their original definitive surgical procedure, and three required subsequent operations.

In the civilian series of 61 arterial injuries reported by Smith and co-workers (1963), approximately two-thirds of the 33 chronic or late lesions were arteriovenous fistulas. They mentioned that the time interval from original injury to treatment varied considerably from a few days to 29 years, the majority of patients, 57 per cent, being treated after one year. Of the six patients with arteriovenous fistulas reported by Patman and colleagues (1964), five did not have initial exploration of the area. The remaining patient did have an initial exploration; however, the arteriovenous fistula was not diagnosed until four hours after injury. The authors stressed that this development demonstrated the rapidity with which an arteriovenous fistula can develop. Both the common and superficial femoral arteries were involved in arteriovenous fistulas. The remaining four fistulas were equally divided among the smaller radial and posterior tibial arteries. There were no deaths, amputations or other significant complications in any of the patients.

Dillard and associates (1968) reported a number of arteriovenous fistulas including: (1) a 29 year old female who was stabbed in the right flank and three years later was found to have severe hypertension; after correction of the renal arteriovenous fistula, the patient's blood pressure returned to normal; (2) a patient with severe leg

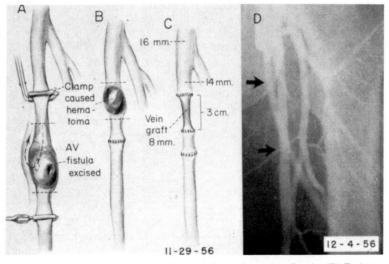

Figure 9–35. (A) Artist's sketch of a superficial femoral arteriovenous fistula. (B) End-to-end anastomosis after excision of the fistula. An intraluminal hematoma developed at the site of a Blalock clamp. (C) Sketch of the vein graft after excision of the hematoma, showing size discrepancies. (D) Postoperative arteriogram with the arrows showing the site of anastomosis. (Hershey, F. B., Am. Surg., 27:33, 1961.)

ulcers which healed only after correction of an arteriovenous fistula in the same extremity between the common femoral artery and vein; (3) a patient with an arteriovenous fistula between the popliteal artery and vein, which resulted in amputation. Two of the nine arteriovenous fistulas reported by Dillard and associates (1968) involved high output failure. One of these fistulas occurred between the subscapular artery and the axillary vein and the other between the right iliac artery and the left common iliac vein.

Sako and Varco (1970) reported corrective procedures in 25 patients with acquired arteriovenous fistulas. Excision of the fistula with arterial and venous repair was performed in more than 50 per cent, or 16 lesions. Quadruple ligation was used in six and multiple ligation in two. Included in the arterial repairs were 13 primary anastomoses, 3 autologous venous grafts and 1 homograft. All of the acquired fistulas were cured by the surgical procedures described without a death.

Gaspard and Gaspar (1972) reported two patients who developed arteriovenous fistulas after Fogarty catheter thrombectomy

in the lower extremity. They emphasized that neither of their patients required immediate operation for limb salvage, nor had either had an operation performed subsequently. They cited the report by Rob and Battle (1971) in which correction of the arteriovenous fistula 26 days after use of the Fogarty catheter was mandatory because the distal extremity was in jeopardy.

Hewitt and co-workers (1973) advocated immediate repair of acute arteriovenous fistulas. This was possible in 13 of the 14 patients in their series, and they reported satisfactory results in all repairs, including resection with end-to-end anastomosis in six, saphenous vein graft in two, saphenous vein patch graft in two and lateral suture repair in three, ligation being required only for one distal internal carotid artery.

In addition to the anticipated complications of cardiac enlargement, cardiac failure, endocarditis and proximal arterial aneurysm formation unusual complications have been reported. Rhodes and colleagues (1973) reported the case of a 53 year old male with a 10 day history of bruising easily, hematuria and bleeding from his tongue. The patient was involved in a

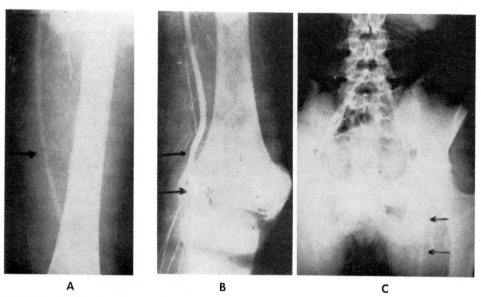

A   B   C

Figure 9–36. (A) Arteriography after excision and anastomosis of the superficial femoral artery shows an excellent lumen. A vein graft inserted into the popliteal artery is demonstrated by angiography approximately six months after operation. Examination of this patient 5½ years after operation showed the vein graft to be functioning perfectly without clinical evidence of dilatation (B). Arteriography was used to demonstrate an arterial homograft which replaced the common femoral artery (C). These angiograms were part of the follow-up of Korean casualties who had repair of arteriovenous fistulas. (Hughes, C. W., and Jahnke, E. J., Jr., Ann. Surg., *148*:790, 1958.)

shooting accident 17 years previously and had acquired an arteriovenous fistula between the left subclavian artery and vein as a result. The authors attributed the local sustained intravascular coagulation that caused the man's symptoms to turbulence from the fistula and stasis from the aneurysm. The coagulopathy and bleeding responded to surgical elimination of the fistula and aneurysm. The authors felt that this was the first report of a consumption coagulopathy resulting from an arteriovenous fistula and false aneurysm.

FOLLOW-UP

Hughes and Jahnke (1958) included a five year follow-up of 148 lesions treated during the Korean Conflict, satisfactory results being obtained in the majority of patients (Fig. 9–36).

The Vietnam vascular registry continues to follow patients included in the report by Rich and associates (1975D). More than one-fourth—149 patients or 29.3 per cent—have been evaluated in the vascular clinic at Walter Reed Army Medical Center. Many of these patients can be expected to live 50 years or more (Fig. 9–37).

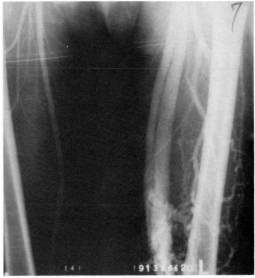

Figure 9–37. This angiogram corroborated the clinical impression of a left femoral arteriovenous fistula. Additional assistance, however, was provided to establish that the communication involved a muscular branch of the superficial femoral artery and the superficial femoral vein. Note the development of collaterals. Also note the proximal arterial dilatation of the superficial femoral artery in this former soldier who had been wounded five years prior to this study. (Rich, N. M., *in* Beebe, H. G. (Ed.), Complications in Vascular Surgery. J. B. Lippincott Company, Philadelphia, 1973.)

Figure 9–38. In this operative photograph aneurysmal dilatation of the superficial femoral artery (A), the narrowed segment (B) where the artery traversed Hunter's canal, and a popliteal aneurysm (C) are demonstrated. This patient had closure of an arteriovenous fistula of 21 years duration which involved the anterior tibial vessels. Fourteen years after the fistula closure, multiple aneurysms of the femoral-popliteal arteries developed. (Sako, Y., and Varco, R. L., Surgery, *67*:40, 1970.)

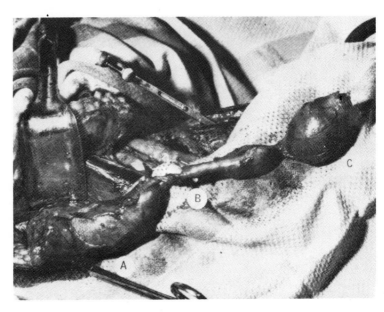

Sako and Varco (1970) reported long term follow-up of 14 of 25 patients with acquired arteriovenous fistulas who were cured of their lesions for 5 to 16 years. Seven additional patients were followed for over two years, and all were cured. One patient in this group had had a portion of the anterior tibial artery repaired after excision of the fistula, but the artery was occluded within the first year. Two were lost to follow-up after the first year, and one had had a quadruple ligation of the subclavian arteriovenous fistula. When last seen, he had symptoms indicating some ischemia of the arm. The other patient lost to follow-up had had a quadruple ligation of the gluteal arteriovenous fistula. The remaining two patients who had had an aneurysmal dilatation in the proximal artery excised and replaced with a prosthetic graft were well 8 and 11 years after the operation (Fig. 9–38). The other two patients with aneurysmal dilatation of the artery proximal to the fistula had not yet had these corrected.

CHAPTER 10

FALSE ANEURYSMS

... he was bled at his own desire by a bleeder who had performed the same operation for him, and generally in the same arm, some 30 or 40 times. Nothing extraordinary occurred, other than he remarked the flow of blood to be greater, and he checked with more difficulty than had usually been the case. This was, however, done by firm compression, and on the day following finding the bandage tight, he removed it, and found the orifice to be completely closed. A short time after this, a small pulsating swelling was observed by him at this point which slowly increased till a day or two previous to my seeing him when after some exertion with his arm he observed a very considerable augmentation of its size.

B. Norris, 1843

HISTORY

Since antiquity, the management of false aneurysms has been closely allied to vascular surgery. It has been repeatedly recorded that Antyllus in the second century treated an arterial aneurysm by ligature above and below the lesion, with incision of the aneurysm and extraction of the clot. Schwartz (1958) reported that Antyllus treated small peripheral traumatic aneurysms by ligating both ends and puncturing the center; however, he advised against this practice in large aneurysms. Figure 10–1 shows some of the early methods of treatment of aneurysms. Hunter electively ligated the femoral artery proximal to a popliteal aneurysm in 1786 to reduce blood loss during subsequent attempts at excision of the aneurysm. Pick (1873) provided an interesting and detailed account of his management of a large femoral false aneurysm by digital compression, which had disastrous final results. This digital com-

pression directly over the pulsating mass was applied fairly continuously initially and then for a considerable period of the waking hours until four days later when the area became so tender that the compression had to be discontinued. Not only did this initiate thrombus formation in the false aneurysm, but also it became evident in less than one week that the distal pulses could not be felt over either the anterior or posterior tibial artery. Gangrene developed approximately three weeks after the initiation of the digital compression, and an amputation was performed at the hip level. The patient had a stormy postoperative course for approximately three hours before he died.

Matas (1888) described his endoaneurysmorrhaphy operation, a method of intrasaccular suture, for the treatment of a brachial arterial aneurysm. Within a few years, Matas (1903) also recommended restoration of circulation through the damaged artery as the ideal treatment for arterial an-

233

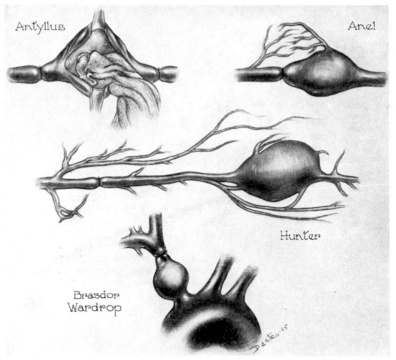

Figure 10–1. Various types of operations employed for treatment of aneurysms prior to the introduction of Matas' endoaneurysmorrhaphy in 1888. (Elkin, D. C., Surg. Gynecol. Obstet., *82*:1, 1946.)

eurysms. He developed a compressor (Fig. 10–2) to test the development of collateral circulation prior to performing his endoaneurysmorrhaphy. His approach—to widely open the aneurysm and to suture the communications into the artery (Fig. 10–3)—was the standard treatment, with minimal modification, for more than 50 years, a period of time which included World War II.

Despite the acceptance of the Matas endoaneurysmorrhaphy during World War I and World War II, interest in preserving arterial continuity was maintained. Lexer (1907) was the first to utilize a segment of saphenous vein as an interposition graft in an arterial defect caused by excision of a traumatic axillary aneurysm. Some of the problems associated with arterial repair have been detailed in Chapter 1. In individual series, successful arterial repair has been reported. Soubbotitch (1913) used suture repair, as has previously been described in Chapter 9. Elkin (1946) emphasized that all of the previous approaches outlined

by Antyllus, Anel, Hunter and Brasdor and Wardrop were frequently followed by infection, hemorrhage, gangrene or failure to cure the false aneurysm. Only the Matas procedure avoided these complications during the World War II experience. The following methods of managing arterial aneurysms were outlined by Freeman and Shumaker (1955):

1. Endoaneurysmorrhaphy of Matas.

2. Measures designed to produce clot in the aneurysmal sac or to induce formation of fibrous tissue about it to prevent further expansion and possible rupture.

3. Obliteration of the sac by closure of the offending vessel.

4. Extirpation of the aneurysm-bearing portion of the artery.

5. Extirpation of the lesion, combined with some procedure to permit maintenance or to re-establish continuity of the affected artery.

The extensive World War II experience is documented in detail by Elkin, by Shumacker and by DeBakey and Elkin (1955).

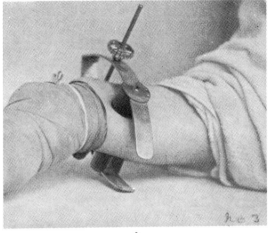

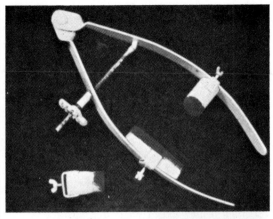

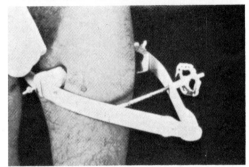

A

Figure 10–2. (A) Matas utilized a contemporary compressor applied to the femoral artery at Hunter's canal to test the collateral circulation in lesions such as this popliteal aneurysm. (Matas, R., *in* Keen's Surgery. Vol. VII. W. B. Saunders Company, Philadelphia, 1921.) (B) In World War II, Elkin found the Matas compressor to be an inexpensive and easily constructed instrument which could compress various arteries to determine the development of collateral circulation. (Elkin, D. C., Ann. Surg., *120*:284, 1944.)

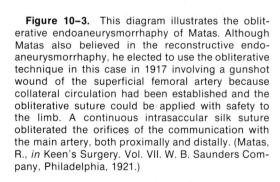

B

Figure 10–3. This diagram illustrates the obliterative endoaneurysmorrhaphy of Matas. Although Matas also believed in the reconstructive endoaneurysmorrhaphy, he elected to use the obliterative technique in this case in 1917 involving a gunshot wound of the superficial femoral artery because collateral circulation had been established and the obliterative suture could be applied with safety to the limb. A continuous intrasaccular silk suture obliterated the orifices of the communication with the main artery, both proximally and distally. (Matas, R., *in* Keen's Surgery. Vol. VII. W. B. Saunders Company, Philadelphia, 1921.)

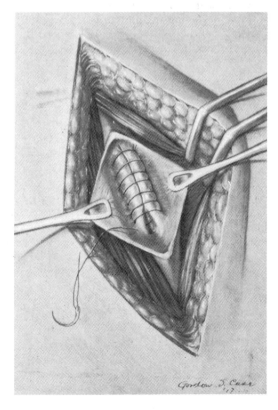

Since the Korean Conflict in which arterial repair was emphasized, vascular reconstruction has become the procedure of choice in restoring arterial continuity in the repair of false aneurysms, in both the military and the civilian situations. Hughes and Jahnke (1958) reviewed the Korean experience and provided a five year follow-up. A similar extensive review has been completed recently for the Vietnam experience (Rich et al., 1975D).

As might be anticipated, a smaller number of false aneurysms have been documented in civilian experience than in recent military experience. Patman and associates (1964) reported 12 patients who developed false aneurysms in their series of 256 patients with civilian arterial injuries in Dallas: an incidence of 4.7 per cent. None of these patients had an initial exploration. Among the major vessels which developed false aneurysms were the aorta (1), subclavian (1), axillary (2), superficial femoral (1) and popliteal (1). There were also three radial artery false aneurysms and single false aneurysms of the profunda femoris, anterior tibial and posterior tibial arteries. The ratio of false aneurysms to arteriovenous fistulas was 2:1 in their series, which was the opposite of the ratio reported by Hughes and Jahnke (1958) from the Korean experience.

INCIDENCE

With the increased interest in primary arterial repair of injured arteries during the past 25 years, many anticipated that there would be a resultant decrease in false aneurysms. This was particularly true in Vietnam (Rich et al., 1975D). However, considering the various etiologic factors, remaining diagnostic problems and priorities of managing a patient with multiple life-threatening injuries, it should be obvious that the treatment of false aneurysms remains an important aspect of vascular surgery.

Similar to the varying incidence of arterial injuries in the injured patient in general (see Chap. 2) and of arteriovenous fistulas (see Chap. 9), there is considerable disparity in the reported incidence of false aneurysms, in both civilian and military experience. One explanation for this is that at times false aneurysms are included in series of arterial trauma and at other times they are not. Also, some series do not distinguish arteriovenous fistulas from false aneurysms in combined reports.

Shumacker and Carter (1946) compared the incidence of arterial aneurysms and arteriovenous fistulas in large caliber peripheral arteries in their World War II experience (Table 10–1). Brachial false aneurysms were more prevalent than brachial arteriovenous fistulas, and the converse was true with femoral arteriovenous fistulas and false aneurysms. Hughes and Jahnke (1958) found that there were approximately twice as many arteriovenous fistulas as false aneurysms in the Korean experience. When major vessel lesions were considered (Table 10–2), they also noted fewer femoral false aneurysms than arteriovenous fistulas. Rich and associates (1975D) reported a somewhat different ex-

TABLE 10–1. COMPARISON OF INCIDENCE OF ARTERIAL ANEURYSMS AND ARTERIOVENOUS FISTULAS IN THE MAIN PERIPHERAL ARTERIES: MAYO GENERAL HOSPITAL—WORLD WAR II*

ARTERY INVOLVED	ARTERIOVENOUS FISTULAS		ARTERIAL ANEURYSM	
	No.	Per Cent	No.	Per Cent
Subclavian	10	4.1	5	4.2
Axillary	12	4.9	15	12.6
Brachial	13	5.3	28	23.5
Common femoral and femoral	66	26.9	17	14.3
Popliteal	42	17.1	21	17.6

*Shumacker, H. B., Jr., and Carter, K. L., Surgery, 20:9, 1946.

TABLE 10–2. TOTAL MAJOR VESSEL LESIONS— KOREAN EXPERIENCE*

VESSEL	ARTERIOVENOUS FISTULAS	FALSE ANEURYSMS	TOTAL
Common carotid	7	2	9
Internal carotid	3	–	3
Subclavian	6	2	8
Axillary	9	11	20
Brachial	10	9	19
Iliac	3	1	4
Common femoral	7	1	8
Superficial femoral	24	7	31
Popliteal	22	10	32
Total:	91	43	134

*Modified from Hughes, C. W., and Jahnke, E. J., Jr., Ann. Surg., *148*:790, 1958.

perience in Vietnam, where there were slightly more false aneurysms than arteriovenous fistulas (Table 10–3).

In the relatively small series of arterial injuries reported by Dillard and associates (1968), false aneurysms (nine injuries) were more common than arteriovenous fistulas (seven injuries) in their civilian experience in St. Louis.

ETIOLOGY

Penetrating injuries are usually responsible for a false aneurysm, or traumatic aneurysm, which is produced by a tangential laceration through all three layers of the wall of an artery. In the military experience fragments from various exploding devices and bullets account for the penetrating missile wounds (Fig. 10–4). In civilian experience stab wounds, in addition to low velocity bullet wounds, are often associated with false aneurysms.

The increased use of fragmenting missiles in combat parallels the relatively high incidence of the development of false aneurysms in a number of wars, particularly prior to the advent of vascular repair. Hughes (1954) noted that 85 per cent of the vascular wounds in Korea resulted

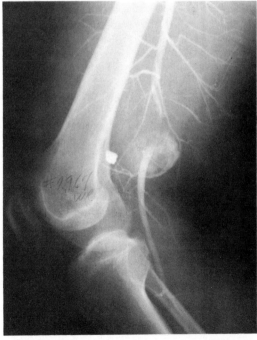

Figure 10-4. Representative of military wounds associated with false aneurysms is this large fragment wound of the popliteal fossa with a large false aneurysm of the popliteal artery demonstrated angiographically. (Vietnam Vascular Registry #2967, NMR, W.R.G.H.)

TABLE 10–3. ARTERIOVENOUS FISTULAS AND FALSE ANEURYSMS—VIETNAM VASCULAR REGISTRY*

LESIONS	NO.	PER CENT
False aneurysms	296	53.1
Arteriovenous fistulas	262	46.9
Total:	558	100.0

*Rich, N. M., Hobson, R. W., II, and Collins, G. J., Jr., Surgery, *78*:817, 1975.

TABLE 10–4. ARTERIOVENOUS FISTULAS AND FALSE ANEURYSMS: ETIOLOGY OF INJURY—VIETNAM VASCULAR REGISTRY*

WOUNDING AGENT		No.	PER CENT
Fragment		487	87.3
Bullet		59	10.6
Blunt		7	1.2
Punji stick		5	0.9
	Total:	558	100.0

*Rich, N. M., Hobson, R. W., II, and Collins, G. J., Jr., Surgery, *78*:817, 1975.

from fragmenting missiles, only 15 per cent being from bullets. Rich and colleagues (1975D) found that a similar percentage—about 87 per cent—of fragment wounds was responsible for 558 false aneurysms and arteriovenous fistulas (Table 10–4).

Diagnostic and therapeutic procedures can result in false aneurysms if the placement of needles and catheters injures the arteries. The first lesions that were successfully treated by Lambert (1759) and Norris (1843) resulted from blood letting. Recently at Walter Reed General Hospital, four false aneurysms developed following catheterization for angiographic procedures (Rich et al., 1975C). Postoperative false aneurysms, other than anastomotic false aneurysms, have been associated with many different operations. Smith and co-authors (1963) cited development of a false aneurysm of the common femoral artery following an inguinal herniorrhaphy. There was sudden profuse arterial bleeding in the course of the herniorrhaphy, and hemostasis was eventually secured by multiple silk sutures. Approximately two weeks after the operation a pulsatile, firm and tender mass, measuring 8 × 6 × 4 cm, was palpated in the area of the left inguinal ligament. Despite the fact that there was a purulent exudate surrounding the area of the 1 cm tear in the common femoral artery where a number of sutures had been placed in the defect, it was elected to excise the traumatized area and perform an end-to-end anastomosis. Five days after this second proce-

dure, severe hemorrhage occurred and it was necessary to ligate the common femoral artery. Nevertheless, viability of the extremity persisted.

The fact that a false aneurysm can develop following the operative removal of a herniated nucleus pulposus was documented by Seeley and co-workers (1954). They mentioned treating a 20 year old patient with a right common iliac artery aneurysm who had been operated upon at the fourth-fifth lumbar intervertebral space one month prior to his admission at Walter Reed General Hospital. Six weeks following the initial disc operation, a second operation was performed and an enormous false sac was found surrounding a right common iliac artery defect (Fig. 10–5). It was necessary to restore arterial continuity by inserting a 2 cm homologous arterial graft. Subsequent complications associated with disruption of the graft necessitated ligation of both the right common iliac artery and vein. Fortunately, viability of the extremity was maintained.

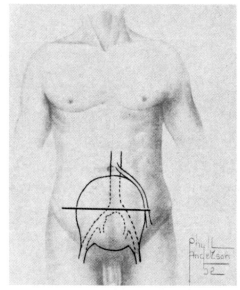

Figure 10–5. An enormous false aneurysm from a defect in the right common iliac artery was operated upon at Walter Reed General Hospital six weeks after the initial disc operation. The right ureter was displaced laterally by the mass. The segment of the artery with the posterior defect was excised, and the hypogastric artery was ligated. A 2 cm homologous arterial graft was used to bridge the defect. (Seeley, S. F., Hughes, C. W., and Jahnke, E. J., Jr., Surgery, *35*:421, 1954.)

Fractures can be associated with false aneurysm formation. Cameron and associates (1972) presented an interesting review of 10 cases of false aneurysms complicating closed fractures in a variety of anatomical locations (Table 10–5). Singh and Gorman (1972) emphasized that the formation of a false aneurysm as a result of closed trauma to the lower extremity was unusual. They presented the case of a 51 year old man who sustained a closed fracture at the junction of the middle and distal thirds of the tibia and fibula when his leg was caught by an encircling boat cable in a shipbuilding yard in 1966. Initially, a closed reduction of the fracture was performed, with immobilization of the limb in a long leg cast. This was replaced by a walking cast, which was kept on for a total of six months before it was determined that the fracture was healed. At that time, the patient noted superficial varicosities. The examining physician stated that his extremity had the typical post-phlebitic syndrome appearance, except that there was a pulsatile mass with a bruit located over the posteromedial aspect of the distal tibia. A femoral arteriogram revealed a large false aneurysm and an arteriovenous fistula of the distal part of the posterior tibial artery and accompanying veins (Fig. 10–6). It was possible to perform a lateral repair of the posterior tibial artery with interruption of the venous component. Six months later the patient was asymptomatic with no extremity edema.

Blunt trauma without an associated fracture can also result in a false aneurysm. Lai and associates (1966) presented an unusual case of a dissecting aneurysm of the cervical carotid artery in a 21 year old male following a hyperextension neck injury sustained in an automobile accident. The patient presented at the Johns Hopkins Hospital with a chief complaint of pain of the left side of his head and neck six months after the car which he was driving collided with a truck. A firm, tender, 4×4 cm mass high in the left cervical area was obvious, and a bruit was heard over the mass. A left carotid angiogram revealed considerable lateral displacement of the internal carotid artery, and the mass promptly filled with contrast media. A 4×6 cm dissecting aneurysm of the internal carotid artery was found at the time of exploration, the hypoglossal nerve, vagus nerve and spinal accessory nerve all being displaced by the aneurysmal sac. Because the superior portion of the aneurysmal sac approached the base of the skull, it was necessary to ligate the internal and external carotid arteries. The patient had an uneventful postoperative recovery with no abnormal neurologic findings other than the cranial nerve deficits present prior to surgery.

TABLE 10–5. REPORTED CASES OF FALSE ANEURYSMS COMPLICATING CLOSED FRACTURES*

AUTHOR	YEAR	ARTERY INVOLVED	FRACTURE
Robson	1957	Fourth lumbar artery	Fractured spinous processes and traumatic spondylolisthesis
Crellin	1963	Anterior tibial artery	Fracture upper third tibia
Meyer	1964	Profunda femoral artery	Subtrochanteric osteotomy
Dameron	1964	Profunda femoral artery	Screw in blade plate
Staheli	1967	Popliteal artery	Fracture distal femoral shaft
Smith	1963	One false aneurysm with closed fracture in 61 arterial injuries; site not stated	
Stein	1958	Anterior tibial artery	Fracture of tibial plateau
Bassett	1964	Profunda femoral artery	Blade plate for subtrochanteric osteotomy
Bassett	1966	Thoracic aorta	Eleventh dorsal vertebra
Harrow	1970	Right internal iliac artery	Pelvis

*Modified from Cameron, H. S., Laird, J. J., and Carroll, S. E., J. Trauma, *12*:67, 1972. Copyright 1972, The Williams & Wilkins Company, Baltimore.

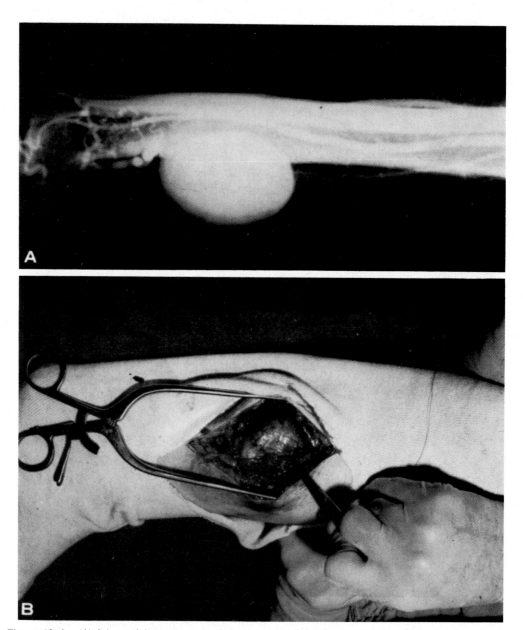

Figure 10–6. (A) A large false aneurysm of the posterior tibial artery and a posterior tibial arteriovenous fistula were demonstrated angiographically in a 51 year old male who sustained a closed fracture at the junction of the middle and distal thirds of the tibia and fibula. (B) The large posterior tibial false aneurysm was demonstrated at the time of surgical exploration. (Singh, I., and Gorman, J. F., J. Trauma, *12*:592, 1972. Copyright 1972, The Williams & Wilkins Company, Baltimore.)

CLINICAL PATHOLOGY

A false aneurysm, or traumatic aneurysm, is caused by trauma which lacerates or ruptures all three layers of the wall of an artery. Arterial flow through the artery is usually maintained, and the extravasated blood through the laceration is contained by surrounding tissues to become a pulsating hematoma and subsequently an encapsulated false aneurysm. The hematoma that is formed compresses and seals the point of injury. Within days to weeks after, the thrombus gradually liquefies. False aneurysms are distinguished from true aneurysms. Whether the true aneurysm is congenital in origin, arteriosclerotic, mycotic, syphilitic or caused by unusual systemic diseases such as polyarteritis nodosa, the true aneurysm has a sac composed of one or more layers of the artery rather than a rupture through all of the walls of the artery, as occurs in the traumatic false aneurysm. Indirect or blunt trauma can actually cause a true aneurysm. True traumatic aneurysms caused by blunt, nonpenetrating trauma form a small group compared to traumatic false aneurysms. Blunt trauma causes a contusion of the arterial wall, the damaged arterial segment progressively dilating and forming a true aneurysm. Early recognition and treatment are rarely possible because the injury will usually not be apparent until the true aneurysm develops to a significant size. Only pathologic evaluation may differentiate a traumatic true aneurysm from a traumatic false aneurysm.

An unrepaired laceration of an artery with an inevitable periarterial hematoma usually has partial liquefaction of the latter, and a communication is established between the artery and the hematoma. A pseudocapsule of connective tissue forms gradually, and the pulsating hematoma becomes a false aneurysmal sac. The lesion will usually continue to expand, often causing pressure symptoms. One of the most easily recognizable results of pressure is a neuropathy, such as the easily recognizable neurologic deficits that develop in the hand from pressure on the median nerve by a false aneurysm (Fig. 10–7). False aneurysms may eventually rupture. The potential for exsanguinating hemorrhage endangers not only the limb but also the patient's life. If there is an associated infection, the threat of rupture is even greater (Fig. 10–8).

The size, configuration and location of false aneurysms can vary greatly. Chapter 9 outlines the frequent association of false aneurysms and arteriovenous fistulas. The false aneurysm can be one single sac (Fig. 10–9), or it can be bilobed (Fig. 10–10). The distribution of 82 false aneurysms

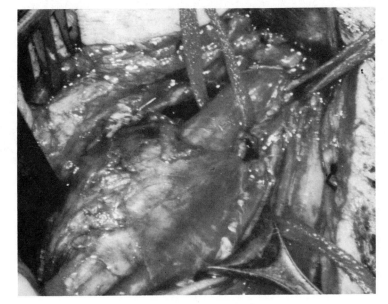

Figure 10–7. Pressure from a false aneurysm can compress an adjacent nerve. Fairly rapid expansion of this false aneurysm of the brachial artery caused external compression of both the median and ulnar nerves with resultant neurologic deficit. (Rich, N. M., *in* Beebe, H. G. (Ed.), Complications in Vascular Surgery. J. B. Lippincott Company, Philadelphia, 1973.)

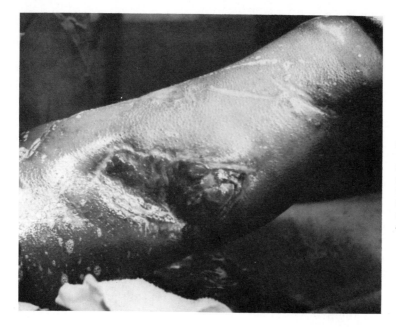

Figure 10-8. A false aneurysm associated with surrounding infection has an increased potential for rupture and exsanguinating hemorrhage. An infected false aneurysm of the superficial femoral artery resulted in intermittent hemorrhage through the open wound of the thigh in a Vietnam casualty. (Vietnam Vascular Registery #837, NMR.)

Figure 10-9. A false aneurysm can exist in a large variety of sizes and configurations. It may be a single sac, as shown in this arteriogram. (Vietnam Vascular Registery, #2590, NMR, W.R.G.H.)

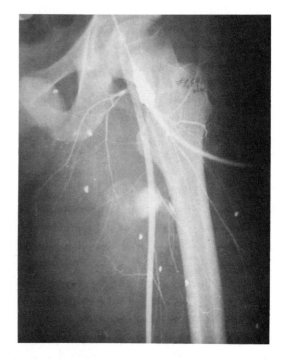

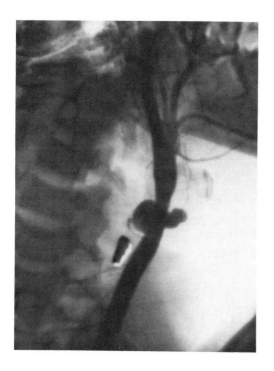

Figure 10-10. Among the variety of configurations of false aneurysms is a double or bilobed sac, as shown in this arteriogram of the common carotid artery. The offending fragment is seen adjacent to the carotid artery. (Vietnam Vascular Registery #826, NMR.)

TABLE 10–6. DISTRIBUTION OF FALSE ANEURYSMS AND ARTERIOVENOUS FISTULAS—MAYO GENERAL HOSPITAL*

ARTERY INVOLVED	ARTERIOVENOUS FISTULAS (NO. OF CASES)			ARTERIAL ANEURYSMS (NO. OF CASES)		
	Operation at M.G.H.	Operation Elsewhere	"Spontaneous Cure"	Operation at M.G.H.	Operation Elsewhere	"Spontaneous Cure"
Aorta	1					
Innominate				1		
Internal carotid	3			2		
External carotid	3					
Common carotid	6		1	1	1	2
Vertebral	4					
Lingual	1					
Occipital	1					
Cirsoid, nose, ear	2					
Superior temporal	2			1		
Transverse cervical	1	1				
Deep cervical				1		
Internal mammary	1					
Subclavian	6	3	1	5		
Axillary	12			13	2	
Branch axillary	4			2		
Brachial	11	1	1	22	5	1
Radial	1	1		2		
Ulnar	4	2		2		
External iliac		1		1		
Hypogastric	1					
Superior gluteal	2			1		
Obturator	1					
Common femoral	3	2				1
Femoral	47	13	1	6	9	1
Profunda femoris	6			2		
Branch profunda	2	2	1	2		
Popliteal	41	1		14	6	1
Geniculate	4					
Posterior tibial	21	5		1	4	2
Anterior tibial	5	1		2	1	
Peroneal	5	1			1	
Branches in calf	5			1		
Total:	206	34	5	82	29	8

*Shumacker, H. B., Jr., and Carter, K. L., Surgery, *20*:9, 1946.

treated in World War II shows that the brachial artery was involved most often, followed by the popliteal artery (Table 10–6). The anat mical region most frequently involved with 558 false aneurysms and arteriovenous fistulas in Vietnam casualties was the lower extremity (Table 10–7). The most frequently involved arteries were the posterior tibial and brachial, followed closely by the superficial femoral and popliteal arteries (Table 10–8). Multiple lesions can exist. Table 10–9 shows that 41 of the 509 Vietnam casualties had two or more lesions, for a total of 90 separate lesions (Fig. 10–11).

TABLE 10–7. ARTERIOVENOUS FISTULAS AND FALSE ANEURYSMS: ANATOMICAL LOCATION—VIETNAM VASCULAR REGISTRY*

LOCATION	No.	PER CENT
Head/neck	42	7.5
Upper extremity	134	24.0
Thorax	17	3.1
Abdomen	22	3.9
Lower extremity	343	61.5
Total:	558	100.0

*Rich, N. M., Hobson, R. W., II, and Collins, G. J., Jr., Surgery, *78*:817, 1975.

TABLE 10–8. ARTERIOVENOUS FISTULAS AND FALSE ANEURYSMS: ARTERIAL INJURIES – VIETNAM VASCULAR REGISTRY*

ARTERY	ARTERIOVENOUS FISTULAS	FALSE ANEURYSMS	TOTAL	PER CENT
Common carotid	6	5	11	2.0
Internal carotid	2	4	6	1.1
External carotid	2	3	5	0.7
Vertebral	6	2	8	1.4
Subclavian	1	7	8	1.4
Axillary	10	8	18	3.2
Brachial	22	33	55	9.9
Radial	2	25	27	4.8
Ulnar	8	15	23	4.1
Innominate	1	1	2	0.4
Thoracic aorta	0	2	2	0.4
Abdominal aorta	0	1	1	0.2
Common iliac	1	1	2	0.4
External iliac	0	6	6	1.1
Internal iliac	0	1	1	0.2
Common femoral	4	7	11	2.0
Superficial femoral	57	31	88	15.8
Deep femoral	17	20	37	6.6
Popliteal	41	28	69	12.4
Posterior tibial	30	33	63	11.3
Anterior tibial	20	18	38	6.8
Peroneal	12	12	24	4.3
Miscellaneous	20	33	53	9.5
Total:	262	296	558	100.0

*Rich, N. M., Hobson, R. W., II, and Collins, G. J., Jr., Surgery, *78*:817, 1975.

Expanding false aneurysms can cause neurologic changes due to direct pressure on major nerves (Fig. 10–12). Shumacker and Carter (1946) emphasized the high frequency of false aneurysms of upper extremity major arteries with associated nerve lesions that required operations (Table 10–10).

Unusual pathologic changes can occur with false aneurysms. Distal embolization of a thrombus (Fig. 10–13) from a false aneurysm (Fig. 10–14) is unusual, but the po-

TABLE 10–9. ARTERIOVENOUS FISTULAS AND FALSE ANEURYSMS – VIETNAM VASCULAR REGISTRY*

PATIENTS	LESIONS	TOTAL
468	1	468
35	2	70
4	3	12
2	4	8
509		558

*Rich, N. M., Hobson, R. W., II, and Collins, G. J., Jr., Surgery, *78*:817, 1975.

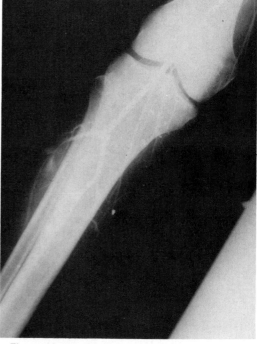

Figure 10–11. Multiple lesions can occur, as evidenced by this Vietnam casualty who had a false aneurysm of the anterior tibial artery, which was obvious, and a false aneurysm of the distal popliteal artery, which was diagnosed only by angiography. (Vietnam Vascular Registry, #5189, NMR.)

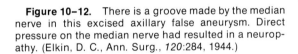

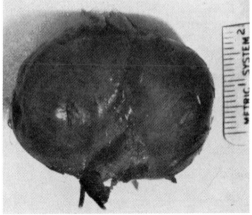

Figure 10-12. There is a groove made by the median nerve in this excised axillary false aneurysm. Direct pressure on the median nerve had resulted in a neuropathy. (Elkin, D. C., Ann. Surg., *120*:284, 1944.)

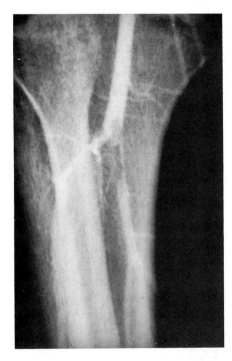

Figure 10-13. Mural thrombus may embolize from either a false aneurysm or an arteriovenous fistula. This angiogram demonstrates an embolus from a proximal popliteal artery false aneurysm to the distal popliteal and proximal posterior tibial arteries. (Rich, N. M., *in* Beebe, H. G. (Ed.), Complications in Vascular Surgery. J. B. Lippincott Company, Philadelphia, 1973.)

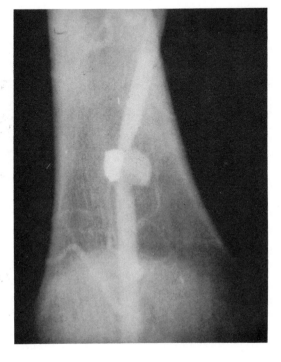

Figure 10-14. Except for 14 per cent of the lesions which were associated with external hemorrhage into open wounds, there were rare preoperative complications associated with arteriovenous fistulas and false aneurysms in this series. One of these was embolization of thrombus from a popliteal arterial false aneurysm, identified in the above arteriogram with its adjacent wounding fragment. In 1968 at Walter Reed Army Medical Center the false aneurysm was resected, the thrombus was removed with a Fogarty catheter, and arterial continuity was re-established by end-to-end anastomosis. (Rich, N. M., Hobson, R. W., II, and Collins, G. J., Jr., Surgery, *78*:817, 1975.)

TABLE 10–10. PERIPHERAL NERVE LESIONS ASSOCIATED WITH ARTERIAL ANEURYSMS*

ARTERY INVOLVED	NERVE LESION REQUIRING OPERATION		NERVE LESION NOT REQUIRING OPERATION		NO NERVE LESION	
	No.	Per Cent	No.	Per Cent	No.	Per Cent
Brachial	24	85.7	1	3.6	3	10.7
Axillary	11	73.3	1	6.7	3	20.0
Subclavian	3	60.0	1	20.0	1	20.0
Popliteal	2	9.5	6	28.6	13	61.9
Femoral	1	6.2	3	18.8	12	75.0
Others	7	13.0	13	24.0	34	63.0
Total:	48	40.3	25	21.0	66	38.7

*Modified from Shumacker, H. B., Jr., and Carter, K. L., Surgery, 20:9, 1946.

tential threat with possible disastrous sequelae always exists. Sachatello and co-workers (1974) described the case of one patient with a false subclavian aneurysm who had distal embolism from a thrombus within a false aneurysm. They managed the problem by resection of the clavicle, resection of the subclavian false aneurysm with vein graft replacement, and brachial arterial embolectomy. Pulses were restored. Rhodes and colleagues (1973) reported the unusual complication of consumption coagulopathy, which developed in a patient with a false aneurysm and an arteriovenous fistula.

CLINICAL FEATURES

The most obvious clinical finding with a false aneurysm is a mass which is usually pulsatile. There is frequently evidence of a penetrating wound (Fig. 10–15). The mass may or may not be painful. On examination, the borders of the mass can be ill-defined because the false aneurysm is beneath the deep fascia. Depending on the amount of thrombus within the false aneurysm, the mass may or may not be pulsatile. There is frequently an associated systolic bruit over the mass, and there can be

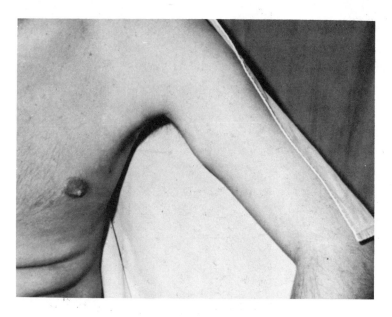

Figure 10–15. The diagnosis of a false aneurysm may be obvious with the physical finding of a pulsating mass. There is usually evidence of a penetrating wound. (Vietnam Vascular Registry, #3273, NMR.)

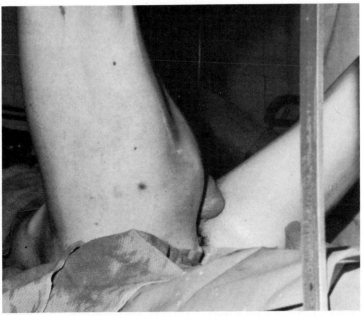

Figure 10–16. Enlargement of a false aneurysm may be gradual, or there may be rapid expansion of a mass. The size of the mass may also be quite variable, as in this large false aneurysm of the profunda femoris artery. The mass may be painful, and there may be warmth and tenderness upon examination. (Vietnam Vascular Registry, #3159, NMR.)

considerable radiation of the bruit into the surrounding anatomy.

Gradual enlargement of the false aneurysm may occur (Fig. 10–16), with the development of a firm, warm, tender area. Confusion with an abscess has occurred in the differential diagnosis. A stable false aneurysm of longer duration can also be confused with a cyst or neoplasm.

If the false aneurysm is associated with an arteriovenous fistula, a continuous bruit and thrill over the site of injury may also be present. As previously noted, pressure on adjacent nerves may result in neurologic deficits, and the first symptom or physical finding may result from a neuropathy. Distal pulses are usually intact and considered to be normal on examination.

DIAGNOSTIC CONSIDERATIONS

Diagnosis is usually made by physical examination of a pulsatile mass. Roentgenograms in the anteroposterior and lateral

views might identify an offending metallic foreign body in the anatomical location of an artery.

Nevertheless, angiography may be necessary to establish the diagnosis (Fig. 10–17). The size of the false aneurysm may be misleadingly small because of the amount of laminated clot filling the sac (Fig. 10–18). Angiography may delineate a clinically unsuspected adjacent arteriovenous fistula (Fig. 10–19) or multiple vascular lesions, as demonstrated in Figure 10–11.

Angiography may be necessary to make the diagnosis of false aneurysms in arteries that are not easily accessible to physical examination, such as those within the chest and abdomen (Fig. 10–20).

Newer investigative techniques, such as sonography, can also be valuable in determining the size and location of false aneurysms. This was recently emphasized by Bole and associates (1976) (Fig. 10–21). The diagnostic value of sonography for both true aneurysms and false aneurysms has been demonstrated with increasing utilization of this modality at Walter Reed General Hospital.

Text continued on page 250

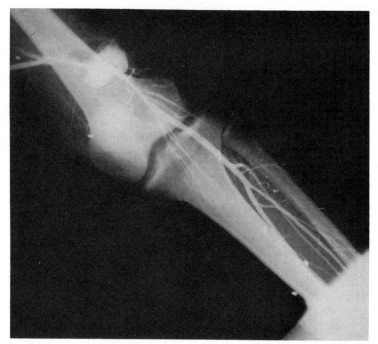

Figure 10–17. Preoperative angiography is helpful in confirming clinical impressions, outlining the site of the vascular defect, and ruling out additional adjacent vascular injuries. When not preoperatively available or practical, angiograms can be obtained easily. This one demonstrates a popliteal arterial false aneurysm seen at Walter Reed Army Medical Center in 1969 prior to resection and end-to-end anastomosis. Similar angiograms in the operating room immediately following repair have helped to establish the status of vascular repair. (Rich, N. M., Hobson, R. W., II, and Collins, G. J., Jr., Surgery, 78:817, 1975.)

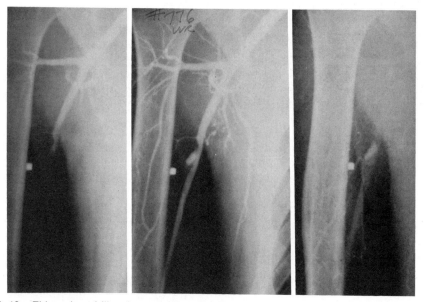

Figure 10–18. This series of films in an angiogram of the right brachial artery demonstrates early filling of the false aneurysm adjacent to the offending fragment (left); the obvious false aneurysm, which was angiographically much smaller than the large palpable mass because of the laminated clot which filled the false aneurysm sac (middle); and residual contrast in the false aneurysm sac (right). (Vietnam Vascular Registry #776, NMR.)

Figure 10–19. A large false aneurysm, such as this one demonstrated angiographically, can cause local arterial compression. In this Vietnam casualty, the large false aneurysm of the popliteal artery compressed the artery sufficiently to nearly obliterate the associated arteriovenous fistula. There was no associated classic "machinery-type" bruit, and the arteriovenous fistula was diagnosed angiographically. Also, the patient had weak pedal pulses because of the compression of the popliteal artery by the large false aneurysm, in contrast to what has previously been described in most patients who have intact distal pulses. (Vietnam Vascular Registry, #2513, NMR.)

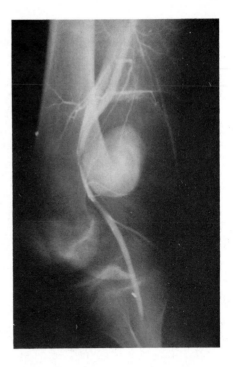

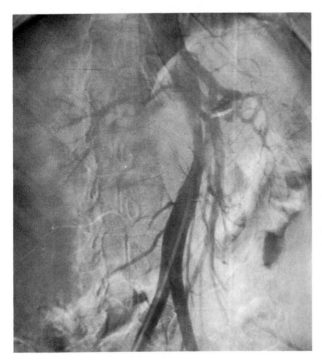

Figure 10–20. Compression and lateral displacement of the abdominal aorta toward the patient's left side are demonstrated in the above subtraction study of an angiogram of the aorta. The offending fragment from an M–26 grenade caused a large false aneurysm of the aorta, which was repaired by lateral suture technique with interrupted sutures at Walter Reed Army Medical Center in 1967. (Rich, N. M., Hobson, R. W., II, and Collins, G. J., Jr., Surgery, *78*:817, 1975.)

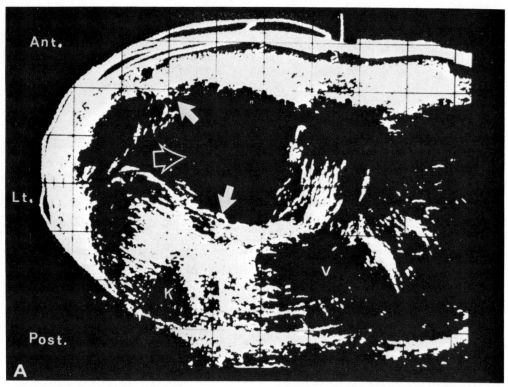

Figure 10–21. Ultrasonic tomography of the upper abdomen in transverse plane showing the pseudo-aneurysm (open arrow) in a patient with nonpulsatile diffuse mass. Thrombus echoes and irregular contour of the aneurysm are noted (solid arrows). Vertebral body (V) and the left kidney (K) are also visualized. (Bole, P. V., Munda, R., Purdy, R. T., Lande, A., Gomez, R., Clauss, R. H., Kazarian, K. K., and Mersheimer, W. L., J. Trauma, *16*:63, 1976. Copyright 1976, The Williams & Wilkins Company, Baltimore.)

SURGICAL TREATMENT

The report of the first operation performed by Matas in 1888 was presented again by Elkin (1946) to emphasize that the Matas operation had stood the test of time for 57 years and had had a profound effect upon the surgery of blood vessels (Fig. 10–22).

On April 6, 1888, I operated upon a young male Negro for a very large traumatic (multiple gunshot) aneurysm of the brachial artery, extending from the armpit to the elbow, which opened my eyes to the possibilities of an entirely new method of conservative treatment which was to revolutionize my previous notions of aneurysmal surgery. In this case, the successive ligation of the main artery on the proximal and distal poles of the aneurysm had been followed by relapse, and it seemed to me, then, that I had no other alternative but to extirpate the sac. When I exposed the sac and emptied its contents, the failure of the ligations to control the circulation was easily explained by the appearance in the bottom of the sac of three large ori-

fices corresponding to the collateral branches which opened into the sac in the segment of the artery included between the ligatures [Fig. 10–22]. It was evident that it was these collateral orifices that fed the sac despite the ligatures that had been placed at each one of its poles. I, at first, intended to secure these collaterals by excising the sac, but the branches of the brachial plexus of nerves were so densely incorporated in its walls that I could not have dissected them out and detached them, without serious damage, thereby paralyzing the arm. It occurred to me then that the easiest way out of this awkward dilemma was to seal the orifices of all the bleeding collaterals by suturing them as we would an intestinal wound, leaving the sac attached and undisturbed in the wound. This procedure was at once put into effect and the hemostasis was so perfect and satisfactory that it seemed to me strange that no one should have thought of so simple an expedient before.

Matas used the intrasaccular suture (Fig. 10–23; see also Fig. 10–3); however, he was also interested in reconstructive endoaneurysmorrhaphy (Fig. 10–24).

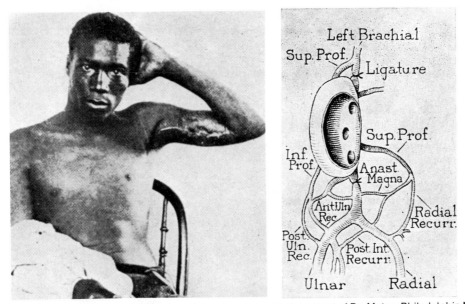

Figure 10–22. The original photograph and drawing shown in the report of Dr. Matas, Philadelphia Medical News, October 27, 1888, when he proposed his endoaneurysmorrhaphy approach to the management of false aneurysms. (Elkin, D. C., Surg. Gynecol. Obstet., *82:*1, 1946.)

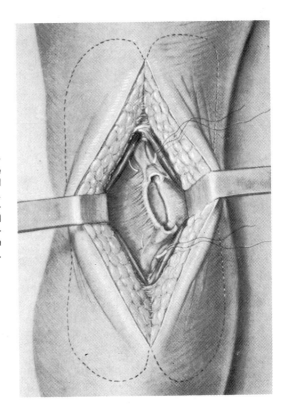

Figure 10–23. The Matas obliterative aneurysmorrhaphy is demonstrated in this intrasaccular suture ligature of a ruptured popliteal aneurysm. The dotted line shows the area of extravasation filled with clot. Arterial reconstruction was considered to be impractical in this specific case, and the distal and proximal popliteal arteries were obliterated with encircling sutures. Collateral circulation was adequate to maintain extremity viability. (Matas, R., *in* Keen's Surgery. Vol. VII. W. B. Saunders Company, Philadelphia, 1921.)

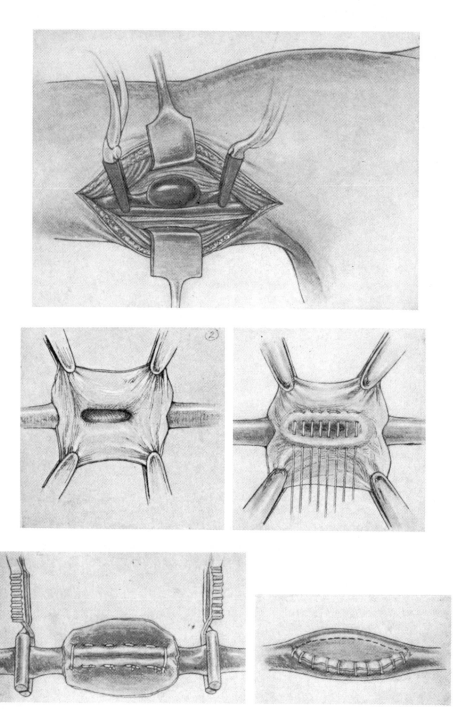

Figure 10–24. In addition to the obliterative aneurysmorrhaphy for the treatment of false aneurysms, Matas encouraged selective reconstructive endoaneurysmorrhaphy, as was utilized in this repair of a false aneurysm of the brachial artery. (Matas, R., *in* Keen's Surgery. Vol. VII. W. B. Saunders Company, Philadelphia, 1921.)

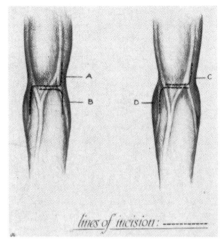

Figure 10–25. Incisions used in exposure of vessels in the antecubital fossa. (A) The usual incision for exposure of brachial vessels in antecubital space. (B) Incision used when lesion is suspected in proximal portion of ulnar vessels. (C) Incision used when brachial vessels are involved just proximal to antecubital crease. (D) Incision used for exploration of distal end of brachial or proximal end of radial vessels. (Shumacker, H. B., Jr., Ann. Surg., *124*:586, 1946.)

In the management of a false aneurysm, repair of the arterial defect is usually the goal that should be sought. An elective incision should be made which will allow adequate exposure for proximal and distal control. Examples were afforded by the extensive World War II experience. Shumacker (1946) described in detail the incisions which could be successfully employed in the surgical approach to aneurysms, especially those in the antecubital (Fig. 10–25) and popliteal (Fig. 10–26) fossae. His report was based on his extensive experience in managing false aneurysms in hundreds of American combat casualties. Specifically, these incisions were devised to replace longitudinal incisions across the popliteal and antecubital creases, which were often associated with heavy scars or keloids, contracture or ulceration.

Although resection of the false aneurysm is often recommended, an alternative plan which is presently employed has several advantages. The laminated clot within the false aneurysm should be evacuated after temporary proximal and distal control is obtained with vascular clamps, but the majority of the sac can usually be left in place. This will shorten the length of the operative procedure and decrease the possibility of damage to associated structures, such as tearing of the popliteal vein which has become closely adherent and attenuated to an adjacent popliteal arterial false aneurysm. If the false aneurysm is inadver-

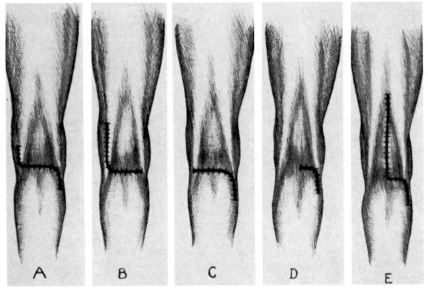

Figure 10–26. Skin incisions used in exploring the popliteal vessels in the surgical approach to false aneurysms in World War II. (A) Incision used when the lesion exists in the popliteal vessels in the mid-popliteal space. (B) Incision used when the lesion is higher in the popliteal fossa. (C and D) Incisions used for exploring the distal popliteal vessels. (E) A modified incision useful when associated nerve lesion requires exploration. (Shumacker, H. B., Jr., Ann. Surg., *124*:586, 1946.)

tently entered prior to obtaining proximal and distal control, digital control will usually suffice as an expedient measure. Unnecessary resection of normal artery can also be avoided if careful dissection of both the proximal and distal artery toward the side of the defect is carried out. In this manner, a more limited resection of artery will be necessary.

Occasionally, lateral suture of a punctate wound of an artery is possible, without constriction of the arterial lumen. However, limited arterial resection and end-to-end anastomosis is usually the procedure of choice. If it is necessary to use an arterial replacement, an autogenous vein graft is usually preferred. This graft should be placed in tissue as normal as possible, which is often difficult because of considerable inflammation and cicatrix. If there is extensive scarring, it might be possible to place a graft in an extra-anatomical area of adjacent tissue in a position away from the usual course of the major vessel. In the case of noncritical arteries, such as the radial artery or distal posterior tibial artery, ligation is usually satisfactory. This is particularly important if there is an infected false aneurysm. However, arterial repair is preferred even in small caliber arteries.

Surgical correction of a false aneurysm should be performed as soon as possible after the diagnosis is made to prevent the complications of rupture or rapid expansion with resultant pressure on adjacent nerves. Immediate surgery should be advocated if neurologic symptoms develop.

Additional information related to specific arterial false aneurysms, such as those of the subclavian artery (Chap. 13), can be found in specific chapters. Details of arterial repair and specific techniques, such as intraluminal control of hemorrhage with a balloon catheter, are to be found in Chapter 5.

RESULTS

Because competent vascular surgeons were chosen to head three centers for vascular surgery during World War II, a large number of arteriovenous fistulas and arterial aneurysms were managed.

Elkin (1946) reported the results of operating on 106 false aneurysms at the Ashford General Hospital Vascular Center in White Sulfur Springs, West Virginia, in a 30 month period. The Matas procedure was employed in 61 of the operations, and some other type of operation, usually complete excision of a small sac, was employed in the remaining 45 cases. There were no deaths in his series, no recurrence of the false aneurysm and no incidence of gangrene. Table 10–11 shows the location and number of injuries treated by endoaneurysmorrhaphy. Elkin and Shumacker (1955) outlined the operative treatment of 209 arterial aneurysms (Table 10–12). Nearly an equal number were treated by endoaneurysmorrhaphy as by excision. Shumacker (1948) reported successful results with vein graft repair of arteries which had false aneurysms (Table 10–13).

de Takats and Pirani (1954) stated that Herlyn, a pupil of Stich in Göttingen, reported he performed 164 ligatures as opposed to 230 reconstructive operations in World War II. This emphasized the trend in German war surgery, and Herlyn felt that the artery should never be ligated for traumatic aneurysm unless it was small or the patient's life was in danger.

Hughes and Jahnke (1958) reported on

TABLE 10–11. LOCATION AND NUMBER OF PATIENTS TREATED BY MATAS ENDOANEURYSMORRHAPHY: ASHFORD GENERAL HOSPITAL VASCULAR CENTER, WHITE SULFUR SPRINGS – WORLD WAR II EXPERIENCE*

ARTERY INVOLVED	CASES
Axillary	5
Brachial	14
Femoral	11
Iliac	2
Peroneal	1
Popliteal	7
Profunda femoris	3
Radial	4
Superior gluteal	1
Tibial, anterior	3
Tibial, posterior	8
Ulnar	2
Total:	61

*Elkins, D. C., Surg. Gynecol. Obstet., *82*:1, 1946.

TABLE 10–12. TECHNIQUES OF OPERATIVE TREATMENT IN 209 ARTERIAL ANEURYSMS— WORLD WAR II EXPERIENCE*

LOCATION	ENDO-ANEURYS-MORRHAPHY	EXCISION	PROXIMAL LIGATION	END-TO-END ANASTOMOSIS	TOTAL CASES
Upper extremity:					
Axillary	10	24	1		35
Brachial	16	30		1	47[1]
Radial	7	5			12
Subclavian	2	10	1		13[2]
Ulnar	3	4			7
Lower extremity:					
Femoral	14	4			18[3]
Gastrocnemius, muscle branch		1			1
Peroneal	2				2
Popliteal	19	2			21[4]
Profunda femoris	6				6
branch	2				2
Tibial, anterior	5				5
Tibial, posterior	7	8			15[5]
Head and neck:					
Carotid		5	8		13[5]
Cervical, deep	1				1
Temporal, superficial		2			2
Trunk:					
Gluteal, superior	2				2
Iliac	2	1	1		4
Innominate	1				1
Thoracic, lateral		1			1
Thoracoacromial		1			1
Total:	99	98	11	1	209

This total does not include—

[1]One aneurysm in which cure occurred spontaneously.

[2]Two aneurysms in which method of management was not stated.

[3]Two aneurysms in which cure occurred spontaneously.

[4]Three aneurysms, 2 in which methods of management not stated and 1 in which spontaneous cure occurred.

[5]Two aneurysms in which cure occurred spontaneously.

*Elkin, D. C., and Shumacker, H. B., Jr., *in* Elkin, D. C., and DeBakey, M. E. (Eds.), Vascular Surgery in World War II. U.S. Government Printing Office, Washington, D.C., 1955.

215 false aneurysms and arteriovenous fistulas treated at Walter Reed Army Medical Center in the early 1950's, mainly in casualties from the Korean Conflict. The various operations used in managing 43 false aneurysms and 91 arteriovenous fistulas in large vessels are reviewed in Table 10–14. Similar data concerning smaller caliber arteries are given in Table 10–15.

Rich and associates (1975D) reported the experience from the recent Vietnam War. There were 296 false aneurysms among 558 arteriovenous fistulas and false aneurysms identified in 509 patients. As might be anticipated by the number of American troops committed in Southeast Asia, the largest number of lesions resulted from wounds during 1968, with a relatively large number of lesions in 1967 and 1969. The time from injury to recognition of the arteriovenous fistulas and false aneurysms was arbitrarily considered to be immediate if recognized within the first 24 hours, early if recognized between the second and thirtieth day, delayed if recognized between the second through the sixth month and remote if recognized after six months. In this study the largest number of lesions—273 or 48.9 per cent—was recognized in the early period (Table 10–16). A nearly equal number of lesions, 228, was recognized in the delayed period. In the immediate group, there were 22 acute lesions operated upon in Vietnam. In the

TABLE 10–13. CASES IN WHICH CONTINUITY OF ARTERY WAS RESTORED BY VEIN TRANSPLANT*

Case No.	Age of Patient	Duration of Lesions in Months	Type of Lesion	Location of Lesion	Pre-operative Sympa-thec-tomy	Length of Vein Graft in cm	Source of Vein Graft	Period of Follow-up in Months	Result
1	26	4.2	AV and saccular aneurysm	Femoral, distal 3rd	0	2	Saphenous	3	Excellent
2	19	5	AV	Femoral, middle 3rd	0	2	Branch of femoral	3	Excellent
3	26	4	AV	Femoral, distal 3rd	+	5	Saphenous	3	Excellent
4	35	?	Saccular aneurysm	Popliteal, middle 3rd	+	2	Small saphenous	4	Excellent
5	36	6 yr	Saccular aneurysm	Femoral, proximal 3rd	0	2.5	Femoral	1.5	Excellent
6	24	5.3	Saccular aneurysm	Brachial, middle 3rd	0	2.5	Saphenous	1.2	Thrombosis; good circulation maintained

*Shumacker, H. B., Jr., Ann. Surg., *127*:207, 1948.

TABLE 10–14. TOTAL OPERATIONS FOR MAJOR VESSEL LESIONS— MILITARY SERIES FROM THE KOREAN CONFLICT*

Vessel	Ligation and Excision	Anasto-mosis	Vein Graft	Artery Graft	Lateral Repair	Division of Fistula	Sponta-neous Closure	Total
Common carotid	—	6	—	—	—	1	2	9
Internal carotid	2	—	—	—	—	1	—	3
Subclavian	3	2	—	1	1	1	—	8
Axillary	4	8	2	1	2	—	3	20
Brachial	6	9	1	1	1	1	—	19
Iliac	—	3	—	1	—	—	—	4
Common femoral	—	3	2	1	—	2	—	8
Superficial femoral	6	14	9	—	—	2	—	31
Popliteal	9	16	3	1	—	2	1	32
Total:	30	61	17	6	4	10	6	134

*Hughes, C. W., and Jahnke, E. J., Jr., Ann. Surg., *148*:790, 1958.

TABLE 10–15. TOTAL MINOR VESSEL LESIONS TREATED—
EXPERIENCE FROM THE KOREAN CONFLICT*

	LESIONS		TREATMENT			
VESSEL	Arterio-venous Fistulas	False Aneurysms	Ligation	Sponta-neous Closure	Anasto-mosis	Total
Occipital	1	1	2	—	—	2
Supraorbital	—	1	1	—	—	1
Superficial temporal	2	1	3	—	—	3
Vertebral	3	—	3	—	—	3
Superior thyroid	—	1	—	1	—	1
Inferior thyroid	2	—	2	—	—	2
Thoracoacromial	2	—	2	—	—	2
Thoracodorsal	2	1	3	—	—	3
Posterior humeral circumflex	1	1	2	—	—	2
Subscapular	1	—	—	—	1	1
Profunda brachii	—	1	1	—	—	1
Radial	2	4	5	—	1	6
Ulnar	2	2	4	—	—	4
Interosseous, posterior	1	—	1	—	—	1
Interosseous, anterior	2	—	2	—	—	2
Digital	—	1	1	—	—	1
Profunda femoris	10	—	10	—	—	10
Muscle branch, femoral	—	1	1	—	—	1
Circumflex femoral, lateral	1	1	2	—	—	2
Genu, inferior	2	1	3	—	—	3
Tibial, posterior	11	2	12	1	—	13
Peroneal	8	1	9	—	—	9
Tibial, anterior	3	3	6	—	—	6
Dorsalis pedis	—	1	1	—	—	1
Plantar, deep	1	—	1	—	—	1
Total:	57	24	77	2	2	81

*Modified from Hughes, C. W., and Jahnke, E. J., Jr., Ann. Surg., *148*:790, 1958.

remote group, all but 7 of the 35 patients had recognition and treatment of their lesions in less than two years. Only two had recognition and treatment of their lesions more than five years following the initial injury, and both were less than six years. Nearly an equal number of operations were performed in the intermediate hospitals, mainly in Japan, and in hospitals in the continental United States (Table 10–17). Several hundred different surgeons were involved in performing the repairs. Table 10–18 outlines the methods of treatment utilized for the various repairs. Arterial ligation was

TABLE 10–16. ARTERIOVENOUS FISTULAS AND FALSE ANEURYSMS: TIME OF DIAGNOSIS—VIETNAM VASCULAR REGISTRY*

TIME	NO.	PER CENT
Immediate (24 hr)	22	3.9
Early (1 to 30 days)	273	48.9
Delayed (1 to 6 mo)	228	40.9
Remote (6 mo)	35	6.3
Total:	558	100.0

*Rich, N. M., Hobson, R. W., II, and Collins, G. J., Jr., Surgery, *78*:817, 1975.

TABLE 10–17. ARTERIOVENOUS FISTULAS AND FALSE ANEURYSMS: HOSPITAL LOCATION FOR REPAIR—VIETNAM VASCULAR REGISTRY*

LOCATION	NO. OF REPAIRS	PER CENT
Vietnam	57	10.2
Japan, etc.	238	42.7
CONUS	251	45.0
No repair	12	2.1
Total:	558	100.0

*Rich, N. M., Hobson, R. W., II, and Collins, G. J., Jr., Surgery, *78*:817, 1975.

TABLE 10–18. ARTERIOVENOUS FISTULAS AND FALSE ANEURYSMS: METHOD OF MANAGEMENT—VIETNAM VASCULAR REGISTRY*

Type		No.	Per Cent
Arterial:			
Ligation		290	52.0
End-to-end anastomosis		143	25.6
Vein graft		57	10.2
Lateral suture		40	7.2
Prosthesis		2	0.3
Miscellaneous		26	4.7
	Total:	558	100.0
Venous:			
Ligation		138	52.7
Suture		79	30.1
Miscellaneous		45	17.2
	Total:	262	100.0

*Rich, N. M., Hobson, R. W., II, and Collins, G. J., Jr., Surgery, *78*:817, 1975.

used in 290 lesions: 52 per cent. The overall mortality rate for the 509 patients was 1.8 per cent: seven deaths (Table 10–19). Only two of these deaths could be directly attributed to the vascular problem. One patient died from a ruptured external iliac arterial false aneurysm. The over-all morbidity included five complications, for a morbidity rate of 6.3 per cent. Hemorrhage occurred in 14, thrombosis in 12 and stenosis in 2.

The numerous reports of the management of false aneurysms from civilian experience range from individual case reports to reports of 20 or 30 lesions. However, the civilian experience has not been as extensive as the warfare experience in this century. Examples of the civilian experience are the reports of Lloyd (1957), Baird and

TABLE 10–19. ARTERIOVENOUS FISTULAS AND FALSE ANEURYSMS: MORTALITY AND MORBIDITY RATES—VIETNAM VASCULAR REGISTRY*

	No.	Per Cent
Deaths	7	1.8
Morbidity:		
Amputations	8	1.7
Complications	35	6.3

*Rich, N. M., Hobson, R. W., II, and Collins, G. J., Jr., Surgery, *78*:817, 1975.

TABLE 10–20. TYPE OF REPAIR—CIVILIAN EXPERIENCE IN NEW YORK CITY*

Resection and end-to-end anastomosis	8
Resection and graft replacement	1
Lateral repair	7
Ligation	5
Spontaneous closure	1
Refused treatment	1
Total:	23

*Bole, P. V., Munda, R., Purdy, R. T., Lande, A., Gomez, R., Clauss, R. H., Kazarian, K. K., and Mersheimer, W. L. J. Trauma, *16*:63, 1976. Copyright 1976, The Williams & Wilkins Company, Baltimore.

Doran (1964), Engelman and associates (1969) and Bole and colleagues (1976). Particularly noteworthy is the recent report of the management of 23 traumatic false aneurysms in 23 patients treated in New York City over a five year period starting in 1968. Table 10–20 outlines the method of management of these false aneurysms, with lateral suture repair, resection and end-to-end anastomosis and ligation being used almost equally. These authors reported no mortality, no recurrence and no distal edema or arterial insufficiency. They did have two patients who continued to have pain, and three wound infections occurred.

SPONTANEOUS CURE

Shumacker and Wayson (1950) evaluated spontaneous cure of false aneurysms and arteriovenous fistulas. They studied 122 aneurysms and 245 arteriovenous fistulas. They felt that thrombosis was responsible for the obliteration of these lesions. Because there were only eight satisfactory spontaneous cures of false aneurysms—6.6 per cent of 122 lesions—these authors felt that there was little merit in awaiting the possibility of this occurrence. This was only slightly better than the 2 per cent spontaneous cure for arteriovenous fistulas (see Chap. 9). Although some case reports have been documented, recent experience has not witnessed a change in the low incidence of spontaneous cure of false aneurysms. This is undoubtedly also affected by early surgical intervention for the mass majority of false aneurysms.

FOLLOW-UP

Hughes and Jahnke (1958) provided a five year follow-up study of 250 arteriovenous fistulas and false aneurysms treated at Walter Reed Army Medical Center. The majority of the patients had been injured during the Korean Conflict. This long term follow-up was one of the first and one of the few extensive follow-up studies to be conducted. This study emphasized the difficulty in evaluating vascular trauma in combat casualties because of the many associated injuries. Neither of the two deaths in this follow-up study were related to vascular problems following repair of false aneurysms. Residual pain, coldness and claudication in the involved extremity were noted; however, no distinction was made between those patients treated for arteriovenous fistulas and those treated for false aneurysms. In the follow-up of the Vietnam casualties through the Vietnam Vascular Registry, more than one-fourth—29.3 per cent—or 149 of the 509 patients with arteriovenous fistulas and false aneurysms have been evaluated at Walter Reed Army Medical Center. In the long term follow-up, which extends to 10 years for many patients, additional problems and symptomatic residuals have been limited. Unfortunately, some of these patients have been lost to the long term follow-up effort because of untimely deaths. One patient was killed in subsequent action during a second tour in Vietnam, and another patient died in an automobile accident.

In the civilian reports, there are very limited data regarding long term follow-up of patients who have had false aneurysms.

CHAPTER 11

CAROTID AND VERTEBRAL ARTERY INJURIES

. . . the critical question . . . when does the patient depart the ischemic and enter the infarct stage . . . [?] The patient's outcome appears to be determined by the severity of the deficit prior to repair. . . .

Dr. Malcolm O. Perry, 1974

In this chapter injuries of the cervical carotid arteries are discussed. Injuries of the intrathoracic left common carotid artery are discussed in Chapter 12.

Carotid artery injuries are unique among the major peripheral artery injuries because of the hazard of irreversible neurological damage, either from the ischemic injury or from temporary interruption of the carotid circulation during arterial reconstruction. The bulk of this chapter concerns penetrating injuries of the carotid arteries. Because of their rarity, injuries of the vertebral artery are of little clinical importance and are mentioned only briefly. In a separate section at the end of this chapter, the interesting subject of nonpenetrating injuries of the carotid artery, perhaps recognized too seldomly, is discussed in some detail.

The first attempt to treat a carotid artery injury probably occurred more than 400 years ago in 1552 when Ambroise Paré successfully arrested a profuse hemorrhage from an épée wound in the left carotid artery (Watson and Silverstone, 1939). Mr. Fleming, aboard the H.M.S. Tonnant, is credited with the first authenticated ligation of a carotid artery for hemorrhage when he treated a patient who had attempted suicide by slashing his throat on October 17, 1803 (Beall et al., 1963). However, as was true with other arterial trauma, most carotid injuries were treated by ligation until the Korean Conflict. In World War I Makins (1919) found that 30 per cent of 128 patients whose carotid artery injuries were managed by ligation had a resultant neurological deficit. This complication prompted a conservative approach to treatment of the acutely injured carotid artery, reserving immediate operation for complications such as secondary hemorrhage, with the hope that collateral circulation would develop and lessen the future hazard of ligation. Only two attempts to repair a carotid injury in World War II were recorded (Lawrence et al., 1948), and only four such repairs were reported from the Korean Conflict (Hughes, 1958). Hence,

TABLE 11–1. INCIDENCE OF CAROTID ARTERY INJURIES

	AUTHOR	TOTAL ARTERIES	COMMON CAROTID	INTERNAL CAROTID	TOTAL CAROTID INJURIES	PER CENT
War Series						
WW I	Makins (1919)	1202	—	—	128	10.7
WW II	De Bakey and Simeone (1946)	2471	—	—	10	0.4
Korean	Hughes (1958)	304	—	—	11	3.6
Vietnam	Rich et al. (1970A)	1000	38	12	50	5.0
Civilian Series						
Houston	Morris et al. (1960)	220	—	—	18	8.2
Atlanta	Ferguson et al. (1961)	200	3	2	5	2.5
Denver	Owens (1963)	70	—	—	—	—
Detroit	Smith et al. (1963)	61	—	—	2	3.3
Dallas	Patman et al. (1964)	271	12	2	14	5.2
Los Angeles	Treiman et al. (1966)	159	.... "Head and Neck (10)"			
St. Louis	Dillard et al. (1968)	85	—	—	—	—
New Orleans	Drapanas et al. (1970)	226	9	3	12	5.3
Dallas	Perry et al. (1971)*	508	24	8	32	6.3
Detroit	Smith et al. (1974)*	127	5	4	9	7.1
Jackson	Hardy et al. (1975)	360	—	—	19	5.3
Denver	Kelly and Eiseman (1975)	116	2	1	3	2.6
Memphis	Cheek et al. (1975)	155	—	—	15	9.7

*This is a sequential study including the earlier report.

the bulk of military experience has evolved from the Vietnam Conflict (Cohen et al., 1970; Rich et al., 1970A).

At least nine separate reports have discussed civilian injuries of the carotid artery (Table 11–1). Beall and co-workers (1963) described experiences with 26 patients, and Perry and associates (1971) found 32 such injuries among 508 arterial injuries in Dallas.

SURGICAL ANATOMY

The origin of the common carotid arteries differs on the two sides. Description of the intrathoracic left common carotid artery, which arises from the arch of the aorta, is covered in more detail in Chapter 12. Because the right common carotid artery begins in the neck behind the sternoclavicular joint at the bifurcation of the innominate artery, a description of the cervical carotid artery will suffice for either side. Each artery passes obliquely upward from beneath the sternoclavicular joint and terminates at the level of the upper border of the thyroid cartilage, where it divides into the external and internal carotid ar-

teries (Fig. 11–1). Although the common carotid artery is the largest artery in the neck, there is a dilatation known as the carotid bulb at its bifurcation. The specialized sensory organ, the carotid body, which is a vascular chemoreceptor, is located at this bifurcation on the posteromedial side.

The two common carotid arteries are separated by a narrow interval, at the lower part of the neck, which contains the trachea. In the upper part of the neck, however, the thyroid gland, larynx and pharynx project forward between the two vessels. The important contiguous structures are the internal jugular vein, lateral to the artery; and the vagus nerve, located between the artery and vein and posterior to both (Fig. 11–2). The common carotid artery, internal jugular vein, and vagus nerve are contained in the carotid sheath, derived from the deep cervical fascia. Inside the carotid sheath, however, each of these structures has a separate fibrous investment. In addition to the integument, superficial fascia, platysma and deep cervical fascia, the common carotid artery is covered by the sternocleidomastoideus muscle. At the lower portion of the neck, the sternohyoideus, sternothyroideus and the superior belly of the omohyoideus muscles all cover the artery. In the

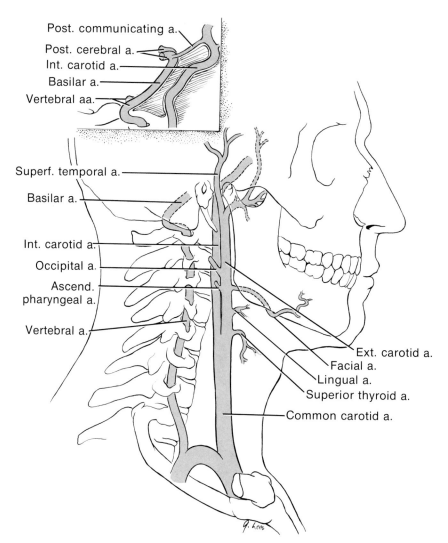

Post. communicating a.
Post. cerebral a.
Int. carotid a.
Basilar a.
Vertebral aa.

Superf. temporal a.

Basilar a.

Int. carotid a.
Occipital a.
Ascend.
pharyngeal a.

Vertebral a.

Ext. carotid a.
Facial a.
Lingual a.
Superior thyroid a.

Common carotid a.

Figure 11–1. Except for the intrathoracic portion of the left common carotid artery, the cervical anatomy of the carotid arteries and the vertebral arteries is bilaterally similar.

more distal portion, the descending branch of the hypoglossus nerve and the ansa hypoglossi are imbedded in the anterior wall of the carotid sheath, and the common facial vein usually crosses the artery near its termination. Posteriorly, the prevertebral fascia and the sympathetic trunk separate the artery from the anterior tubercles of the transverse processes of the lower four cervical vertebra and the scalenus anticus, longus capitus, and longus colli muscles.

Although there is more anatomical variation in the left common carotid artery, the right common carotid artery occasionally arises above the level of the upper border of

the sternoclavicular articulation. It may also arise as a separate branch from the arch of the aorta. Anomalies are rare. The common carotid artery may ascend without any subdivision, either the external or internal artery being absent. Also, the common carotid may be absent, the external and internal carotids arising directly from the arch of the aorta.

There are usually no branches from the common carotid artery prior to its bifurcation. However, the superior thyroid and the ascending pharyngeal arteries may occasionally originate from the distal common carotid artery. The inferior thyroid artery

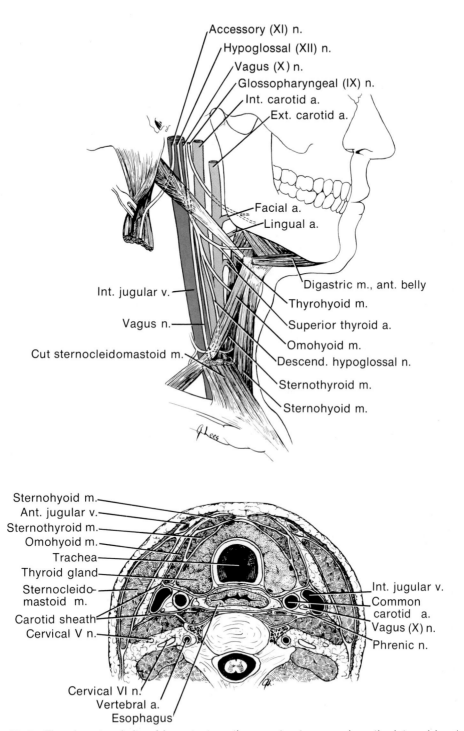

Figure 11–2. The close proximity of important contiguous structures, such as the internal jugular vein and the vagus nerve is emphasized. The cross-section shows the contents of the carotid sheath and the associated surrounding structures.

and, more rarely, the vertebral artery may also arise from the more proximal common carotid artery.

The internal carotid artery supplies the anterior part of the brain, and the eye and its appendages and sends branches to the forehead and the nose. It is usually the larger of the two terminal branches of the common carotid artery. It passes into the carotid canal of the temporal bone from its origin at the upper border of the thyroid cartilage and terminates intracranially by dividing into the anterior and middle cerebral arteries. Curvatures in its course are remarkable. An important relationship in surgical anatomy is the crossing of the hypoglossal nerve on the anterior surface of the internal carotid artery near its origin. To avoid confusion with the external carotid artery, a potentially serious error, several features should be remembered: (1) For practical purposes, the internal carotid has no extracranial branches (occasionally a small branch, the ascending pharyngeal artery, may occur near its origin); (2) the artery usually is not internal but is posterolateral to the external carotid artery; and (3) as the internal carotid artery ascends, it passes to the medial side of the external carotid toward the lateral wall of the pharynx. The carotid sinus, an important associated structure, is usually located at the origin of the internal carotid artery. Stimulation of this sinus, which is a pressoreceptor, causes a reduction of blood pressure and a slowing of the heart rate.

The external carotid artery, usually the smaller of the two terminal branches of the common carotid artery, extends from the upper portion of the thyroid cartilage to the neck of the mandible and divides into two terminal branches: the superficial temporal and the maxillary artery. This carotid is called "external" because of its extracranial distribution. An important feature involves the enclosure of a portion of the external carotid artery by the parotid gland. There are eight branches. Five of these are below the digastric muscle: the superior thyroid, lingual, facial, ascending pharyngeal, and occipital arteries. The other three branches are above the digastric muscle: the previously described two terminal branches— superficial temporal and the internal maxillary arteries—and the posterior auricular artery.

There are many significant collateral anastomoses which provide adequate circulation in the majority of instances after ligation of either the internal or external carotid arteries. These anastomotic connections exist between the arteries of the ophthalmic region of the internal carotid artery and the facial branch of the external carotid artery. There are also communications between the external carotid artery and the thyrocervical trunk. A very important communication exists between the vertebral and the internal carotid arteries via the posterior communicating artery of the circle of Willis. Communications between the various branches of the two external carotid arteries are numerous, and the internal carotid arteries communicate across the base of the brain by the anterior communicating artery and the basilar trunk.

The vertebral artery is the first and largest branch of the subclavian artery (Fig. 11–1); also see Chap. 13), and is divided into four parts. The first segment passes upward and backward through the foramen in the transverse process of the sixth cervical vertebra. It is contiguous to the vertebral and internal jugular veins. The second, and longest part, ascends through the foramina in the transverse processes of the upper sixth cervical vertebra. The third part passes almost horizontally backward and medially behind the lateral portion of the atlas. The fourth part is intracranial, passing through the foramen magnum to form the circle of Willis with the internal carotid arteries after it joins the vertebral artery from the opposite side to terminate as the basilar artery. Although the circle of Willis is the best potential source of collateral circulation between the two internal carotid arteries, or between either carotid artery and the basilar artery (Fig. 11–3), there is considerable variability in nearly one-half of all individuals (Strandness, 1969). Hypoplasia of the various segments, such as the anterior communicating, anterior cerebral or posterior communicating arteries, is usually not associated with inadequate circulation unless there is interruption of the carotid artery with an inadequate collateral circulation through the circle of Willis caused by the small caliber of one of its components. An important collateral circulation can be established between muscular branches of the vertebral and the occipital

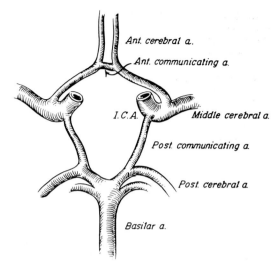

Ant. cerebral a.

Ant. communicating a.

I.C.A.

Middle cerebral a.

Post. communicating a.

Post. cerebral a.

Basilar a.

Figure 11–3. This is the standard model of the circle of Willis. Although normal variations within the circle are common, hypoplasia of various segments may be particularly significant with interruption of either internal carotid artery (ICA). This may result in an inadequate collateral flow. (Strandness, D. E., Jr., Collateral Circulation in Clinical Surgery. W. B. Saunders Company, Philadelphia, 1969.)

branch of the external carotid artery. There are also intraspinal vertebral-to-vertebral anastomoses and communications with the ascending cervical artery. The most common anomaly of practical significance is origin of the left vertebral artery from the aortic arch.

INCIDENCE

Carotid injuries represent about 5 per cent of all arterial injuries (Table 11–1). In 1919 Makins reported a frequency of nearly 11 per cent among 1202 injuries, probably including injuries of the external carotid artery. In World War II, less than one per cent of the patients had carotid injuries (DeBakey and Simeone, 1946), while the incidence in the Korean Conflict was about 4 per cent (Hughes, 1958). In the interim report from the Vietnam Vascular Registry of 1000 acute major arterial injuries, the frequency was 5 per cent (Rich et al., 1970A). Among civilian injuries, Morris and associates reported 18 injuries among 220 arterial injuries in 1960, an

incidence of 8 per cent. In a comparable series from Atlanta, however, Ferguson and co-workers documented a frequency of only approximately 3 per cent. In 1971, Perry and co-authors described 32 carotid injuries among 508 arterial injuries in Dallas, an incidence of approximately 6 per cent. Among the more recent series, Cheek and associates (1975) documented an incidence of nearly 10 per cent of 155 arterial injuries in Memphis. Reasons for the comparative rarity of carotid injuries were discussed by Lichenstein in 1947 and included the small size of the neck in relation to the total body surface area exposed, and the fact that many such injuries are promptly fatal because of exsanguination or asphyxiation. The recent increasing incidence, however, is emphasized by the following reports. Bradley (1973) described a series of 31 patients with penetrating carotid trauma in Atlanta. DiVincenti and Weber (1974) documented carotid artery injuries in 28 patients in New Orleans. Larger series came from Dallas (Thal et al., 1974) and Houston (Rubio et al., 1974): 60 and 81 carotid artery injuries, respectively.

Twenty to 30 per cent of carotid artery injuries involve the internal carotid (Table 11–1). Injuries of the external carotid artery are seldom reported because of negligible disability associated with ligation of the external carotid artery. Apparently external carotid injuries represent about 1 per cent of all arterial injuries. DeBakey and Simeone (1946) mentioned three external carotid injuries among 2471 cases in World War II. In civilian injuries, a total of 10 such cases has been recorded in three separate reports which taken together described 979 arterial injuries; again, this is a frequency of about 1 per cent. Rubio and associates (1974) found the external carotid artery injured in association with the common carotid artery in ten patients.

ETIOLOGY

As mentioned earlier, nonpenetrating injuries are discussed in a separate section at the end of this chapter. In military injuries, the majority of penetrating trauma resulted from fragments from different ex-

TABLE 11–2. ETIOLOGY OF CAROTID ARTERY INJURIES INTERIM VIETNAM EXPERIENCE*

Wounding Agent	Carotid Injuries	Per Cent
Fragment wound	44	88.0
Gunshot wound	4	8.0
Questionable	2	4.0
Total	50	100.0

*From Rich, N. M., Baugh, J. H., and Hughes, C. W., J. Trauma, 10:359, 1970. Copyright 1970, The Williams & Wilkins Co., Baltimore.

TABLE 11–3. ETIOLOGY OF CAROTID ARTERY INJURIES, EARLY CIVILIAN EXPERIENCE IN HOUSTON*

Wounding Agent	Carotid Injuries	Per Cent
Stab wounds	12	46.1
Gunshot wounds	10	38.5
Shotgun blasts	2	7.7
Auto accidents	2	7.7
Total	26	100.0

*From Beall, A. C., Jr., Shirkey, A. L., and DeBakey, M. E., J. Trauma, 3:276, 1963. Copyright 1963, The Williams & Wilkins Co., Baltimore.

ploding devices, such as grenades, mortars, rockets and mines. Fragment wounds accounted for 88 per cent of the carotid artery injuries in the Vietnam experience (Table 11–2) (Rich et al., 1970A). Probably most carotid injuries from high velocity gunshot wounds are fatal because of exsanguination. In civilian injuries, about one-half of carotid injuries were due to stab wounds and one-half to gunshot wounds, represented by a series from Houston (Beall et al., 1963) (Table 11–3 and Fig. 11–4).

In a subsequent review from Houston, Rubio and co-workers (1974) emphasized the marked contradistinction during the most recent 10 years of the 25-year study period. Only 17 per cent of the injuries were stab wounds, with the remainder being missile wounds. As a result, three of four wounds in the Houston experience were missile wounds. The experience in Dallas was similar (Thal et al., 1974) (Fig. 11–4).

In a series of 24 patients from Chicago, Monson and co-workers (1969) found that 17 were due to gunshot wounds and only seven from stab wounds. This corresponds with a recent increase in the use of guns rather than knives in the civilian community. Risley and McClerkin (1971) reported a patient who survived despite transection of both common carotid arteries from a .22 caliber bullet. Only one similar surviving case could be found in the literature (Haller, 1962) (Fig. 11–5).

Carotid artery injuries following percutaneous puncture of the carotid artery for cerebral angiography have been reported with increasing frequency. Such injuries may be due to dislodgement of an intimal flap or to inadvertent injection of contrast media into the arterial wall. At least three such problems have been seen at Walter Reed General Hospital during the past few years (Fig. 11–6).

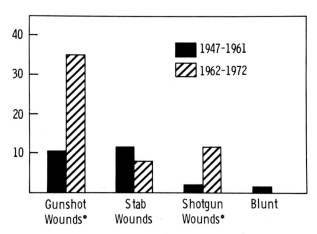

Figure 11–4. Etiology of carotid artery injuries, cumulative experience in Houston (25 years). (Rubio, P. A., Renl, G. J., Beall, A. C., Jr., Gordan, G. L., Jr., and DeBakey, M. E., J. Trauma, 14:967, 1974. Copyright 1974, The Williams and Wilkins Co., Baltimore.)

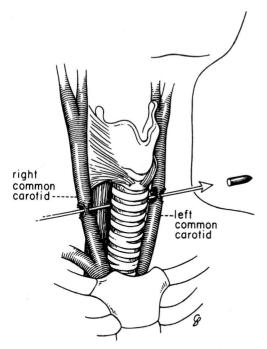

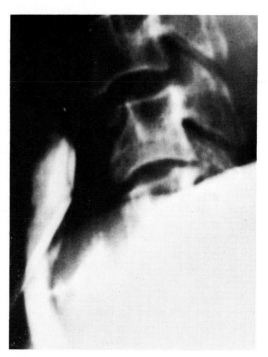

Figure 11-5. The through-and-through perforation of both common carotid arteries by a .22 caliber bullet which passed between the esophagus and trachea without perforation of either. (Haller, J. A., Amer. J. Surg., *103*:532, 1962.)

Figure 11-6. This angiogram reveals an intimal flap caused by the tip of a needle during a percutaneous carotid artery puncture. Developing cerebral symptomatology necessitated an emergency carotid thromboendarterectomy. (Rich, N. M., Hobson, R. W., II, and Fedde, C. W., Am. J. Surg., *128*:715, 1974.)

Among the 11 cases of major vascular injury occurring during the course of elective operative procedures, Lord and associates (1958) documented two carotid artery injuries, one during an emergency tracheostomy and the other during a radical neck dissection.

CLINICAL PATHOLOGY

Most injuries in surviving patients are lacerations. Of 50 carotid injuries in Vietnam, the great majority were lacerations and perforations (Rich et al., 1970A). Two patients had a transection with thrombosis of the severed ends, three had contusion of the carotid artery and two had an acute arteriovenous fistula. Among 18 civilian injuries reported by Beall and associates (1963), approximately two-thirds were lacerations, and five resulted in arteriovenous fistulas. Transection occurred only twice, and one patient had thrombosis of a

false aneurysm. Thal and co-authors (1974) found lacerations in 70 per cent of 60 carotid artery injuries.

Early recognition of an acute arteriovenous fistula involving the carotid or vertebral vessels may not be possible because the classic continuous murmur may not be audible for several days, probably evolving as surrounding clot is resorbed. In the classic fistula, a continuous thrill is readily felt, and dilated regional veins may visibly pulsate. The diagnosis can be further substantiated by obliterating the continuous bruit with digital pressure and noting a concomitant slowing of the heart rate (Branham-Nicaladoni sign).

CLINICAL FEATURES

Bright red bleeding from a neck wound, or a rapidly expanding hematoma, both suggest injury to the carotid artery. However, the simple presence of a penetrating neck wound in proximity to the carotid vessels should suggest the diagnosis, because tangential injuries may be temporarily sealed by a thrombus. Absence of distal pulsations with penetrating wounds is not very useful clinically, because large hematomas often make accurate palpation difficult. When head injuries are also present, a neurological deficit may be due to the head trauma or to the ischemia from injury to the carotid artery. If the patient is fully conscious despite the presence of a severe neurological deficit, the likelihood of the cause being an ischemic injury is great. However, the absence of neurological injury is not a particularly helpful sign in excluding carotid injury, for neurological injuries may be present in only approximately one-third of all carotid artery injuries.

Roentgenograms of the neck and skull should be obtained in any patient with injuries of the head and neck. With penetrating injuries, foreign bodies may be recognized and the path of the missile may be projected. Kapp and associates (1973) reported two patients with hemiplegia who underwent successful carotid reconstruction; subsequent removal of metallic emboli from the middle cerebral artery was eventually followed by neurological recovery. Angiograms are not indicated in most patients with penetrating injuries, especially when overt hemorrhage makes the diagnosis obvious. In obscure cases, usually those in which a small laceration has become sealed by thrombus, elective angiography may be of value (Fig. 11–7).

SURGICAL TREATMENT

An important concept in the treatment of penetrating injuries of the neck is that the vast majority of such injuries should be surgically explored whether symptoms are present or not. This concept has been gradually recognized in the last several years in both civilian and military injuries. With such an approach, clinically undetectable lacerations of a carotid artery, temporarily sealed by thrombus, may be identified and repaired and the subsequent development of a false aneurysm or secondary hemorrhage avoided.

Often penetrating neck injuries with hemorrhage must be treated with great urgency. Control of hemorrhage may be particularly difficult because tourniquets or pressure dressings cannot be applied without obstructing the trachea. Direct pressure with a finger may be the only effective method while the patient is being taken to the operating room.

Intubation of the trachea should be quickly performed because airway obstruction frequently evolves rapidly, either from an expanding hematoma or from edema of the vocal cords. Even if hemorrhage or airway obstruction does not force immediate operation, surgical exploration should be done promptly because an expanding hematoma may further decrease cerebral blood flow and produce irreversible neurological injury.

At operation the best incision is a diagonal one along the medial border of the sternocleidomastoideus muscle (Fig. 11–8).

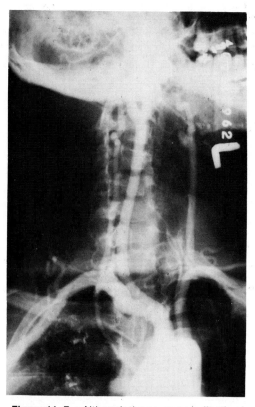

Figure 11–7. Although there was no indication by history or physical examination, complete occlusion of the left internal carotid artery was demonstrated by an arch aortogram in this patient following a gunshot wound of the neck. (W.R.G.H.)

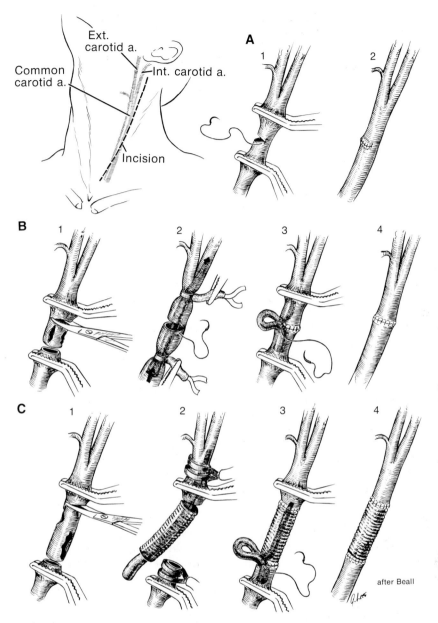

Figure 11-8. The approach and various methods which can be successfully utilized in repairing carotid artery injuries. Refer to the text for the full discussion of the use of a shunt during carotid reconstruction. Most patients who are neurologically intact following carotid artery injury tolerate the arterial reconstruction without benefit of a shunt. (After Beall, et al., 1963.)

General anesthesia should be used. Once the incision has been made, the hematoma should be quickly evacuated and the area of injury identified, controlling hemorrhage and obtaining proximal and distal control of the artery. Appropriate débridement of associated soft tissue injuries should be performed, combined with liberal irrigation with saline.

The different methods of repair of carotid artery injuries in a civilian series are shown in Tables 11-4 and 11-5. A lateral suture may be performed in many patients, especially when injury has been produced by

TABLE 11–4. OPERATIVE PROCEDURES EMPLOYED IN RELATION TO LOCATION OF CAROTID ARTERY INJURIES, EARLY EXPERIENCE IN HOUSTON*

| METHOD OF REPAIR | LOCATION OF CAROTID INJURY | | | TOTAL |
	Common	Internal	External	
Ligation	1	2	3	6
Lateral Arteriorrhaphy	5	0	1	6
End-to-end anastomosis	4	2	0	6
Excision of arteriovenous aneurysm				
with lateral arteriorrhaphy	3	1	0	4
with end-to-end anastomosis	1	0	0	1
Total	14	5	4	23

*From Beall, A. C., Jr., Shirkey, A. L., and DeBakey, M. E., J. Trauma, *3*:276, 1963. Copyright 1963, The Williams & Wilkins Co., Baltimore.

a small fragment. A patch of autogenous vein may be used to avoid constriction of the lumen. With a localized extensive injury, excision of the traumatized segment followed by an end-to-end anastomosis may be done. This latter method was utilized in 22 per cent of the Vietnam injuries included in the interim report from the Vietnam Vascular Registry (Table 11–6) (Rich et al., 1970A). Otherwise, a vascular graft, preferably from the greater saphenous vein, should be used. Prosthetic material is best avoided in contaminated wounds. Alternative methods of repair are illustrated in Figure 11–9.

A major unsettled question with carotid injuries is whether a shunt, either internal or external, should be used during the time of repair to maintain blood flow to the brain through the carotid artery. Abundant data are available from operations performed for arteriosclerotic stenosis of the carotid artery under local anesthesia, and these data indicate that many patients tolerate temporary occlusion of the carotid very well because of abundant collateral circulation. However, a small but significant minority do not, and serious neurological injury can result in this group. In the current Vietnam experience, most patients have been treated without shunts (Cohen et al., 1970; Rich et al., 1970A; Buchman et al., 1972). Cohen and associates emphasized that they were unable to relate morbidity or mortality to interruption of cerebral flow and did not believe that shunts were necessary. In their series, 90 per cent of their patients had no neurological abnormalities, and in the postoperative period there were no problems that could be related to temporary occlusion without shunts, even occlusion lasting up to 60

TABLE 11–5. OPERATIVE PROCEDURES EMPLOYED IN RELATION TO LOCATION OF CAROTID ARTERY INJURIES, CUMULATIVE HOUSTON SERIES*

| METHOD OF REPAIR | LOCATION OF CAROTID INJURY | | | TOTAL |
	Common	Internal	External	
Arteriorrhaphy	33	1	1	35
Anastomosis	19	6	0	25
Vein graft or Dacron interposition	4	1	0	5
Vein patch graft	1	0	0	1
Ligation	1	2	9	12
None	3	0	0	3
Total	61	10	10	81

*Modified from Rubio, P. A., Ruel, G. J., Jr., Beall, A. C., Jr., Jordon, G. L., Jr., and DeBakey, M. E., J. Trauma, *14*:967, 1974.

TABLE 11–6. MANAGEMENT OF CAROTID ARTERY INJURIES VIETNAM VASCULAR REGISTRY*

Method	Number	Per Cent
Lateral suture	19	38.0
Autogenous vein graft	14	28.0
End-to-end anastomosis	11	22.0
Miscellaneous	6	12.0
Totals	50	100.0

*From Rich, N. M., Baugh, J. H., and Hughes, C. W., J. Trauma, *10*:359, 1970. Copyright 1970, The Williams & Wilkins Co., Baltimore.

minutes. Fitchett and associates (1969) reported a similar experience with nine patients in whom occlusion time exceeded 55 minutes. Obviously, effective collateral circulation existed in these patients.

There remains, however, the well established fact that a small percentage of patients will not tolerate occlusion of the carotid artery. How to identify this small group is uncertain. In all likelihood patients who have no neurological abnormalities but who have sustained a complete interruption of the carotid flow may be safely operated upon without a shunt. In patients with small tangential lacerations, however, occlusion for a prolonged period would seem an unwarranted risk without some method of protection from cerebral ischemia. Some type of shunt would seem preferable in these circumstances, the simplest being an intraluminal shunt with the artery reconstructed around the shunt. An alternate guideline, not fully established, is to measure the arterial pressure in the distal carotid artery, which will represent the degree of collateral circulation. A mean

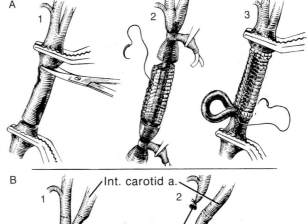

Figure 11–9. A variety of alternative methods may be a necessary part of the surgeon's armamentarium in repair of carotid artery injuries. Three such methods are illustrated.

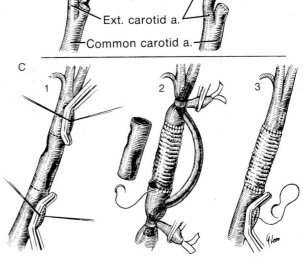

arterial pressure of above 50 to 60 mm Hg probably indicates that collateral circulation is adequate and that a shunt is unnecessary. The presence of bright red retrograde arterial flow from the distal end of the carotid injury also usually indicates the presence of good collateral circulation. Clinical results when neurological injury is present beforehand are particularly difficult to evaluate because the postoperative neurological defect may be due to irreversible changes before operation or, alternately, may have been intensified by ischemic injury at the time of operation.

A second unsettled question is the possible adverse effect of restoration of carotid artery flow in patients with abnormal neurological findings following carotid artery trauma. Cohen and co-workers (1970) emphasized that arterial repair in these patients resulted in a significant mortality and morbidity in Vietnam. They noted the clinical similarity between this type of patient and those patients undergoing immediate or early operation for acute stroke, with the probable conversion of an anemic infarction to hemorrhagic infarction after increase in carotid blood flow. The question arises whether ligation of the carotid artery in this group of patients is preferable. Although this question remains unanswered, ligation of the carotid artery in this situation may be the safest procedure.

Following carotid reconstruction, adjacent soft tissues should be closed over the repair site. Most cervical incisions can be closed primarily. However, with extensive contamination of the wound, the skin and subcutaneous tissues may be left open for delayed primary suture in three to six days.

Concomitant venous injuries, usually to the internal jugular vein, can be safely ligated, though a small laceration of a jugular vein can be sutured. If there is any question regarding the adequacy of the arterial repair at operation, an operative arteriogram is useful in identifying technical faults, distal thrombi or additional sites of injury.

POSTOPERATIVE CARE

Careful neurological monitoring of the patient in the immediate postoperative period is extremely important. As soon as the patient is reactive, a complete neurological examination should be performed and documented. The development of any new neurological deficits could herald a possible catastrophe. Reoperation, with or without a postoperative arteriogram, may be mandatory in the early postoperative period. An example of this problem is a case cited by Buchman and associates (1972), in which a 20 year old soldier underwent a saphenous vein graft for a severed right common carotid artery. Despite the fact that the patient had a good distal pulse following the repair, he developed a left hemiplegia three hours postoperatively. Reoperation was performed and a thrombectomy accomplished, and the patient recovered completely from his neurological deficit. If this problem had not been recognized in the early postoperative period, the hemiplegia might have become permanent.

Although postoperative arteriograms are not generally performed, valuable information can be obtained. The unsuspected find-

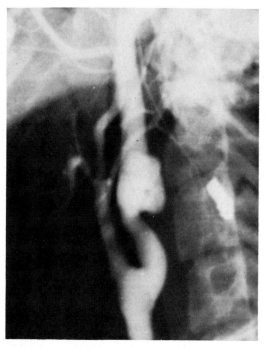

Figure 11-10. This postoperative arch study revealed an unexpected false aneurysm of the left internal carotid artery at the site of a recent repair in a Vietnam casualty. (Courtesy Dr. Kenneth E. Thomas.)

ing of a false aneurysm at a recent repair site in one Vietnam casualty is an example (Fig. 11–10).

COMPLICATIONS

Beall and co-workers (1963) in their series of 26 patients emphasized that two deaths and all major complications were related to neurological ischemic injury. This problem remains a principal one with reconstruction, but is difficult to correlate with results of repair.

Because of the rich blood supply in the neck, infection is seldom seen. One particularly unusual patient with infection after operation was treated at Walter Reed General Hospital. He was a 19 year old soldier who was injured in February, 1968, and had had aphasia and hemiplegia from the time of wounding. The severed left carotid was repaired with an autogenous vein graft. A wound infection followed, with drainage of purulent material. One month later, in an evacuation hospital in Japan, brisk arterial hemorrhage occurred from the neck wound. At surgical exploration a small defect in the middle of the vein graft was found and the surgeon elected to wrap this defect with a split 8 mm Dacron prosthesis. An arteriogram performed in the early postoperative period showed patency of the carotid artery (Fig. 11–11). Subsequently the patient was transferred to Walter Reed General Hospital where all physicians anticipated additional bleeding from the previously infected wound with the Dacron prosthesis. To everyone's surprise, with massive doses of antibiotics, the wound healed uneventfully and no further operation was necessary. *Pseudomonas aeruginosa* had been cultured from the wound (Fig. 11–12). This is the only known instance in the Vietnam experience where a prosthetic arterial repair remained functional despite the fact that the foreign material in an infected vascular repair was not removed.

Although thrombosis of the carotid ar-

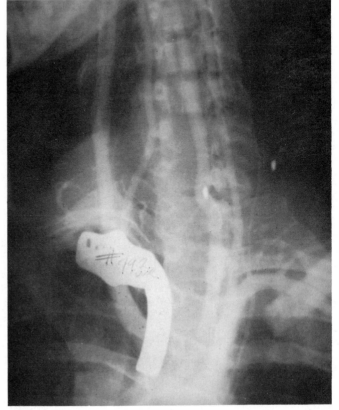

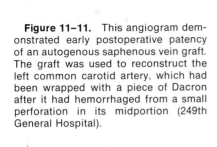
Figure 11–11. This angiogram demonstrated early postoperative patency of an autogenous saphenous vein graft. The graft was used to reconstruct the left common carotid artery, which had been wrapped with a piece of Dacron after it had hemorrhaged from a small perforation in its midportion (249th General Hospital).

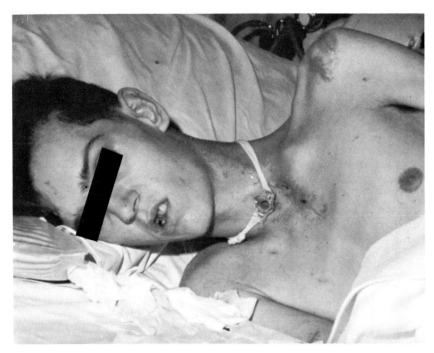

Figure 11-12. Healing of the left neck took place in this patient despite the presence on culture of *Pseudomonas aeruginosa*. The infection occurred after a piece of Dacron had been used to wrap a perforated saphenous vein graft that had originally been used in reconstruction of a left common carotid artery (see Fig. 11-11). (W.R.G.H.)

tery repair could lead to late cerebral infarction, four patients seen at Walter Reed General Hospital with occlusion of the reconstructed artery had no neurological defects. An arch arteriogram is probably the only method to determine if an arterial repair has failed if pulses cannot be felt (Fig. 11-13).

A separate question is the significance of stenosis of an arterial repair. Stenosis is probably not significant unless more than 80 per cent of the lumen is occluded. Two patients seen at Walter Reed General Hospital had audible, high pitched carotid artery bruits, but they remained asymptomatic. Vague dizziness developed in one patient following a gunshot wound repaired by an end-to-end anastomosis of the common carotid artery to the internal carotid artery using an internal shunt. An arch arteriogram showed marked stenosis (Fig. 11-14), and an elective reconstruction with a vein graft was performed.

Although lateral repair of the common carotid is frequently employed, several complications have been reported. At Valley Forge General Hospital, Buchman and

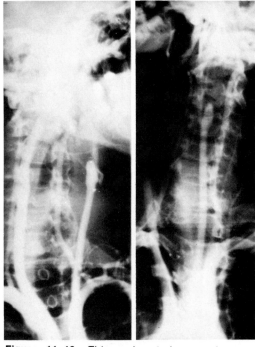

Figure 11-13. This arch arteriogram demonstrated total occlusion of the internal carotid artery; however, the patient had only vague symptomatology and no physical findings to confirm this diagnosis clinically. (W.R.G.H.)

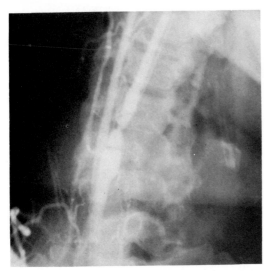

Figure 11–14. Arch aortogram. There is involvement, including marked stenosis, at several sites where an end-to-end anastomosis of the common carotid artery to the internal carotid artery was completed over an internal shunt. (W.R.G.H.)

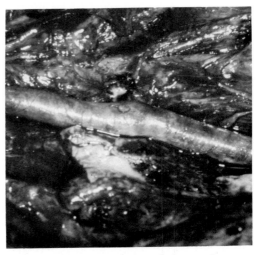

Figure 11–16. At the time that an autogenous saphenous vein bypass graft was utilized to reconstitute this thrombosed right common carotid artery, the site of the original repair was visualized. The original repair had taken place in Vietnam and had been accomplished with a vein patch graft. (W.R.G.H.)

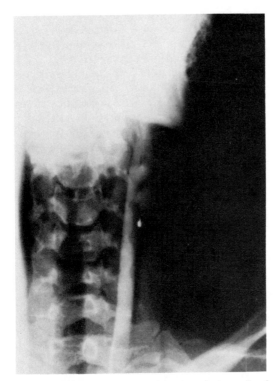

Figure 11–15. Following an attempted repair of the left common carotid artery by lateral suture, this patient developed a left carotid to internal jugular arteriovenous fistula with a small false aneurysm, which is demonstrated angiographically. (Buchman, R. J., Thomas, P. A., Jr., and Park, B., Angiology, 23:97, 1972.)

associates (1972) reported one patient with an arteriovenous fistula and false aneurysm that had developed after a lateral repair (Fig. 11–15). A patient who returned to Walter Reed General Hospital was found to have thrombosed the right common carotid artery after a lateral repair with an autogenous vein patch (Fig. 11–16).

RESULTS

In World War I Makins (1919) reported a neurological deficit in 30 per cent of 128 carotid artery injuries. In World War II Lawrence and co-workers (1948) reported a 47 per cent mortality among 17 cases, including one patient in whom lateral suture was successfully employed and another patient with an unsuccessful anastomosis and thrombosis of a Blakemore tube. In their review of 2471 American casualties, DeBakey and Simeone (1946) recorded a 30 per cent morbidity—three of ten patients developed cerebral complications. In the Korean Conflict, Inui and co-authors (1955) reported hemiparesis developing in two patients after ligation of the carotid artery, but three subsequent patients with primary repairs had no neurological problems. Hughes (1958) recorded only four carotid artery repairs among 11 injuries. The repairs included two by lateral suture, one by end-to-end anastomosis and one by autogenous vein graft. Five patients with pulsating hematomas or arteriovenous fistulas did not require emergency operation and were evacuated to be operated upon at a later time. Two patients were treated by ligation with resulting hemiplegia.

Experiences with 50 patients in the Vietnam Conflict are tabulated in Table 11–6. Lateral suture was used more than any other method, being employed in 19 repairs. End-to-end anastomosis and autogenous vein grafts were used with almost equal frequency. Only three patients required ligation. Four of the 14 vein grafts were known to have thrombosed. In a series of 85 carotid artery injuries, including both Vietnamese and American casualties, Cohen and associates (1970) reported a mortality rate of 15 per cent among 82 patients. This mortality was only 6 per cent if death from associated injuries is excluded. Eight of the 82 patients had neurological deficits on admission. Two of the eight became normal, two became worse, one remained unchanged and three patients died following arterial repair.

As previously mentioned, seven patients have been seen at Walter Reed General Hospital with complications following carotid artery repair in Vietnam; one had infection, four had thrombosis and two had stenosis (Rich et al., 1970C). The complications could be related to inadequate arterial reconstruction. Fortunately, significant neurological complications have not developed in the majority of these patients.

In reporting a relatively large civilian series, Beall and co-authors (1963) reported definitive operations in 22 of 25 patients with carotid injuries (Table 11–4). Three of the group died before definitive therapy could be performed. Over-all mortality was 20 per cent, but only two of the 22 patients in whom carotid artery repair was possible died—a mortality of 9 per cent—and both deaths were related to cerebral

TABLE 11–7. RESULTS OF MANAGING CAROTID ARTERY INJURIES IN HOUSTON*

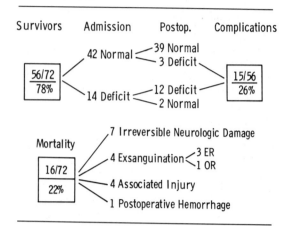

*Rubio, P. A., Reul, G. J., Jr., Beall, A. C., Jr., Jordon, G. L., Jr., and DeBakey, M. E., J. Trauma, *14*:967, 1974. Copyright 1974, The Williams & Wilkins Co., Baltimore.

damage evident at the time of admission. Among 20 long term survivors, 16 were asymptomatic and four had neurological deficits following operation. In one of these four patients the deficit was hemiplegia, and this was present before operation and remained unchanged following operation. Hemiparesis followed operation in the other three patients. In one of these three patients, thrombosis of the anastomosis occurred, while another had the common carotid artery occluded for 70 minutes. The cummulative results from Houston were similar for 81 carotid artery injuries (Rubio et al., 1974). Details are outlined in Table 11–7. Thal and co-workers (1974) found an overall mortality rate of 8.3 per cent among 60 patients with carotid arterial trauma.

FOLLOW-UP

Among patients with thrombosis of a repaired carotid artery seen at Walter Reed General Hospital (Rich et al., 1970C), elective reconstruction was performed in five patients who had minimal symptoms of cerebral ischemia. A representative patient was a 22 year old soldier who sustained a

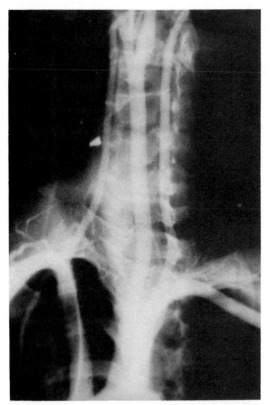

Figure 11–17. This arch aortogram demonstrates complete occlusion of the right common carotid artery following a vein patch graft repair in a Vietnam casualty. Reconstitution of the internal carotid artery is demonstrated in Fig. 11–18. (Rich, N. M., Baugh, J. H., and Hughes, C. W., Arch. Surg., *100*:646, 1970. Copyright 1970, American Medical Association.)

gunshot wound of the right side of the neck in Vietnam in September, 1968. A saphenous vein patch graft was used to repair an incomplete transection of the right common carotid artery. At Walter Reed General Hospital three weeks later, an arteriogram demonstrated thrombosis of the repair (Fig. 11–17). Distal patency could be seen, however (Fig. 11–18), and the occluded artery was reconstructed with a saphenous vein bypass graft. No neurologic defect was present at any time.

Buchman and colleagues (1972) reported 15 patients seen at Valley Forge General Hospital over a six year period following carotid artery injuries in Vietnam (Table 11–8). There were 13 patients who had carotid artery reconstruction, and there

were good immediate results in nine of these. Two who were hemiparetic before arterial reconstruction had similar neurological deficits afterward. Additional operations were required in 5 of the 15 patients, including two aortocarotid bypasses, one thrombectomy, one closure of an arteriovenous fistula and one ligation of the internal carotid artery. Preoperatively, both patients treated with a bypass had complained of dizziness and one had recurrent syncope. Both became asymptomatic after reconstruction. Twelve of the 13 patients eventually had a good result. This excludes the two patients who were hemiparetic immediately following injury.

One month after bilateral carotid artery repair by end-to-end anastomosis, approximately 1 inch proximal to the bifurcation, Haller (1962) obtained a retrograde aortic

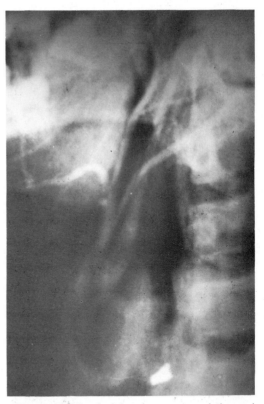

Figure 11–18. A delayed exposure of the arch study described in Fig. 11–17 reveals reconstitution of both the right internal and external carotid arteries. (Rich, N. M., Baugh, J. H., and Hughes, C. W., Arch. Surg., *100*:646, 1970. Copyright 1970, American Medical Association.)

TABLE 11-8. CAROTID ARTERY INJURIES IN VIETNAM WITH FOLLOW-UP EVALUATION AT VALLEY FORGE GENERAL HOSPITAL*

VESSEL	ADMISSION CNS STATUS	PROCEDURE	EARLY RESULT	REOPERATION	FINAL RESULT
CC	normal	anastomosis	good	—	good
IC	normal	lateral suture	good	—	good
CC	right hemiparesis	anastomosis	right hemiparesis	—	right hemiparesis
IC	right hemiparesis	anastomosis	right hemiparesis	—	right hemiparesis
CC	normal	anastomosis	good	—	good
CC	normal	vein graft	left hemiparesis	thrombectomy	good
CC	paraplegia	anastomosis	ischemia	aortocarotid bypass	ischemia relieved
CC	normal	ligation	ischemia	aortocarotid bypass	good
CC	normal	vein graft	good	—	good
CC	normal	lateral suture	good	—	good
CC	unconscious	vein graft	partial hemiparesis	—	good
CC	normal	anastomosis	good	—	good
IC	normal	vein graft	good	—	good
CC	normal	lateral suture	good	closure A-V fistula	good
IC	paresis VII, X, XII	—	paresis VII, X, XII	ligation	right hemiplegia

*Modified from Buchman, R. J., Thomas, P. A., Jr., and Park, B., Angiology, *23*:97, 1972.

arch study which revealed patent common carotid arteries bilaterally, and a single small vertebral artery on the left (Fig. 11-19). His patient was able to return to work as a heavy laborer approximately six weeks after injury and had experienced no subsequent difficulty up to the time of the report. An unusual complication of carotid artery obstruction was reported by Carrasquilla and Weaver (1972), who found aneurysmal dilatation of a saphenous vein graft which had been used to repair the common carotid artery of a Vietnam casualty (Fig. 11-20).

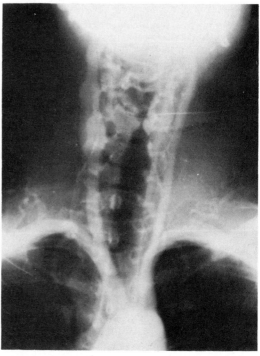

Figure 11-20. Fusiform aneurysmal dilatation of a greater saphenous vein graft in the right common carotid artery is demonstrated in this retrograde arch study 25 months following the original injury in a Vietnam casualty. (Carrasquilla, C., and Weaver, A. W., Vasc. Surg., *6*:66, 1972.)

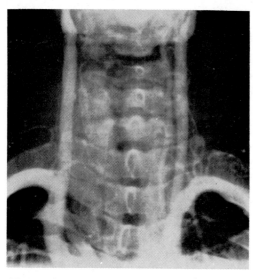

Figure 11-19. One month following immediate repair of both common carotid arteries, this retrograde femoral aortic arteriogram revealed patent carotid arteries and a single left vertebral artery. (Haller, A. C. Amer. J. Surg., *103*:532, 1962.)

NONPENETRATING INJURIES OF THE CAROTID ARTERIES

There are an increasing number of reports of carotid injuries from blunt trauma to neck. In 1967 Yamada and co-authors reported one case and found 52 cases reported by others of carotid occlusion following acute nonpenetrating trauma. Similarly, in 1968 Fleming and Petrie reported two cases and found reports of 90 similar cases. Towne and associates (1972) presented four patients with thrombosis of the internal carotid artery following blunt cervical trauma seen in a four year period in Omaha. This increased recognition is probably due to the increasing frequency of carotid angiography and also of postmortem examination of the carotid artery.

The exact mechanism of injury to the carotid artery by nonpenetrating trauma is not completely understood. The etiology of 52 cases reviewed in the literature is outlined in Table 11–9. Fleming and Petrie (1968) suggested four possible mechanisms:

1. A direct blow.
2. Stretching of the carotid artery by hyperextension and lateral flexion of the neck.
3. Trauma to the peritonsillar area by a foreign object in the mouth.
4. Injury to the intrapetrous portion of the carotid artery in association with a basilar skull fracture.

Injuries with intraoral foreign bodies occur particularly in children when they fall with a foreign object, such as a pencil, stick or toothbrush, in the mouth (Pitner, 1966).

Extrinsic compression of the internal carotid artery is an unusual mechanism of trauma. Mandlebaum and Kalsbeck (1970) reported a 20 year old nurse injured in an automobile accident. Hemorrhagic infarction of a group of lymph nodes subsequently compressed the left internal carotid artery at the level of the first cervical vertebra (Fig. 11–21). Excision of the constricting mass of lymph nodes released the compression, which was subsequently confirmed by a normal angiogram.

The first known report of traumatic carotid artery thrombosis was made by Hirshfeld in 1858. In 1872 Verneuil reported a similar patient in whom thrombosis

TABLE 11–9. SUMMARY OF HISTORY AND ADMISSION FINDINGS IN 52 CASES OF CAROTID ARTERY OCCLUSION DUE TO NONPENETRATING INJURY*

	NUMBER	PER CENT
Source of Trauma		
Vehicular accidents	27	52
Fighting (brawl)	8	15
Fall	8	15
Object striking neck	4	8
Boxing	2	4
Objects striking head	2	4
Diagnostic carotid compression	1	2
History and Admission Diagnosis		
History of head injury	39	75
History of cervical region injury	19	37
Admission diagnosis of head injury	46	88
Admission diagnosis of carotid artery injury	3	6
Actual significant head injury	12	23
Signs of Trauma to the Neck		
Present	25	48
Absent	26	50
Unknown	1	4

*Modified from Yamada, S., Kindt, G. W., and Youmans, J. R., J. Trauma, 7:333, 1967.

followed forced rotation of the head (Javid, 1963). Hockaday (1969) noted that in most patients with traumatic thrombosis of the internal carotid the site of obstruction was about 2 cm above the bifurcation of the common carotid artery. In his review, 9 of 10 cases with autopsy findings showed injury to the intima and media with localized thrombus formation. Distal intracranial extension of thrombus, extending even to the origin of the middle cerebral artery, was common. Distal embolism from the intraluminal thrombus was thought to account for the sudden delayed onset of hemiplegia and aphasia in some patients.

In a case report by Yamada and co-authors (1967), a 39 year old patient was injured in a fight in a bar. Symptoms evolved slowly, with a left hemiparesis becoming obvious 19 hours after injury. A carotid arteriogram revealed almost a complete block of the right internal carotid artery about 1.5 cm above the common carotid bifurcation (Fig. 11–22). A thromboendarterectomy was performed under

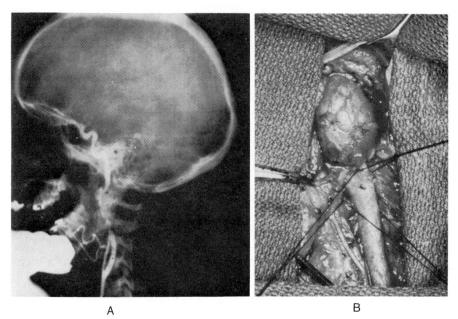

A   B

Figure 11–21. (A) This preoperative carotid angiogram shows narrowing of the internal carotid artery. Blunt cervical trauma caused a hemorrhagic infarction in adjacent lymph nodes which resulted in an extrinsic compression of the internal carotid artery. (Mandlebaum, I., and Kalsbeck, J. E., Ann. Surg., *171*:434, 1970.)

(B) The photograph taken during surgery reveals a 2 × 3 cm mass lying upon the internal carotid artery and adherent to it. Extrinsic compression of the artery was caused by this mass of lymph nodes with hemorrhagic infarction. (Mandlebaum, I., and Kalsbeck, J. E., Ann. Surg., *171*:434, 1970.)

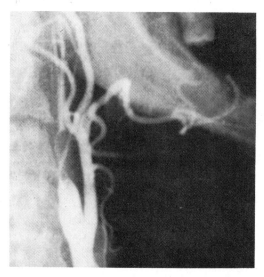

Figure 11–22. This preoperative arteriogram reveals nearly total occlusion of the internal carotid artery, about 1.5 cm above the right common carotid bifurcation, after a nonpenetrating injury to the neck during a fight. (Yamada, S., Kindt, G. W., and Youmans, J. R., J. Trauma, 7:333, 1967. Copyright 1967, The Williams & Wilkins Co., Baltimore.)

general anesthesia, and a small amount of thrombus was removed from the internal carotid artery immediately above a fractured atheromatous plaque (Fig. 11–23). The postoperative arteriogram revealed that the internal carotid artery patency was restored (Fig. 11–24). These authors also summarized the report of pathological findings in 52 patients reported in the literature (Table 11–10). Most lesions were near the bifurcation of the common carotid artery, but nearly one-third were between the carotid bifurcation and the base of the skull. A definite tear of the intima was demonstrated in 40 per cent of the cases. The variable location contrasts with the rather uniform location of atheromatous plaques, which are most frequently found at the carotid bifurcation. Atheromata were present, however, in several of the patients in this series and may have increased the susceptibility to injury.

Pitner (1966) stated that children who died of internal carotid occlusion following

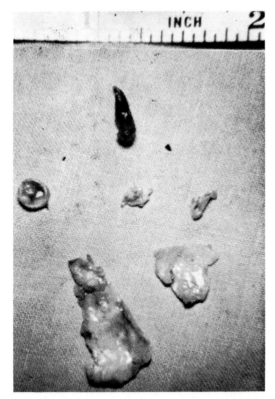

Figure 11–23. Thrombus that nearly occluded the internal carotid artery (see Fig. 11–22) is located at the top of this picture. Also shown is the atheroma which was removed during a thromboendarterectomy of the right carotid artery following occlusion secondary to nonpenetrating trauma. (Yamada, S., Kindt, G. W., and Youmans, J. R., J. Trauma, 7:333, 1967. Copyright 1967, The Williams & Wilkins Co., Baltimore.)

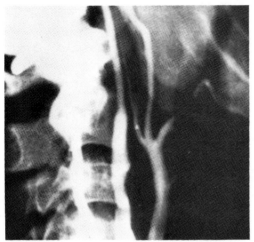

Figure 11–24. Postoperative arteriogram shows a patent internal carotid artery following a thromboendarterectomy for acute occlusion due to a nonpenetrating cervical injury. (Yamada, S., Kindt, G. W., and Youmans, J. R., J. Trauma, 7:333, 1967. Copyright 1967, The Williams & Wilkins Co., Baltimore.)

TABLE 11–10. SUMMARY OF PATHOLOGICAL FINDINGS IN 52 CASES OF CAROTID ARTERY OCCLUSION SECONDARY TO NONPENETRATING INJURY*

	NUMBER	PER CENT
Site of Occlusion		
Common carotid	3	6
At or just above bifurcation	29	56
Between bifurcation and base of skull	15	29
Base of skull	5	9
Type of Damage to Vessel Wall		
No damage apparent	8	15
Intimal tear	21	40
Intramural hemorrhage	2	4
Scarring of wall (fibrosis)	3	6
Status unknown	18	35
Presence of Atheroma		
Present	8	15
Known to be absent	21	40
No evidence on angiogram	9	17
Not discussed in protocols	14	28

*Modified from Yamada, S., Kindt, G. W., and Youmans, J. R., J. Trauma, 7:333, 1967.

blunt intraoral trauma had a constant pathological finding of extension of thrombus from the internal carotid artery distally into the major intracranial arteries, with subsequent massive infarction of the hemisphere.

An unusual clinical feature of nonpenetrating injuries is the delayed appearance of symptoms (Yamada et al., 1967). Only three of 52 patients were admitted to the hospital with a diagnosis of carotid artery injury. Significant head injuries were present in 23 per cent of the patients, and this may have obscured the correct diagnosis. However, only one-half of the patients had signs of injury to the neck, such as a bruise or abrasion of the skin (Table 11–9). This delay in the development of symptoms is a particularly critical clinical feature. Only 10 per cent of the patients had their initial serious symptoms within one hour of injury, and half were asymptomatic after 10 hours (Table 11–11). Once symptoms appeared, they were typical of carotid insufficiency — loss of consciousness, aphasia, hemiparesis and paresthesias. Monoparesis or hemiparesis was present in all but one of the 52 reported patients.

TABLE 11–11. TIME AND ONSET OF SYMPTOMS IN 52 CASES OF CAROTID ARTERY OCCLUSION DUE TO NONPENETRATING INJURY*

INITIAL SERIOUS SYMPTOMS Time	No.	%
0–1 hour	5	10
1–4 hours	12	23
4–10 hours	11	21
10–24 hours	15	29
Over 24 hours	9	17

ONSET OF PARTICULAR SYMPTOMS

Time	Lowered Conscious Level No.	%	Aphasia No.	%	Seizures No.	%	Paresthesia No.	%	Monoparesis or Hemiparesis No.	%
0–1 hour	2	4	2	4	1	2	4	8	5	10
1–4 hours	9	17	4	8	1	2	6	11	11	21
4–10 hours	3	6	4	8	0	0	2	4	9	17
10–24 hours	15	29	7	13	1	2	13	25	17	33
Over 24 hours	8	15	6	11	3	6	7	13	8	15
Not present	14	27	24	46	45	86	3	6	1	2
Unknown	1	2	5	10	1	2	17	33	1	2

*Modified from Yamada, S., Kindt, G. W., and Youmans, J. R., J. Trauma, 7:333, 1967.

The reason for the frequent delay in appearance of symptoms is uncertain. It may be due to the gradual development of a thrombus at the site of the intimal injury, or possibly a subintimal dissection of the hematoma. A useful guideline in management is to consider a possible evolving thrombus of the carotid artery in any patient with a head injury with late appearance of hemiparesis.

Similarly, in children with internal carotid thrombosis following blunt intraoral trauma, the delayed appearance of symptoms makes early diagnosis difficult (Pitner, 1966). Awareness of the late appearance of lethal carotid artery thrombosis is one of the best aids in establishing the correct diagnosis.

Jernigan and Gardner (1971), in documenting two cases and reviewing the literature, stated that Horner's syndrome was reported on the initial examination in many patients prior to any other neurological deficit. They felt that trauma to the superior sympathetic chain and first ganglion sufficient to cause Horner's syndrome was also likely to injure the internal carotid artery because of the close anatomical proximity of these structures (Table 11–12).

Once suspected, the diagnosis of carotid artery thrombosis can be readily established by angiography (Table 11–13). Surgical exploration with thrombectomy should be performed promptly in most patients if there is not a complete hemiplegia. A Fogarty balloon catheter may be helpful for removal of distal propagating thrombus (Fleming and Petrie, 1968). Towne and associates (1972) have emphasized that nonoperative treatment is the best choice for the patient with thrombosis of the internal carotid artery following blunt

TABLE 11–12. EARLY CLINICAL FEATURES OF CAROTID ARTERY INJURY SECONDARY TO BLUNT CERVICAL TRAUMA*

1. Hematoma lateral neck
2. Horner's syndrome
3. Transient ischemic attacks
4. Lucid interval
5. Hemiplegia or hemiparesis in an alert patient

*Modified from Jernigan, W. R., and Gardner, W. C., J. Trauma, *11*:429, 1971.

TABLE 11–13. SUMMARY OF DIAGNOSTIC PROCEDURES IN 52 PATIENTS WITH CAROTID ARTERY OCCLUSION DUE TO NONPENETRATING TRAUMA*

METHOD OF DIAGNOSIS	NUMBER	PER CENT
Autopsy only	6	11
Autopsy following trephining or craniotomy	4	8
Craniotomy angiogram	5	10
Exploration only	1	2
Angiography	36	69

*Modified from Yamada, S., Kindt, G. W., and Youmans, J. R., J. Trauma, 7:333, 1967.

cervical trauma when there has been a resultant hemiplegia. They feel that the clinical situation is similar to that of acute stroke, where the restoration of blood flow to a softened ischemic brain often results in hemorrhagic infarction. According to Towne and co-workers, efforts should be directed toward aiding the collateral blood flow and preventing propagation and embolization of thrombus. They advocate the use of heparin, dextran and steroids.

At present the results of treatment of carotid artery occlusion secondary to nonpenetrating trauma are poor. In the review by Yamada and associates in 1967, 21 pa-

TABLE 11–14. RESULTS OF TREATMENT OF CAROTID ARTERY OCCLUSION SECONDARY TO NONPENETRATING TRAUMA*

	NUMBER	PER CENT
No Carotid Operation		
Died	17	55
Severe deficit (unable to work)	14	45
Total	31	100
Carotid Operation		
Died	3	14
Severe deficit (unable to work)	12	58
Moderate deficit	1	5
Minimal deficit	1	5
No deficit	4	18
Total	21	100

*From Yamada, S., Kindt, G. W., and Youmans, J. R., J. Trauma, 7:333, 1967. Copyright 1967, The Williams & Wilkins Co., Baltimore.

tients were operated upon; 3 died, 12 had a remaining serious neurological deficit, 2 had moderate deficits and only 4 were asymptomatic (Table 11–14). In 31 patients who were not operated upon, 17 died and 14 remained with a severe deficit. The over-all mortality was approximately 40 per cent and a severe neurological residual occurred in 52 per cent of patients with such injuries. In the latest report by Towne and co-authors (1972), two of three patients operated upon died and none of the three was improved. The fourth patient, who was treated by nonoperative management, recovered without neurological residuals. Earlier diagnosis and treatment will possibly alter this dismal record in the future.

VERTEBRAL ARTERY INJURIES

Penetrating injuries of the vertebral artery are fortunately rare and of little clinical significance. Most have been treated by ligation (Fig. 11–25). As shown in Table

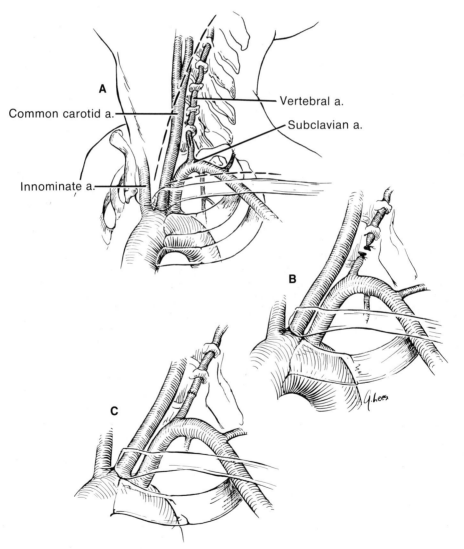

Figure 11–25. Laceration of the proximal left vertebral artery and two methods of management, either by end-to-end anastomosis or by ligation.

TABLE 11-15. INCIDENCE OF VERTEBRAL ARTERY INJURIES

	AUTHOR	TOTAL ARTERIES	VERTEBRAL	PER CENT
War Series				
WW I	Makins (1919)	1202	3	0.2
WW II	De Bakey and Simeone (1946)	2471	—	—
Korean	Hughes (1958)	304	—	—
Vietnam	Rich et al. (1970A)	1000	—	—
Civilian Series				
Houston	Morris et al. (1960)	220	—	—
Atlanta	Ferguson et al. (1961)	200	1	0.5
Denver	Owens (1963)	70	—	—
Detroit	Smith et al. (1963)	61	1	1.6
Dallas	Patman et al. (1964)	271	2	0.7
Los Angeles	Treiman et al. (1966)	159	—	—
St. Louis	Dillard et al. (1968)	85	—	—
New Orleans	Drapanas et al. (1970)	226	—	—
Dallas	Perry et al. (1971)*	508	4	0.8
Denver	Kelly and Eiseman (1975)	116	1	0.9
Memphis	Cheek et al. (1975)	155	3	1.9

*This is a sequential study including the earlier report.

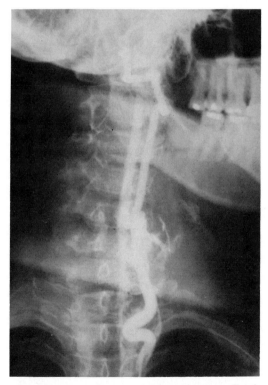

Figure 11-26. This vertebral arteriovenous fistula resulted from trauma from a percutaneous carotid artery puncture during angiographic studies 16 years previously. The patient had been told erroneously that she had a congenital vertebral arteriovenous malformation. (W.R.G.H.)

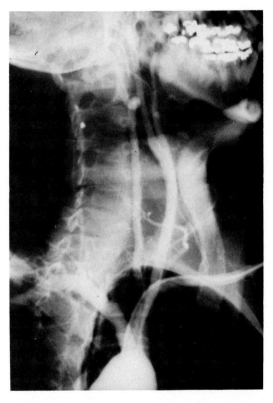

Figure 11-27. An unsuspected right vertebral artery occlusion was demonstrated during this arch study, which was performed to confirm occlusion of the right carotid artery without reconstitution of the internal carotid artery. (Rich, N. M., Baugh, J. H., and Hughes, C. W., Arch. Surg., *100*:646, 1970. Copyright 1970, American Medical Association.)

11–15, three such injuries were reported in World War I, and none from World War II or the Korean or Vietnam Conflicts. A total of eight such injuries have been recorded among eight different series of civilian arterial injuries. Nonpenetrating injuries have also been reported to cause thrombosis of the vertebral artery. Murray (1957) cites thrombosis of the right vertebral artery in a 16 year old boy following nonpenetrating trauma. Gurdjian and associates (1963) reported thrombosis of the vertebral artery in two of five patients with cervical trauma in association with thrombosis of the carotid arteries.

Trauma to the vertebral artery has rarely occurred with percutaneous angiography. One unusual patient at Walter Reed General Hospital was seen 16 years after percutaneous puncture, when the correct diagnosis of a vertebral arteriovenous fistula was made (Fig. 11–26). Until that time the condition was erroneously diagnosed as a congenital malformation.

In the long term follow-up of patients through the Vietnam Vascular Registry, unsuspected vertebral artery occlusion has been discovered in patients with previously documented cervical trauma (Fig. 11–27).

CHAPTER 12

INJURIES OF THE INTRATHORACIC BRANCHES OF THE AORTIC ARCH

Intrathoracic injuries of arteries originating from the aortic arch are infrequently reported in both civilian and military practice despite the recent increase in the number of patients sustaining trauma to major vessels. The arteries include the innominate, the left common carotid and the left subclavian (Fig. 12–1). Anatomically, the injuries to these arteries have variously been located in the base of the neck, the thoracic outlet, the upper thorax, the superior anterior mediastinum and the cervico-mediastinal area. Cervical injuries of the common carotid artery and its two main branches deserve special emphasis, and they are discussed in Chapter 11. Cervical injuries of the subclavian arteries are discussed in Chapter 13.

The dominant problem with injuries of the intrathoracic great vessels is massive hemorrhage, with death from exsanguination. Because most injuries are immediately fatal, there are few reports of the results of treatment. Probably less than 20 successful repairs of acute injuries of the intrathoracic great vessels have been reported in the English literature. Therefore, in this chapter attention will be focused on the problems of prompt diagnosis and control of hemorrhage. The problems of neurologic injury are considered in more detail in Chapter 11. The problems of ischemia in

the arm are discussed in more detail in Chapter 13.

Because of the complex anatomical relationships in the upper mediastinum, which contains many vital structures crowded together as they emerge from the thoracic outlet, the search for the best surgical incision has occupied the attention of many surgeons. The ideal incision needs to be made promptly to control hemorrhage and similarly to provide wide exposure. In addition, it should be possible to extend the incision in different directions, depending upon the type of injury encountered. Greenough (1929), in a comprehensive review, detailed 17 different operative approaches which had been described for the innominate and subclavian vessels. He credited Mott with performing the first ligation of the innominate artery in 1818 by using a supraclavicular approach. He also gave Cooper credit for first adopting the principle of increasing the exposure by removal of bony structures through resection of a portion of the clavicle. Halsted (1892) resected the medial two-thirds of the clavicle to perform the first successful excision of a subclavian aneurysm. Lindskog (1946) stated that Burrell of Philadelphia was the first to resect a portion of the sternum to expose the innominate artery in 1895. Sencert (1918), following his World War I experi-

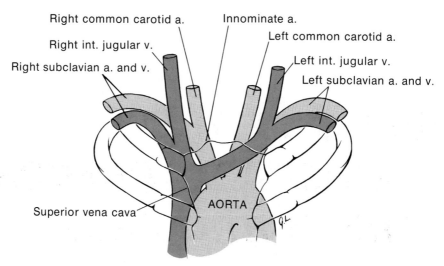

Figure 12–1.   This is an artist's conception of the aortic arch and its intrathoracic branches. The branches include the innominate or the brachiocephalic trunk, the left common carotid and the left subclavian arteries.

ence in the French Army, described an extensive incision employing resection of part of the clavicle and incision of the costal cartilages and manubrium (Fig. 12–2). Following World War II, Elkins described operative approaches in 1945 and 1946, and Shumacker (1947) described his preferred technique of sternotomy combined with resection of the inner third of the clavicle (Fig. 12–3). In more recent years different approaches have been described by Steenburg and Ravitch (1963) (Fig. 12–

4), Mansberger and Lindberg (1965) and Amato and associates (1969) (Fig. 12–5), all of whom are concerned with civilian trauma in large metropolitan areas. Bricker and co-workers (1970) published a technique involving a "trapdoor" incision, which permitted progressive enlargement of the incision at operation. This was employed in a patient who had a penetrating gunshot wound of the left common carotid artery about 3 cm distal to its origin (Fig. 12–6).

Only in the present decade has extensive

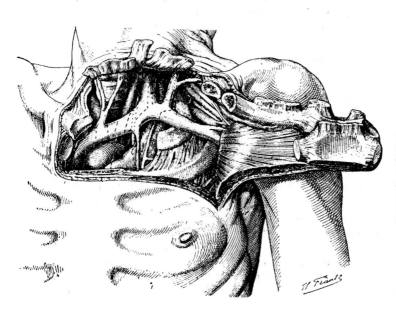

Figure 12–2. From his experience in the French Army, Sencert described his use of an extensive incision employing resection of part of the clavicle and incision of the costal cartilages and manubrium. (Steenburg, R. W., and Ravitch, M. M., Ann. Surg., *157*:839, 1963.)

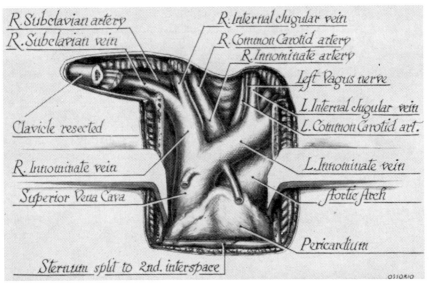

Figure 12–3. Following World War II, Shumacker described his preferred technique of sternotomy combined with resection of the inner third of the clavicle. (Shumacker, H. B., Jr., Ann. Surg., *127*:464, 1948.)

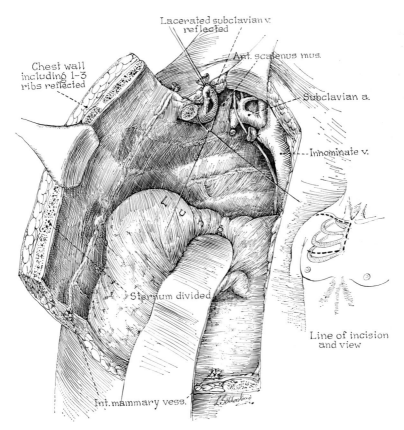

Figure 12–4. Another recent exposure which has been advocated connects the intercostal incision and the transverse cervical incision with a median sternotomy. (Steenburg, R. W., and Ravitch, M. M., Ann. Surg., *157*: 839, 1963.)

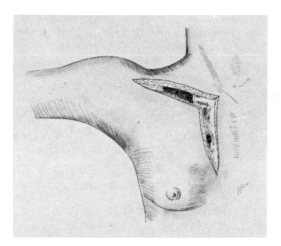

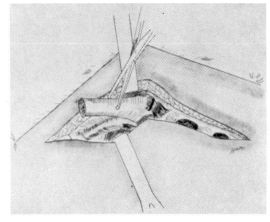

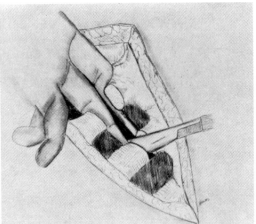

Figure 12–5. This series of sketches demonstrates one of the latest approaches for exposing the branches of the aortic arch, which involves extending the original supraclavicular incision downward to the third intercostal space. A knife is used to transect the first two costal cartilages, while the underlying structures are protected. (Amato, J. J., Vanecko, R. M., Yao, S. T., and Weinberg, M., Jr., Ann. Thorac. Surg., *8*:537, 1969.)

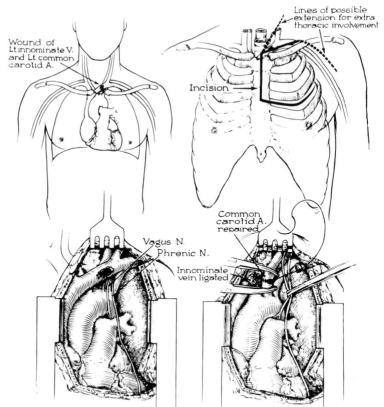

Figure 12-6. These drawings show the progressive management of a gunshot wound of the left common carotid artery. A "trapdoor" type of incision permitted progressive enlargement to obtain satisfactory exposure of the injured artery. (Bricker, D. L., Noon, G. P., Beall, A. C., Jr., and DeBakey, M. E., J. Trauma, *10*:1, 1970. Copyright 1970, The Williams & Wilkins Co., Baltimore.)

experience been gained with elective operations upon the intrathoracic aorta and its branches, often by employing techniques with cardiopulmonary bypass. Previously, experience was quite limited. Greenough's collective review in 1929 included only 91 patients in whom operative procedures had been performed upon the innominate artery, who showed a mortality of 56 per cent. In Lindskog's review in 1946, only 18 additional cases were added. He stated that since 1900 the mortality rate was 31 per cent in 61 cases following innominate arterial ligation or suture.

SURGICAL ANATOMY

Three major arteries—the innominate, the left common carotid and the left subclavian—arise from the aortic arch (Fig. 12-1).

The innominate artery originates in front of the trachea and passes upward, backward and to the right. Anteriorly, the left innominate vein crosses the artery near its origin. Usually, a remnant of the thymus is also found between the innominate artery and the manubrium. The right innominate vein and superior vena cava lie to the right between the innominate artery and the right pleural cavity. The left common carotid artery and the trachea are to the left. Posteriorly, the innominate artery lies on the trachea near its origin and on the long cervical muscle above.

Beneath the posterior aspect of the right sternoclavicular joint, the innominate divides into the right subclavian and the right common carotid arteries. Occasionally, the innominate artery arises from the aortic arch far to the left of the midline and makes a small indentation on the anterior trachea (Strandness, 1969).

The left common carotid artery arises from the aortic arch to the left and adjacent to the innominate artery. These two arteries lie side by side at their origin but diverge as they ascend. The left innominate vein crosses anteriorly to the left common carotid artery, and the thymic remnant intervenes between it and the manubrium. Posteriorly, the arteries are in contact with the trachea, the esophagus and the left recurrent laryngeal nerve. The left subclavian artery, the left phrenic and vagus nerves and the left pleural cavity are on its left.

Passing upward to the left, the left common carotid artery enters the neck behind the left sternoclavicular joint and continues in the neck beneath and parallel to the left sternocleidomastoid muscle.

The left subclavian artery arises from the aortic arch to the left and slightly behind the left common carotid artery (see Chap. 13).

INCIDENCE

As mentioned earlier, there are probably less than 20 reported successful repairs of acute injuries of the intrathoracic great vessels in the English literature. Kemmerer and associates (1961) state that only 11 of 38 patients with injuries to major arteries and veins at the base of the neck reached the hospital alive. The true incidence of in-

nominate arterial trauma is undoubtedly higher than reported; however, the majority of the patients exsanguinate prior to receiving treatment. The limited experience with injuries of the innominate artery in both civilian and military trauma is shown in Table 12–1.

In World War I (Makins, 1919), World War II (DeBakey and Simeone, 1946) and the Korean Conflict (Hughes, 1958), no innominate arterial injuries were treated. In the interim report of 1000 acute major arterial injuries in the Vietnam Conflict (Rich et al., 1970A), treatment of three innominate arterial injuries was found. This represents an incidence of less than 1 per cent.

In reports of civilian trauma, innominate arterial injuries are similarly rare. Neither Morris and associates (1960), in a report of 220 arterial injuries, nor Patman and co-authors (1964), in a report of 271 injuries, treated a patient with innominate arterial trauma. Ferguson and co-authors (1961) found only one innominate arterial injury among 200 patients with arterial trauma in Atlanta over a 10-year period starting in 1950. Owens (1963) had one innominate arterial injury in his Denver series of 70 cases. Pate and Wilson (1964) reported only one innominate injury in a total of 21

TABLE 12–1.   INCIDENCE OF INNOMINATE ARTERIAL INJURIES

	AUTHOR	TOTAL ARTERIES	INNOMINATE	PER CENT
War Series				
WW I	Makins (1919)	1191	0	0.0
WW II	DeBakey and Simeone (1946)	2471	0	0.0
Korean	Hughes (1958)	304	0	0.0
Vietnam	Rich et al. (1970)	1000	3	0.3
Civilian Series				
Houston	Morris et al. (1960)	220	0	0.0
Atlanta	Ferguson et al. (1961)	200	1	0.5
Denver	Owens (1963)	70	1	1.4
Detroit	Smith et al. (1963)	61	0	0.0
Dallas	Patman et al. (1964)	271	0	0.0
Los Angeles	Treiman et al. (1966)	159	1	0.6
St. Louis	Dillard et al. (1968)	85	0	0.0
New Orleans	Drapanas et al. (1970)	226	0	0.0
Dallas	Perry et al. (1971)*	508	1	0.2
Denver	Kelly and Eiseman (1975)	116	0	0.0
Jackson	Hardy et al. (1975)	360	0	0.0
Memphis	Cheek et al. (1975)	155	2	1.3
New York	Bole et al. (1976)	126	4	3.2

*This is a sequential study including the earlier report.

arterial injuries at the base of the neck at the City of Memphis Hospital over a period of 12 years. Treiman and associates (1966) recorded one innominate arterial injury among 159 major arterial injuries at the Los Angeles County General Hospital over a 15-year period from 1948 to 1963. Amato and co-workers (1969), in discussing the emergency approach to the subclavian and innominate vessels, reviewed the management of 25 patients with subclavian injuries but they did not include any patients with innominate injuries. Bricker and associates (1970) described 27 patients with 38 injuries of major intrathoracic vessels in Houston from 1955 to 1966; however, they did not have any patients with innominate arterial injuries. Drapanas and associates (1970) did not report any innominate arterial trauma among 226 patients with arterial injuries treated from 1942 through 1969 in New Orleans. Perry and co-workers (1971) found only one innominate arterial injury among 508 significant arterial injuries in a combined series from Dallas. Later, Flint and co-workers (1973) found seven in the same institution. Hewitt and associates (1974) reported 46 arterial injuries of the thoracic outlet including two of the innominate and one of the aortic arch in their New Orleans Series. Symbas and co-authors (1974) treated three innominate artery injuries in Atlanta. Smith and associates (1974) had no innominate artery injuries in Detroit from 1961 through 1973 when 127 arterial injuries were treated. In recent large civilian series, there were no injuries in Denver (Kelly and Eijeman, 1975) or in Jackson (Hardy et al., 1975). However, two injuries of the innominate artery were reported from Memphis (Cheek et al., 1975) and four from New York (Bole et al., 1976), with the latter representing the highest incidence of any series: 3.2 per cent (4 of 126 arterial injuries).

The incidence of injuries of the intrathoracic carotid artery is uncertain because most reports include both the cervical and intrathoracic carotid arterial injuries together. Bricker and associates (1970) did report four intrathoracic injuries of the common carotid artery, three on the left and one on the right near the origin from the innominate. At that time, they stated that they could not find a previous detailed report of successful repair of an injury of

an intrathoracic carotid artery. Similarly, there are only a few scattered reports of treating injuries to the intrathoracic left subclavian artery, such as those by Symbas and co-authors (1969) and Rojas and co-workers (1966).

ETIOLOGY

Because of the infrequent reports of treatment of injuries of major vessels at the base of the neck, accurate documentation of the wounding agent is difficult to establish. Many patients with these injuries caused by high speed accidents or by high velocity missiles exsanguinate prior to receiving any medical attention. As a result, the most frequent forms of injuries seen include stab wounds and injuries from low velocity missiles. Pate and Wilson (1964) found that 13 of 21 arterial injuries at the base of the neck were caused by knife wounds. This included the one innominate arterial injury in their series. In the report by Bricker and associates (1970) of 27 vascular injuries in the thoracic outlet, 11 were due to stab wounds and 16 to gunshot wounds, including one by shotgun. Among 29 patients with cervicomediastinal injury reported by Imamoglu and associates (1967) from the Detroit General Hospital, 18 were injured with a knife. A recent switch from the use of the knife to the use of the gun is evident in many of our urban crimes. This is emphasized by the report of Symbas and co-workers (1974) from the Grady Memorial Hospital in Atlanta: all three of their patients with innominate arterial trauma were the victims of gunshot wounds. The case outlined in Figure 12–6 represented a 33 year old man with a .22 caliber gunshot wound involving the intrathoracic left common carotid artery. Monson and associates (1969) reported two patients with gunshot wounds involving the innominate artery in their experience at Cook County Hospital in Chicago.

Of the three injuries of the innominate artery in the Vietnam Conflict, two were due to shell fragments, and one resulted from a gunshot wound (Rich et al., 1970A). No injuries of the intrathoracic carotid artery were reported from the Vietnam Vascular Registry among the 50 carotid arterial injuries in the interim report.

Although they are still unusual, there is an increasing number of case reports involving blunt trauma to the intrathoracic branches of the aortic arch. Bosher and Freed (1967) reported the case of a 20 year old woman who had a crushing injury to the chest when she was pinned beneath the steering wheel of her automobile which had overturned. There was rupture of both the innominate and left common carotid arteries. In their review of the literature they found seven other cases of traumatic rupture or avulsion of the innominate artery. Symbas and associates (1969) reported the case of a patient with traumatic rupture of the aortic arch between the left common carotid and left subclavian arteries with avulsion of the left subclavian artery. This occurred in a 27 year old woman involved in a major automobile accident. Piwnica and co-workers (1971) reported successful management of a 45 year old male, involved in an automobile accident, who had a traumatic rupture of the aortic arch with disinsertion of the innominate artery.

An unusual form of injury of the innominate artery is erosion from a tracheostomy tube, usually a combination of infection and improper placement of the tube. Silen and Spieker (1965) (Fig. 12–7) reviewed the problem of fatal hemorrhage from the innominate artery after tracheostomy and added four proved and two suspected cases from the San Francisco General Hospital. Although erosion of the innominate artery was originally thought to be caused by the tip of the long tracheostomy tube, the most frequent mechanism of vascular erosion in the San Francisco series was believed to be the constant pounding of the vessel against the inferior concave border of the rigid tracheostomy tube placed low in the trachea. In a patient with a similar injury reported by Imamoglu and associates (1967), a tracheostomy tube which had been in place for only five days had eroded through the trachea into the innominate artery. Although the artery was repaired, the patient died. Myers and associates (1972) added four cases of tracheal–innominate arterial fistula from

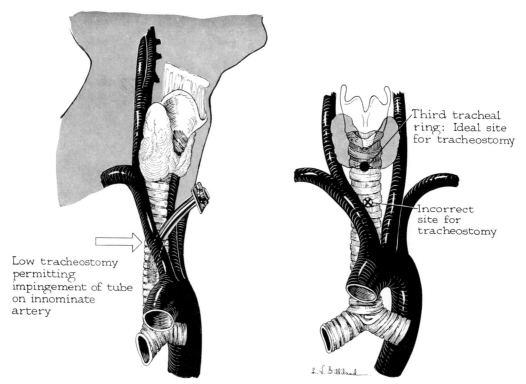

Figure 12–7. Fatal hemorrhage can occur after tracheostomy. This illustration shows how the low-lying tracheostomy tube can impinge on the innominate artery and cause vascular erosion and a tracheal-innominate fistula. (Silen, W., and Spieker, D., Ann. Surg., *162*:1005, 1965.)

TABLE 12–2. VESSEL OF ORIGIN OF MAJOR VESSEL HEMORRHAGES: COMPLICATION OF TRACHEOSTOMY

SITE	PRESENT SERIES (1950–1971)		SCHLAEPFER (TO 1924)	
	Number	*Per Cent*	*Number*	*Per Cent*
Innominate artery	53	78	83	72
Anomalous vessel*	12	18	–	–
Unknown	7	10	17	15
Carotid artery	5	7.5	5	4.3
Lowest thyroid artery	1	1.5	–	–
Thyroid artery	1	1.5	4	3.5
Common trunk	1	1.5	–	–
Innominate vein	1	1.5	4	3.5
Aortic aneurysm			2	1.7
Total:	81†		115	

*"Anomalous vessel" is an overlapping category.
†In the original source, the total is given as 68.
Modified from Brantigan, C. O., J. Trauma, *13*:235, 1973. Copyright 1973, The Williams & Wilkins Co., Baltimore.

their experience at the Marshfield Clinic in Wisconsin. Table 12–2 shows the innominate artery involvement according to Brantigan's review (1973). Stemmer and co-authors (1976) reported three deaths from arterial hemorrhage following tracheostomy.

CLINICAL PATHOLOGY

Almost all injuries in surviving patients have been either lacerations or smaller perforations. Transections are usually promptly fatal. All three injuries of the

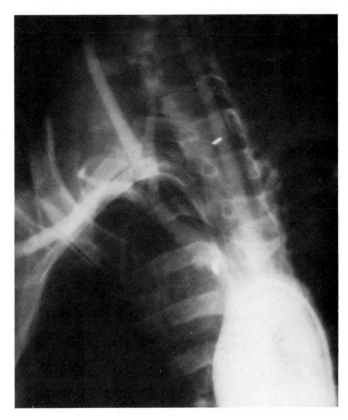

Figure 12–8. The offending fragment from a mortar wound which penetrated the neck in the suprasternal notch of this patient is seen opposite a small, false aneurysm of the mid-innominate artery, which is demonstrated by this retrograde femoral angiogram of the aortic arch and its major branches taken two weeks after injury. Although the arterial injury was initially suspected, the patient's stable condition prompted the surgeons to follow a conservative approach by delaying a definitive reconstruction. (W.R.G.H., 1969.)

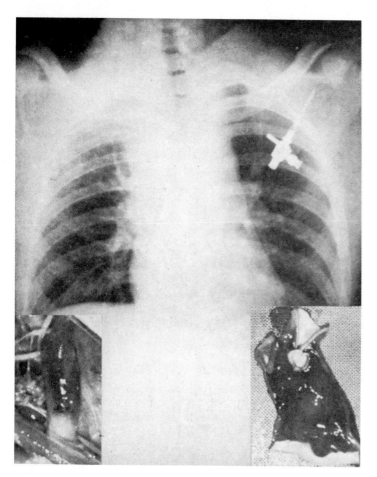

Figure 12–9. As in vascular injuries in other arteries, blunt trauma can fracture the intima of the innominate artery. Widening of the mediastinum with a central venous catheter in the left subclavian vein can be seen in this 19 year old male. The insert to the left shows the hematoma of the adventitia of the innominate artery. The insert to the right is the sectioned innominate artery with the contained thrombus and the intimal tear. (Owens, J. C., Surg. Clin. North Am., 43:371, 1963.)

innominate artery in Vietnam were small lacerations less than 1 cm in length (Rich et al., 1970A). If these injuries are not managed at the time of acute trauma, false aneurysms and arteriovenous fistulas may result (Fig. 12–8).

Blunt trauma can cause disruption of the intima and the media, with only the adventitia remaining intact (Bosher and Freed, 1967). Intimal tears and subintimal hematomas associated with intraluminal thrombosis can also occur (Fig. 12–9).

CLINICAL FEATURES

Hemorrhage and shock usually dominate the clinical findings, in association with the penetrating injury near the base of the neck with signs of arterial bleeding. In one series, 17 of 27 patients, about 63 per cent, were in shock at the time of hospitalization (Bricker et al., 1970). A hemothorax may also be present. A pulsating tracheostomy tube should alert one to the juxtaposition of the innominate artery, and bleeding around the tube may herald the catastrophe of innominate arterial erosion.

Localized neurologic findings may be present with injury of an intrathoracic carotid artery. Absence of pulse in either arm may indicate involvement of the corresponding subclavian artery. These findings are discussed in considerably more detail in Chapter 11 on carotid arterial injuries and in Chapter 13 on subclavian arterial injuries.

Concomitant injuries are usually present and complicate the diagnosis. These include a flail chest, tracheal compression, hemopneumothorax and respiratory insufficiency.

DIAGNOSTIC CONSIDERATIONS

In most patients prevention of impending death from hemorrhage dominates all consideration, and operative intervention must be performed quickly. In less urgent circumstances, a chest roentgenogram provides valuable information. This may demonstrate a hemothorax or pneumothorax. A mediastinal hematoma with widening of the mediastinum or displacement of the trachea is a frequent finding. This is demonstrated by a through-and-through .38 caliber gunshot wound of the proximal left common carotid artery, which caused a hemomediastinum with deviation of the trachea to the right (Fig. 12–10).

In elective circumstances, aortography can be employed to demonstrate the presence or absence of injuries of the aortic arch branches. This is of particular value in the case of a mediastinal hematoma without signs of active bleeding. Prompt per-formance of aortography can resolve the question of whether immediate operative intervention should be performed. Angiographically, there may be an aneurysmal widening, as shown in Figure 12–11, or there may be total occlusion, as shown in Figure 12–12.

SURGICAL TREATMENT

The numerous approaches, which have been well described, indicate the problems encountered by different surgeons with injuries of this type. The increasing use of median sternotomy for elective cardiac operations in recent years has indicated the simplicity and safety of this procedure. This is undoubtedly the incision of choice in the vast majority of patients in whom the site of injury is uncertain and control of hemorrhage is the immediate consideration. In urgent circumstances a sternotomy can be properly and quickly performed within five

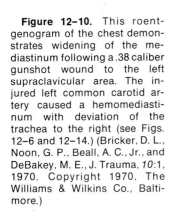

Figure 12–10. This roentgenogram of the chest demonstrates widening of the mediastinum following a .38 caliber gunshot wound to the left supraclavicular area. The injured left common carotid artery caused a hemomediastinum with deviation of the trachea to the right (see Figs. 12–6 and 12–14.) (Bricker, D. L., Noon, G. P., Beall, A. C., Jr., and DeBakey, M. E., J. Trauma, *10*:1, 1970. Copyright 1970, The Williams & Wilkins Co., Baltimore.)

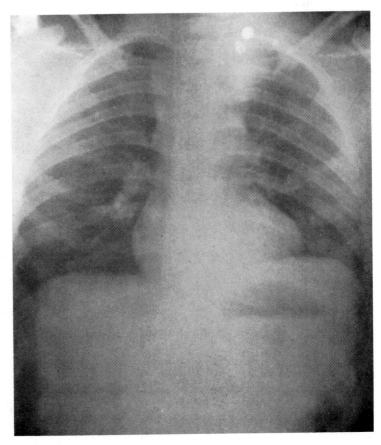

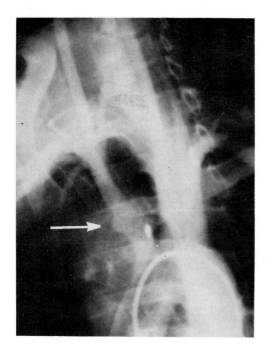

Figure 12–11. This angiogram of the innominate artery (brachiocephalic trunk) demonstrates aneurysmal widening (arrow). The wounding fragment is adjacent to the site of arterial trauma (Vietnam Vascular Registry #2626, NMR).

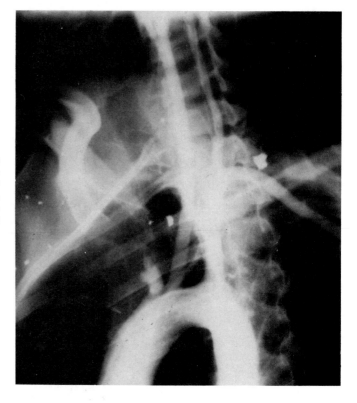

Figure 12–12. Total occlusion of the innominate artery is shown in the arteriogram above. This Vietnam casualty sustained multiple fragment wounds. Lateral suture repair of the innominate artery was unsuccessful in Vietnam (see Figs. 12–17 and 12–21). (W.R.G.H.)

minutes, giving access not only to the great vessels but also to the entire mediastinum and the heart. Cardiac tamponade can be relieved, and direct cardiac massage can be performed if necessary. The adequacy of transfusion of blood can quickly be estimated by noting the degree of cardiac filling. Immediate performance of a median sternotomy should probably supersede all other types of incision if circumstances are urgent. Exposure of the great vessels in the neck will require extension of the sternotomy in an appropriate direction (Fig. 12–13). In the neck, the incision can be curved to the right or the left, depending on the site of injury, transecting the sternocleidomastoid and strap muscles initially, then the underlying anterior scalene muscle, and preserving the phrenic nerve if possible. Division of these muscles widely exposes the carotid arteries and most of the subclavian arteries. Further exposures can be obtained by subperiosteal excision of the mid-portion of the clavicle, followed by transverse division of the clavicular periosteum to obtain full exposure of the distal subclavian and proximal axillary arteries (see Chap. 13).

When control of hemorrhage is not the dominant consideration, an alternative method to complete median sternotomy is

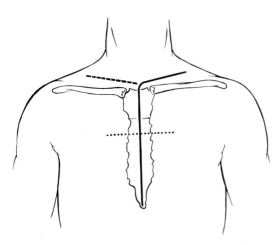

Figure 12–13. For rapid proximal control of the aortic arch branches, median sternotomy is the incision of choice. This will allow further extension into the neck in the appropriate direction if additional exposure of the great vessels is required. (See Chapter 13 for information concerning subclavian arterial trauma, especially Fig. 13–15.)

a sternotomy to the level of the second or third interspace, followed by transverse division of the sternum at this level. When this incision is combined with an appropriate cervical incision, excellent exposure of the vessels in the upper mediastinum is obtained. The transverse division of the sternum, carrying the incision a short distance into either pleural cavity if necessary, is preferable to the "trapdoor" incision, in which a long intercostal incision is made into one pleural cavity.

As previously indicated, a great number of modifications have been suggested, including resection of costal cartilages among other variants. Most of these are the result of lack of familiarity with the simplicity and safety of median sternotomy. When sternotomy is used as previously described, most of the modified incisions are simply of historical interest.

A left thoracotomy provides excellent exposure of the left subclavian artery, but it is virtually an elective approach because exposure of remaining portions of the mediastinum and aortic arch is limited. Hence, such an incision is employed only when the definitive diagnosis of isolated injury of the proximal left subclavian artery has been established, usually by arteriography.

Once hemorrhage has been controlled and the surrounding hematoma evacuated, most injuries are found to be lacerations which can be repaired by lateral suture. Bricker and associates (1970) reported one patient in whom an injury of the intrathoracic left common carotid artery was repaired by end-to-end anastomosis (Fig. 12–14). After proximal and distal arterial control have been secured, a partial occluding clamp on the arch of the aorta may be required; adequate debridement of the traumatized arterial wall, as well as of the surrounding devitalized tissue, is necessary. This debridement may be possible with minimal loss of the arterial wall in knife wounds and low velocity missile wounds. Although arteriorrhaphy is frequently possible without compromising the lumen, a patch graft can be utilized to eliminate the problem of stenosis in some injuries. In other cases, end-to-end anastomosis similar to that mentioned above may be possible. However, a replacement or bypass occa-

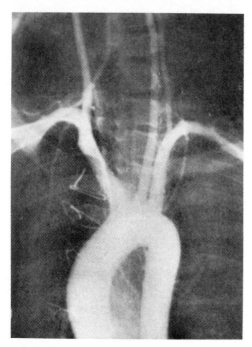

Figure 12–14. This follow-up angiogram demonstrates patency of the proximal left common carotid artery after resection and end-to-end anastomosis (see Figs. 12–6 and 12–10). (Bricker, D. L., Noon, G. P., Beall, A. C., Jr., and DeBakey, M. E., J. Trauma, *10*:1, 1970. Copyright 1970, The Williams & Wilkins Co., Baltimore.)

sionally may be required. Beall and co-workers (1963) have outlined a method for bypassing a through-and-through gunshot wound of the proximal left common carotid artery (Fig. 12–15). Extracorporeal bypass may be needed in unusual cases, such as that outlined by Piwnica and associates (1971) in the management of traumatic rupture of the aortic arch and rupture of the innominate artery in their patient.

Utley and co-workers (1972) emphasized the value of occlusion of the innominate artery by digital pressure against the sternum when hemorrhage occurs as a complication of the tracheostomy tube eroding the innominate artery (Fig. 12–16). These authors noted that after adequate resuscitative measures the innominate artery could be approached by median sternotomy with the divided ends over-sewn. They recommended that a bypass graft should not be used in the contaminated area. Myers and associates (1972) advocated axillo-axillary bypass in some

unusual situations as a method to avoid the contaminated area and still provide adequate arterial perfusion distal to the ligated innominate artery.

The question of the safety of ligation of the innominate artery or of the left common carotid artery cannot be answered with certainty. Langley (1943) presented the case of a 23 year old rear gunner wounded in World War II with a through-and-through wound of the bifurcation of the innominate artery. There was resultant hemiplegia from cerebral ischemia. Suture of the wounds was unsuccessful, and ligation of the innominate, subclavian and common carotid arteries was followed by death. Although it is not ideal, certainly the left subclavian artery could be electively ligated in its intrathoracic portion in the majority of patients because of excellent distal circulation. This, of course, is routinely done in the Blalock operation for subclavian-pulmonary anastomosis for tetralogy of Fallot. Obviously, repair of the innominate or left common carotid arteries is preferable, but with multiple associated injuries the hazard of simply ligating the vessel cannot be stated with certainty. Neurologic injuries are a common component of such vascular injuries, but these are often due to shock in association with initial injury and may have occurred before the patient can be treated. Innominate aneurysms have often been treated successfully by simple excision, because of the excellent collateral circulation between the carotid and subclavian arteries. Similarly, in most patients collateral circulation would probably be adequate to maintain function after ligation of the left carotid artery. A technique whose reliability is not yet entirely certain is the measurement of intra-arterial pressure in an intrathoracic artery while the artery is temporarily occluded at its origin. A mean arterial pressure, back pressure or "stump" pressure above 50 mm Hg, indicative of good collateral circulation, is almost surely compatible with normal function. Of eight injuries of the common carotid artery reported by Pate and Wilson (Table 12–3), ligation was done in one patient, who subsequently died. Repair was performed in five patients, one of whom died and two of whom had significant neurologic disability.

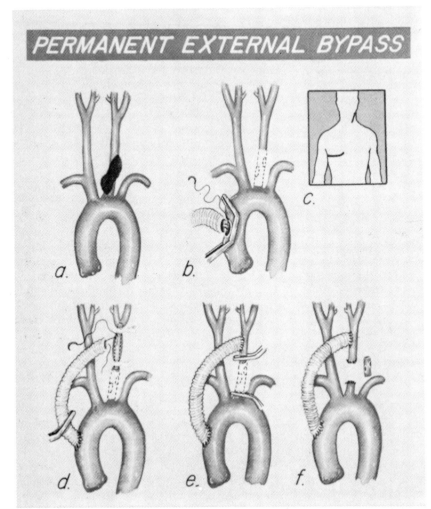

Figure 12–15. These drawings illustrate repair of a common carotid injury located in a poorly accessible area of the intrathoracic left common carotid artery. This method of bypassing the area of injury can be successful. (Beall, A. C., Jr., Shirkey, A. L., and DeBakey, M. E., J. Trauma, 3:276, 1963. Copyright 1963, The Williams & Wilkins Co., Baltimore.)

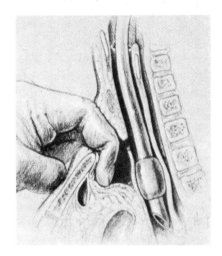

Figure 12–16. This drawing illustrates the technique of occlusion of the innominate artery by digital pressure against the sternum. The procedure requires blunt dissection of the artery away from the anterior wall of the trachea. (Utley, J. R., Morley, M., Singer, M. D., Roe, B. R., Fraser, D. G., and Dedo, H. H., J.A.M.A., 220:577, 1972.)

TABLE 12–3. COMMON CAROTID ARTERY INJURIES AT THE BASE OF THE NECK: RESULTS OF SURGERY*

	NUMBER	RESULTS
Ligation	1	Died, 1 day
None	2	A-V fistulas
Prostheses	1	Died, 7 days
Primary repair	4	2 Normal
		2 Residual neurologic damage

*Modified from Pate, J. W., and Wilson, H., Arch. Surg., *89*:1106, 1964. Copyright 1964, American Medical Association.

A serious technical problem with intra-thoracic injuries is that of laceration of the superior vena cava. This may be temporarily sealed by hematoma because of low pressure, but massive or fatal hemorrhage can result when the hematoma is removed during a surgical exploration of the mediastinum. This possibility should be carefully considered in planning surgical exploration. The best adjunct in such a procedure is the use of partial cardiopulmonary bypass with the disposable pump oxygenator. Such equipment is available in most hospitals and can be readily employed. If the patient is heparinized and an arterial cannula is inserted, blood can be aspirated and returned by the pump into the patient. Hence, hemorrhage can be more expeditiously controlled because massive transfusions of blood are unnecessary.

POSTOPERATIVE CARE

Careful observation in the immediate postoperative period is essential to insure the adequacy of arterial flow. Details are outlined in Chapters 11 and 13.

COMPLICATIONS

Avoidable errors may be responsible for immediate thrombosis of the repair. A major problem would include inadequate resection of the damaged artery during debridement or marked stenosis caused by a constricting lateral suture repair.

Inadequate hemostasis and hematoma formation in the immediate postoperative period can cause pressure on the repair site and subsequent loss of distal pulses.

Bleeding from the suture line is most likely associated with wound infection and occurs between four and 10 days after operation. Acute hemorrhage from a disrupted arterial suture line is a dramatic event that is a threat to the patient's life. Subsequent ligation of the artery is usually required. Collateral circulation, fortunately, is usually sufficient to prevent more serious complications of distal gangrene. Complications associated with carotid arterial ligation are discussed in detail in Chapter 11.

Stenosis of the repair site will usually have no associated symptoms. Even if occlusion of the artery occurs, the patient may remain asymptomatic. With proximal left subclavian or innominate arterial occlusion, a symptomatic subclavian steal syndrome can occur (Fig. 12–17).

RESULTS

The small number of surviving patients limits the conclusions currently available. No single surgeon has managed more than a few injuries to the major arteries at the base of the neck. However, repair rather than ligation has been practiced in most situations in the past 15 years. Pate and Wilson (1964) reported a successful primary repair of an innominate artery which was lacerated by a knife. Imamoglu and co-workers (1967) documented a successful innominate arterial repair following a gunshot wound of the thorax. Silen and Spieker (1965) suggested that direct replacement by vein graft or prosthesis of the friable infected innominate artery eroded by the tracheostomy tube usually could not be performed. They stated that a bypass graft in noncomminuted and noninfected tissues might be necessary if the patient could not tolerate ligation of the innominate artery. After failing in two surgical attempts to correct tracheal–innominate arterial fistulas, Myers and associates (1972) successfully treated one patient with an axillo-axillary bypass associated with innominate arterial ligation intrapericardially and in the supraclavicular fossa.

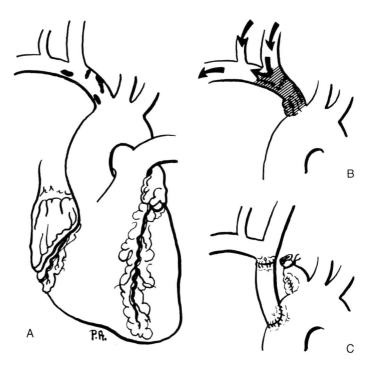

Figure 12–17. These drawings demonstrate occlusion of the innominate artery in a Vietnam casualty who had unsuccessful lateral repair of multiple small lacerations. The patient had dizziness from a subclavian steal syndrome (see Figs. 12–12 and 12–21). (W.R.G.H.)

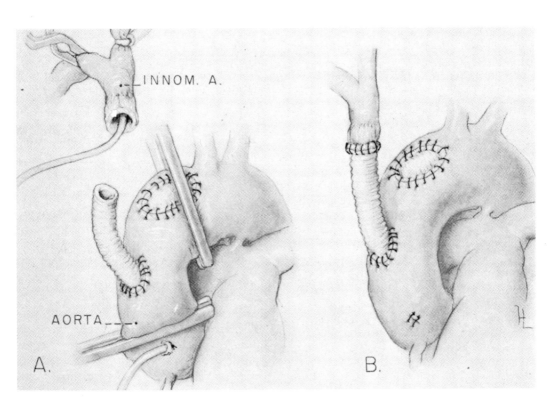

Figure 12–18. Although it is infrequently reported, the innominate artery can be bypassed successfully. These drawings show carotid and coronary perfusion under deep hypothermia and temporary circulatory arrest. A patch graft was used to repair the aortic defect, and a Dacron prosthesis was used as a bypass from the ascending aorta to the distal innominate artery. (Bosher, L. H., and Freed, T. A., J. Thorac. Cardiovasc. Surg., 54:732, 1967.)

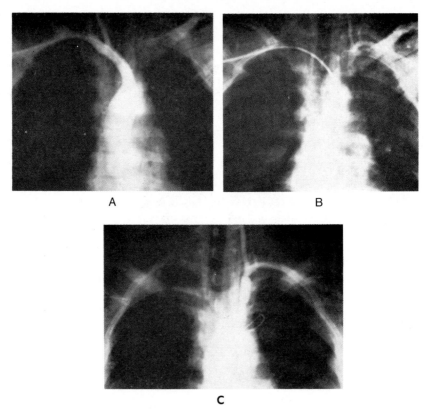

A

B

C

Figure 12–19. This series of angiograms demonstrates successful management of a traumatic subclavian steal syndrome. (A) Occlusion of proximal left subclavian artery. (B) Retrograde flow in the left vertebral artery. (C) Postoperative study eight days after repair with a Dacron prosthesis interposition, showing a patent repair and filling of the left vertebral artery in an antegrade fashion. (Rojas, R. H., Levitsky, S., and Stansel, H. C., J. Thorac. Cardiovasc. Surg., *51*:113, 1966.)

Symbas and associates (1974) revealed that two of their three patients with gunshot wounds of the innominate artery did not regain consciousness after repair and one died three and the other nine days postoperatively. In more elective situations, there are individual case reports of successful management of difficult problems. This is emphasized by the report of Bosher and Freed (1967), who bypassed the avulsed innominate artery and repaired the aortic arch (Fig. 12–18).

One of the three patients with innominate arterial lacerations treated in Vietnam subsequently suffered occlusion of the innominate artery and developed a subclavian steal syndrome (Rich et al., 1970A). The operations in the other two patients had good results.

Of the eight patients with injuries of the common carotid artery reported by Pate and Wilson (1964), only two had satisfactory results when treated by primary repair (Table 12–2). Of the four patients reported by Bricker and co-workers (1970), two patients died and two had successful repairs of the intrathoracic carotid artery.

The results of management of trauma to the intrathoracic left subclavian artery are usually included with those of injury to the cervical subclavian arteries. Again, individual reports such as that by Rojas and associates (1966) can be found (Fig. 12–19).

FOLLOW-UP

Because there have been so few documented injuries to the intrathoracic branches of the arch of the aorta, long term follow-up of most of these cases would be valuable. The long term results should also be known following major arterial ligations.

Bricker and associates (1970) demonstrated a patent end-to-end anastomosis of the intrathoracic left common carotid artery (Fig. 12–14). This angiogram was performed in subsequent follow-up to the

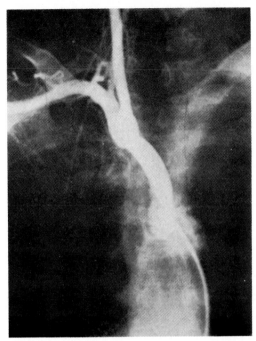

Figure 12–20. An 18-month follow-up was possible in the patient whose angiogram is shown above. The innominate artery had been ruptured as a result of nonpenetrating chest trauma incurred during an automobile accident. The angiogram reveals patency of the innominate arterial repair, which was performed using a Dacron prosthesis. (Carlsson, E., and Silander, T., Acta Chir. Scand., *125*:294, 1963.)

patient's short hospitalization of five days following arterial repair. Similar relatively short follow-ups have been reported in isolated civilian cases. Carlsson and Silander (1963) obtained an 18-month follow-up on one of their patients, a 35 year old male involved in an automobile accident (Fig. 12–20).

At least two patients listed in the Vietnam Vascular Registry have developed symptomatic subclavian steal syndromes. One of these patients was included in the interim report of 1000 acute major arterial injuries (Rich et al., 1970A). An additional operative procedure was performed utilizing a Dacron bypass from the ascending aorta to the innominate artery bifurcation in the patient mentioned. Another patient developed reversal of flow in the right common carotid artery, as well as in the right vertebral artery, following thrombosis of the innominate arterial repair that had been attempted by lateral suture of multiple lacerations (Fig. 12–21). In this case a second operative procedure performed at Walter Reed Army Medical Center through the original sternotomy was successful in restoring arterial flow in the proper direction, utilizing an

Figure 12–21. Reversal of flow occurred in the right common carotid artery as well as in the right vertebral artery following thrombosis of the innominate artery, which had been repaired in Vietnam by lateral suture of multiple lacerations. Successful reconstruction was carried out at Walter Reed Army Medical Center using a saphenous vein bypass graft from the ascending aorta to the innominate artery bifurcation (see Figs. 12–12 and 12–17). (W.R.G.H.)

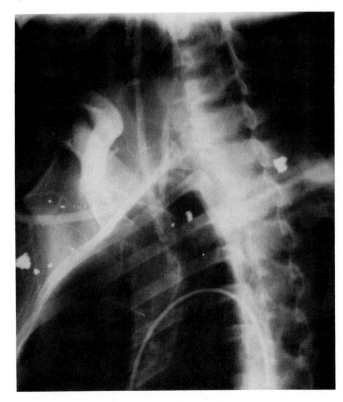

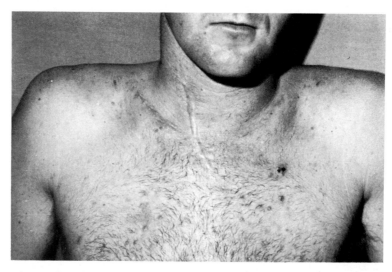

Figure 12–22. A returning Vietnam casualty had had a successful repair by end-to-end anastomosis of the right common carotid artery; however, the finding of a murmur at the base of the neck on physical examination upon arrival at Walter Reed Army Medical Center prompted an angiogram, which revealed an unsuspected right vertebral false aneurysm. (W.R.G.H.)

autogenous greater saphenous vein bypass graft from the ascending aorta to the innominate arterial bifurcation.

Although the initial management of injuries of major arteries at the base of the neck remains the most significant problem, occasionally later reconstruction of the arterial repair may be necessary. Also, additional vascular injuries may be diagnosed at a later time. After the right common carotid

artery was successfully repaired by lateral suture adjacent to its origin from the innominate artery, a returning Vietnam casualty was found to have a continuous murmur at the right base of the neck. An arteriogram performed at Walter Reed Army Medical Center revealed the presence of a second vascular lesion, a right vertebral arteriovenous fistula (Fig. 12–22).

CHAPTER 13

SUBCLAVIAN ARTERY INJURIES

There was an alarming rush of blood from the wound as soon as I withdrew my finger from it, and the cavity of the wound refilled with blood in an instant after it was sponged out with absorbent wool. I made repeated attempts to discover the bleeding point, but the blood flow was so profuse as to render this impossible. Fortunately, on passing a finger into the wound I was able to find an opening in the subclavian artery behind the scalenus anticus muscle, and this stopped the bleeding by making pressure upon this opening. The man's condition was now desperate, he being pale and unconscious from loss of blood; and any further attempt to tie the artery at the seat of injury was clearly inadmissible, attended as this must have been by still further loss of blood. An attempt to seize the artery with Spencer Wells' forceps guided by touch only failed, as other structures beside the artery became engaged within the forceps. There was not time for much deliberation and I decided to tie the common carotid and innominate arteries . . . explained to his friends the hopeless character of the case, feeling convinced that as I spoke he was either dead or dying. But he did not die. . . .

J. Lewtas, 1889

Injuries of the subclavian artery in patients surviving trauma in this area are uncommon because the arteries are well protected by the overlying sternum and clavicles. Massive trauma which disrupts the chest wall and the underlying branches of the aortic arch is often immediately fatal. Considerable progress has been made in managing subclavian artery trauma since the above description was written. However, associated complex problems continue to make management of these injuries stimulating challenges. Because of the infrequent occurrence of subclavian injuries, few surgeons have seen more than two or three such patients. Hughes (1958) found only three subclavian injuries among 304 major arterial injuries in the Korean Conflict (Table 13–1). Rich and associates (1970A) found only eight such patients in an interim report of 1000 acute major arterial injuries recorded in the Vietnam Vascular Registry.

The complex anatomical relationship surrounding the subclavian artery as it traverses the root of the neck, combined with the hazard of exsanguination immediately following injury, has led to the

TABLE 13–1. INCIDENCE OF SUBCLAVIAN ARTERY INJURIES

	AUTHOR	TOTAL ARTERIES	SUBCLAVIAN	PER CENT
War Series				
WW I	Makins (1919)	1191	45	3.8
WW II	DeBakey and Simeone (1946)	2471	21	0.9
Korean	Hughes (1958)	304	3	1.0
Vietnam	Rich et al. (1970A)	1000	8	0.8
Civilian Series				
Houston	Morris et al. (1960)	220	combined with axillary	
Atlanta	Ferguson et al. (1961)	200	8	4.0
Denver	Owens (1963)	70	1	1.4
Detroit	Smith et al. (1963)	61	0	0.0
Dallas	Patman et al. (1964)	271	11	4.0
Los Angeles	Treiman et al. (1966)	159	4	2.5
St. Louis	Dillard et al. (1968)	85	4	4.7
New Orleans	Drapanas et al. (1970)	226	16	7.1
Dallas	Perry et al. (1971)*	508	23	4.5
Memphis	Cheek et al. (1975)	155	16	10.3
Denver	Kelly and Eiseman (1975)	116	0	0.0
Jackson	Hardy et al. (1975)	360	12	3.3
New York	Bole et al. (1976)	126	2	1.6

*This is a sequential study including the earlier report from Dallas.

description of many different incisions to facilitate rapid and extensive exposure of the many vital structures merging from the thorax at the thoracic inlet. Numerous surgical exposures have been utilized since Halsted (1892) resected the medial two-thirds of the clavicle when he performed the first successful resection of a subclavian aneurysm at the Johns Hopkins Hospital. As a result of his experience with French casualties in World War I, Sencert (1917) advocated the sternoclavicular flap, which provided wide subclavian exposure (Fig. 13–1). Greenough (1929) described a total of 17 different approaches which have been used; additional details are discussed in Chapter 12. Shumacker (1947, 1948) emphasized the value of subperiosteal resection of the medial portion of the clavicle and combined this with extension of the incision into a portion of the sternum (Fig. 13–2). Median sternotomy, supraclavicular incision, anterior thoracotomy, and modifications and preferences in sur-

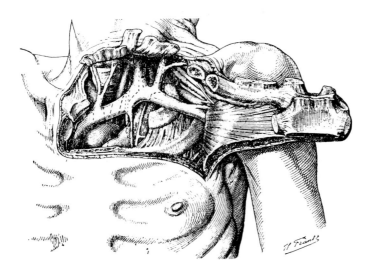

Figure 13–1. Sternoclavicular flap as described by Sencert in his 1917 monograph War Wounds of the Blood Vessels, based on his experience in treating French wounded. (Steenburg, R. W., and Ravitch, M. M., Ann. Surg., *157*:839, 1963.)

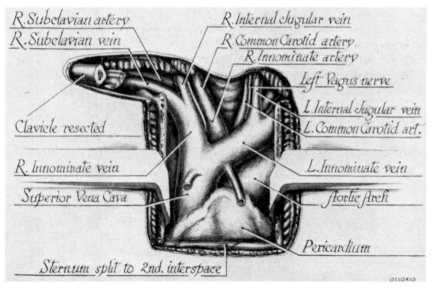

Figure 13–2. This is one of the numerous approaches to the subclavian arteries. Shown is resection of the inner third of the clavicle with the sternum split to the second inner space. (Shumacker, H. B., Jr.; Ann. Surg., *127*:464, 1948.)

gical approach are outlined in Table 13–2.

Additional discussion regarding injuries to the intrathoracic left subclavian artery is found in Chapter 12.

SURGICAL ANATOMY

The right subclavian artery originates from the innominate artery and courses through the base of the neck in a gentle curve behind the right sternoclavicular joint. The left subclavian artery arises directly from the aortic arch and courses in the mediastinum for one to two inches before entering the neck behind the left sternoclavicular joint (Fig. 13–3). The subclavian artery terminates at the lateral border of the first rib, where it becomes the axillary artery. In the mediastinum, the left subclavian artery is parallel to the esophagus and trachea for a short distance. At the point of entry of the subclavian arteries into the neck, the common carotid arteries are located anteriorly. On the left side, the innominate vein lies between the subclavian artery and the sternoclavicular

TABLE 13–2. SUBCLAVIAN ARTERY TRAUMA SURGICAL EXPOSURE*†

Year	Author	Method
1818	Mott	V-shaped cervical incision
1859	Cooper	removal of medial clavicle and part of manubrium
1892	Halsted	removal of medial clavicle
1917	Sencert	sternoclavicular flap
1929	Greenough	reviewed 17 approaches
1948	Shumacker	subperiosteal excision of inner clavicle with partial sternal split
1962	Cook and Haller	median sternotomy combined with partial resection of clavicle
1963	Steenburg and Ravitch	connecting intercostal incision and transverse cervical incision with median sternotomy
1965	Mansberger and Lindberg	first rib resection for distal exposure
1967	Imamoglu et al.	emphasized value of median sternotomy
1969	Amato et al.	extension of supraclavicular incision to 3rd intercostal space through two costal cartilages

*Adapted from Rich, N. M., Hobson, R. W., II, Jarstfer, B. S., and Geer, T. M., J. Trauma, *13*:485, 1973. Copyright 1973, The Williams & Wilkins Co., Baltimore.

†Emphasis is given to historical development and recent contributions.

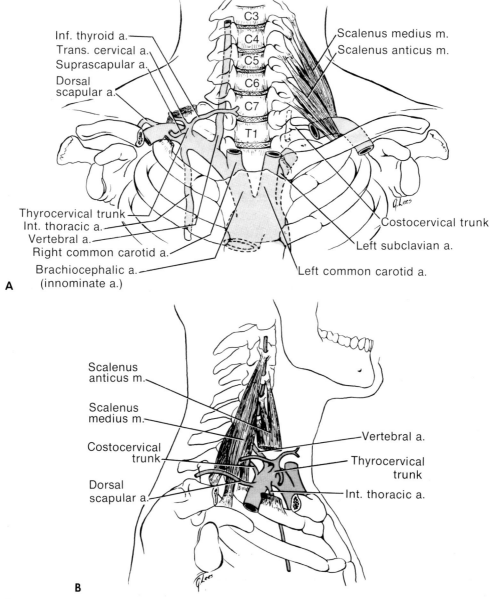

Figure 13–3. Relationships of the subclavian artery. (A) Anterior view with branches of the subclavian artery arising from the right side. (B) The right lateral view illustrating the branches of the subclavian artery with potential collateral anastomoses.

joint, while on the right side only the two infrahyoid muscles are between the joint and the artery.

Anomalous subclavian arteries are unusual. The most frequent is the right subclavian artery originating from the descending thoracic aorta and traveling posteriorly to the esophagus to the right side.

Classically, the relationship between the scalenus anticus muscle and the subclavian artery divides the subclavian artery into three parts. The scalenus anticus muscle lies anterior to the artery, separating it from the subclavian vein (Fig. 13–4). The first portion of the subclavian artery is that portion between its origin and the medial border of the scalenus anticus muscle. Contiguous structures include the common

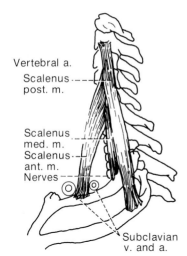

Figure 13–4. Separation of the subclavian artery and vein by the scalenus anticus muscle as viewed from the left side.

carotid artery, the vagus nerve, the internal jugular vein and the cervical dome of the pleura. Three branches are usually found, the most important of which is the vertebral artery arising from the posterior superior portion. The internal mammary artery arises inferiorly. The location of origin of the thyrocervical trunk, the most important collateral pathway to the arm, is variable.

The second portion of the subclavian artery lies behind the scalenus anticus muscle, adjacent to the pleura and brachial plexus. One important tributary, the costo-cervical trunk, arises from its posterior aspect. Occasionally, the transverse cervical artery also originates in this portion rather than from the thyrocervical trunk.

In the third portion, the subclavian artery extends from the lateral border of the scalenus anticus muscle to the outer border of the first rib. Usually no tributaries arise from this segment.

INCIDENCE

As mentioned earlier, injuries of the subclavian artery are uncommon, both in military and civilian trauma. Reports from different groups, representing most of the reported experiences with subclavian injuries in both military and civilian trauma, are tabulated in Table 13–1. In World War I, the classic report of Makins (1919) analyzed experiences with arterial injuries in the British Army. Forty-five subclavian artery injuries were found, representing 4 per cent of the total group. In World War II, DeBakey and Simeone (1946) reviewed 2471 injuries in American soldiers; of these, there were only 21 subclavian injuries, an incidence of less than 1 per cent. The report by Hughes (1958) of 304 injuries in the Korean Conflict included only three subclavian injuries, again less than 1 per cent of the total group. Similarly, in an analysis of 1000 major acute arterial injuries in the Vietnam Conflict (Rich et al., 1970A), only eight subclavian artery injuries were found, an incidence of less than 1 per cent. Rich and colleagues (1973) later reported a total of 65 subclavian artery injuries among approximately 7500 wounded American servicemen whose records are included in the Vietnam Vascular Registry. Although some records are incomplete, the incidence remains less than 1 per cent. Table 13–3 outlines the reports generated by the management of subclavian artery injuries in Vietnam. Nearly two-thirds of the injuries were treated in 1968 and 1969. At least 21 hospitals in Vietnam, three other hospitals in the Far East and four hospitals in the United States have been responsible for the management of these patients. Moreover, at least 48 different surgeons have experienced the challenge of managing these injuries; only two surgeons operated on more than one patient, and each of these surgeons performed two operations (Rich et al., 1973).

Civilian experience with subclavian arterial trauma parallels the relatively uncommon combat injury incidence. The true incidence is probably significantly larger because traumatized patients who exsanguinate soon after injury are seldom reported. In 1960 Morris and co-workers reported from a total of 220 arterial injuries over a period of ten years only 19 patients with injuries of the axillary and subclavian arteries (Table 13–1). Ferguson and co-authors (1961) found eight subclavian injuries in a total of 200 arterial injuries in Atlanta over a ten year period. Similar figures were described by Patman and associates (1964), who found 11 subclavian injuries in a series of 271 arterial

TABLE 13–3. INCIDENCE OF SUBCLAVIAN ARTERY TRAUMA
VIETNAM VASCULAR INJURIES*

Author	Year	Arteries	Subclavian	Per Cent
Fisher	1967	108	1	< 1
Chandler and Knapp	1967	118	1	< 1
Levitsky et al.	1968	56	1	~ 2
Williams et al.	1968	90	0	0
Rich and Hughes	1969	500	1	< 1
Hewitt et al.	1969	62	0	0
Gorman	1969	106	5	~ 5
Bizer	1969	63	0	0
Rich et al.	1970	1000	8	< 1
Rich et al.	1973	7500	65	< 1

*Adapted from Rich, N. M., Hobson, R. W., II, Jarstfer, B. S., and Geer, T. M., J. Trauma, 13:485, 1973. Copyright 1973, The Williams & Wilkins Co., Baltimore.

injuries in Dallas over a 12 year period. In a sequential study from the same city, Perry and co-authors (1971) found the number of subclavian injuries increased to 23 in a series of 508 significant arterial injuries. This emphasizes the increase in subclavian artery trauma: 12 cases in a six year period compared to only 11 cases in a previous 12 year period. Treiman and associates in 1966 at Los Angeles County General Hospital found only four subclavian injuries among 159 patients in a 15 year period between 1948 and 1963, a frequency of approximately 3 per cent. The highest incidences were 7.1 per cent reported by Drapanas and co-authors from New Orleans in 1970 and 10.3 per cent reported by Cheek and associates from Memphis in 1975. In addition to the reports found in Table 13–1, there are other valuable references from the past 10 years which describe the management of subclavian artery trauma.

Table 13–4 cites civilian series which are specifically concerned with injuries of the subclavian artery. Pate and Wilson (1964) described experiences with 12 subclavian injuries among a total of 21 arterial injuries in the base of the neck seen at the City of Memphis Hospital over a period of 12 years. At Cook County Hospital in Chicago, Amato and co-workers (1969) described 25 patients with acute subclavian vessel injury, which included 14 subclavian artery injuries. Bricker and associates (1970) described experiences with 14 subclavian artery injuries treated in Houston between 1955 and 1968. Hermreck and co-workers (1974) found five cases of subclavian artery injuries in Kansas City in their more recently reported series. Schaff and Brawley (1977) had 11 cases at Johns Hopkins Hospital.

TABLE 13–4. SUBCLAVIAN ARTERY TRAUMA CIVILIAN REPORTS*†

City	Year	Author	Injuries
Louisville	1962	Cook and Haller	3
Memphis	1964	Pate and Wilson	12
Rochester	1968	Matloff and Morton	3
Chicago	1969	Amato et al.	14
Houston	1970	Bricker et al.	14
Baltimore	1970	Brawley et al.	11

*Adapted from Rich, N. M., Hobson, R. W., II, Jarstfer, B. S., and Geer, T. M., J. Trauma, 13:485, 1973. Copyright 1973, The Williams & Wilkins Co., Baltimore.
†Particular emphasis is given to trauma involving the subclavian artery, in contrast to arterial trauma in general, as outlined in Table 13–1.

ETIOLOGY

Subclavian artery injuries which are not promptly fatal are usually penetrating wounds from a knife, low velocity gunshot wounds in civilian life, or low velocity fragments from various exploding devices in military injuries. Historically, injuries from knives, spears, arrows and bayonets have been described. A stab wound from a knife remains one of the common forms of injury (Figs. 13–5 and 13–6).

Pate and Wilson (1964) found that 6 of 12 injuries resulted from knife wounds, while

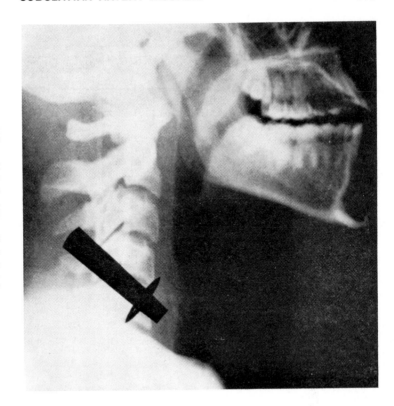

Figure 13-5. Subclavian artery trauma can result from a stab wound. Roentgenogram shows the offending agent causing a stab wound of the right side of the neck at the level of the sixth cervical vertebra. Venous bleeding was evident and shock was presumed due to external blood loss from trauma to the jugular vein. Initially, a massive left hemothorax caused by trauma to the right subclavian and vertebral arteries was overlooked. (Hunt, T. K., Blaisdell, F. W., and Okimoto, J., Arch. Surg., *98*:586, 1969. Copyright 1969, American Medical Association.)

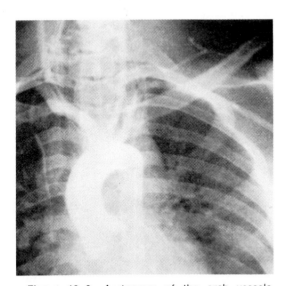

Figure 13-6. Aortogram of the arch vessels showing occlusion of the left subclavian artery about 3 cm from its aortic origin. The patient sustained a knife wound of the neck. There is also displacement of the trachea to the right and of the left vertebral artery to the left, indicating a hematoma in this area. (Brawley, R. K., Murray, G. F., Crisler, C., and Cameron, J. L., Surg. Gynecol. Obstet., *131*:1130, 1970.)

the others were from gunshot wounds (Table 13–5). Amato and associates (1969), in a review of 25 subclavian vessel injuries at Cook County Hospital, found 13 produced from stab wounds and 12 from gunshot wounds. In a report of 14 subclavian artery injuries in Houston by Bricker and associates (1970), only four resulted from stab wounds, while 10 were produced by gunshot wounds. In Kansas City there were two gunshot wounds, two knife wounds and one injury from an automobile accident (Hermreck et al., 1974).

In eight subclavian artery injuries reported in the Vietnam Conflict, six were produced by fragments from different exploding devices, and only two were caused by gunshot wounds (Rich et al., 1970A). When the series was expanded, the number of gunshot wounds, 27, was nearly equal to the number of fragment wounds, 32 (Table 13–6) (Rich et al., 1973).

Blunt trauma rarely injures a subclavian artery. Two such injuries, reported by

TABLE 13–5. SUBCLAVIAN ARTERY INJURIES, CITY OF MEMPHIS HOSPITALS 12 YEAR PERIOD PRIOR TO 1964*

Age	Weapon	Incision	Operation	Postoperative Course	Result	Comment
32	knife	thoracic	artery ligated	cardiac arrest, cerebral infarction	died	poor control of hemorrhage
34	knife	local	artery and vein ligated	—	died	poor control of hemorrhage
24	shotgun	local	artery ligated	viable, paralyzed arm	poor	plexus injury
37	shotgun	none	fistula resected, 6 wks.; artery repair	marked causalgia, paralyzed arm	poor	plexus injury, misdiagnosis of hemothorax
30	shotgun	none	amputation, 1 wk.; quad. ligation, 2 mos.	useless, swollen stump	poor	plexus injury, vein ligation
30	pistol	local	artery and vein ligated	viable, but paralyzed painful arm	poor	plexus vein ligated, hemothorax
37	pistol	none	quad. ligation, 2 wks.	swollen, ischemic hand	poor	artery and vein ligated
23	knife	local	artery and vein ligated	marked edema and causalgia at 1 yr.	poor	ischemic swollen arm
29	rifle	suture	none	developed A-V fistula 1 mo., normal arm	accept.	misdiagnosis
27	knife	thoraco-clavicular	repair artery and vein	uneventful; normal arm	good	artery and vein repaired
60	knife	thoraco-clavicular	repair artery and vein multiple	uneventful; normal arm	good	artery and vein repaired
22	knife	thoraco-clavicular	repair artery	normal arm	good	artery repaired

*Modified from Pate, J. W., and Wilson, H., Arch. Surg., *89*:1106, 1964.

Matloff and Morton in 1968, had resulted from automobile accidents. Three of 12 subclavian artery injuries reported by Hardy and associates (1975) were caused by blunt trauma. Rarely, blunt trauma may produce an avulsion injury of the subclavian artery with rupture of the intima and subsequent thrombosis. One such patient was reported by Yao and associates (1970) (Fig. 13–7).

Bony spicules from a fracture of the first rib or clavicle may lacerate the artery, but such an event is surprisingly infrequent, probably because of protection of the overlying scalenus anticus muscle. One such

TABLE 13–6. SOURCE OF WOUNDING AGENT 65 SUBCLAVIAN ARTERY INJURIES VIETNAM EXPERIENCE*

	Number	Per Cent
Fragment wounds	32	54
Gunshot wounds	27	46
Total	59†	100

*Adapted from Rich, N. M., Hobson, R. W., II, Jarstfer, B. S., and Geer, T. M., J. Trauma, *13*:485, 1973. Copyright 1973, The Williams & Wilkins Co., Baltimore.

†Incomplete records for six injuries.

patient was reported by Penn (1964) (Fig. 13–8); another, described by Fisher and Rienhoff (1966), had a 1 cm laceration of the left subclavian artery resulting from a fractured rib. The latter study also cited a previous report by Watson-Jones of a patient with subclavian artery thrombosis produced by repeated contusion from a fractured clavicle. Klingensmith and co-workers (1965) illustrated the manner in which the subclavian artery was punctured by clavicular fragments (Fig. 13–9). Guilfoil and Christiansen (1967) described subclavian artery thrombosis as a sequela of nonunited fracture of the clavicle (Fig. 13–10).

Subclavian artery laceration as a complication of left subclavian puncture for central venous pressure monitoring has also been reported (Goldman et al., 1971). Four days after the procedure, fatal hemorrhage ensued. At autopsy a laceration of the left subclavian artery was demonstrated (Fig. 13–11).

Lord and associates (1958), in reviewing their management of 11 cases of major vascular injury arising during the course of elective operative procedures, reported trauma to the subclavian artery in one patient during a radical neck dissection.

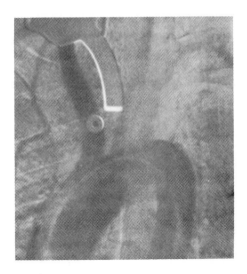

Figure 13–7. Aortic arteriogram outlining a normal arch, right brachiocephalic vessels and left common carotid artery. The proximal segment of the left subclavian artery is opacified, with faint visualization above that level and filling of the distal segment from retrograde flow in the vertebral artery. (Yao, J. K. Y., Suri, R., Patt, N. L., Fielden, R. H. N., and Baker, C. B., J. Trauma, *10*:176, 1970. Copyright 1970, The Williams & Wilkins Co., Baltimore.)

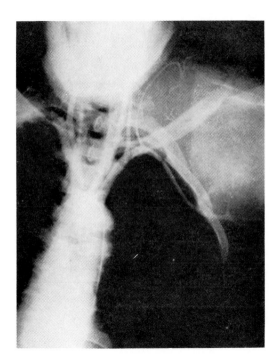

Figure 13–8. Arch aortogram shows marked downward displacement of the subclavian artery and medial displacement of the thyrocervical trunk. The subclavian artery trauma with a resulting false aneurysm was caused by a closed, nonunited fracture of the left clavicle from a heavy blow on the left shoulder. (Penn, I., J. Trauma, *4*:819, 1964. Copyright 1964, The Williams & Wilkins Co., Baltimore.)

Figure 13–9. Fracture of the clavicle has caused laceration, contusion and thrombosis with intimal rupture and complete transection of the subclavian artery. Diagram shows the relationship of the subclavian artery to the clavicle and first rib. The artery is held in a fixed position as it crosses the rib and may be punctured by the clavicular fragments. (Klingensmith, W., Oles, P., and Martinez, H., Am. J. Surg., *110*:849, 1965.)

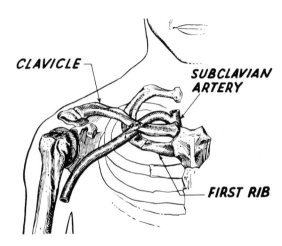

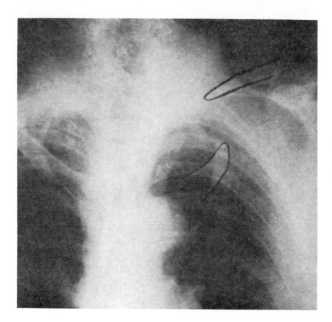

Figure 13–10. Roentgenogram demonstrates nonunion of a fractured left clavicle (outlined) which resulted in thrombosis of the subclavian artery. (Guilfoil, P. H., and Christiansen, T., J.A.M.A., *200*:178, 1967.)

Figure 13–11. At autopsy a small laceration of the left subclavian artery was demonstrated. This resulted as a complication of an attempt to place a central venous pressure monitoring catheter in the left subclavian vein. The patient had a short episode of hypovolemic shock that was treated with transfusions, and he died four days later when a second episode of severe bleeding ensued. (Goldman, L. I., Maier, W. P., Drezner, A. D., and Rosemond, G. P., J.A.M.A., *217*:78, 1971.)

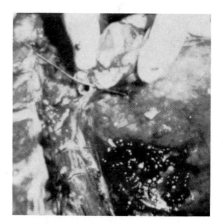

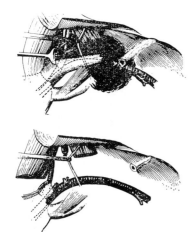

Figure 13–12. These drawings demonstrate complete transection of the left subclavian artery caused by a widely displaced fracture of the left clavicle and fracture of four ribs posteriorly. The clavicle was resected, the scalenus anticus muscle was transected, and an end-to-end anastomosis of the subclavian artery was carried out. (Gryska, P. F., New Engl. J. Med., *266*:381, 1962.)

CLINICAL PATHOLOGY

The most common injury to the subclavian artery is a laceration. Transection of the vessel is found less frequently, perhaps because such injuries may promptly result in exsanguination. Gryska (1962) recorded the case of a patient in whom a clavicular fracture was complicated by complete transection of the subclavian artery (Fig. 13–12). In eight subclavian injuries in the Vietnam Conflict, five were lacerations and three were transections (Rich et al., 1970A). The lacerations were caused by low velocity fragments. Of the three transections, two were associated with extensive soft tissue destruction from high velocity gunshot wounds. Table 13–7 documents the most recent figures from the Vietnam experience, showing that slightly more than two-thirds of the injuries resulted in laceration. In this study of 65 subclavian artery injuries in Vietnam, 91 per cent (59) were acute injuries, and 9 per cent were chronic injuries, with six false aneurysms and one arteriovenous fistula (Rich et al., 1973).

The subclavian artery is relatively thin compared to the more muscular arteries in the lower extremities. As a result, lacerations may readily extend during manipulation of the injured artery at the time of surgical repair. Untreated lacerations may subsequently produce a false aneurysm, or an arteriovenous fistula if the subclavian vein is also injured.

Contusion and thrombosis of the subclavian artery is unusual, probably because of the protection from the overlying bony structures. One such patient was reported

TABLE 13–7. TYPE OF CLINICAL PATHOLOGY SUBCLAVIAN ARTERY INJURIES*

	NUMBER	PER CENT
Laceration	44	68
False aneurysm	(5)	
A-V fistula	(1)	
Transection	10	15
Undetermined	7	11
Contusion	4	6
Total	65	100

*Adapted from Rich, N. M., Hobson, R. W., II, Jarstfer, B. S., and Geer, T. M., J. Trauma, *13*:485, 1973. Copyright 1973. The Williams & Wilkins Co., Baltimore.

by Guilfoil and Christiansen (1967). Avulsion injuries with stretching of the artery and disruption of the intima are also uncommon but may result from fractures of the clavicle and scapula. One such instance was reported by Yao and colleagues (1970).

More than 100 specimens of injured arteries from the Vietnam Conflict have been studied by microscopic examination. One of these, from a lacerated subclavian artery, is shown in Figure 13–13. After minimal débridement of the area of gross injury, successful end-to-end anastomosis was performed. Microscopic sections made at the proximal and distal margin of the debrided artery did not show any pathological changes. MacLean (1961) provided a clear illustration of intimal rupture in a subclavian artery when the external surface of the artery appeared fairly normal (Fig. 13–14).

Figure 13–13. Resected segment of a subclavian artery shows a tangential laceration that was caused by a fragment from an exploding device in Vietnam. The margins of resection revealed no microscopic evidence of trauma. An end-to-end anastomosis was possible. (Rich, N. M., Manion, W. C., and Hughes, C. W., J. Trauma, 9:279, 1969. Copyright 1969, The Williams & Wilkins Co., Baltimore.)

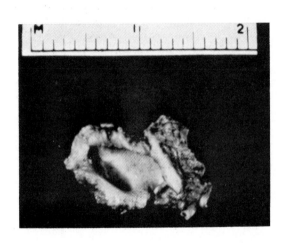

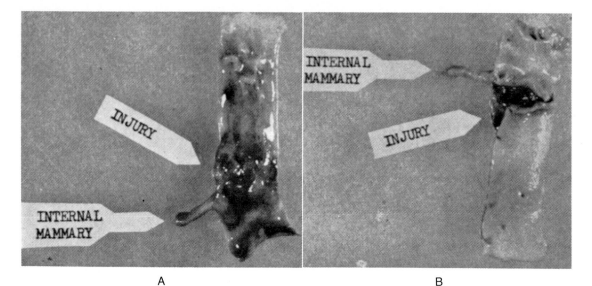

A   B

Figure 13–14. (A) The external appearance of the subclavian artery in a patient without a palpable radial pulse on the injured side did not suggest the serious nature of the arterial injury.

(B) Although spasm had been entertained as the initial diagnosis, it was proved by exploration and resection of the injured portion of the subclavian artery that intimal rupture was the cause of the arterial obstruction. (MacLean, L. D., J. Can. Med. Assoc., *88*:1091, 1963.)

CLINICAL FEATURES

Massive hemorrhage and shock often dominate the clinical picture. In the 14 patients reported by Bricker and associates (1970), shock was present in over 50 per cent of the group. From the records of 58 patients in Vietnam, it was possible to determine that 24 of them (41 per cent) reached the hospital in severe shock in Vietnam (Rich et al., 1973). For 40 patients in whom it was possible to determine accurately the blood replacement, an average of 6663 cc were used. The replacement ranged from no blood replacement in two patients to a total of 18,000 cc in one patient. The possibility of injury of a subclavian artery should be promptly considered in any patient with massive hemorrhage following a penetrating injury at the base of the neck.

The classic signs of an arterial injury may be present in the involved extremity—absent pulses, a cool, pale hand, paresthesias, and even motor paralysis. Collateral circulation is often so effective, however, that signs of ischemia may be minimal or absent. The Blalock operation for tetralogy of Fallot, in which the first portion of the subclavian artery is divided and anastomosed to the pulmonary artery, provides an excellent example of the effectiveness of collateral circulation because significant ischemia in the arm is almost unknown following operation.

There are commonly injuries of adjacent structures, including the brachial plexus, subclavian vein, clavicle, ribs, and contiguous pleural cavity and lung. Severe dyspnea may be present from an expanding hematoma in the base of the neck with displacement of the trachea and a hemothorax (Fig. 13–6). Associated injuries are particularly common in subclavian artery trauma caused

TABLE 13–8. CONCOMITANT INJURIES
58 SUBCLAVIAN ARTERY INJURIES IN VIETNAM*

	NUMBER	PER CENT
Veins	39	67
Nerves	39	67
Lung	25	43
Bone	21	36
Artery	13	22
Thoracic duct	3	5
Esophagus	2	3

*Modified from Rich, N. M., Hobson, R. W., II, Jarstfer, B. S., and Geer, T. M., J. Trauma, *13*:485, 1973. Copyright 1973, The Williams & Wilkins Co., Baltimore.

by high velocity missiles. Concomitant venous injuries are most frequently encountered. In two series, 50 per cent of the subclavian artery injuries were associated with venous injuries (Bricker et al., 1970; Rich et al., 1970A). Table 13–8 outlines the high percentage of concomitant injuries associated with 58 subclavian artery injuries in Vietnam: two-thirds had concomitant venous trauma and an equal number had associated nerve damage.

Patients initially examined weeks or months after an untreated injury of the subclavian artery may show the physical findings of a false aneurysm or an arteriovenous fistula. The latter may be easily recognized from the characteristic continuous murmur. False aneurysms initially appear as firm, ill-defined masses which gradually enlarge and eventually become pulsatile.

DIAGNOSIS

The diagnosis may be obvious with a penetrating wound at the base of the neck combined with absent pulses and a cool, pale extremity. On the other hand, with good collateral circulation, decreased pulse volume and blood pressure in the involved extremity may be the only clinical findings. When shock from extensive hemorrhage dominates the clinical picture, the diagnosis may be impossible until the blood pressure has been returned to normal levels by appropriate transfusion of blood. Reduced blood pressure in one arm compared to the other arm may be indicative of subclavian artery occlusion, and comparison of wrist pressures may be helpful.

Chest roentgenograms frequently show a hematoma at the base of the neck, often with hemothorax or widening of the mediastinum. In obscure cases, angiography may be needed. Rarely, the diagnosis is first made during emergency thoracotomy for massive hemothorax, especially on the left, at which time a laceration of the subclavian artery is discovered.

SURGICAL TREATMENT

With massive hemorrhage, immediate operation is often required to prevent exsanguination. An incision which promptly and widely exposes an actively bleeding subclavian artery, protected by the clavicle, sternum, costal cartilages and ribs, is not easy and has challenged the ingenuity of many surgeons. In Chapter 12 and in Figure 13–2, historical summaries of different types of incisions which have been employed are presented. Greenough reported 17 of these incisions in 1929.

For the intrathoracic left subclavian artery, a left thoracotomy is the incision of choice, usually employing an anterolateral approach in the third intercostal space (Fig. 13–15). Injuries of the right subclavian artery and of the distal left subclavian artery may initially be approached through supraclavicular incisions, with or without subperiosteal excision of the medial portion of the clavicle. With the supraclavicular approach, division of the sternocleidomastoideus and scalenus anticus muscles provides good exposure of the distal subclavian artery, and the origin of the right subclavian from the innominate artery can usually be seen. With distortion and displacement of the adjacent structures from a massive hematoma, resection of the medial part of the clavicle facilitates distal exposure. In urgent circumstances with massive hemorrhage, a median sternotomy down to the third interspace, combined with transection of the sternum at this level, gives excellent exposure of the mediastinum with the innominate artery and adjacent structures (see Chap. 12, Surgical Treatment). If necessary, the transverse sternotomy incision can be extended into either pleural cavity, but this is usually unnecessary. In the majority of patients, the cervical incision combined with upper median sternotomy and resection of the clavicle as needed will provide adequate exposure (Fig. 13–16). An alternative approach for the surgeons' armamentarium is shown in Figure 13–17, where resection of the first rib is carried out to provide distal exposure of the subclavian vessels.

Once proximal and distal control of the injured artery has been obtained, débridement of the lacerated edges can be done. This must be done gently, because the subclavian artery is thin and tears easily. Ligation of adjacent tributaries may be necessary for mobilization of the injured artery. Preservation of the vertebral artery

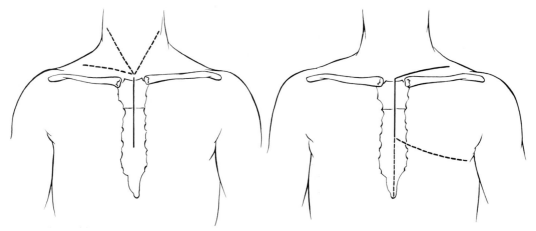

Figure 13–15.   Various incisions that can be used to approach the subclavian arteries, either electively or in an emergency situation. A combination of median sternotomy with extension into the supraclavicular area can provide wide exposure of the right subclavian and distal left subclavian arteries. A left anterolateral thoracotomy in the third intercostal space is ideal for exposure of the intrathoracic left subclavian artery (see Chap. 12).

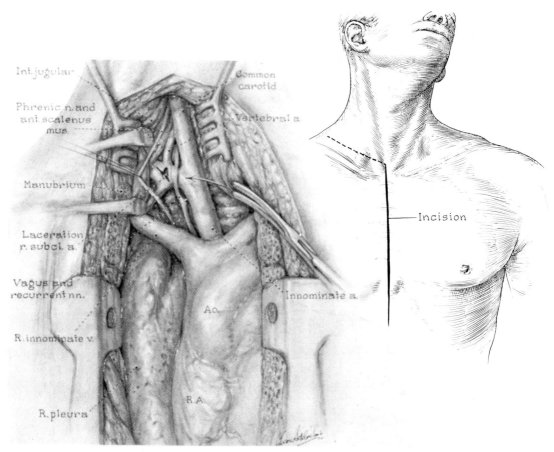

Figure 13–16.   Exposure of an injured right subclavian artery by means of a median sternotomy with extension of the incision into the soft tissues of the right side of the neck. There is excellent exposure of the ascending aorta; the proximal part of the aortic arch; the innominate, subclavian and common carotid arteries; the innominate veins; and the superior vena cava (Brawley, R. K., Murray, G. F., Crisler, C., and Cameron, J. L., Surg. Gynecol. Obstet., *131*:1130, 1970.)

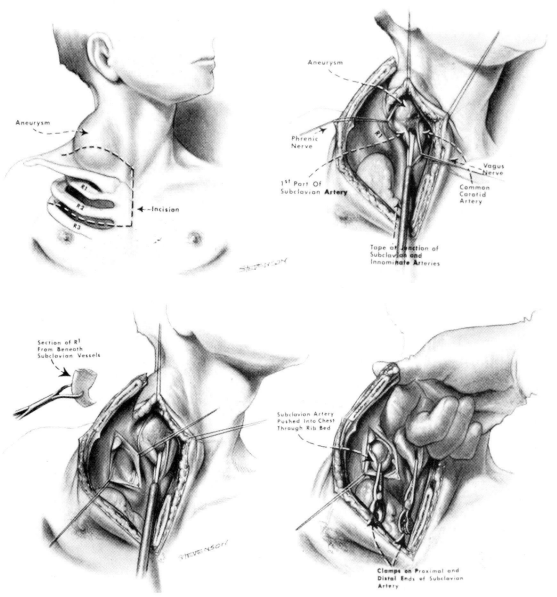

Figure 13–17. Drawings made at the time of an operation for resection of a false aneurysm resulting from blunt trauma to the sternum. This is an alternative method which can be used to manage subclavian artery injuries; first rib resection is used to obtain distal exposure of the subclavian vessels. (Mansberger, A. R., Jr., and Linberg, E. J., Surg. Gynecol. Obstet., *120*:579, 1965.)

is desirable, but in the majority of patients it can be ligated safely.

Following débridement, most injuries can be repaired with an end-to-end anastomosis. Only a few can be repaired by lateral suture, and a vein patch graft may be helpful in preventing stenosis at the repair site. If direct anastomosis is not possible, a vein graft, preferably from the greater saphenous vein, is the next best choice. Synthetic vascular prostheses, such as a Dacron prosthesis, should be avoided if possible because of the hazards of infection in contaminated wounds. Before the vascular repair is completed, a Fogarty catheter should be inserted into the distal artery to remove any thrombi which may have developed from stasis. This is an important

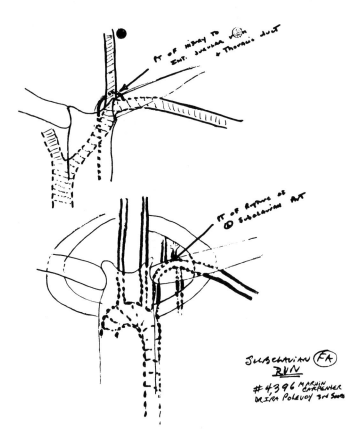

Figure 13–18. Drawings made in Vietnam by Dr. Ira Polevoy of Denver while on active duty at the 3rd Surgical Hospital. Not only is this brief and concise outline of great value for surgeons in their understanding of the extent of injury, but it also provides a notation of associated injuries to the internal jugular vein and the thoracic duct. Documentation of these concomitant injuries, as well as of the associated fractures and nerve injuries, is extremely important. (Rich, N. M., Hobson, R. W., II, Jarstfer, B. S., and Geer, T. M., J. Trauma, *13*:485, 1973. Copyright 1973, The Williams & Wilkins Co., Baltimore.)

adjunct because the development of distal thrombi is highly variable, depending on the collateral circulation, the blood pressure and the time lag between injury and arterial repair.

Following completion of the arterial repair, adjacent soft tissues should be approximated over the area. The skin and subcutaneous tissues, however, may be left open for delayed primary closure in three to six days if significant contamination is present.

Following reconstruction, a radial or ulnar pulse, or both, should soon be palpable. Otherwise, an operative arteriogram is indicated to be certain that the repair is satisfactory. Routine use of operative angiography should be considered to insure the best results.

Ligation of the injured artery should rarely be performed. There is little risk of gangrene if collateral circulation is intact, but normal collateral circulation may have been destroyed to a variable extent. In World War II, ligation of the subclavian artery resulted in gangrene in 28.6 per cent of the cases.

Antibiotics should be used routinely as soon as possible after injury. Postoperative fasciotomy is rarely necessary in muscles of the upper extremity but can be considered if the arm or forearm muscles become turgid and hard. Concomitant fractures are usually managed by external methods because internal fixation is hazardous in contaminated wounds. Primary nerve repairs are usually not performed, but severed nerves are noted and identified for delayed reconstruction (Fig. 13–18). Small lacerations of the subclavian vein may be sutured, but more extensive injuries usually require ligation.

POSTOPERATIVE CARE

The two immediate questions following operation are whether the extremity is viable and whether arterial circulation has been sufficiently restored. A palpable radial

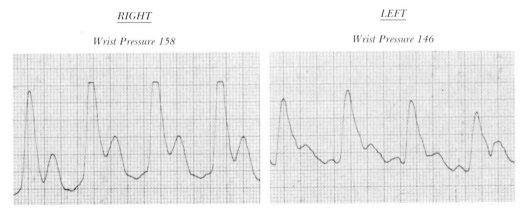

Figure 13–19. Routine plethysmographic and Doppler tracings have been utilized in the follow-up of patients at Walter Reed Army Medical Center. The above thumb tracings reveal an adequate curve and pressure on the left side distal to the subclavian artery repair, as compared to the right side. Although it is smaller, there is also a dicrotic notch on the left. (Rich, N. M., Hobson, R. W., II, Jarstfer, B. S., and Geer, T. M., J. Trauma, *13*:485, 1973. Copyright 1973, The Williams & Wilkins Co., Baltimore.)

pulse is a welcome and reliable sign of adequate repair, while its continued absence is a cause for serious concern. An absent pulse may be due to thrombosis of the arterial repair from stenosis or tension, or to thrombi in the distal arterial tree. If the extremity is viable, as indicated by normal muscle turgor and normal motor and sensory function, further procedures may be delayed in seriously ill patients. As long as sensation and motor function are intact, there is little risk of gangrene. With a numb, paralyzed extremity, however, the presence of adequate arterial flow must be determined quickly. When concomitant injuries of the brachial plexus eliminate the valuable clinical guide of neurological function, other methods of evaluation must be used. An ultrasonic sounding device (Doppler) has given encouraging early results in substantiating the presence of adequate arterial blood supply in the absence of peripheral pulses, but further data are needed (Fig. 13–19). Arteriography should usually be performed promptly if pulses are absent and viability of the extremity is uncertain.

When viability of the extremity is questionable despite adequate peripheral pulses, the muscles should be observed for edema and rigidity, and this may require fasciotomy. However, this is not required nearly as often, as with comparable injuries in the lower extremities. Sympathetic blocks, cervical sympathectomy and anticoagulants are of little value.

RESULTS

Representative series describing the management of subclavian injuries are outlined in Table 13–9. In recent years, with the exception of the report of Pate and Wilson in 1964 (Table 13–5), ligation has rarely been necessary. Most repairs have been by lateral suture or direct anastomosis. Three vein grafts were employed in the early

TABLE 13–9. MANAGEMENT OF SUBCLAVIAN ARTERY INJURIES

AUTHOR	YEAR	TOTAL INJURIES	LATERAL SUTURE	END-TO-END ANASTOMOSIS	VEIN GRAFT	DACRON PROSTHESIS	LIGATION	NONE
Pate and Wilson	1964	12	"3 primary arterial repairs"			0	5	4
Matloff and Morton	1968	3	1	0	0	0	0	2
Amato et al.	1969	14	5	7	1*	0	1	0
Bricker et al.	1970	14	3	6	1	0	1	3
Rich et al.	1970A	8	2	2	3	0	1	0
Total		51	11	15	5	0	8	9

*Vein patch graft.

TABLE 13-10. SUBCLAVIAN ARTERY TRAUMA SURGICAL APPROACH*†

Resection clavicle	33
Thoracotomy	21
Median sternotomy	13
Supraclavicular	3
Split clavicle	2
"Trap door"	2

*Adapted from Rich, N. M., Hobson, R. W., II, Jarstfer, B. S., and Geer, T. M., J. Trauma, *13*:485, 1973. Copyright 1973, The Williams & Wilkins Co., Baltimore.

†Combinations and modifications of these incisions were made in some patients.

TABLE 13-11. MANAGEMENT OF SUBCLAVIAN ARTERY INJURIES*

METHOD	NUMBER	PER CENT
End-to-end anastomosis	17	26
Lateral suture	13	20
Autogenous vein graft	11	17
Ligation	10	15
Undetermined	7	11
Exploration	5	8
Prosthesis	2	3
Total	65	100

*Modified from Rich, N. M., Hobson, R. W., II, Jarstfer, B. S., and Geer, T. M., J. Trauma, *13*:485, 1973. Copyright 1973, The Williams & Wilkins Co., Baltimore.

Vietnam experience (Rich et al., 1970A). It is of some interest that no prostheses were used in the 51 subclavian artery injuries tabulated in these different reports.

Some of the most recent details from the Vietnam experience provide valuable information which has not previously been available. In 40 patients it was possible to determine the lag time from injury until the patient reached the operating room (Rich et al., 1973). The range was from 15 minutes to 10 hours, with an average lag time of 3 hours and 15 minutes. Helicopter evacuation made it possible for nearly two-thirds of these patients to reach the operating room of a definite surgical center in two hours or less. Hostile fire or inclement weather prolonged the evacuation for only a small number of casualties.

A list of the incisions that were utilized in approaching the subclavian artery injuries is outlined in Table 13-10. In some of the patients a combination of these procedures was used. It is important to emphasize that an isolated supraclavicular incision was employed in only three patients. Also, neither splitting the clavicle nor use of the "trap door" incision was very popular.

End-to-end anastomosis was used in managing one-fourth of the subclavian artery injuries (Table 13-11). The 17 end-to-end anastomoses represented approximately 40 per cent of the known subclavian artery injuries. Surprisingly, lateral suture was possible in 13 of the injuries. Autogenous vein grafts, usually from the greater saphenous vein, were used in 11 repairs. Dacron prostheses were used to bridge the gap of the missing segment of subclavian artery in two patients.

Of the five subclavian artery explorations, contusion was believed to be insignificant in three and no further therapy was instituted. The remaining two patients expired on the operating table before repair could be completed. The subclavian artery was ligated in 10 patients, representing an incidence of 15 per cent of the total injuries, and no extremities were lost following these ligations. In the remaining seven patients, the exact nature of the management of the subclavian artery trauma could not be determined from the available information.

In a number of reports complications were unusual following arterial repair (Table 13-12). Bricker and associates (1970)

TABLE 13-12. RESULTS OF SUBCLAVIAN ARTERY REPAIR

AUTHOR	YEAR	INJURIES	REPAIRS	COMPLICATIONS	AMPUTATIONS	DEATHS
Amato et al.	1969	14	13	0	0	0
Bricker et al.	1970	14	11	0	0	3
Rich et al.	1970A	8	7	1	0	0
Drapanas et al.	1970	16	0	0	1	4
Perry et al.	1971	23	0	0	0	1

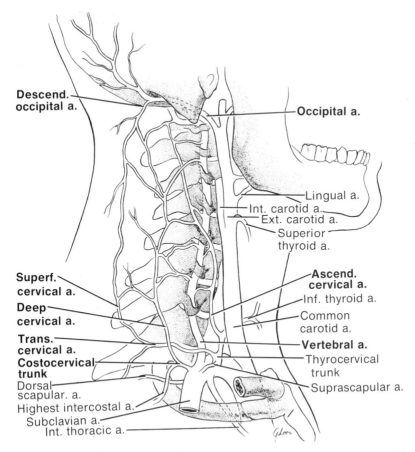

Descend. occipital a.

Occipital a.

Lingual a.
Int. carotid a.
Ext. carotid a.
Superior thyroid a.

Superf. cervical a.

Ascend. cervical a.
Inf. thyroid a.

Deep cervical a.

Common carotid a.

Trans. cervical a.

Vertebral a.
Thyrocervical trunk

Costocervical trunk
Dorsal scapular. a.
Highest intercostal a.
Subclavian a.
Int. thoracic a.

Suprascapular a.

Figure 13–20. There is usually excellent development of collateral circulation following either ligation of the subclavian artery or thrombosis of an attempted repair. This results in a relatively low amputation rate compared to similar situations in some other major extremity arteries (see also Figs. 13–3 and 13–21).

Figure 13–21. Collateral circulation in the shoulder region. Important collateral vessels are the thoracoacromial, lateral thoracic, subscapular, and anterior and posterior humeral circumflex arteries. (Levin, P. M., Rich, N. M., and Hutton, J. E., Jr., *Arch. Surg.*, *102*:392, 1971. Copyright 1971, American Medical Association.)

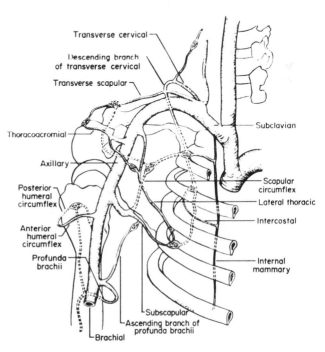

Transverse cervical
Descending branch of transverse cervical
Transverse scapular
Subclavian
Thoracoacromial
Axillary
Scapular circumflex
Lateral thoracic
Posterior humeral circumflex
Intercostal
Anterior humeral circumflex
Internal mammary
Profunda brachii
Subscapular
Ascending branch of profunda brachii
Brachial

recorded no complications following repair of 11 subclavian artery injuries. In Vietnam, Rich and colleagues (1970A) found thrombosis in only one of seven subclavian artery repairs associated with interposed cephalic vein graft. In addition to early thrombosis, another major complication to consider in the postoperative course is infection of the wound with associated risk of secondary hemorrhage. Fortunately, with the combination of antibiotics, wound débridement and delayed primary suture, infection is unusual. If infection occurs with secondary hemorrhage, ligation of the subclavian artery should be done promptly. Gangrene in these circumstances is unusual because of collateral circulation (Figs. 13–20 and 13–21). Stenosis and occlusion of the artery may occur from progressive fibrosis and constriction, or from intimal hypoplasia at the suture line. In such patients, the extremity often remains asymptomatic.

Among 46 Vietnam casualties whose records were complete with adequate follow-up established, the complication rate (nine known complications) was higher than that previously recorded (Table 13–13). Thrombosis was the most frequent compli-

TABLE 13–13. ACUTE SUBCLAVIAN ARTERY TRAUMA SURVIVOR COMPLICATIONS 46 PATIENTS*†

COMPLICATION	NUMBER
Thrombosis	4
Technical	2
Infection	1
False aneurysm	1
Stenosis	1
Total	9 (20%)†

*Modified from Rich, N. M., Hobson, R. W., II, Jarstfer, B. S., and Geer, T. M., J. Trauma, *13*:485, 1973. Copyright 1973, The Williams & Wilkins Co., Baltimore.

†Additional operations were required in three patients.

cation, representing almost 50 per cent of the total. Three of the patients who had thrombosis of the attempted subclavian artery repair have remained essentially asymptomatic. Two patients' operations were listed as technical complications because the surgeon in Vietnam had attempted a repair which was not possible and ultimately had to ligate the subclavian artery. Only one patient developed wound infection with asso-

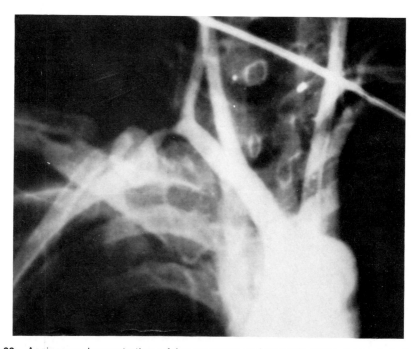

Figure 13–22. Angiogram demonstrating a false aneurysm and stenosis of the right subclavian artery just distal to the origin of the vertebral artery. Previous repair had been done in Vietnam by lateral suture of two lacerations of the right subclavian artery. (Rich, N. M., Hobson, R. W., II, Jarstfer, B. S., and Geer, T. M., J. Trauma, *13*:485, 1973. Copyright 1973, The Williams & Wilkins Co., Baltimore.)

ciated hemorrhage from a disrupted suture line; despite additional attempts at repair, ligation was ultimately necessary. The patient with an established stenosis at the repair site remains asymptomatic. Another patient developed a false aneurysm at the suture line (Fig. 13–22). Only three patients required additional operations: one for infected repair, one for false aneurysm and one for thrombosis.

Only one amputation was necessary in the cases described in recent reports (Table 13–12). This amputation was recorded in the series by Drapanas and co-workers (1970) and represented 6.2 per cent of the 16 subclavian artery injuries. In World War II the amputation rate was approximately 29 per cent in the group of 21 patients treated by ligation (DeBakey and Simeone, 1946). In the Korean Conflict, one amputation was reported following ligation and the remaining two injuries were successfully repaired (Hughes, 1958). Pate and Wilson (1964) also documented one amputation following subclavian artery ligation (Table 13–5). Again, it is important to emphasize that there have been no amputations associated either with the 10 subclavian artery ligations or with the repair failures.

The mortality rate associated with subclavian artery injuries has been variable. Bricker and co-workers (1970) documented three deaths among 14 patients with subclavian artery injuries. Perry and co-authors (1971) also reported the mortality of a single patient who had concomitant trauma to the innominate vein. The highest mortality rate from subclavian artery injury was reported by Drapanas and associates (1970): they noted the death of four patients in their series of 16, representing a 25 per cent mortality. Of those patients who were included in the early Vietnam experience, none died from this injury (Rich et al., 1970A). However, in the more complete evaluation of the Vietnam experience, the mortality rate was approximately 10 per cent for the 59 patients with acute arterial injuries (Rich et al., 1973). All six of the patients who died arrived at the hospital in severe shock with exsanguinating hemorrhage, and cardiac arrest usually ensued fairly rapidly. It was possible, however, to surgically manage the subclavian artery injuries in four of these patients (Table 13–14).

TABLE 13–14. ACUTE SUBCLAVIAN ARTERY TRAUMA MORTALITY RATE VIETNAM EXPERIENCE*

PATIENTS	DEATHS	PER CENT
59	6	10

*Modified from Rich, N. M., Hobson, R. W., II. Jarstfer, B. S., and Geer, T. M., J. Trauma, *13*:485, 1973. Copyright 1973, The Williams & Wilkins Co., Baltimore.

FOLLOW-UP

There is a paucity of long term follow-up evaluation of patients with subclavian injuries. None of the reported eight patients from the Vietnam series (Rich et al., 1970A) had additional problems in a subsequent two year period of observation. However, in several other patients seen at

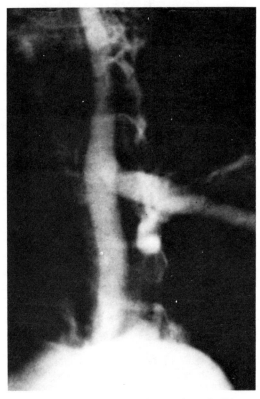

Figure 13–23. To control hemorrhage in this patient in Vietnam, constricting lateral sutures were placed in the left subclavian artery. The arteriogram demonstrates occlusion of the subclavian artery near its origin. Reconstruction was performed with a greater saphenous vein bypass between the left common carotid artery and the left axillary artery. (W.R.G.H.)

A

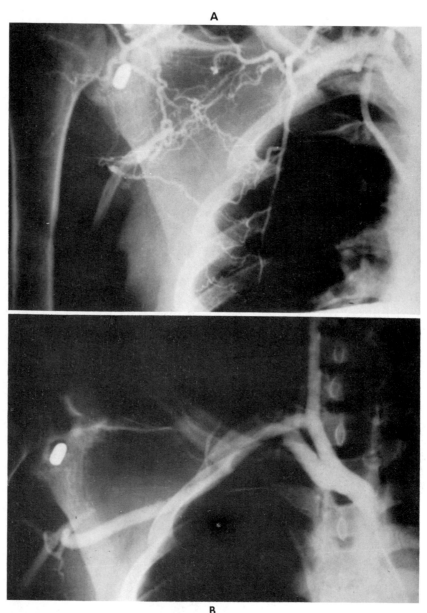

B

Figure 13–24. (A) Subclavian arterial and venous ligation had been performed in the initial treatment of an axillary arteriovenous fistula caused by a low velocity pistol bullet. (B) Postoperative arteriogram demonstrating a patent autogenous greater saphenous vein bypass graft between the right carotid and axillary arteries. Four such operations have been performed at Walter Reed Army Medical Center to relieve symptoms of ischemia following post-traumatic subclavian artery occlusion. (Rich, N. M., Hobson, R. W., II, and Collins, G. J., Jr., Am. J. Surg., *130*:712, 1975.)

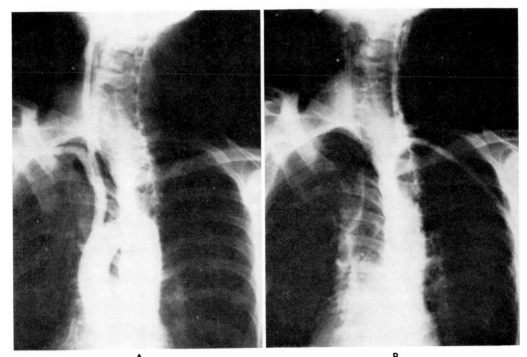

A   **B**

Figure 13–25. (A) The arch aortogram shows filling of the innominate artery and its branches, but there is no visualization of the left carotid or subclavian artery.

(B) With a 1.5 second delay, the second film reveals retrograde filling of the left vertebral and subclavian arteries, creating a subclavian steal. (Sweetman, W. R., Am. Surg., *31*:463, 1965.)

Walter Reed General Hospital, occlusion of the subclavian artery caused moderate symptoms of ischemia with repetitive motion. Constricting lateral sutures used to provide hemostasis at the original operation in Vietnam effected a ligation of the second portion of the subclavian artery (Fig. 13–23). Reconstruction was performed with a bypass greater saphenous vein graft between the left common carotid artery and the left axillary artery. This was performed through a supraclavicular incision, avoiding the necessity of a repeat thoracotomy. The result was excellent. This experience stimulated three additional carotid-axillary bypasses at Walter Reed General Hospital in patients with post-traumatic subclavian artery occlusion (Fig. 13–24) (Rich et al., 1975C).

An interesting problem associated with subclavian artery trauma is the development of a subclavian steal syndrome, which may either be symptomatic or asympto-matic. Sweetman (1965) presented the case of a 44 year old man who suffered a severe crushing injury when he was carried on a saw mill conveyor belt. For the next 23 months the patient noticed dizziness of increasing frequency when he turned his head, associated with roaring in his ears. This became so severe that he felt he would fall if he did not sit down immediately. The episodes were usually transient, but occasionally they lasted up to six hours. He also had aching and numbness in the left arm. Angiograms revealed an occlusion of the left subclavian artery (Fig. 13–25). A Teflon prosthesis was used successfully to re-establish continuity in the left subclavian artery.

Hence, in summary, the outlook for repair of subclavian artery injuries is excellent. The major problem is early recognition following injury when the risk of massive hemorrhage and exsanguination is great.

CHAPTER 14

AXILLARY ARTERIAL INJURIES

Trauma to the axillary artery occurs frequently enough to require management on any busy trauma service. In recent combat experience, axillary injuries occurred in about 6 per cent of major arterial injuries (Hughes, 1958; Rich et al., 1970A). A similar frequency is found in reported civilian experience, with an incidence between 5 and 9 per cent (Table 14–1).

Because of the high frequency of concomitant injuries to adjacent veins, bones and nerves which lie in close proximity to the artery, special attention must be given to a well-organized system of management. Functional demands and the role of collateral circulation in the upper extremity differ from those in the lower extremity. Following axillobrachial arterial injuries, particularly when associated with nerve injuries, impaired use of the hand may constitute the most severe permanent disability.

Certain types of trauma should alert the surgeon to the possibility of injury to the

TABLE 14–1. INCIDENCE OF AXILLARY ARTERIAL INJURIES

	AUTHORS	TOTAL ARTERIES	AXILLARY	PER CENT
War Series				
WW I	Makins (1919)	1191	108	9.0
WW II	DeBakey and Simeone (1946)	2471	74	2.9
Korean	Hughes (1958)	304	20	6.6
Vietnam	Rich et al. (1970A)	1000	59	5.9
Civilian Series				
Houston	Morris et al. (1960)	220	Combined with subclavian	
Atlanta	Ferguson et al. (1961)	200	10	5.0
Denver	Owens (1963)	70	10	14.3
Detroit	Smith et al. (1963)	61	3	4.9
Dallas	Patman et al. (1964)	271	24	8.9
Los Angeles	Treiman et al. (1966)	159	Combined with brachial	
St. Louis	Dillard et al. (1968)	85	6	7.1
New Orleans	Drapanas et al. (1970)	226	12	5.2
Dallas	Perry et al. (1971)*	508	38	7.5
Denver	Kelly and Eiseman (1975)	116	2	1.7
Jackson	Hardy et al. (1975)	360	23	6.4
New York	Bole et al. (1976)	126	2	1.6

*This is a sequential study including the earlier report.

axillary artery. These include fractures of adjacent bones, dislocation of the shoulder and the unusual but challenging "crutch thrombosis." The recent increased utilization of percutaneous transaxillary arterial catheterization for angiographic studies also has created a unique form of iatrogrenic arterial trauma.

SURGICAL ANATOMY

The axillary artery, approximately six inches in length, is a continuation of the subclavian artery. It starts at the lateral border of the first rib and ends at the inferior border of the teres major muscle, where it becomes the brachial artery (Fig. 14–1).

Similar to the subclavian artery, the axillary artery is divided into three parts proximal, beneath and distal to the pectoralis minor muscle. The second part beneath the muscle is the shortest, and the third portion, which is distal to the muscle, represents the longest part. Usually, the first part has one branch, the superior thoracic artery. Part two has two branches, the thoracoacromial and the lateral thoracic arteries. The third part has three

arteries, the subscapular and the anterior and posterior circumflex humeral arteries.

The superior thoracic artery is a small artery from the first part of the axillary artery, which courses medially to supply the muscles of the first two intercostal spaces.

The thoracoacromial artery, an important branch for collateral circulation, arises as a short trunk from the second part of the axillary artery. It divides into four branches to supply the deltoid muscle, some of the pectoral muscles and the acromioclavicular region. The lateral thoracic artery, the second branch of the second part of the axillary artery, travels along the lower border of the pectoralis minor muscle to the chest wall. A significant variant is its origin from the thoracodorsal branch of the subscapular artery (Fig. 14–2).

The subscapular artery, the largest branch, originates in the third part of the axillary artery at the level of the glenoid fossa and descends along the lower border of the subscapular muscle and scapula to the muscles of the posterior axillary wall. Excellent collateral blood supply is possible through its anastomosis with the descending branch of the deep brachial artery beneath the triceps muscle (Fig. 14–3). The

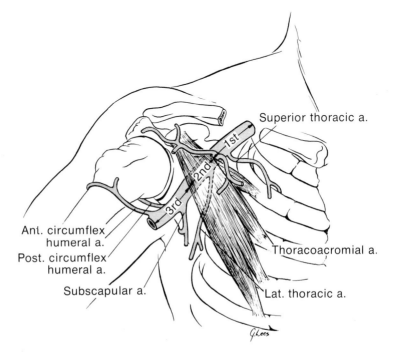

Figure 14–1. Surgical anatomy of the axillary artery with the usual configuration of six branches coming from the three parts of the artery.

Superior thoracic a.

Ant. circumflex humeral a.

Post. circumflex humeral a.

Subscapular a.

Thoracoacromial a.

Lat. thoracic a.

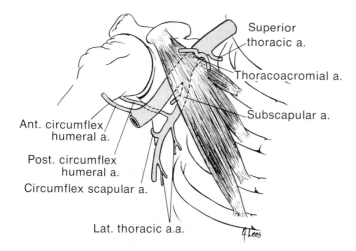

Figure 14–2. The second most frequent site of origin of the branches of the axillary artery. Note that the large subscapular artery originates from the second part of the axillary artery. (Drawn after Standness, D. E., Jr. Collateral Circulation in Clinical Surgery. W. B. Saunders Co., Philadelphia, 1969.)

last two branches of the axillary artery are the anterior and posterior circumflex humeral arteries, which form an arterial ring around the cervical neck of the humerus. Anastomosis of the posterior circumflex humeral artery with the ascending branch of the deep brachial artery constitutes another important collateral connection. The major variation of the branches of the third part include a common origin of all three

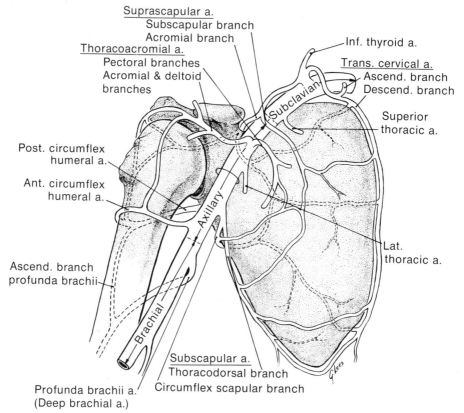

Figure 14–3. Diagrammatic representation of the collateral arterial system surrounding the shoulder. Circuitous pathways traversing several collateral systems create an important arterial network supplying the upper extremity.

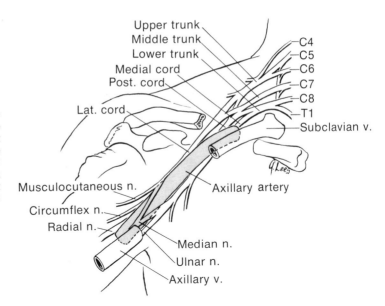

Figure 14–4. The close proximity of the brachial plexus to the cord adjacent to the second part of the axillary artery and the branches surrounding the third part demonstrate why there is a high incidence of concomitant nerve injuries with axillary arterial trauma, as shown above.

branches from one trunk, where the posterior circumflex humeral artery may arise from the deep brachial artery.

There is a fairly constant configuration of the axillary artery and its branches, but each branch may not always arise directly from the artery. Strandness (1969) reviewed the variations in this complex network of arterial branches, which vary in number from four to 11. He noted that the second most frequent configuration was a large subscapular artery arising from the second portion (Fig. 14–2). He summarized 12 variations of the arterial patterns in the upper extremities originally reported by Keen. These numerous anastomoses of the branches of the axillary artery create an excellent collateral blood supply in the thoracic-scapular-humeral collateral system (Fig. 14–3).

The axillary vein is formed by the joining of the two venae comitantes of the brachial artery, the brachial veins, with the basilic vein. The axillary vein usually exists in a single trunk, covering the axillary artery when the arm is abducted. This intimate relationship contributes to the frequency of arteriovenous fistulas following penetrating injuries. A similar close relationship exists with branches of the brachial plexus (Fig. 14–4). Proximally, the plexus lies lateral to the artery. Distally, the three cords of the plexus virtually surround the second

and third parts of the artery. The close proximity of these structures explains the high incidence of concomitant nerve injuries in axillary arterial trauma.

INCIDENCE

Representative military and civilian experiences with axillary arterial trauma are outlined in Table 14–1. Such injuries occur in about one patient in 15 with major arterial injuries.

Makins (1919) reported British experiences in World War I with arterial trauma. He found 108 axillary arterial injuries, 9 per cent of a total of 1191 arterial injuries. DeBakey and Simeone's (1946) review of 2471 arterial injuries in World War II found only a 3 per cent incidence of axillary injuries: 74 cases. Both of these series included many smaller arteries in the total number reviewed. In the more recent combat experience, only injuries to large arteries were included. Hughes (1958) documented 20 axillary arterial injuries among 304 arterial injuries in the Korean Conflict, an incidence of about 7 per cent. Interim statistics from Vietnam reveal almost equal incidence, 6 per cent, with 59 axillary injuries included in 1000 acute major arterial injuries (Rich et al., 1970A).

Representative civilian series show an

incidence similar to that of military injuries except for the relatively high incidence — about 14 per cent, 10 of 70 arterial injuries — reported by Owens (1963) in Denver. Ferguson and associates (1961) found 10 axillary arterial injuries among 200 large and small arterial injuries in Atlanta. The lowest percentage, about 5 per cent, in the series reviewed was reported by Smith and colleagues (1963) in a report of three axillary injuries among 61 arterial injuries in Detroit. Patman and associates (1964) recorded 24 axillary injuries in 271 arterial injuries, about 9 per cent, in Dallas. In a sequential series from this same city published in 1971, there were 38 axillary injuries among 508 arterial injuries, 7.5 per cent (Perry et al., 1971). Among 85 major arterial injuries in St. Louis, Dillard and associates (1968) found six axillary injuries, about 7 per cent. Drapanas and co-workers (1970) reported approximately a 5 per cent incidence with 12 axillary injuries among 226 arterial injuries in New Orleans. Kelly and Eiseman (1975) documented only two axillary arterial injuries in Denver, and Hardy and associates (1976) found only two in New York City in two civilian series of 116 and 126 arterial injuries, respectively.

In a few large series, injuries to the axillary artery were not independently reported. Treiman and co-workers (1966) combined axillary and brachial injuries for a total of 54 in a group of 159 major arterial injuries in Los Angeles. It is understandable how difficult it might be to identify the exact anatomical location of the arterial injury in the area of the lower border of the teres major muscle where the axillary artery becomes the brachial artery. In another large series of 220 arterial injuries, axillary injuries were combined with subclavian injuries for a total of 19 cases (Morris et al., 1960).

Smith and co-authors (1963), in reporting 54 arterial injuries of the upper extremity, found six axillary injuries, 11 per cent, in this anatomical region. Kleinert and Kasdan (1963) found only three axillary injuries in a series of 79 arterial injuries of the upper extremity, an incidence of 4 per cent. These two reports included injuries to the smaller arteries, such as the radial artery. Brawley and associates (1970) reviewed seven axillary injuries among a total of 20 innominate, subclavian and axillary arterial injuries.

ETIOLOGY

In civilian life most injuries of the axillary artery result from lacerations due to broken glass, knives or low velocity missiles. In several large series of arterial injuries reviewed, the wounding agent could not be determined because the axillary artery was grouped with other arterial injuries in the upper extremity. Smith and associates (1963) reported 36 lacerations, 16 of which were caused by broken glass, windows or bottles. Seven resulted from gunshot wounds. Kleinert and Kasdan (1963) reported that, in a group of 79 patients, 41 injuries were caused by broken glass, nine by knife wounds, seven by bullets and three by gunshot blasts. Brawley and co-workers (1970) reported four axillary arterial injuries from stab wounds, two from gunshot wounds and one from glass when a child fell through a plate glass window.

Axillary arterial injuries have also resulted from percutaneous transaxillary arterial catheterization for angiography, a procedure being used with increasing frequency. In an extensive experience at Walter Reed Army Medical Center, acute axillary thrombosis has occurred in about 1 per cent of these catheterizations.

Rupture of the axillary artery is an unusual well-recognized complication of anterior shoulder dislocation or fracture of the neck of the humerus. Arterial injury can also occur during reduction of a shoulder dislocation, a fact with significant medical-legal implications. Rob and Standeven (1956) recorded an example of each type of injury. One involved a young man, injured in a road accident, with an unstable fracture of the proximal humerus and a contusion and thrombosis of the axillary artery. The other involved anterior dislocation of the shoulder in an elderly patient. McKenzie and Sinclair (1958) reported two patients with axillary arterial occlusion complicating shoulder dislocation. They demonstrated marked displacement of the axillary artery as the head of the humerus impinged on the subscapular artery (Fig. 14–5). Johnson and associates (1962) reported a woman with arterial trauma caused by anterior dislocation of the shoulder and reviewed previous reports, finding less than 100 cases described since 1825. Owens (1963) reported the case of a young male, involved

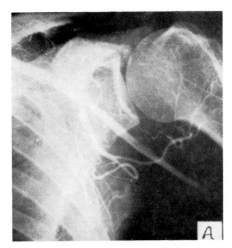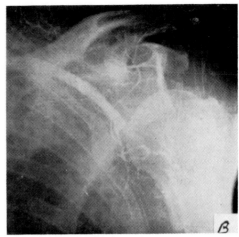

Figure 14–5. (A) This arteriogram shows normal axillary and subscapular arteries, with the common variant of the posterior circumflex originating from the subscapular artery. (B) In the same patient with the shoulder dislocated anteriorly, there is marked displacement of the axillary artery, with the humeral head impinging on the subscapular artery. (McKenzie, A. D., and Sinclair, A. M., Ann. Surg., *148*:139, 1958.)

in an automobile accident, who sustained fractures of the clavicle and scapula with intimal fracture of the axillary artery and subsequent thrombosis. A similar unreported patient, in whom an avulsing injury to the shoulder stretched the artery enough to rupture the intima, has been treated by one of the authors (F.C.S.). Following resection of the thrombosed segment, an end-to-end anastomosis was easily performed. Gibson (1962) reported two patients with traumatic rupture of the axillary artery in the absence of anterior dislocation of the shoulder or fracture of the neck of the humerus. He felt that hyperabduction of the arm could stretch and tear an atheromatous axillary artery anchored at the origin of the subscapular branch. He also suggested that temporary subluxation of the head of the humerus could produce an injury similar to that resulting from anterior dislocation of the shoulder. Stein and associates (1971) documented the rare and unusual case of a 19 year old male, involved in an automobile accident, who had disruption of the axillary artery associated with a closed fracture of the neck of the scapula. Inahara (1962) described another unusual case of complete disruption of the axillary artery associated with subluxation of the right sternoclavicular joint in a 44 year old woman who was thrown out of a car at the time of an accident.

Injury to the axillary artery can occur during a variety of operations. Lord and associates (1958), in documenting 11 cases of major vascular injury that occurred during the course of elective operative procedures, included two cases of axillary arterial injury. One injury occurred during a radical mastectomy and the other during a Z-plasty of a contracture of the axilla. Trauma to the axillary artery can occur during resection of the first rib through the transaxillary approach for thoracic outlet syndrome, as demonstrated in the case of a patient treated at Walter Reed Army Medical Center (Fig. 14–6).

An interesting and unusual injury may develop over a period of time if an improperly adjusted crutch impinges repeatedly on the axilla. Rob and Standeven (1956) reported four patients who developed an axillary thrombosis or aneurysm following use of an axillary crutch for many years. Smith and associates (1963) also reported a case of "crutch thrombosis." Brooks and Fowler (1964) added three additional cases of axillary thrombosis following prolonged use of axillary crutches and found eight previously reported cases in the English literature. Wholey and Bocher (1967) radiographically demonstrated occlusion of the axillary artery at the circumflex humeral branch during application of a crutch (Fig. 14–7). Abbott and

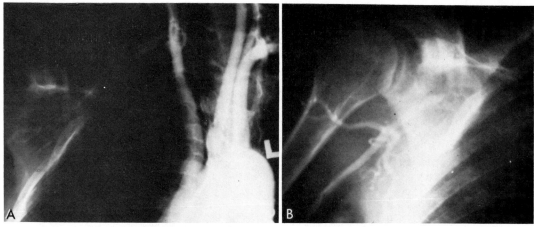

Figure 14–6. This angiogram demonstrates occlusion of the right subclavian artery (A) with reconstitution near the axillary-brachial junction (B). There was an accidental laceration of the right axillary artery during first rib resection through the transaxillary approach, and it was necessary to ligate the subclavian artery to control the hemorrhage. The patient was later referred to Walter Reed Army Medical Center for vascular reconstruction because of easy fatigability in the upper extremity. (N.M.R., W.R.G.H., 1973.)

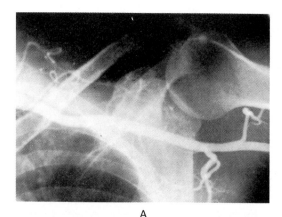

A

Figure 14–7. This axillary arteriogram reveals a normal axillary artery prior to application of a crutch (A). There is, however, occlusion of the axillary artery at the circumflex humeral branch (B) shortly after crutch application, with the crutch visible in the lower corner. (Wholey, M. H., and Bocher, J., Surg. Gynecol. Obstet., *125*:730, 1967.)

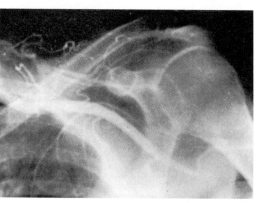

B

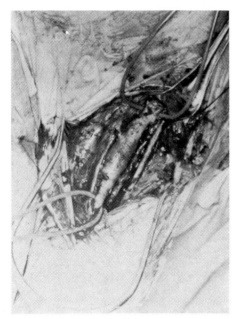

Figure 14–8. Aneurysmal formation can also occur in the axillary artery following prolonged use of a crutch. This finding is demonstrated in the above photograph taken in the operating room. (Abbott, W. M., and Darling, R. C., Am. J. Surg., *125*:515, 1973.)

associates (1973) at Massachusetts General Hospital have reported the largest and most recent series of this type of injury that included axillary aneurysmal formation (Fig. 14–8).

In the Vietnam injuries, Rich and co-workers (1970A) found that slightly more than 50 per cent of the 59 axillary injuries were due to high velocity bullets (Table 14–2). Most other injuries (in 28 patients) resulted from fragment wounds due to mortars, rockets and booby traps. One patient sustained contusion and thrombosis of the axillary artery from blunt trauma in a helicopter crash.

TABLE 14–2. SOURCE OF 59 AXILLARY ARTERIAL INJURIES — VIETNAM EXPERIENCE

	NUMBER	PER CENT
Gunshot wounds	30	50.8
Fragment wounds	28	47.5
Blunt trauma	1	1.7
Total	59	100.0

CLINICAL PATHOLOGY

All types of traumatic injury, ranging from thrombosis due to blunt trauma to complete rupture caused by a high velocity bullet, have been documented for axillary arterial injuries. Laceration is the most common type. Although axillary arteries were not separated from other injuries in the upper extremity, Smith and associates (1963) found lacerations from knives and broken glass in 36 of 54 patients, and Kleinert and Kasdan (1963) reported lacerations from glass and knives in 50 of 79 injuries. In the latter series 25 of 41 arteries injured by broken glass were completely severed.

Smith and colleagues (1963) reported an avulsion of the axillary artery from anterior dislocation of the shoulder. In a similar injury, McKenzie and Sinclair (1958) found a small laceration of the subscapular artery at its origin in one patient and partial avulsion of the subscapular artery from the axillary artery in another patient, both associated with contusion and thrombosis of the axillary artery. Both the subscapular and posterior circumflex humeral arteries are vulnerable during either dislocation or reduction of the shoulder and may incur a laceration, avulsion or thrombosis.

In two patients with axillary arterial rupture reported by Gibson (1962), atheromatous plaques were found in one. Rob and Standeven (1956) reported sudden occlusion of the axillary artery, with no overt evidence of generalized arterial disease, in two patients who used crutches. A third patient had an arterial embolism, and a fourth had an aneurysm at the site of pressure of the axillary crutch with a probable associated embolism. Abbott and co-workers also documented the formation of aneurysms in the axillary artery in patients who used crutches (Fig. 14–8). Owens (1963) described disruption of the intima of the axillary artery with subsequent thrombosis in a young man who had fractures of the clavicle and scapula. Thrombosis may also occur after catheter angiography, often in association with elevation of a strip of intima.

Rich and co-workers (1970A) found that lacerations of the axillary artery were usually associated with fragment wounds in the Vietnam conflict. Transections and avulsions were more frequent following gunshot wounds. Blunt trauma produced contusion and thrombosis in one patient. In 100 segments from injured arteries that were studied microscopically, the abnormalities from five axillary arteries were similar to those of other arteries (Rich et al., 1969C) (see Chap. 4).

CLINICAL FEATURES

A steadily expanding hematoma in the axilla may be a dramatic finding in an axillary arterial injury (Fig. 14–9). This may occur in a penetrating injury with a small point of entry, or in closed injuries from blunt trauma. Bright, pulsatile bleeding is seen with larger wounds. Shock often results.

Absent distal brachial and radial pulses with unobtainable blood pressure, a cool, pale hand and a numb upper extremity are common findings in acute axillary injuries. However, a palpable radial pulse does not exclude arterial injury, because lacerations may seal and permit distal flow of blood. Also, excellent collateral circulation may

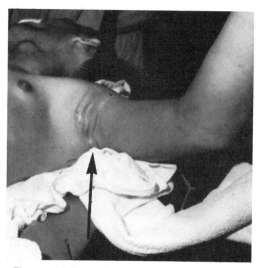

Figure 14–9. A large and rapidly expanding hematoma can develop in the axilla following trauma that results in axillary arterial injury. This is emphasized in the above photograph (arrow): the young man developed a pulsating hematoma as a result of an automobile accident. (Rich, N. M., Hobson, R. W., II, and Collins, G. J., Jr., Am. J. Surg., *130*:712, 1975.)

exist. Owing to the proximity of the axillary vein, an arteriovenous fistula may be produced. Distal pulses are present, but the characteristic thrill and continuous bruit establish the diagnosis.

Peripheral nerve injuries with loss of sensory and motor function are frequent and complicate diagnostic considerations. Other associated injuries, such as fractures of the scapula, clavicle and humerus, are also frequent. There should be a high degree of suspicion in symptomatic patients who have had an anterior dislocation of the shoulder or recent percutaneous transaxillary angiographic studies, or who have used an axillary crutch for many years.

DIAGNOSTIC CONSIDERATIONS

Diagnosis is often obvious, because of either a penetrating injury spurting bright red arterial blood or a cold, numb extremity with absent pulses. Roentgenograms may aid the diagnosis by disclosing fractures of the clavicle, scapula or humerus and by demonstrating retained foreign bodies in the region of the neurovascular bundle. Arteriography is the most precise diagnostic measure and can be performed with adequate facilities, but it has been of limited value in military injuries. Angiography has been of particular value when the question of arterial injury is associated with blunt trauma and associated fracture or with dislocation (Fig. 14–10).

Other diagnostic adjuncts, such as plethysmography, ultrasonic sounding devices and oscillometry, have been of limited value. In some patients with a penetrating injury, the simplest approach is careful examination of the axillary artery during operative débridement of the wound.

SURGICAL TREATMENT

The success rate following repair of axillary injuries should approach 100 per cent because the artery is a large one which can be readily mobilized for repair without tension (Fig. 14–11). Failures are almost always due to preventable errors in technique, such as inadequate débridement, stenosis or residual distal thrombi. Al-

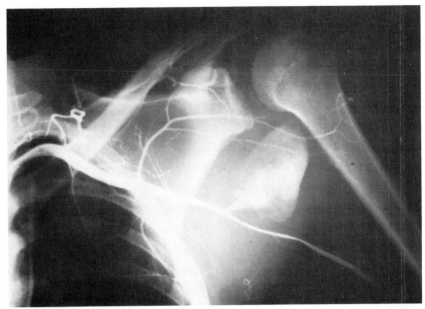

Figure 14–10. When there is a question of arterial trauma associated with blunt trauma, fracture of the humerus or clavicle, or shoulder dislocation, angiography can be of great value in localizing the lesion. A contrast medium is seen passing from a defect in the wall of the artery into a large false aneurysm. (Rich, N. M., Hobson, R. W., II, and Collins, G. J., Jr., Am. J. Surg., *130*:712, 1975.)

though collateral circulation is excellent in this area, ligation is a poor second choice. Gangrene after ligation has been reported in only 9 per cent of cases (Bailey, 1944), but DeBakey and Simeone (1946) found a

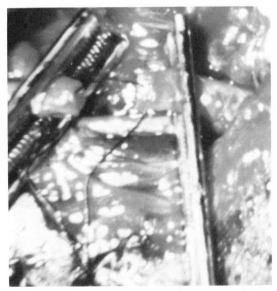

Figure 14–11. After adequate débridement of the artery, end-to-end anastomosis can frequently be carried out without undue tension on the suture line and without sacrificing major collateral vessels. (N.M.R., 2nd Surgical Hospital, 1966.)

frequency of about 43 per cent in 74 arterial injuries in World War II. The hazard of gangrene varies with the degree of concomitant destruction of the collateral circulation. Hence, the injuries most difficult to repair because of the extensive tissue destruction are, at the same time, those in which repair is most urgently needed.

Adequate transfusion of blood is routinely necessary because serious hemorrhage and shock are common with axillary arterial injuries. Antibiotics should be started promptly and continued for several days after operation. Control of hemorrhage may be a significant technical problem in some patients because direct pressure is difficult and a tourniquet cannot be applied. Packing the wound with a large amount of gauze may be a temporary satisfactory expedient. Clamps should almost never be applied because of the proximity of the brachial plexus. Adequate surgical exposure is essential because a large hematoma in the axilla, with hemorrhage into adjacent fat, conceals and distorts associated vital structures, such as the brachial plexus (Fig. 14–12). A curved incision over the cephalic vein in the deltopectoral groove is ideal (Fig. 14–13). An S-shaped incision centered over the axilla will also provide

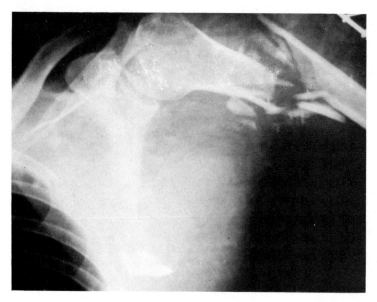

Figure 14–12. It is mandatory to develop adequate exposure of the axillary artery, which is often distorted and concealed by a large hematoma. Other vital structures in juxtaposition must be protected. The large soft tissue density seen on this roentgenogram represents a large hematoma in the axilla and shoulder caused by massive hemorrhage from a severed axillary artery. The wounding agent, a large artillery shell fragment in the mid-lower area, also caused a comminuted fracture of the humerus (Rich, N. M., Metz, C. W., Jr., Hutton, J. E., Jr., Baugh, J. H., and Hughes, C. W., J. Trauma, *11*:463, 1971. Copyright 1971, The Williams & Wilkins Co., Baltimore.)

the exposure needed. Usually the tendon of the pectoralis major muscle is transected to provide prompt access to the proximal portion of the artery. The pectoralis minor tendon can be severed if necessary. Once the pectoral tendons have been divided, the axilla is widely exposed, and hemorrhage can be quickly arrested by isolating the artery just distal to its exit from beneath the clavicle. Occasionally, only a medial longitudinal incision along the course of the proximal brachial artery, but not carried across the axillary crease, is adequate for certain distal lesions, such as thrombosis of

the distal axillary artery after catheterization for angiographic studies.

Once the injured artery has been isolated and the injured edges debrided, the ends should be gently dilated and the lumen irrigated with saline to carefully inspect the intima for unrecognized fractures and disruptions. Significant areas of contusion should usually be resected. Routine insertion of a Fogarty balloon catheter into the distal arterial tree is valuable because of the unpredictable occurrence of distal thrombi from stasis. Further development of thrombi during repair can be minimized

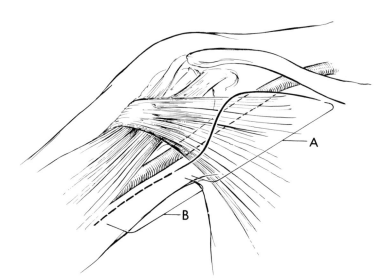

Figure 14–13. (A) An S-shaped incision centered over the axilla will provide needed exposure of the axillary artery. The tendon of the pectoralis major muscle may be transected to augment visualization. (B) For distal axillary arterial lesions, a longitudinal incision along the course of the proximal brachial artery may be all that is needed.

by distal instillation of 10 to 15 mg of heparin solution or by using 1 to 2 mg of heparin per kg intravenously.

Rarely repair can be done by lateral suture, usually in the case of small puncture wounds or tiny, clean lacerations (Fig. 14–14). Lateral repair is tempting to the novice but is notoriously unsuccessful in more extensive injuries because of stenosis and immediate or late occlusion. An alternate choice is a vein patch graft to prevent these potential complications.

Usually a direct anastomosis or a vein graft is necessary. In 57 injuries in the Vietnam Conflict, direct anastomosis was performed in 14 and autogenous vein grafts in 38 (Rich et al., 1970A). The elasticity of the axillary artery should be remembered, because retraction of the severed ends of the vessel creates the impression that a great loss of artery has occurred (Fig. 14–15). Preservation of major branches, such as the subscapular artery, should be managed if possible to maintain the pathway of important collateral systems.

Direct anastomosis with fine synthetic vascular suture is preferred unless undue tension results. Otherwise, an autogenous vein graft, preferably using the greater saphenous vein, should be employed. The cephalic vein can also be used but is less satisfactory. Synthetic materials such as

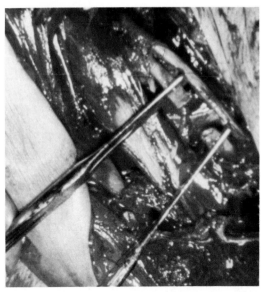

Figure 14–15. Following transection of the axillary artery, retraction of the severed ends may give an impression of a much greater loss than has actually occurred. It is important to keep in mind the elastic nature of the extremity arteries. (Rich, N. M., Metz, C. W., Jr., Hutton, J. E., Jr., Baugh, J. H., and Hughes, C. W., J. Trauma, *11*:463, 1971. Copyright 1971, The Williams & Wilkins Co., Baltimore.)

Dacron prostheses should be avoided if possible because of the hazard of infection in contaminated wounds.

Following reconstruction, adjacent soft tissues must be approximated over the site of repair. With extensive contamination, the skin and subcutaneous tissues should be left open for delayed primary suture in three to six days (Fig. 14–16).

If distal pulses are not readily palpable after the arterial reconstruction, an operative arteriogram is indicated. This not only will outline the possible technical failure of the repair but also will identify residual distal thrombi and possible additional lesions, such as a coexisting brachial arterial injury.

With prolonged preoperative ischemia, the muscles of the upper extremity should be carefully observed for the appearance of progressive rigidity, indicating the need for fasciotomy. Such circumstances are infrequent, however, as compared to their occurrence in the lower extremity.

Concomitant fractures are usually managed by external immobilization because of the danger of infection that accompanies

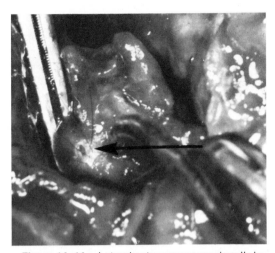

Figure 14–14. Lateral suture may occasionally be possible and acceptable for a small puncture wound similar to that seen in this photograph (arrow) taken in the operating room. A venous patch graft can be utilized to prevent constriction at the repair site. (N.M.R., W.R.G.H., 1969.)

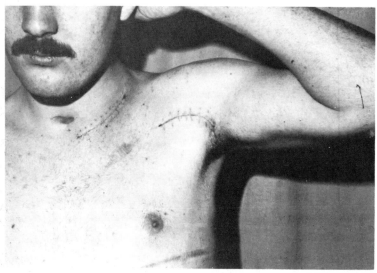

Figure 14–16. In an attempt to avoid infection, a delayed primary closure of the skin at approximately three to six days has been carried out in the management of axillary arterial trauma (W.R.G.H.)

internal fixation in contaminated wounds. If internal fixation is performed, it should be done before the arterial repair is completed to prevent later disruption of the arterial repair during fracture manipulation. Nerve injuries should be documented, but primary nerve repair is seldom indicated. Small venous lacerations may be repaired by lateral suture; venous insufficiency following ligation of the axillary vein, however, has not been a significant problem.

POSTOPERATIVE CARE

Brachial and radial pulses should be palpable soon after reconstruction. Sufficient edema to obscure peripheral pulses, a frequent problem in lower extremities, usually does not occur in the upper extremities. With absent pulses, possible causes include thrombosis of the anastomosis, residual thrombi in the distal arterial tree, an additional arterial injury and vasospasm. Vasospasm of sufficient degree to eliminate distal pulses for several hours is unusual and is an erroneous diagnosis made too often by the inexperienced. In almost all patients, continued absence of the peripheral pulse is due to mechanical obstruction, which can be corrected only by reoperation. Arteriography is the simplest approach to establishing the diagnosis. If arteriography

cannot be satisfactorily performed, surgical reexploration of the anastomosis, combined with exploration of the distal artery with a Fogarty catheter, should be performed. In military casualties, in whom multiple injuries of other organs are frequent, the stress of an additional operative procedure may be significant. The alternatives should be carefully weighed in deciding for or against the operation. If motor and sensory function are intact in the extremity despite absence of pulses, there is little risk of gangrene. A better choice may be to delay attempts at arterial reconstruction until more favorable circumstances occur. Concomitant nerve injuries may, however, eliminate this valuable clinical guide of sensory and motor function. Early experience with the ultrasonic sounding device (Doppler) has been encouraging in substantiating the clinical impression of adequate blood supply in the absence of palpable peripheral pulses (Fig. 14–17).

Sympathetic blocks and cervical sympathectomy are of dubious value and are not recommended for most patients. Systemic heparinization is usually contraindicated because it is of limited value and entails the serious hazard of bleeding into the wound. The dominant principle of repair of injured axillary arteries is that the success rate after arterial reconstruction should approach 100 per cent, because the injured

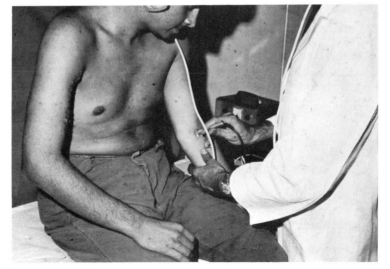

Figure 14–17. If distal pulses are absent following axillary arterial trauma, the ultrasonic sounding device (Doppler) can be utilized to help determine the extent and quality of the collateral circulation. (Photograph taken in the Vascular Laboratory at Walter Reed General Hospital, N.M.R., 1969.)

arteries are usually free of intrinsic disease and are of adequate size for repair. Errors are almost always due to technical failures because of inexperience and are correctable by reoperation. If this principle is adopted, the role of different adjuncts to increase flow of blood is very limited.

If no signs of infection are present in the operative wound, wounds left open initially can be sutured in four to seven days. In complex injuries, especially those involving fracture and nerve injuries, physical therapy should be started soon after operation to maintain proper hand and shoulder function. Stiffness of the interphalangeal joints of the fingers to a disabling degree can develop within a surprisingly short period of time.

COMPLICATIONS

Early thrombosis of axillary arterial repairs is usually secondary to avoidable technical errors, as previously discussed. Inadequate hemostasis and hematoma formation may cause pressure on the repair site. Distal pulses may disappear until the

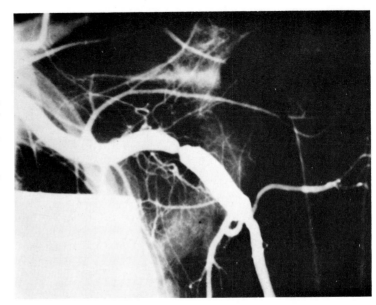

Figure 14–18. Stenosis followed by occlusion may occur within weeks to months after axillary arterial repair. This angiogram reveals marked stenosis at the proximal suture line of an interposition autogenous saphenous vein graft repair of the axillary artery in a returning Vietnam casualty. N.M.R., W.R.G.H., 1967.)

pressure is relieved by hematoma evacuation.

Serious wound infection with secondary hemorrhage from disruption of the arterial repair fortunately is an unusual event. In such circumstances, ligation of the injured artery should be performed. Gangrene at this time, usually several days after injury, is infrequent because of the excellent collateral circulation available.

A late stenosis and subsequent occlusion of the axillary artery may occur weeks or months after operation (Fig. 14–18). Such patients often remain asymptomatic because of the concomitant development of collateral circulation. In some circumstances no further treatment is needed.

RESULTS

The largest series of repaired injuries of the axillary artery is from the Vietnam Conflict. In the interim report from the Vietnam Vascular Registry of 1000 acute major arterial injuries, the axillary artery was involved in 59 patients (Rich et al., 1970A). Ligation was performed in two patients with massive soft tissue injuries, both of whom subsequently required amputation. An arterial repair was performed in 57 patients, three of whom subsequently required amputation (Table 14–3). One of these three amputations was performed a long time after the injury was incurred and did not result from failure of the arterial repair but rather from the uselessness of the upper extremity, which had no motor or sensory function. Concomitant nerve in-

TABLE 14–3. AMPUTATION RATE FOR AXILLARY ARTERIAL INJURIES

AUTHORS	ARTERIES	AMPUTATED	PER CENT
Following Ligation			
Makins (1919)	108	5	4.6
Bailey (1944)	–	–	9.0
DeBakey and Simeone (1946)	74	32	43.2
Hughes (1958)	5	1	20.0
Following Repair			
Hughes (1958)	15	1	6.7
Rich et al. (1970A)	57	3	5.3

juries occurred in about 92 per cent of the patients, vein injuries in 34 per cent and fractures in 29 per cent. Arterial repair was accomplished by lateral suture in only five patients. An end-to-end anastomosis was done in 14 and a vein graft in 38, or about 67 per cent of the total (Table 14–4). The use of a vein graft in two-thirds of the injuries is unusual and may be due to erroneously interpreting the traction of the ends of the severed artery as due to loss of arterial substance rather than to elastic recoil. Also, it must be remembered that many of the wounds were caused by high velocity missiles creating massive destruction. The greater saphenous vein was used for repair in nearly all of the patients. The cephalic vein was utilized twice, and the azygos vein was unsuccessfully used once. Complications occurred in 19 patients, one-third of the group, usually as postoperative thrombosis. This developed in 14 of the vein grafts, in four of the direct anastomoses and in one lateral suture repair. Additional vascular operations were performed on 18 of these 19 patients with satisfactory results. Additional data from the preliminary report from the Registry (Rich and Hughes, 1969) revealed that one acute axillary arteriovenous fistula was repaired in Vietnam, but two arteriovenous fistulas were recognized and repaired only after evacuation. Three patients with axillary arterial trauma had additional brachial arterial injuries in the same extremity.

In the Korean Conflict, Hughes (1958) reported only one failure requiring amputation among 15 repairs of injured axillary arteries (Table 14–3). A direct anastomosis was performed in nine of the 15 patients and vascular grafts in five (Table 14–4). A transverse suture was possible in one patient.

Although Bailey stated in 1944 that ligation of the axillary artery resulted in gangrene in only 9 per cent of the patients, DeBakey and Simeone (1946) found an amputation rate of approximately 43 per cent in 74 patients with axillary injuries, in almost all of whom the injured artery was ligated (Table 14–3). In Korea only five axillary arteries were ligated, one of which resulted in gangrene.

In reports from civilian series, results

TABLE 14–4. METHOD OF AXILLARY ARTERIAL REPAIR

AUTHORS	ARTERIES	END-TO-END ANASTOMOSIS	VEIN GRAFT	ARTERY GRAFT	DACRON PROSTHESIS	LATERAL SUTURE
Hughes (1958)	15	9	3	2	0	1
Rich et al. (1970A)	57	14	38	0	0	5

from axillary arterial repairs are difficult to evaluate because such injuries are often combined with injuries of the brachial artery or of other upper extremity arteries (Treiman et al., 1966; Morris et al., 1960). Also, the axillary arterial injuries are often included in the general discussion of upper extremity injuries (Smith et al., 1963; Kleinert and Kasdan, 1963). Certain reports are of specific interest. The patient who had an end-to-end anastomosis for a right axillary arterial injury during the course of a radical mastectomy in 1949, reported by Lord and associates (1958), continued to have good distal pulses during a 6½-year follow-up period. Gibson (1962) discussed the problem of arteriosclerotic plaques causing failure of an end-to-end anastomosis. Treiman and co-workers (1966) reported the necessity for amputation following blunt trauma to the axillary artery after an unsuccessful thrombectomy and reoperation. Greenfield and Ebert (1967) demonstrated a patent vein graft following repair of an injured axillary artery (Fig. 14–19). Smith and associates (1963) reported a successful thrombectomy in a patient with "crutch thrombosis." They also reported another interesting case of a patient who had massive bleeding from the axillary wound following repair of an acute axillary arteriovenous fistula. At the time of reoperation, a second arterial injury, a laceration of the subclavian artery, was found and repaired.

FOLLOW-UP

In civilian series of axillary arterial injuries, there is little long term follow-up

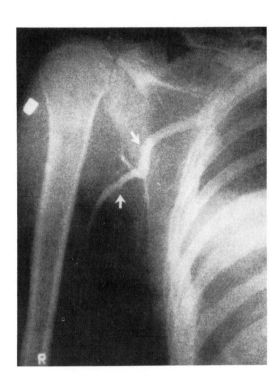

Figure 14–19. Successful results have been reported following axillary arterial repair. This angiogram shows a patent vein graft which was used as an interposition graft in the repair of an injured axillary artery. (Greenfield, L. J., and Ebert, P. A., J. Trauma, 7:606, 1967. Copyright 1967, The Williams & Wilkins Co., Baltimore.)

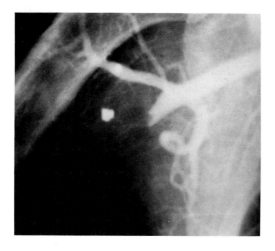

Figure 14–20. Arteriogram of one of six patients with axillary arterial repair failure seen during the long term follow-up in the Vietnam Vascular Registry at Walter Reed Army Medical Center. All six patients have remained asymptomatic. (Rich, N. M., Baugh, J. H., and Hughes, C. W., Arch. Surg., *100*:646, 1970. Copyright 1970, American Medical Association.)

information available. The durability of reported successful repairs of axillary arteries, as well as the results after ligation, is uncertain. Hence, data from the Vietnam injuries represent the largest amount of information available.

Of the 59 patients known to have axillary arterial injuries treated in Vietnam, 21 subsequently have been evaluated at Walter Reed Army Medical Center (Rich et al., 1970A). Six patients with thrombosis of the repaired axillary artery remained asymptomatic (Fig. 14–20). Two others with ligation of an axillary artery were asymptomatic, and four with stenosis of a repaired axillary

artery also remained asymptomatic. A more recent patient not included in the previously described interim report has a 10-mm Dacron sleeve used to repair his left axillary artery after failure of a cephalic vein graft in Vietnam. Because he remained asymptomatic after thrombosis of the Dacron prosthesis, the thrombosed prosthesis was excised without additional arterial reconstruction at the time of exploration of the injured brachial plexus (Fig. 14–21).

Residual neuropathy from concomitant nerve injuries is the most disabling factor in most patients following injuries of the axillary artery. Fractures of the humerus,

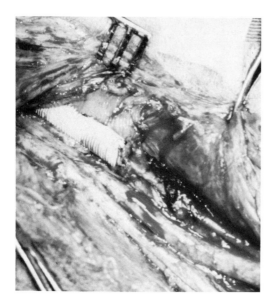

Figure 14–21. In Vietnam an unsuccessful attempt was made to reconstruct the left axillary artery with a Dacron prosthesis. The thrombosed prosthesis was removed later, as shown in this operating room photograph, at Walter Reed General Hospital. No additional vascular repair was considered, because the patient was asymptomatic and the wound was contaminated. (Rich, N. M., and Hughes, C. W., J. Trauma, *12*:459, 1972. Copyright 1972, The Williams & Wilkins Co., Baltimore.)

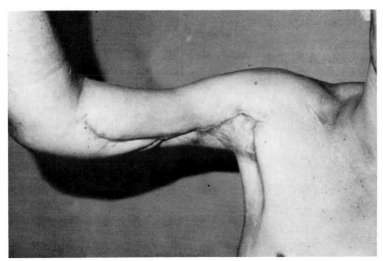

Figure 14-22. In addition to axillary arterial trauma, this Vietnam casualty also had permanent injury of the median, radial and ulnar nerves. (Rich, N. M., Baugh, J. H., and Hughes, C. W., J. Trauma, *10*:359, 1970. Copyright 1970, The Williams & Wilkins Co., Baltimore.)

soft tissue loss and disruption of major venous return are additional contributing factors. Figure 14–22 shows a patient, wounded in Vietnam, who had massive soft tissue loss and disruption of three major nerves. Significant permanent disability is all too frequent following injuries of the brachial plexus and constitutes the most significant problem for future study. It is hoped that improvement in methods of management of peripheral nerve injuries will decrease its frequency.

Chapter 15

BRACHIAL ARTERY INJURIES

In numerous reports of arterial injuries from either civilian or military trauma, the brachial artery is the most frequently injured, constituting one-third to one-fourth of all peripheral arterial injuries (Table 15–1). The frequency of injury is nearly the same for the superficial femoral artery; some reports document a slightly higher incidence of trauma to the superficial femoral artery, followed closely by the brachial artery. Both arteries are long and located in vulnerable positions in the extremity. In the experience from both Korea (Hughes, 1958) and Vietnam (Rich et al., 1970A), nearly 30 per cent of all arterial injuries involved the brachial artery.

Certain anatomical characteristics are particularly important with regard to brachial artery injuries. As with the femoral artery, there is marked difference in the

TABLE 15–1. INCIDENCE OF BRACHIAL ARTERY INJURIES

	AUTHOR	TOTAL ARTERIES	BRACHIAL	PER CENT
War Series				
WW I	Makins (1919)	1191	200	16.8
WW II	DeBakey and Simeone (1946)	2471	601	26.5
Korean	Hughes (1958)	304	89	29.3
Vietnam	Rich et al. (1970A)	1000	283	28.3
Civilian Series				
Houston	Morris et al. (1960)	220	55	25.0
Atlanta	Ferguson et al. (1961)	200	29	14.5
Denver	Owens (1963)	70	14	20.0
Detroit	Smith et al. (1963)	61	13	21.3
Dallas	Patman et al. (1964)*	271	46	17.0
St. Louis	Dillard et al. (1968)	85	26	30.6
New Orleans	Drapanas et al. (1970)	226	39	17.3
Dallas	Perry et al. (1971)*	508	78	15.4
Detroit	Smith et al. (1974)	127	28	22.0
Memphis	Cheek et al. (1975)	155	21	13.5
Denver	Kelly and Eiseman (1975)	116	37	31.9
Jackson	Hardy et al. (1975)	360	75†	20.8
New York	Bole et al. (1976)	126	14	11.1

*Continuing series.
†Number includes brachial artery and branches.

TABLE 15–2. ANATOMICAL LOCATION
OF THE BRACHIAL ARTERY INJURY
AS IT AFFECTS THE AMPUTATION
RATE FOLLOWING LIGATION
FOR ACUTE TRAUMA*

	ARTERIES	AMPUTA-TIONS	PER CENT
Brachial Total	601	159	26.5
Above profunda	97	54	55.7
Below profunda	209	54	25.8

*From DeBakey, M. E., and Simeone, F. A., Ann. Surg., *123*:534, 1946.

degree of ischemia resulting from injuries proximal and distal to the profunda brachii branch. Accordingly, the hazard of gangrene is approximately twice as great following ligation of the common brachial as compared to the superficial brachial (Table 15–2). As described in the subsequent section on surgical anatomy, the brachial artery is surrounded by important peripheral nerves—the median, ulnar and radial—and also parallels the humerus and associated veins. Because of this, associated nerve and bone injuries are frequent and residual neuropathy from such nerve injuries is often the main source of permanent disability. In the lower extremity, weight bearing is the principal consideration in rehabilitation; however, in the upper extremity functional use of the hand is the most important objective.

The brachial artery distal to the profunda brachii branch is the least critical of the major extremity arteries, according to Bailey (1944). He stated that distal gangrene would occur in only 3 per cent of the patients following ligation of the brachial artery. However, DeBakey and Simeone (1946) showed that 25.8 per cent required amputation, and Hughes (1958) in a small series of only nine patients from the Korean Conflict found this figure to be 33.3 per cent. Repair of brachial artery injuries is recommended except in an exceptional situation, such as when there is an absence of soft tissue coverage.

SURGICAL ANATOMY

Although the brachial artery is subject to striking anatomical variations, it is consid-

ered to be a continuation of the axillary artery arbitrarily originating at the lower border of the teres major muscle. It leaves the axilla medially and deep to the median nerve and courses distally in a lateral direction to a position anterior to the humerus and posterior to the bicipital aponeurosis. It terminates about one inch below the transverse skin crease in the antecubital fossa, where it divides into two branches. Of these branches, the ulnar artery is larger than the radial artery. The brachial artery pulsation is palpable along the medial bicipital groove in the arm and beneath the lacertus fibrosus near its termination when the elbow is extended.

The brachial artery lies successively on three muscles, has three major branches, is in contact with three important nerves and is associated with three veins (Thorek, 1962) (Fig. 15–1).

The long head of the triceps, the coracobrachialis and the brachialis muscles make up the floor (from above, downward) for the brachial artery. As it courses downward, the artery follows the inner border of the biceps muscle.

Of the three main branches, the large profunda brachii artery arises as the first branch from the upper portion of the brachial artery, sometimes originating as high as the teres major muscle. It is the companion vessel of the radial nerve and it passes downward, backward and outward between the medial and long heads of the triceps muscle. An important collateral anastomosis is made with the axillary artery through its ascending branch and the posterior humeral circumflex artery. The profunda brachii artery has two branches: the anterior branch anastomoses with the radial recurrent artery, and the posterior branch anastomoses with the posterior interosseous recurrent artery; both branches form additional important collateral pathways. The second main branch of the brachial artery is the superior ulnar collateral artery, also called the inferior profunda artery. The superior ulnar collateral artery is the companion vessel of the ulnar nerve after the vessel originates near the middle of the arm. After passing behind the medial epicondyle, this branch anastomoses with the posterior ulnar recurrent artery. The third and last main branch of the brachial artery is the inferior ulnar

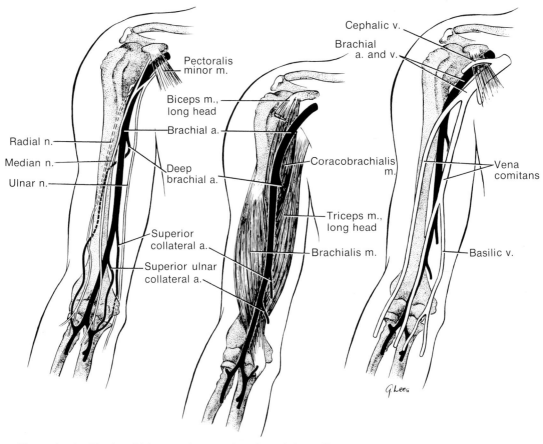

Figure 15–1. The brachial artery is a continuation of the axillary artery at the lower border of the teres major muscle. It terminates approximately 1 inch below the transverse skin crease in the antecubital fossa, where it divides into two branches. Important anatomical relationships include three associated nerves, three associated veins and three main branches with the brachial artery lying successively on three muscles.

collateral artery, also called the anastomotica magna because of its connections to the rich collateral anastomoses around the elbow joint. It anastomoses with the anterior ulnar recurrent artery.

The median nerve is closely related to the brachial artery throughout its entire course. The radial nerve is associated only with the proximal portion of the artery, and the ulnar nerve leaves the artery in the middle of the arm.

Two venae comitantes, the brachial veins, pass on either side of the artery and make many venous contacts around the artery throughout its course. They are joined at varying levels by the basilic vein, which becomes intimately associated with the brachial artery in the middle of the arm.

Strandness (1969) has summarized the numerous variations in the configuration of the brachial artery and its branches. He stated that the principal variants of the proximal brachial artery involved the profunda brachii artery. He also noted that major variations of the brachial artery involve its terminal configuration in approximately 15 to 20 per cent of the patients. The most common of these variants include types of a "superficial brachial artery" which lies superficial to the median nerve and serves as a "high origin" for either the radial artery or the ulnar artery (Fig. 15–2). This variability makes it dangerous to assume that the brachial artery lies deep to the median nerve or that it represents the major blood supply to the upper extremity. Also, the brachial artery may occasionally bifurcate in the upper arm and encircle the

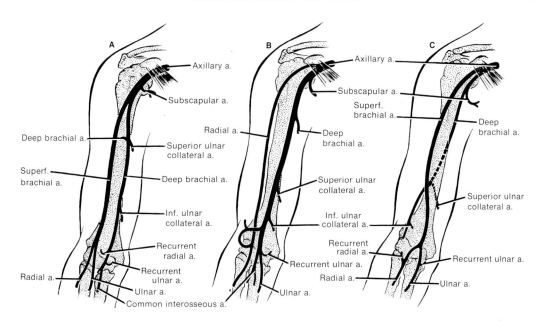

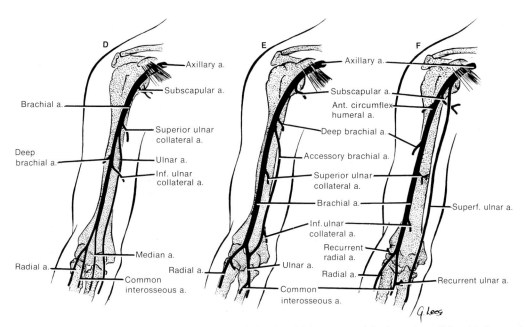

Figure 15–2. Variations in the configuration of the brachial artery and its branches. (After McCormack, L. J., Cauldwell, E. W., and Anson, B. J., Surg. Gynec. Obstet., *96*:43, 1953.)

median nerve, appearing as a double brachial artery.

INCIDENCE OF INJURIES

As stated earlier, about one patient of three who sustains major arterial trauma has involvement of the brachial artery. The frequency of occurrence in a total of 1173 brachial injuries in the major military conflicts of this century involving the United States Armed Forces (World Wars I and II, Korea and Vietnam) are shown in Table 15–1. The frequency ranges from 17 to 29 per cent. However, it must be emphasized that in Makins's World War I report (1919) covering the British experience and in DeBakey and Simeone's review (1946) of 2471 acute arterial injuries in American combat casualties in World War II, there were many smaller arteries included in the total number reviewed. In the more recent combat experience, only injuries to large arteries were considered. Hughes (1958) documented 89 brachial artery injuries among 304 arterial injuries collected from the Korean Conflict, for a 29.3 per cent incidence. The interim statistics from the experience in Vietnam revealed almost an equal incidence of 28.3 per cent, representing 283 brachial artery injuries among 1000 acute major arterial injuries (Rich et al., 1970A).

A similar frequency is shown in 13 separate reports of civilian arterial injuries, representing a total of 300 brachial injuries among 1641 arterial injuries (Table 15–1). The lowest frequency of brachial artery injuries was reported by Bole and colleagues (1976) from New York; they found only 14 brachial artery injuries among 126 arterial injuries, for an incidence of 11.1 per cent. Kelly and Eiseman (1975) reported the highest frequency of 31.9 per cent, with 37 brachial artery injuries among 116 arterial injuries. The largest number of brachial artery injuries (78) was reported by Perry and co-workers (1971) in their series of 508 arterial injuries, for an incidence of 15.4 per cent.

The frequency of involvement of brachial artery trauma among the major civilian series of arterial injuries shown in Table 15–1 varied from 11 to 32 per cent. Some of the variation is due to terminology; that is, the axillary injuries occasionally were not clearly separated from the brachial injuries, since the axillary artery becomes the brachial artery after crossing the lower border of the teres major muscle. In Los Angeles, Treiman and associates (1966) combined axillary artery and brachial artery injuries for a total of 54 of 159 major arterial injuries. Similarly, the frequency reported may be influenced by inclusion of smaller distal arteries such as the radial and ulnar arteries. Kleinert and Kasdan (1963), in reviewing a series of 79 arterial injuries including small arteries such as the radial artery in the upper extremity, found 14

brachial artery injuries. Smith and co-workers (1963) found the brachial artery most frequently involved—30 arterial injuries, or more than 50 per cent of the total—in reviewing 54 acute arterial injuries of the upper extremity.

ETIOLOGY OF INJURIES

Most injuries are caused by low velocity missiles or by lacerations from knives or broken glass, especially in civilian trauma. Ashbell and co-workers (1967) thoroughly reviewed the problem of vascular injuries about the elbow. Although they included radial and ulnar arteries injuries along with 36 brachial artery injuries, the latter trauma representing more than 50 per cent of the total, the list of the wounding agents in Table 15–3 is fairly representative of the causes of brachial artery injuries in civilian experience. This list even includes a most unusual arrow wound. In two previously cited series of upper extremity arterial injuries, Smith and associates (1963) recorded 36 lacerations, noting that 16 were caused by broken glass windows or bottles. They also treated seven gunshot wounds and five fractures associated with acute arterial injuries of the upper extremity. Kleinert and Kasdan (1963) recorded 41 arterial injuries caused by knife lacerations, seven injuries caused by bullets, and three injuries caused by shotgun blasts.

In Vietnam, 250 of 283 injuries resulted from either fragments or missiles (Table 15–4). Rich and co-authors (1970A) found that nearly 50 per cent of the brachial artery injuries were due to fragments from various exploding devices, and that approximately 40 per cent of the patients sustained gunshot wounds (Fig. 15–3). In contrast to the high incidence of brachial artery injuries from broken glass in civilian experience, there was only one such injury of this type in the combat experience. Of the three patients who sustained blunt trauma, one patient was injured in a helicopter crash and another patient had a tree fall on him.

With the increasing frequency of cardiovascular diagnostic procedures, usually angiographic or cardiac catheterization, there has been a sharp increase in the frequency of subsequent brachial artery throm-

TABLE 15-3. CAUSES OF CIVILIAN ARTERIAL TRAUMA VASCULAR INJURIES ABOUT THE ELBOW*

INJURING AGENT	CASES	PER CENT	LACERATION	DESTRUCTION OF SEGMENT	THROMBOSIS	SPASM
Glass	19	29	17	2	—	—
Knife	13	20	12	1	—	—
Shotgun	8	12	1	7	—	—
Car accident	6	9	2	—	2	—
Bullet	5	8	3	—	1	1
Machinery	5	8	4	2	—	1
Crushing injury	4	6	4	—	—	—
Power saw	2	3	2	—	—	—
Fracture or dislocation	2	3	1	—	—	1
Arrow	1	2	1	—	—	—
Total	65	100	47	12	3	3
Percentage of total			72	18	5	5

*Ashbell, T. S., Kleinert, H. E. and Kutz, J. E., Clin. Orthop., *50*:107, 1967.

bosis (Fig. 15-4). At Walter Reed General Hospital, thrombosis of either the axillary or brachial artery has been found to occur in approximately 1 per cent of the studies performed. If thrombosis is promptly recognized, repair is usually satisfactory. However, the potential gravity of such problems should not be underestimated. In one particularly tragic case at New York University, a series of complications developed after brachial thrombosis subsequent to retrograde cardiac catheterization for coronary angiography. A number of operative procedures were performed over the following three months because of recurrent thrombosis, but eventually amputation of the hand and lower forearm became necessary. It was thought that the unusual severity of this problem was caused by diffuse distal embolization of thrombotic

material with widespread occlusion of the peripheral vascular bed.

Fractures or dislocations of the humerus often injure the brachial artery. Such injuries with supracondylar fractures of the humerus have resulted in the ischemic syndrome of Volkmann's contracture; fortunately, this is now rare because of a better

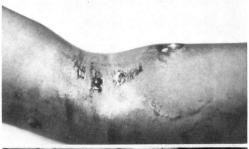
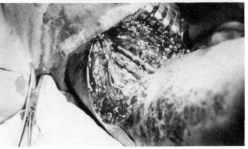

Figure 15-3. Low velocity gunshot wound in Vietnam which traumatized the brachial artery. A successful end-to-end anastomosis was possible (Rich, N. M., Surg. Clin. North Amer., *53*:1367, 1973.)

TABLE 15-4. CAUSES OF BRACHIAL ARTERY TRAUMA IN VIETNAM

AGENT	ARTERIES	PER CENT
Fragment wound	135	47.7
Gunshot wound	115	40.6
Blunt trauma	3	1.1
"Cut down"	2	0.7
Glass	1	0.35
Saw	1	0.35
Unknown	26	9.2
Total	283	100.0

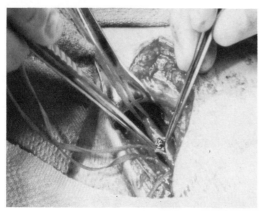

Figure 15–4. There has been an associated increase of brachial artery thrombosis secondary to the increasing use of cardiovascular diagnostic procedures, including angiographic and cardiac catheterization. This photograph taken during surgery demonstrates thrombus in the proximal brachial artery. (Rich, N. M., Hobson, R. W., II, and Collins, G. J., Jr., Am. J. Surg., *128*:715, 1974.)

understanding of etiology and prompt treatment. MacLean (1963) reported an unusual example of a four year old boy who sustained a supracondylar fracture; the radial pulse was absent even after reduction of the fracture. An angiogram (Fig. 15–5) demonstrated traumatic occlusion of the brachial artery. Fortunately, however, collateral circulation was sufficient to prevent ischemia. Kilburn and colleagues (1962) reported an unusual example of posterior dislocation of the right elbow with rupture of the brachial artery in a 13 year old girl (Fig. 15–6). Klingensmith and co-authors (1965A) emphasized that damage to an artery most likely occurs where the artery is in close approximation to bone and is held more or less fixed by muscle or another bone. They noted that the brachial artery was particularly vulnerable where it is closely adjacent to the humeral shaft or distorted at the site of a supracondylar fracture.

Rarely, blunt trauma directly over the brachial artery can cause thrombosis. Rob and Standaven (1956) reported two such instances. One patient received a blow from the edge of a locker in a fall, and the second patient slipped and struck the inner aspect of his arm against the edge of a large wooden box. A large hematoma may also rarely compress the brachial artery; when

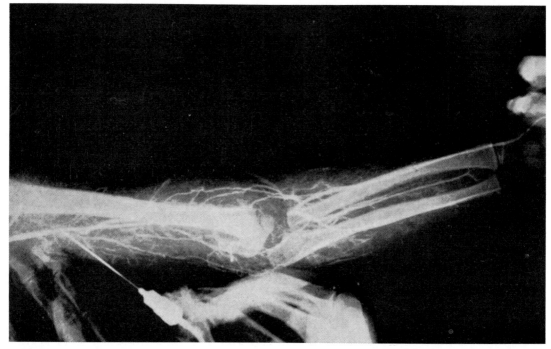

Figure 15–5. Angiogram reveals a block in the brachial artery with reconstitution of the distal blood supply to the hand through excellent collaterals. This was an unusual case of a 4 year old boy with a supracondylar fracture who had an absent radial pulse, even after reduction of the fracture. (MacLean, L. D., Can. Med. Assoc. J., *88*:1037, 1963.)

associated with arterial spasm, the hematoma may occlude the artery. One such example was reported by Ashbell and associates (1967) when they documented an extravascular compression in a patient who suffered a contusion to the right antecubital fossa in an automobile accident (Fig. 15–7). Exploration of the large hematoma revealed severe arterial spasm. This was effectively treated by evacuation of the hematoma, stripping of the arterial adventitia and infiltration of lidocaine. Finally, in the category of unusual injuries, at least two patients in Vietnam had injury of the brachial artery during a rapid cut-down under combat conditions.

Accidental intra-arterial injection of drugs by drug addicts has been an increasing contributor to the damage of arteries. Gaspar and Hare (1972) reported the injection of a drug, usually secobarbitol (Seconal), into the brachial artery in 13 of 20 patients in the series. Intense pain with cyanosis and mottling of the forearm and hand and swelling and induration of the entire hand were prominent features (see Chap. 26).

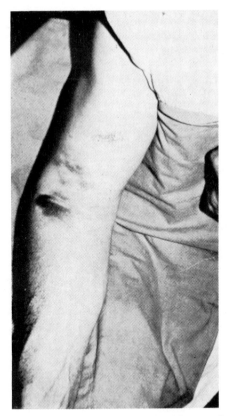

Figure 15–7. Contusion and hematoma of the right antecubital fossa caused by a car accident. Because of a cold, numb hand with a barely perceptible radial pulse, the antecubital fossa was explored. A large hematoma, which had compressed the brachial artery with resultant spasm, was evacuated. Release of the compression, adventitial stripping and periarterial infiltration of Lidocaine relieved the spasm, and distal pulses returned. (Ashbell, T. S., Kleinert, H. E., and Kutz, J. E., Clin. Orthop., *50*:107, 1967.)

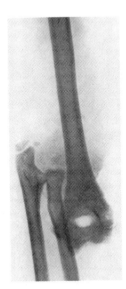

Figure 15–6. Unusual example of posterior dislocation of the right elbow in a 13 year old girl with associated rupture of the brachial artery. Although the artery was ligated at the time that the dislocation was reduced, there was a palpable radial pulse on the fourth postoperative day because of excellent collateral flow. (Kilburn, P. K., Sweeney, J. G., and Silk, F. F., J. Bone Joint Surg., *44-B*:119, 1962.)

CLINICAL PATHOLOGY

Although all varieties of arterial trauma, ranging from thrombosis after blunt trauma to destruction of a segment of the artery from a high velocity bullet, have been described with brachial injuries, laceration is the most common. Ashbell and associates (1967) found laceration in 72 per cent of a series of 65 arterial injuries in the elbow region; the report did not separate radial and ulnar artery injuries from the 36 brachial artery injuries. They also found destruction of a segment of the artery in 12 cases, thrombosis in three and spasm in three. Smith and co-authors (1963), who did

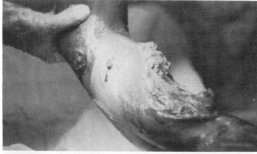

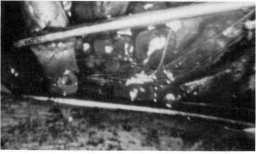

Figure 15–8. Vietnam casualty demonstrates two high velocity gunshot wounds caused by 7.62 mm. bullets which severed the brachial artery. Note also the relatively small entrance wounds above the elbow and the much larger proximal exit wound with massive soft tissue destruction. Below, end-to-end anastomosis was possible, shown partially completed, after adequate débridement. (Rich, N. M., J. Cardiovasc. Surg., *11*:368, 1970.)

not separate axillary artery injuries from the brachial artery injuries, found lacerations from knives and broken glass in 36 of 54 patients. On the other hand, Kleinert and Kasdan (1963) documented a considerable difference in their results when they reported a total of 61 completely severed arteries of a series of 79 cases which included injury to all arteries of the upper extremity. There were only 16 lacerated arteries and two with thrombosis.

In a series of 100 arterial segments removed following arterial trauma in Vietnam, study of the 26 segments of the brachial artery revealed findings very similar to those of arterial injuries in other areas (Rich et al., 1969C) (see Chap. 2).

What was once an unusual form of injury but was seen more frequently in Vietnam is thrombosis caused by the temporary cavitational effect of a high velocity missile passing near but not touching the artery. One example from Vietnam is shown in Figure 15–8, which demonstrates thrombosis of the brachial artery following a high velocity gunshot wound of the upper extremity. Therapy consisting of resection of the thrombosed segment and insertion of

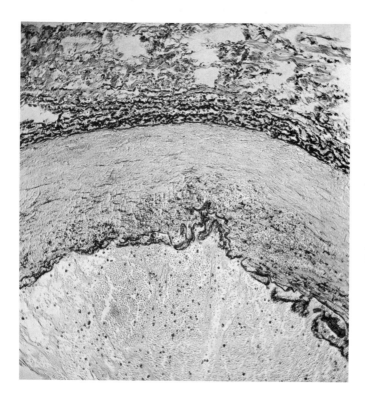

Figure 15–9. Microscopic evaluation of one end of the traumatized brachial artery segment shown in Fig. 15–8 demonstrates disruption of the media and intima with hemorrhage and infiltration of polymorphonuclear cells. There is also thrombus within the lumen, as noted above the disrupted intima. (Vietnam Vascular Registry Study at Armed Forces Institute of Pathology.)

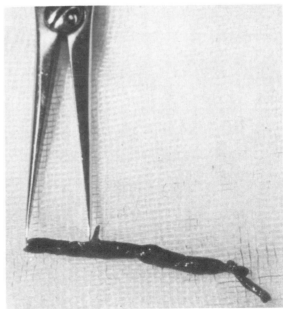

Figure 15–10. Segmental thrombosis may develop in the proximal brachial artery after retrograde catheterization for angiographic studies, particularly when associated with elevation of a strip of intima. This postoperative photograph is a typical example of relatively fresh thrombus that was removed by Fogarty catheter through a small arteriotomy in the brachial artery. (W.R.G.H.)

a saphenous vein graft was successful despite the fact that there were microscopic changes at one end of the resected segment (Fig. 15–9).

Thrombosis may develop after retrograde catheterization if a strip of intima has been detached and subsequently prolapses into lumen or acts as a nidus for thrombus formation (Fig. 15–10).

Because of the proximity of the humerus and peripheral nerves to the brachial artery, concomitant injuries of these structures are frequent. In the 283 brachial artery injuries studied in Vietnam, a peripheral nerve injury occurred in 204 (72 per cent), a fracture in 98 (35 per cent) and trauma to adjacent major veins in 65 (23 per cent) (Table 15–5).

CLINICAL FINDINGS

The usual clinical findings are a cool, pale hand with an absent radial pulse and im-

TABLE 15–5. BRACHIAL ARTERY TRAUMA, 283 INJURIES, IN VIETNAM CONCOMITANT INJURIES

NERVE INJURY	FRACTURE	VEIN TRAUMA
204	98	65
72.1%	34.6%	23.0%

paired sensation and motor function. Paresthesias or pain are frequent findings. A palpable radial pulse, however, does not exclude arterial injury. The laceration may be temporarily sealed by thrombus without obstructing the distal flow of blood. Also, collateral circulation within a few days is often adequate to maintain a weak but definite radial pulse. Distal pulses may also be present when a brachial artery injury results in the formation of a false aneurysm or an arteriovenous fistula. These lesions should be recognized by a thrill and bruit: the arteriovenous fistula can usually easily be recognized by the presence of prominent veins, a characteristic thrill and a continuous bruit. Jeresaty and Liss (1968) reviewed the effects of brachial artery catheterization on arterial pulse and blood pressure in 203 patients undergoing retrograde cardiac catheterization by means of a brachial arteriotomy. Occlusion or stenosis of the brachial artery associated with an obtainable auscultatory blood pressure occurred in 57 patients (28 per cent). Of these 57 patients, eight (3.9 per cent of the total series) had no radial pulse.

Obvious brachial artery trauma might be associated with bright red, pulsatile bleeding in an open wound. However, if the brachial artery trauma was caused by a closed injury from blunt trauma or from a small, low velocity missile, the hematoma should be viewed with suspicion as possibly associated with an arterial injury.

The occurrence of peripheral nerve injuries in nearly 70 per cent of patients with brachial artery trauma complicates evaluation and makes it necessary to use other clinical findings to evaluate the degree of ischemia present.

DIAGNOSTIC MEASURES

The use of plethysmography or the ultra-sonic sounding device (Doppler) can help

substantiate the clinical impression. Figure 15–11 demonstrates the lower pressure and the relatively flattened curve on the plethysmographic tracing in the upper extremity where the brachial artery was occluded following a percutaneous angiographic study.

Roentgenograms of the upper extremity may be helpful in disclosing fractures or dislocations or in demonstrating retained missiles, particularly when they are found in the area of the brachial artery. If uncertainty exists about the diagnosis, angiography can be performed. Angiography is

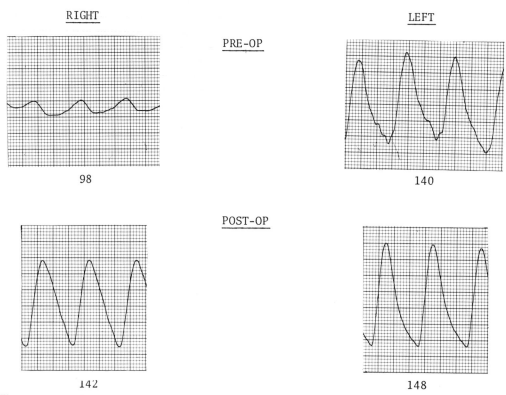

Figure 15–11. Compared to plethysmographic tracings from the upper extremity of the normal side, these tracings demonstrate the relatively lowered pressure and flattened curve from the upper extremity in which the brachial artery was occluded following a percutaneous angiographic study. Within two hours post-thrombectomy, studies from both upper extremities were essentially equal. (W.R.G.H.)

particularly helpful in patients who have had blunt trauma or in patients where there is suspected arterial trauma associated with fractures and dislocations. Actually, this diagnostic tool has seldom been necessary in military experience because the diagnosis has usually been obvious in the open wounds. The simplest approach in uncertain instances is careful exploration of the brachial artery during operative débridement of the wound.

SURGICAL MANAGEMENT

With the ease of diagnosis and the superficial location of the brachial artery, a high frequency of successful arterial repair can be anticipated. However, complications and failures are not unusual, probably because of the small size of the artery in some patients and the frequency with which significant arterial spasm develops, seemingly much more commonly than in the arteries of the lower extremity. Routine preoperative management includes adequate blood and fluid replacement and early administration of broad spectrum antibiotics.

Hemorrhage can usually be controlled by direct pressure. With distal injuries, a pneumatic tourniquet near the axilla can be used temporarily. Surgical exposure is best with a longitudinal incision along a course of the brachial artery extended as an S-curve across the axilla proximally or across the antecubital fossa distally, as needed (Fig. 15–12). The median nerve is the structure most vulnerable to injury because it must be separated and retracted from the artery to expose the artery properly. The brachial veins often form a network around the artery and can cause troublesome bleeding if hemostasis is not precise.

Following débridement of devitalized tissue and profuse irrigation to remove foreign debris, the traumatized artery can be debrided of all grossly injured arterial wall. Careful inspection of the intima near the margins of resection should be made. Although grossly normal artery walls should not be sacrificed, areas of contusion with the probability of intimal fracture or of a subintimal hematoma should be excised.

Before arterial repair is performed, a Fogarty catheter should be advanced down the distal artery to the hand to remove any distal thrombus. If feasible, selective passage of the catheter down both the radial and the ulnar arteries should be done.

Lateral repair of brachial artery injuries should rarely, if ever, be done. On initial inspection of the laceration, repair by lateral suture may seem simple and attractive, but such repairs have a high frequency of both immediate thrombosis and late stenosis, probably because of the relatively small size of the artery. Infrequently, an autogenous vein patch graft may be used. The only exception to the above comments might involve trauma to the brachial artery caused by a needle or catheter.

The safest method of management is excision of the area of injury followed by direct repair by end-to-end anastomosis. With transections, elastic recoil of the two ends of the artery may initially simulate substantial loss of arterial tissue. Following application of vascular clamps, however, gentle traction can usually be made and the ends approximated satisfactorily for anastomosis. As the brachial artery has a long, straight course without significant branches, mobilization for a few centimeters both proximally and distally is often possible. With an associated fracture of the humerus, arterial repair is actually facilitated because the humerus may be shortened to a slight degree. If a vascular graft is needed, the reversed autogenous greater saphenous vein is preferable, even though the cephalic vein is theoretically more accessible and some reports have emphasized that its use is equally successful. Synthetic grafts, such as Dacron, should be avoided, particularly in contaminated wounds. Ligation of the brachial artery rarely may be necessary with multiple injuries which threaten survival of a patient, or with destructive wounds associated with massive soft tissue loss.

In Table 15–6 are shown methods of arterial repair employed in 80 brachial artery injuries treated in the Korean Conflict and 273 treated in Vietnam. An end-to-end anastomosis was possible in the majority of arterial reconstructions in the Korean injuries, while autogenous vein grafts were used in almost 40 per cent of the 273 arterial injuries in Vietnam.

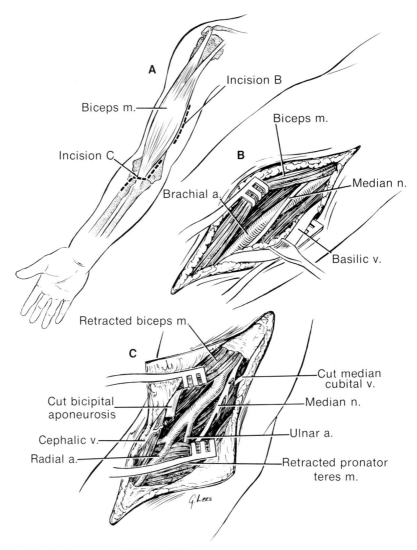

Figure 15–12. Surgical exposure of the brachial artery is rapidly obtained by a longitudinal incision along the course of the artery with an extension as an S-curve either across the axilla proximally or across the antecubital fossa distally, as needed. The median nerve and basilic veins are in close proximity to the artery.

TABLE 15–6. AMPUTATION RATE FOR BRACHIAL ARTERY INJURIES

Author	Arteries	Amputated	Per Cent
Following Ligation			
Hughes (1958)	9	3	33.3
Rich et al. (1970A)	7	3	42.9
Following Repair			
Hughes (1958)	80	0	0.0
Rich et al. (1970A)	276	13	4.7

Soft tissue coverage after reconstruction is usually not difficult unless there has been massive destruction of associated structures. Further wound closure is usually best delayed three to six days unless contamination is minimal. A fasciotomy is needed much less frequently than in the lower extremity, probably because the smaller muscles are much less vulnerable to ischemia. However, muscle turgor should be carefully followed and a fasciotomy performed if serious edema evolves. Also, in the absence of concomitant nerve injuries, development of paresthesia might indicate the need for fasciotomy.

Anticoagulants do not play a significant role in operative treatment, although a frequent practice is to inject 10 to 20 mg of heparin solution into the distal artery at the time of reconstruction. This is primarily to prevent the formation of distal thrombi during reconstruction.

If distal pulses are not readily palpable after reconstruction, possible causes include distal thrombi, stenosis at the anastomosis or, rarely, a separate distal arterial injury. In such instances an operative angiogram is of great value.

Concomitant fractures are usually treated by external fixation. Although internal fixation is commonly used in civilian trauma, it is best avoided in contaminated wounds from military trauma. Associated nerve injuries should be noted and the location of the nerve ends marked for repair at a later time. Repair of injuries to major veins may be done if simple lacerations are present, but more complex repairs are probably superfluous since venous insufficiency following ligation in the upper extremity is virtually unknown.

Although beyond the scope of this discussion, the possibility of replantation of a severed extremity should be kept in mind. A recent report by Malt and associates (1972) presented convincing data that in ideal circumstances useful extremities can be obtained by replantation.

POSTOPERATIVE CARE

Immediately following reconstruction, distal pulses, usually the radial, should be palpable. These are detected more simply than in the lower extremity, where edema occurs more commonly. An absent pulse following repair is always a cause for serious concern. The physical factors to be considered are thrombi in the distal artery or thrombosis of the anastomosis. Thrombosis may result from inadequate débridement of the injured arterial wall, stenosis of the anastomosis from a constricting suture, or

excessive tension on the suture line following excision of the injured arterial segment. An additional arterial lesion should not be overlooked. There may be concomitant trauma to the axillary artery or additional injuries to the radial and ulnar arteries. Arteriography may indicate the best method of treatment, with surgical exploration at the site of anastomosis as an alternate possibility. If the extremity is warm, with intact sensation and motor function, the risk of gangrene is almost negligible, and operation may be delayed for an indefinite period of time. If there has been significant wound contamination, reoperation has an increased risk of infection; therefore, delay may be wise. However, the high frequency of concomitant nerve injuries often eliminates the valuable clinical guides of loss of sensation or motor function in determining the severity of ischemia present. In some patients without palpable pulses, the ultrasonic sounding device (Doppler) has been helpful in confirming adequate peripheral blood flow. Sympathetic blocks, sympathectomy, anticoagulants or dextran will have limited, if any, value in postoperative care. Fasciotomy, seldom needed, should be performed promptly if increasing turgor develops in muscles of the forearm.

If there are no signs of wound infection, secondary closure can be done four to five days after the initial operation. Physical therapy is particularly important and should be started early in the postoperative period, with particular attention to maintenance of shoulder motion as well as function of the hand.

Wound infection followed by wound disruption of the anastomosis and secondary hemorrhage is the most feared postoperative complication, constituting a threat to the patient's life as well as to the extremity. Ligation of the artery is most often necessary. Fortunately, collateral circulation is usually adequate to permit survival of the arm, especially in the absence of extensive soft tissue injuries (Fig. 15–13). In some unusual instances in Vietnam, as many as six attempts, all unsuccessful, were made to repair an infected brachial artery. This example is mentioned only to indicate the futility of attempted repair in the presence of infection.

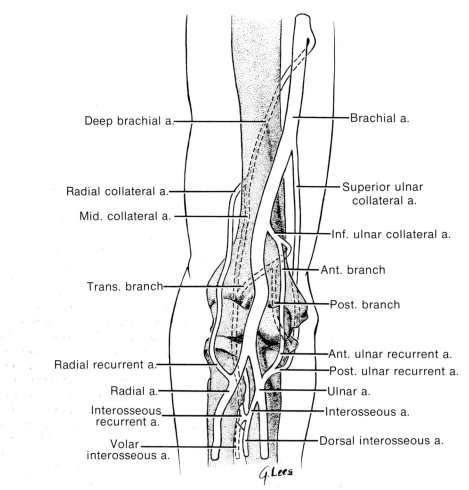

Figure 15–13. Excellent collateral circulation of the arm and elbow. The important collateral vessels are the deep brachial, the radial and ulnar recurrent, and the ulnar collateral arteries.

RESULTS

In the treatment of 283 brachial artery injuries in Vietnam, ligation was necessary in seven patients, three of whom subsequently required amputation (Table 15–6). Among the 276 treated by arterial reconstruction, only 13 (4.7 per cent) required amputation. Of the 13 amputations necessary following repair, seven had been done with an end-to-end anastomosis and six were repaired with vein grafts.

Fifty per cent of the 276 repairs were done by end-to-end anastomosis, approximately 44 per cent with vein grafts and a small number (18 patients) by lateral suture (Table 15–7). The saphenous vein was used in almost all of the vein graft repairs per-

TABLE 15–7. METHOD OF BRACHIAL ARTERY REPAIR

AUTHOR	ARTERIES	END-TO-END ANASTOMOSIS	VEIN GRAFT	ARTERY GRAFT	DACRON PROSTHESIS	LATERAL SUTURE
Hughes (1958)	80	59	9	4	0	8
Rich et al. (1970A)	276	138	120	0	0	18

formed. In the Korean Conflict, Hughes (1958) reported that no amputations were necessary following repair of brachial artery injuries. Fifty-nine of the 80 repairs were done by direct anastomosis, while autogenous vein grafts were used in nine, lateral suture repair in eight and artery grafts in four.

Complications occurred in almost 24 per cent of the patients following brachial artery reconstruction. Thrombosis was the most frequent, while hemorrhage subsequent to infection and disruption of the anastomosis were the most serious in this interim Registry report from the Vietnam Vascular Registry (Rich et al., 1970A).

Amputation has rarely been necessary following civilian brachial artery trauma. In 1960, Morris and associates described 49 brachial injuries among a series of 220 over-all arterial injuries. Three amputations were necessary in the group of 49. Two amputations were necessary following direct repair, and one amputation was necessary in a brachial artery repair using a graft. Patman and co-workers (1964) reported amputation in two patients in a series of 46 brachial artery repairs, and Treiman and associates (1966) similarly described amputation in two patients in a group of 54 brachial artery injuries. Ashbell and co-workers (1967) reported one amputation after 34 brachial artery reconstructions, and Dillard and co-workers (1968) reported no amputations after 26 brachial artery reconstructions. Bole and associates (1976) had no amputations following 14 brachial artery repairs. One vein graft failed in a 7 year old child; however, the extremity remained viable and functional.

FOLLOW-UP

Detailed follow-up of arterial repairs for civilian injury has been minimal. It is noteworthy that late ischemic symptoms are almost unknown. In all likelihood, thrombosis that does occur is usually associated with sufficient collateral circulation to prevent symptoms. There are a few illustrative and interesting cases which warrant documentation in civilian series. Beall and co-authors 1966 presented a case of a patient with a gunshot wound of the right brachial artery; the wound was successfully repaired by end-to-end anastomosis, with both the injury and the postoperative patency radiographically demonstrated (Fig. 15–14).

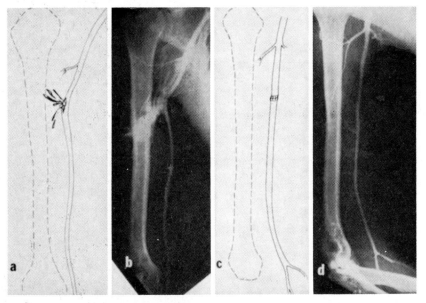

Figure 15–14. Gunshot wound of the brachial artery. (A) Drawing and (B) arteriogram demonstrating injury with extravasation of contrast media. (C) Drawing and (D) arteriogram demonstrating end-to-end repair following excision of the wound. (Beall, A. C., Jr., Diethrich, E. B., Morris, G. C., Jr., and DeBakey, M. E., Surg. Clin. North Am., *46*:1001, 1966.)

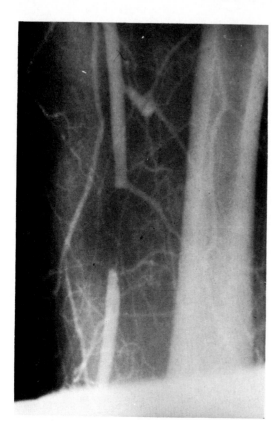

Figure 15–15. Arteriogram demonstrates a short segmental thrombosis in the mid-left brachial artery following a lateral arteriorrhaphy performed in Vietnam. Although there were no distal pulses palpable, the patient had a viable hand and was limited only by neurologic deficits. (Rich, N. M., Baugh, J. H., and Hughes, C. W., Arch. Surg., *100*: 646, 1970. Copyright 1970, American Medical Association.)

Figure 15–16. This angiogram demonstrates severe stenosis of the proximal anastomosis of an autogenous saphenous vein graft to the right brachial artery. Although prominent collateral circulation was evident between the humeral circumflex and the deep brachial arteries, the patient developed discomfort in his forearm muscles with repetitive motions. (Rich, N. M., Baugh, J. H., and Hughes, C. W., Arch. Surg., *100*:646, 1970. Copyright 1970, American Medical Association.)

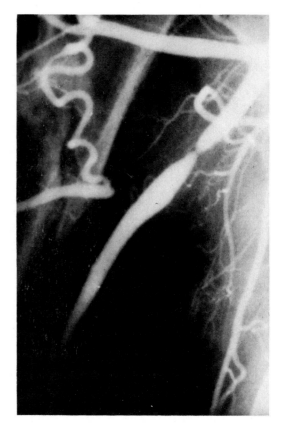

Hershey and Spencer (1960) reported proximal and distal arteriosclerotic narrowing that resulted in the late occlusion of a brachial artery vein graft which had been used in repairing an arteriovenous fistula. They mentioned that the brachial pulse returned and that the patient was able to perform manual labor with no disability.

Ninety-one patients who had brachial artery injuries repaired in Vietnam have been evaluated by one of the authors (NMR) at Walter Reed General Hospital. This group represents nearly one-third of the 283 patients sustaining acute brachial artery trauma reported in the interim review from the Vietnam Vascular Registry (Rich et al., 1970A). Some of the patients with complete thrombosis of the brachial artery repair site have remained asymptomatic (Fig. 15–15). Usually, neurological deficits have constituted the principal disability. One unusual problem developed in a patient whose radial pulse gradually weakened as a loud systolic bruit developed over the site of arterial repair five months after operation. Angiography showed stenosis of the proximal anastomosis of the saphenous vein graft (Fig. 15–16). At operation it was possible to excise the short segment of stenosis and re-establish arterial continuity by direct anastomosis between the proximal brachial artery and the saphenous vein graft.

CHAPTER 16

RADIAL AND ULNAR ARTERY INJURIES

In both military and civilian experience, trauma to the radial and ulnar arteries frequently has been overlooked or given only brief mention in numerous series reviewing the management of arterial trauma. In both World War I (Makins, 1919) and World War II (DeBakey and Simeone, 1946), the incidence of radial and ulnar artery trauma was in the range of 5 per cent (Table 16–1). There were no statistics regarding radial and ulnar artery trauma available from the Korean Conflict (Hughes, 1958) or from the recent experience in Vietnam (Rich et al., 1970A). Although some recent civilian series do report an incidence of approximately 20 per cent (Drapanas et al., 1970; Perry et al., 1971), there are only minimal details regarding the management and results (Table 16–1).

Because either the radial or ulnar artery frequently can be ligated without any resultant symptoms, far too often these injuries are considered insignificant. Occasionally, however, when both the radial and ulnar arteries are simultaneously injured, the magnitude of the vascular deficit can rapidly change from minor to major and threaten loss of viability of the hand. If more

TABLE 16–1. INCIDENCE OF RADIAL AND ULNAR ARTERY INJURIES

	AUTHOR	TOTAL ARTERIES	RADIAL-ULNAR	PER CENT
War Series				
WW I	Makins (1919)	1202	59	4.9
WW II	DeBakey and Simeone (1946)	2471	168	6.1
Korean	Hughes (1958)	304	–	–
Vietnam	Rich et al. (1970A)	1000	–	–
Civilian Series				
Houston	Morris et al. (1960)	220	33	15.0
Atlanta	Ferguson et al. (1961)	200	54	27.0
Denver	Owens (1963)	70	4	5.7
Detroit	Smith et al. (1963)	61	7	11.5
Dallas	Patman et al. (1964)	271	51	18.8
Los Angeles	Treiman et al. (1966)	159	–	–
St. Louis	Dillard et al. (1968)	85	–	–
New Orleans	Drapanas et al. (1970)	226	46	20.4
Dallas	Perry et al. (1971)*	508	97	19.1
New York	Bole et al. (1976)	126	9	7.1

*This is a sequential study including the earlier report.

interest is taken in repair of these injuries, success in repair may be more easily obtained when it is particularly important. If one has to choose between repair of one or the other artery, the radial artery might be selected because more attention is given to it during physical examination. However, the ulnar artery is generally larger and might be repaired more readily.

Additional attention recently has been given to trauma to the radial and ulnar arteries because of the increased use of intra-arterial monitoring and intra-arterial drug injections; both of these procedures occasionally produce distal ischemic problems.

With continued refinement of techniques in hand surgery, successful repair of digital arteries has been accomplished. However, this material is presently beyond the scope of our presentation. Replantation of hands has received increased interest in the past five years, with some long term data becoming available at a few medical centers.

SURGICAL ANATOMY

After the brachial artery passes through the cubital fossa beneath the lacertus fibrosus, it divides into the radial and ulnar arteries at the level of the coronoid process of the ulna and the neck of the radius. Additional description and diagrams can be found in Chapter 15, Brachial Artery Injuries, regarding the usual anatomy as well as the aberrant variations in the origin of the radial and ulnar arteries. Also included in Chapter 15 is consideration of the rich collateral blood supply around the elbow.

The ulnar artery is the larger of the two terminal branches of the brachial artery; however, the difference in size becomes somewhat less apparent near the wrist (Fig. 16–1). The artery takes its origin in the cubital fossa at the level of the neck of the radius and passes obliquely downward and medially before it proceeds straight down to the wrist. Although the ulnar artery is the larger terminal branch, the radial artery is the more direct continuation of the brachial artery. The anterior and posterior ulnar recurrent arteries arise near the elbow as the first branches and anastomose

with branches of the brachial artery on the front and back of the medial epicondyle. About one inch below the origin of the ulnar artery and immediately below the origin of the recurrent branches, the common interosseous artery originates and passes backward to the upper margin of the interosseous membrane, where it divides into the volar, or anterior, and the dorsal, or posterior, interosseous arteries (Fig. 16–1). Below the bifurcation of the short common interosseous artery, there are four parallel arterial trunks with numerous segmental intercommunications which provide excellent collateral circulation. There is also a recurrent interosseous artery which contributes to the collateral blood supply around the elbow. The slender median artery can also be a branch of the anterior interosseous artery. The ulnar artery terminates in the superficial palmar, or volar, arch, with the arch continuing into one of three branches of the radial artery: superficial palmar, princeps pollicis or radialis indicis arteries (Fig. 16–2). According to the review by Strandness (1969), the superficial palmar arch has never been found to be absent; however, it is incomplete in about 20 per cent of cases. He also mentioned that the diverse and complex nature of the different patterns of the arterial supply to the hand have been studied in detail, and attempts to classify them by type have been abandoned. Alternate pathways to various portions of the hand are known and can be dominated by either the superficial or deep arches.

The ulnar artery passes through the deep fascia immediately above the flexor retinaculum and then passes on to the front of it. It is accompanied by two venae comitantes throughout its entire course. It runs deep to the forearm muscles arising from the mesial epicondyle. In the oblique upper portion it is crossed by both heads of the pronator teres and the flexor carpi radialis, the palmaris longus, the flexor digitorum sublimis and the median nerve (Fig. 16–3). In its lower vertical part, it is covered by the flexor carpi ulnaris, but near the wrist it comes closer to the surface and lies between the deep fascia in the interval between the tendon of the flexor carpi ulnaris and the tendons of the flexor sublimis. In the proximal portion, the median nerve crosses in

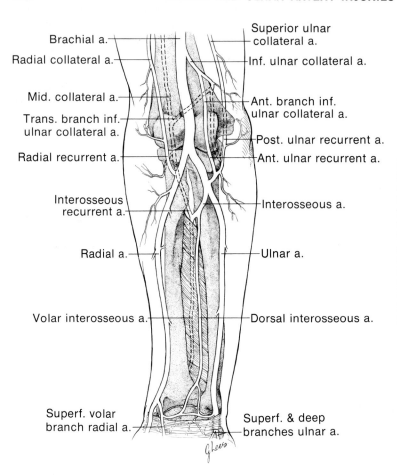

Brachial a.
Radial collateral a.
Mid. collateral a.
Trans. branch inf. ulnar collateral a.
Radial recurrent a.
Interosseous recurrent a.
Radial a.
Volar interosseous a.
Superf. volar branch radial a.

Superior ulnar collateral a.
Inf. ulnar collateral a.
Ant. branch inf. ulnar collateral a.
Post. ulnar recurrent a.
Ant. ulnar recurrent a.
Interosseous a.
Ulnar a.
Dorsal interosseous a.
Superf. & deep branches ulnar a.

Figure 16–1. As the brachial artery divides into the radial artery (its more direct continuation) and the ulnar artery (the larger of the two branches) in the forearm, there are important collateral branches which help form the rich anastomosis around the elbow. The common interosseous is also an important branch of the ulnar artery. Figure 16–2 illustrates the continuation of the circulation beyond the wrist level to the hand.

Figure 16–2. The contribution of the radial and ulnar arteries to the circulation of the hand. The ulnar artery that terminates in the superficial volar arch provides the majority of the blood supply to the fingers; however, the radial artery that terminates in the deep volar arch provides the blood supply to the thumb and the thenar side of the index finger, as well as important collateral pathways to the superficial volar arch.

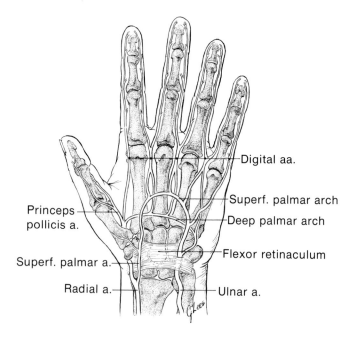

Digital aa.
Superf. palmar arch
Deep palmar arch
Flexor retinaculum
Princeps pollicis a.
Superf. palmar a.
Radial a.
Ulnar a.

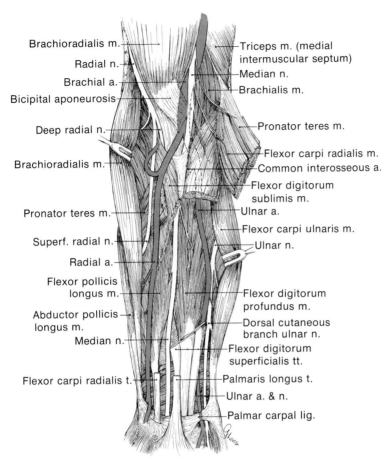

Figure 16-3. The relationship of the radial and ulnar arteries to the important nerves, major muscle groups and tendons. Particularly note the crossing of the proximal ulnar artery by the median nerve and the close approximation of the ulnar nerve to the distal two-thirds of the ulnar artery. The cross section through the upper third of the forearm emphasizes the relatively deep location of the ulnar artery compared with the more superficial radial artery.

front of the ulnar artery, but these two structures are separated from each other by the ulnar head of the pronator teres muscle. The ulnar nerve is adjacent to the ulnar artery when the artery begins its straight descent in the middle third of the forearm, and the two structures are closely related at the wrist.

Although the radial artery is the smaller of the two terminal branches of the brachial artery, it is the more direct continuation of the latter in the forearm (Fig. 16–1). It originates in the cubital fossa opposite the neck of the radius and descends in the lateral part of the front of the forearm to the wrist level. The radial artery is unique in that no muscles cross over it, and it is different from the ulnar artery in that no

motor nerve crosses over it. It lies superficial to the skin, although it is covered by the brachioradialis in the upper forearm. Throughout its entire length it is closely accompanied by venae comitantes. The radial nerve lies along its lateral side in the middle third of the arm, and distally the nerve turns away from the artery (Fig. 16–3).

The radial recurrent artery originates near the beginning of the radial artery. It contributes to the rich anastomosis around the elbow by uniting with the anterior branch of the profunda brachii artery. The radial artery gives off numerous branches to muscles at irregular intervals, mainly in the upper course of the forearm; however, there are no major branches, such as the common interosseous from the ulnar artery. Near its termination at the wrist level, the radial artery gives rise to a superficial palmar artery and continues into the hand to form the deep palmar arch (Fig. 16–2). This arch is also joined to the deep branch of the ulnar artery.

There are several anatomic variations, according to Strandness (1969), which are worthy of consideration. The radial and ulnar arteries are almost never absent, but when they are, the arterial supply is taken over by the anterior interosseous artery. Another variation which can be seen is a persistent median artery, which is distinguished from the anterior interosseous artery because of its intimate association with the median nerve.

INCIDENCE

The incidence of trauma to the ulnar and radial arteries is undoubtedly much higher than reported. Often these injuries are felt to be of minor significance. Even in series identifying trauma to the ulnar and radial arteries, the injuries are frequently mentioned in combination.

In World War I, 59, or 4.9 per cent, of the injuries reported by Makins (1919) involved the radial and ulnar arteries (Table 16–1). In the American World War II experience, DeBakey and Simeone (1946) reported that the radial artery was involved in 99 patients and the ulnar artery in 69 patients. This total of 168 radial and ulnar artery injuries represented 6.1 per cent of the 2471 acute arterial injuries. Combined radial and ulnar artery injuries were present in 28 patients. In a summary of the results from the Korean Conflict, Hughes (1958) described 304 arterial injuries without including trauma to the radial and ulnar arteries. In the initial report from the Vietnam Vascular Registry, Rich and Hughes (1969) did not document any details regarding radial and ulnar artery injuries, and the interim Registry report (Rich et al., 1970A) involved 1000 acute arterial injuries of larger caliber. Although the Registry statistics remain incomplete, a total of 375 radial artery injuries and 320 ulnar artery injuries are included. Although the true incidence cannot yet be calculated,

it is conceivable that it will be higher than in previous wars because of a greater interest in documenting these injuries.

Among the major civilian series reviewing the management of arterial trauma, the incidence of radial and ulnar artery injuries has ranged from a low of 5.7 per cent, or 4 of 70 injuries, reported by Owens (1963), to a high of 27.0 per cent, or 54 of 200 injuries, reported from Atlanta by Ferguson and co-workers (1961) (Table 16–1). In one major report from New Orleans, Drapanas and co-authors (1970), in reporting 226 arterial injuries, found that a combined total of 46 radial and ulnar artery injuries represented the site most frequently involved (Fig. 16–4). The relatively high incidence of these injuries compared to other arterial injuries in their series is emphasized in Figure 16–5.

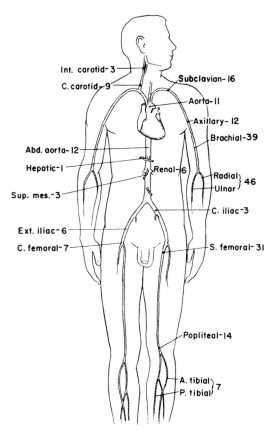

Figure 16–4. The distribution of 226 acute arterial injuries in New Orleans is outlined above. The largest number of injuries involves a combined total of 46 radial and ulnar arterial injuries (see Fig. 16–5). (Drapanas, T., Hewitt, R. L., Weichert, R. F., and Smith, A. D., Ann. Surg., *172:*351, 1970.)

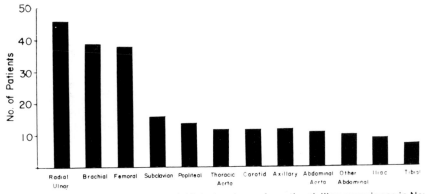

Figure 16–5. The frequency of various arterial injuries drawn from the civilian experience in New Orleans is presented above. A total of 46 radial and ulnar arterial injuries (see Fig. 16–4) represents the highest incidence of injury. (Drapanas, T., Hewitt, R. L., Weichert, R. F., and Smith, A. D., Ann. Surg., *172*:351, 1970.)

In considering the relative incidence of radial compared to ulnar artery injuries, the majority of civilian reports are similar to the World War II experience (DeBakey and Simeone, 1946) in documenting a higher incidence of radial artery injuries. Smith and associates (1963) stated that the radial artery was traumatized in five patients and the ulnar artery in two patients. Patman and co-authors (1964) found the radial artery was involved more than twice as often as the ulnar artery: 35 radial artery injuries in the combined total of 51. Perry and co-workers (1971) reported 58 radial artery injuries and 39 ulnar artery injuries. Only Ferguson and co-authors in Atlanta (1961) reported a reversal of these statistics when they found the radial artery was involved only 50 per cent as often as the ulnar artery, with 18 radial artery injuries in a combined total of 54.

ETIOLOGY

Trauma to the radial and ulnar arteries ranges from a small fragment wound of a single vessel to a much larger wound involving both the radial and ulnar arteries, as well as soft tissue, nerves, tendons and bone (Figs. 16–6 and 16–7).

In civilian life low velocity gunshot wounds and stab wounds, as well as blunt trauma from a variety of agents, can contribute to ulnar and radial artery injuries. The following quotation emphasizes that recognition of problems associated with expanding subfascial hematomas was cited as early as 1914 by Murphy:

In our cases it is fairly clear that hemorrhage beneath the aponeurosis of the upper forearm following fracture or injuries of the deep structures can cause myositis or subsequent contraction even when splints or bandages have not been used. These are the internal compression variety. The splints cause the external compression.

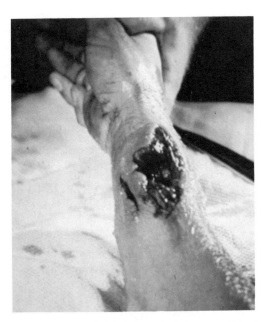

Figure 16–6. A large fragment from an 8-inch artillery round caused this wound proximal to the right wrist, which severed both the radial and ulnar arteries as well as the major nerves and tendons. (N.M.R., 2nd Surgical Hospital, 1966.)

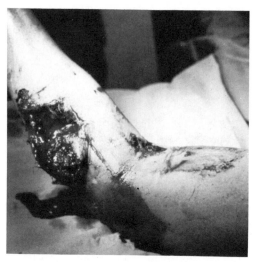

Figure 16–7. This high velocity gunshot wound of the forearm caused massive soft tissue and osseous damage, as well as disruption of numerous tendons, nerves and the ulnar artery and vein. (N.M.R., 2nd Surgical Hospital, 1966.)

Bennett (1965) emphasized that even minor-appearing injuries, such as a stab wound or puncture wound of the volar aspect of the forearm, may produce signs of neurovascular compression due to an expanding subfascial hematoma. He presented a case of a 23 year old man who punctured the volar surface of his left mid-forearm while opening a carton with a sharp knife. When first seen in the emergency room, only a small laceration at the location mentioned was noted. However, five hours later the patient returned to the emergency room complaining of pain and swelling in the left forearm. Examination showed the forearm to be tense and swollen with the fingers held in flexion. Radial and ulnar pulses were normal. After extensive forearm fasciotomy with expression of a massive hematoma, the patient regained full use of his forearm and hand. Great care must be taken to insure that no lacerations of the radial and ulnar arteries have occurred with puncture-type injuries.

There are several types of injury to the radial and ulnar arteries which present particular challenges. Bergan and associates (1971) named the traumatic thrombosis of the superficial palmar arch of the ulnar artery, which often results when the hand has been repeatedly used as a hammer, the hypothenar hammer syndrome. Invariably, the hypothenar eminence strikes the blow with a maximum force in the area of

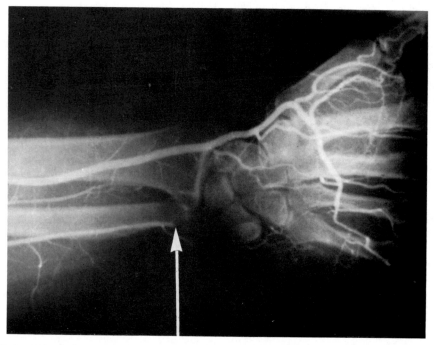

Figure 16–8. This angiogram demonstrates thrombosis of the terminal ulnar artery (arrow) in a woman who used her hand as a hammer over a three-year period while doing ceramic work. This is similar to the hypothenar hammer syndrome, as described by Bergan and associates (1971.) (W.R.G.H.)

the hook of the hamate. The superficial palmar arch of the ulnar artery lies directly over the hook of the hamate or to its ulnar side. Little and Ferguson (1972) emphasized that occlusion of the superficial palmar branch of the ulnar artery can occur among workers in mechanical workshops who use their hands as hammers. They reported that among 79 such habitual hammerers, 11 patients, or 14 per cent, demonstrated evidence of ulnar artery occlusion in one or both hands. Occlusion of the superficial palmar arch of the ulnar artery was reported in 13 hands of 11 patients from a group of 127 men who worked in a vehicle maintenance shop using their hands as hammers. Seventy-nine of the 127 men examined, or 62 per cent, habitually used their hands as hammers. A woman seen at Walter Reed Army Medical Center had sustained a similar injury and had used her hand as a hammer over a three-year period in her ceramic work (Figs. 16–8). Another patient was a young soldier who used his right hand to pound a pinball

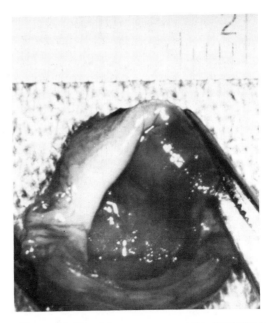

Figure 16–10. A true aneurysm of the distal ulnar artery was part of the hypothenar hammer syndrome illustrated in Fig. 16–9. (N.M.R.)

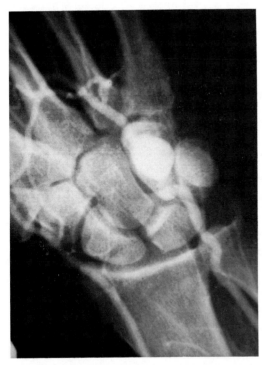

Figure 16–9. This angiogram outlines a true aneurysm of the ulnar artery in a young soldier who used his right hand to repeatedly pound a pinball machine (see also Fig. 16–10). (W.R.G.H., courtesy of Dr. George P. Bogumill.)

machine and subsequently developed a true aneurysm of the ulnar artery (Figs. 16–9 and 16–10).

Accidental intra-arterial injection of drugs, usually secobarbitol (Seconal) by drug addicts, has resulted in gangrenous changes in the extremity distal to the injection. Gaspar and Hare (1972) reported 20 such patients, including six who had an injection into either the radial or ulnar artery and had experienced intense pain, intense swelling, induration, cyanosis and mottling (Fig. 16–11).

The radial artery has occasionally been lacerated in a suicidal attempt. However, laceration or transection of the radial or ulnar arteries probably occurs more frequently when the hand is shoved, either accidentally or purposely, through a glass window or door.

There is increasing interest in the hazards of radial artery pressure monitoring. Complications can be mild (Fig. 16–12) or can result in gangrene requiring amputation. Saaman (1971) emphasized these hazards in describing three cases of ischemia of the hand following the use of the radial artery for prolonged pressure monitoring with ligature of the distal end

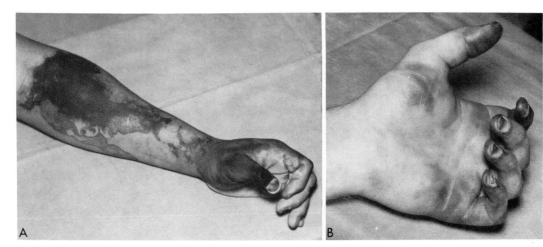

Figure 16–11. Intense swelling of the hand and flexion of fingers associated with intense pain, cyanosis and mottling are demonstrated above following injection of sodium secobarbital into the radial artery; these are typical findings associated with accidental intra-arterial drug injections. (Gaspar, M. R., and Hare, R. R., Surgery, 72:573, 1972.)

of the radial artery. Even without distal ligature, there have been five patients at Walter Reed Army Medical Center over the last eight years who have had ischemic changes in the hand associated with intra-arterial monitoring. Obviously, evaluation of patency of the ulnar artery and the palmar arches can also be of value in attempting to avoid this complication. Ischemia from this type of injury has occasionally required amputation (Fig. 16–13).

CLINICAL PATHOLOGY

Lacerations and transections of the radial and ulnar arteries are most frequently recorded. Contusion with intimal flaps and thrombosis from blunt trauma are also possible. Trauma can occur when associ-

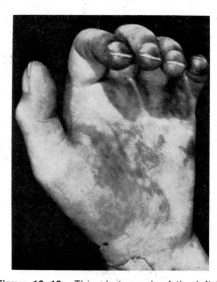

Figure 16–13. This photograph of the left hand shows pallor, edema and color changes on the skin of the fingers and the hand following radial artery pressure monitoring utilizing a plastic catheter with ligation of the distal radial artery. Ischemic changes progressed to gangrene in 48 hours, and an above-the-wrist amputation was required. (Samaan, H. A., J. Cardiovasc. Surg., 12:342, 1971.)

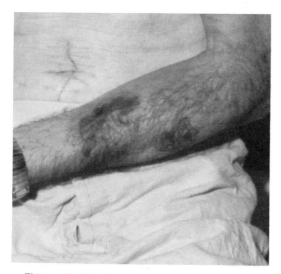

Figure 16–12. Local gangrenous skin changes can occur with radial arterial monitoring, or more extensive distal gangrene can develop and require subsequent amputation. (W.R.G.H.)

ated with fractures of the radius or ulna. Hull and Hyde (1967) noted that two of four radial and ulnar artery injuries were associated with fractures or dislocations.

Erskine (1964) documented the case of a 35 year old male mechanic who sustained a severe blow to the volar aspect of the right wrist when a wrench slipped. The patient developed a true aneurysm of the radial artery (Fig. 16–14). Pathologically it was found that the wall of the artery was weakened and dilated; however, there was no evidence of total disruption of the artery at any point. (See also Figs. 16–9 and 16–10.)

In the previously described hypothenar hammer syndrome, some of the pathologic problems associated with thrombosis of the superficial palmar arch are revealed. Because the superficial palmar arch of the ulnar artery provides the main source of blood for most of the fingers, digital ischemia and gangrene have been frequent findings with occlusion of this artery. Al-

though the superficial palmar arch is completed on the radial side, the communication is often quite small.

Concomitant venous trauma to the venae comitantes has not presented the problems it has in the lower extremities. On the other hand, frequent injuries to associated nerves occur, and residual disability is often caused by the nerve trauma rather than by the arterial trauma. Associated tendon injuries can also cause residual disability.

CLINICAL FEATURES

Early recognition of trauma to the ulnar and radial arteries can prevent serious complications. Cold sensitivity in the affected hand is a frequent complaint in patients with significant arterial insufficiency. Intermittent coldness, numbness, paresthesias and color change without exposure to cold can occur, as well as absence of pulses at the wrist. It must be remembered, however, that interruption of either the radial or ulnar artery frequently will have no adverse effect on the extremity circulation, particularly when the palmar arches are complete and intact.

Intense swelling and hematomas, as well as wounds and fractures in the forearm and hand, should alert one to the possibility of arterial trauma. Bennett (1965) presented the case of a 42 year old man who sustained a puncture wound of the volar surface of the right forearm with an electric drill (Fig. 16–15). Blood was seen to spurt from the wound, and the right forearm rapidly became tense with tingling of the fingers of the right hand. Although the radial pulse was interpreted as normal, one hour later in the emergency room the ulnar pulse was diminished. The patient was taken to the operating room where a forearm fasciotomy was carried out with evacuation of a moderate amount of hematoma. Exploration revealed incomplete transection of the ulnar artery. It was possible to repair the artery with 6–0 silk. This case, as well as a previously described case by Bennett (1965), emphasizes the potentially dangerous complications of puncture wounds of the extremity. Incomplete transection of an artery may

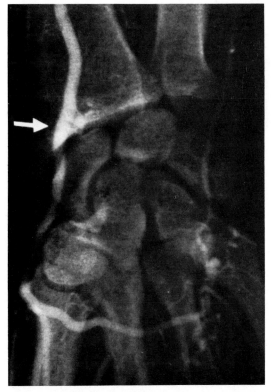

Figure 16–14. The above angiogram demonstrates a true aneurysm of the radial artery (arrow) caused by blunt trauma. (Erskine, J. M., J. Trauma, *4*:530, 1964. Copyright 1964, The Williams & Wilkins Co., Baltimore.)

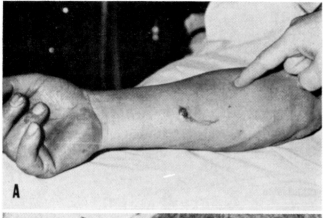

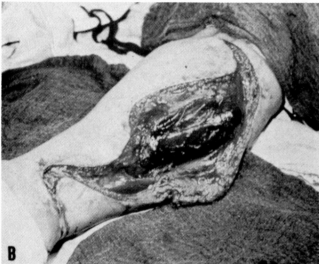

Figure 16–15. (A) A puncture wound of the volar surface of the forearm caused by a power drill is shown one hour after injury. The hand and fingers were hypoesthetic, particularly over the ulnar nerve distribution. (B) Decompression of the superficial flexor compartment was carried out through an extensive fasciotomy with evacuation of a moderate amount of hematoma. A partially transected ulnar artery was also repaired. (Bennett, J. E., Plast. Reconstr. Surg., *36*:622, 1965. Copyright 1965, The Williams & Wilkins Co., Baltimore.)

result in continuous bleeding and hematoma formation in a fairly rigid fascial compartment. Increased pressure within this compartment caused by the expanding hematoma may subsequently compress nerves, cause venous stasis and contribute to arterial spasm. The final outcome may be the development of Volkmann's ischemic contracture of the extremity. Physical signs that should alert the examiner to the possibility of an expanding hematoma in the forearm include marked tension in the fascial compartments, the development of superficial venous engorgement and the appearance of neuromuscular deficits in the hand, including numbness and tingling, as well as flexion of the fingers.

Little and Ferguson (1972) reported that symptoms of vascular insufficiency existed in all 11 patients with blocked ulnar arteries associated with the hypothenar hammer syndrome. The patients who used their hands as hammers in mechanical workshops were found to be older and to have had longer employment in the hammering jobs than those patients who used their hands as hammers but had intact ulnar arteries.

DIAGNOSTIC CONSIDERATIONS

The Allen test and a variation of this test can be invaluable in determining patency of the radial and ulnar arteries by utilizing compression of the opposite artery. In our follow-up of Vietnam casualties, we have frequently demonstrated occlusion of the proximal or midradial artery, when the patient had a strong radial pulse, by oc-

DOPPLER TRACING

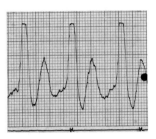

Recording over Ulnar Artery Distal to Repair
Ipsilateral Radial Artery Occluded

VVR# 815
20 August 1968

Figure 16–16. The ultrasonic sounding device (Doppler) has been valuable in determining the presence or absence of blood flow in the radial, ulnar and digital arteries. With the ipsilateral radial artery occluded, the above tracing demonstrates good flow through the repaired ulnar artery. (W.R.G.H.)

clusion of the distal ulnar artery, which also caused loss of the strong radial artery pulse at the wrist.

Roentgenograms of the upper extremities are also helpful in outlining fractures or dislocations which may have caused arterial trauma. Moreover, foreign bodies adjacent to the neurovascular bundles may be identified. In unusual cases, such as the two mentioned by Kleinert (1971), intra-arterial foreign bodies from missile embolization can be identified.

Use of the ultrasonic sounding device (Doppler) has been of value in evaluating patients (Figs. 16–16 and 16–17). Use of the Doppler was even extended to measuring flow in the digital arteries in the Walter Reed experience (Lavenson et al., 1970). Little and Ferguson (1972) found the Doppler of use in evaluating patients

PLETHYSMOGRAPHIC TRACINGS

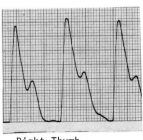

Right Thumb

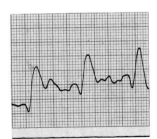

Left Thumb

Right Fifth Finger

Left Fifth Finger

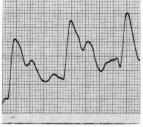

Wrist Pressure 150

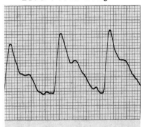

Wrist Pressure 120

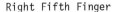

Figure 16–17. Plethysmographic tracings as well as Doppler tracings can give a graphic record of arterial flow in the digits. Wrist pressures can also be obtained. (W.R.G.H.)

with hypothenar hammer syndrome. They used the Doppler flow detector if an Allen test suggested ulnar artery occlusion. The Doppler test was performed with the probe over the digital arteries between the little and ring fingers, with a pulse tracing made on a chart recorder. The radial artery was then compressed at the wrist. It was assumed that ulnar artery circulation was deficient if the pulse wave form was dampened or eliminated. They found that this test correlated well with the findings of angiography when it substantiated the clinical evidence of occlusion of the superficial palmar arch of the ulnar artery.

In uncertain situations angiography can assist in documenting trauma to the radial and ulnar arteries; however, this usually would not be indicated with open wounds in which débridement and exploration were already indicated.

SURGICAL TREATMENT

Pressure can usually control hemorrhage in the majority of radial and ulnar artery injuries. Tourniquets usually are not warranted, because potential complications from their use far outweigh any advantages. The usual supportive measures should be instituted, fractures must be stabilized, and adequate wound débridement should be performed.

Exposure of the proximal portions of both arteries can be accomplished through an S-shaped incision in the cubital fossa, as diagrammed in Figure 15–12, showing the exposure of the brachial artery bifurcation. Although the ulnar artery is deeper than the radial, both can be approached from the volar aspect of the forearm through the longitudinal incisions (Fig. 16–18). Elective incisions should be used where necessary, and exposure should not be compromised by attempting to perform débridement through an entrance or exit wound away from the vessels.

Bleeding from the venae comitantes can frequently be troublesome. Ligation of these small veins will usually be helpful in obtaining a dry field. It is of paramount importance that all nerve and tendon injuries should also be noted and documented.

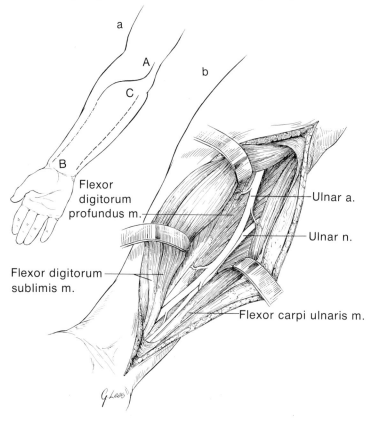

Flexor digitorum profundus m.

Flexor digitorum sublimis m.

Ulnar a.

Ulnar n.

Flexor carpi ulnaris m.

Figure 16–18. Elective incisions that can be utilized for approach to the radial and ulnar arteries. An S-type incision starting along the course of the distal brachial artery, carried through the antecubital fossa and continued down on the forearm will give excellent exposure of the proximal ulnar and radial arteries as well as the origin of the common interosseous artery (A). Additional details can be found in Chapter 15 regarding exposure of the distal brachial artery. An extension of this incision (B) along the course of the radial artery can be used for exposure to the wrist level. A separate incision can be used over the course of the ulnar artery (C); the companion drawing demonstrates exposure of the ulnar neurovascular bundle within the deep muscle layers which have been split proximally. No effort is made to demonstrate the exposure of the palmar arches, and the interested reader is referred to a text on hand surgery.

Frequently, concomitant tendon repair can be carried out; however, repair of major nerves, particularly in contaminated wounds, is usually best deferred for three to four weeks. The nerve ends can either be "marked" with small loops of wire, or the ends of the nerves can be very loosely approximated with several sutures through the epineurium to prevent retraction.

Because of the relatively small size of the radial and ulnar arteries, particularly in their medial and distal portions, reconstruction is frequently not feasible with extensive injuries. However, if there is a small laceration or defect, end-to-end anastomosis (Fig. 16–19) after adequate débridement may be performed easily and successfully. Lateral suture repair should be reserved essentially for puncture wounds following thrombectomy. If the patient's condition will permit, reconstruction with autogenous veins may be occasionally considered. The lower portion of the greater saphenous vein may be utilized to approximate more nearly the diameter of the artery, or the cephalic vein can provide an acceptable substitute. Fine synthetic vascular suture of either 6–0 or 7–0 size should be utilized. Frequently, interrupted sutures will help prevent anastomotic stenosis. Optical magnification may be of considerable value with the smaller vessels. The

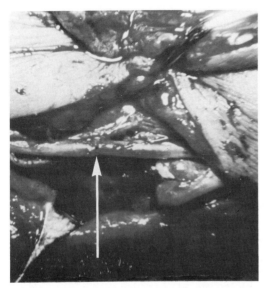

Figure 16–19. End-to-end anastomosis (arrow) was possible in the above successful ulnar arterial repair (see Figs. 16–6, 16–21, 16–22 and 16–23). (N.M.R., 2nd Surgical Hospital, 1966.)

Fogarty catheter, which should be passed to insure there is no residual intra-arterial thrombus, can also be used for careful intraluminal arterial dilatation. As was mentioned under Surgical Anatomy, the ulnar artery is usually larger than the radial artery and should be selected if a choice must be made (see Chapter 15, regarding repair of arterial injuries at the brachial artery bifurcation). At the wrist level, it is frequently possible to overcome a significant segmental loss of the ulnar artery with ulnar deviation of the hand and flexion of the wrist. The advantages of this maneuver are not as easily accomplished with the small radial artery. Additional comments regarding the repair of small arteries can be found in Chapter 5.

An aggressive approach should be utilized in managing fractures that are associated with large hematomas and distal ischemia. Not only should the fracture be adequately stabilized, but also exploration of the arteries should be carried out and decompression by fasciotomy achieved. Fasciotomy is not an important consideration in dealing with open wounds, because a limited type of fasciotomy is already accomplished. On the other hand, with closed wounds fasciotomy may be necessary. If fasciotomy is not performed, very careful and repeated observation should be carried out to insure that distal ischemia does not develop or that neurologic deficits do not occur. When fasciotomy is indicated, the deep fascia should be incised on the volar surface of the forearm from the wrist to the elbow. The lacertus fibrosus also should be incised to help decompress the distal brachial artery and the median nerve.

Intraoperative angiography is of importance for two reasons: to insure adequate patency of the repair site and to demonstrate distal patency. If there is residual thrombus in the palmar arches or digital arteries, distal ischemia of the fingers or hands may be present despite successful arterial repair in the forearm.

POSTOPERATIVE CARE

The usual supportive measures should be carried out as for any patient with upper

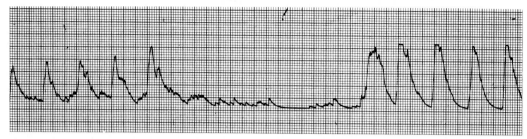

Figure 16–20. The ultrasonic sounding device (Doppler) can be of value in confirming the clinical impression of success or failure of repair of radial or ulnar arterial injuries. In the above tracing, radial arterial flow is demonstrated to come through the ulnar artery. This disproved the clinical impression that a palpable radial pulse meant there had been a successful end-to-end anastomisis of the mid-radial artery. (W.R.G.H.)

extremity injury. Particular attention should be given to the development of any edema or changes in neurologic status, particularly if fasciotomies have not been performed during the operation. If the wound was closed and there was no operation, fasciotomies may be necessary in the early postinjury period.

The ultrasonic sounding device (Doppler) can be of extreme value in determining flow distal to the repair of either the radial or ulnar arteries, particularly when combined with compression of the opposite artery (Fig. 16–20). These examinations would usually preclude the necessity for performing early postoperative angiograms. Nevertheless, these adjunctive measures are only supportive in the early postoperative period, when clinical evaluation of viability and function is the most important consideration.

In the absence of infection, as with other peripheral arterial injuries, delayed primary closure of the wound four to seven days later will usually provide good wound healing.

COMPLICATIONS

Thrombosis of relatively small arteries which are repaired is frequent. Although statistics remain incomplete in the Vietnam Vascular Registry, the clinical impression of repair thrombosis has often been made on follow-up examination. If thrombosis involves only one artery and the opposite artery is patent, the significance is usually unimportant and often probably not recognized. On the other hand, thrombosis in the immediate postoperative period of one artery when the opposite is also occluded, combined with questionable viability of the

hand, will necessitate a return to the operating room for an additional attempt at reconstruction.

Infection with possible disruption of the suture line and resultant hemorrhage is always a dreaded problem. In a contaminated wound, particularly if only one of the two arteries has been involved, the safest approach is ligation of the artery.

With unsuspected arterial trauma and the development of a compartment compression syndrome, Volkmann's ischemic contracture may result.

The development of false aneurysms and arteriovenous fistulas may also occur if the initial trauma to the radial and ulnar arteries is not recognized. False aneurysms, in turn, can cause pressure on adjacent nerves. This should be kept in mind particularly if a patient begins to develop a neurologic deficit within the first several weeks after the initial injury.

RESULTS

In the World War II series, DeBakey and Simeone (1946) reported an amputation

TABLE 16–2. AMPUTATION RATE FOLLOWING LIGATION— WORLD WAR II*

	ARTERY INJURIES	AMPUTA- TIONS REQUIRED	PER CENT AMPUTA- TIONS
Radial artery	99	5	5.1
Ulnar artery	69	1	1.5
Radial and ulnar arteries	28	11	39.3

*Modified from DeBakey, M. E., and Simeone, F. A., Ann. Surg., *123*:534, 1956.

TABLE 16–3. RADIAL ARTERY INJURIES—VIETNAM VASCULAR REGISTRY (TOTAL 375*)

Ligation	138	59%
Repair	97	41%
Total	235	100%

*In studies which are incomplete, 235 of 375 injuries had a known mode of therapy. The majority of the repairs were by lateral suture or end-to-end anastomosis.

TABLE 16–4. ULNAR ARTERY INJURIES—VIETNAM VASCULAR REGISTRY (TOTAL 320*)

Ligation	148	75%
Repair	49	25%
Total	197	100%

*From this study, which remains incomplete, the exact method of management has been determined in only 197 of the 320 injuries. The majority of the repairs were by lateral suture or end-to-end anastomosis.

rate of 5.1 per cent following radial artery ligation for 99 injuries and only 1.5 per cent following 69 ulnar artery ligations; however, there was a marked increase in the amputation rate when both the radial and ulnar arteries had to be ligated following injury, as they were in 11 of 28 patients, or in 39.3 per cent (Table 16–2).

Although statistics from Vietnam remain incomplete in the Registry, repair of 41 per cent of the radial artery injuries was carried out in the group about which details are known (Table 16–3). Repair was also carried out in 25 per cent of the ulnar artery injuries (Table 16–4). The vast majority of these repairs were by end-to-end anastomosis or lateral suture of a punctate wound. Specific follow-up has been possible for some injuries through the Registry

effort, and the results have been encouraging. One soldier was treated at the 2nd Surgical Hospital in Vietnam in 1966 (Fig. 16–21). The original injury is shown in Figure 16–22 and the operative photograph of the ulnar artery injury shown in Figure 16–23. He was followed at Walter Reed for the next 2½ years. Approximately one year after repair, it was noted during reconstructive hand surgery that the radial artery repair site had become occluded; however, the ulnar artery repair remained patent.

In civilian series, details regarding the results of the management of trauma to the radial and ulnar arteries are minimal. Morris and associates (1960) stated that immediate pulses developed in 13 of 14 suture repairs and one graft repair; how-

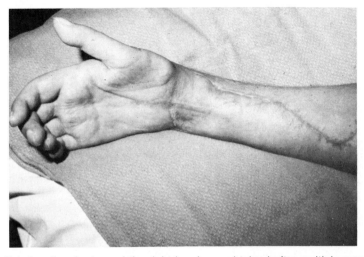

Figure 16–21. Fair functional return of the right hand was obtained after multiple reconstructive procedures in this patient approximately two years after wounding (see Fig. 16–6). There was thrombosis of the right radial arterial repair; however, the right ulnar arterial end-to-end anastomosis continued to function well. (W.R.G.H., 1968.)

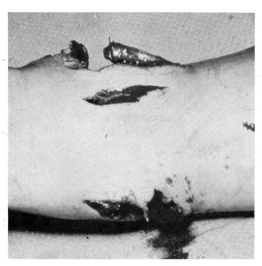

Figure 16–22. The entrance and exit wounds of the distal forearm are obvious in this casualty in Vietnam (see Figs. 16–6, 16–19 and 16–23). (N.M.R., 2nd Surgical Hospital, 1966.)

ever, follow-up was not noted. Perry and associates (1971) reported occlusion of four radial and ulnar artery repairs with successful reoperation in one patient. They also noted that an amputation was required in one of eight patients with combined radial and ulnar artery injuries.

Morton and associates (1966) emphasized what is generally known, that ligation of either the radial or ulnar artery was frequently well tolerated in their experience with several patients.

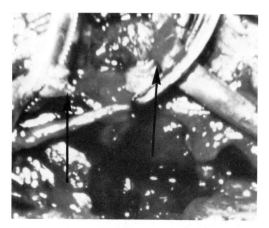

Figure 16–23. Transection of the ulnar artery (arrows) was caused by a large fragment from an exploding artillery shell (see Figs. 16–6 and 16–22). (N.M.R., 2nd Surgical Hospital, 1966.)

FOLLOW-UP

From the minimal information that is available regarding the success of radial and ulnar artery repair, it is obvious that efforts such as those through the Vietnam Vascular Registry should be continued to provide meaningful statistics. Although successful repair of an isolated injury is usually relatively unimportant, these repairs are important, particularly in combined injuries, when viability of the hand may depend upon successful repair.

The following case emphasizes the importance of reconstruction after the initial injury. A 19 year old male sustained a severe laceration of his right wrist from a broken plate glass door with resultant laceration of the flexor tendons, the median nerve and the radial and ulnar arteries. He was treated initially with ligation of the ulnar artery and an attempted end-to-end anastomosis of the radial artery. However, the arterial repair did not function. In the immediate postoperative period, it was noted that there was marked marginal viability of the right hand. Pregangrenous changes were noted, particularly over the tip of the index finger. He was transferred to Walter Reed Army Medical Center for evaluation of his vascular status, as well as for reconstruction of his tendons and median nerve.

In his evaluation, an angiogram (Fig. 16–24) revealed segmental loss of the right ulnar artery in the area of previous ligation and thrombosis of the right radial artery repair site. There was some reconstitution in the palmar arches; however, the question of additional thrombus in portions of the digital arteries was of concern. At the time of re-exploration of the wound, it was possible to identify the two ends of the severed right ulnar artery. Following additional débridement and gentle intraluminal dilatation of the ulnar artery segments with a Fogarty catheter, an end-to-end anastomosis was possible with interrupted 6–0 vascular sutures. The angiogram taken immediately after the anastomosis was completed revealed a patent repair (Fig. 16–25). All of the flexor tendons were repaired; however, it was elected to defer repair of the median nerve for

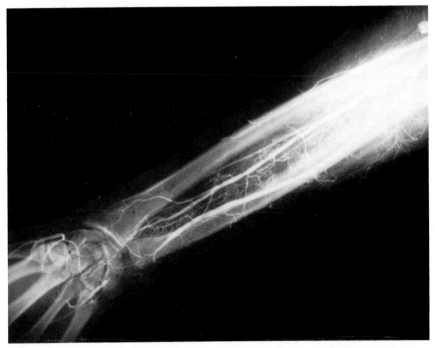

Figure 16–24. Following a severe laceration caused by fragments from a broken plate glass door, the ulnar artery was ligated and an attempted end-to-end anastomosis of the radial artery failed in a 19 year old male. The above angiogram was obtained when he was transferred to Walter Reed Army Medical Center. The very marginal supply to his hand is demonstrated. Upon reexploration, it was possible to reconstruct the ulnar artery by end-to-end anastomosis. Patency was insured angiographically, as shown in Figure 16–26. (W.R.G.H.)

several additional weeks. The hand was positioned with ulnar deviation and wrist flexion in a cast for 21 days to insure that there was no tension on the suture line. The Doppler ultrasonic sounding device assisted in the postoperative care by assuring that there was good circulation throughout the digital arteries. This had not been present prior to ulnar artery repair. There was notable improvement in the warmth and color of the hand, emphasizing the importance of the ulnar artery repair.

Figure 16–25. Patency of an end-to-end anastomosis (arrow) is demonstrated by this angiogram performed immediately after ulnar arterial repair at the wrist. The patient's preoperative angiogram is shown in Figure 16–24. (W.R.G.H.)

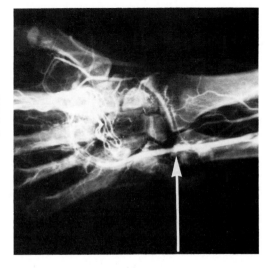

CHAPTER 17

WOUNDS OF THE HEART

Pericentesis of the pericardium is an operation which, in my opinion, approaches very closely to that kind of intervention which some surgeons would term a prostitution of the surgical art and other madness.

Billroth, 1875

The surgeon who should attempt to suture a wound of the heart would lose the respect of his colleagues.

Billroth, 1883

HISTORY

The heart has always been regarded as the sustainer of life, and its wounds have been approached through the ages with awe and apprehension. Homer provided antique literature with many references to heart wounds. Their fatality is clear.

The insulting victor with disdain bestrode
The prostrate prince and on his bosom trod;
Then drew the weapon from his panting heart,
The reeking fibers clinging to the dart;
From the wide wound gush'd out a stream of blood
And the soul issued in the purple flood.
Quoted by Beall et al., 1971

Attempts to treat wounds of the heart have been recorded as early as the first century A.D., when Galen wrote of therapy based on anatomical and experimental study through surgery of the pericardium (Siegel, 1970). Ambroise Paré tried to dispel the general belief that cardiac injuries were usually fatal in his sixteenth century reports. Yet even in 1709, Boerhaave wrote that all heart wounds resulted in death.

Larry is often credited with the first successful decompression of the pericardium in 1810 during the Napoleonic Wars, but it is only the last 80 years that treatment of heart wounds has been repeatedly beneficial to the patient. Until 1896, pericardiocentesis, either alone or combined with phlebotomy, was the only method of surgical treatment for heart wounds. Those treated were usually small penetrating wounds of the pericardium. In 1896, however, Cappelen attempted to repair a heart by suturing a myocardial laceration. Though this operation failed, in the same year Rehn (1897), in Frankfurt, was successful in relieving the cardiac tamponade and in suturing a knife wound of the heart. Rehn's accomplishment is generally regarded as the first actual repair of the heart wound, although in 1908 Matas reported that Farina had performed a similar operation, also in 1896. In a textbook of that time, Paget wrote:

The surgery of the heart has probably reached the limits set by nature to all surgery; no new method and no new discovery can overcome the natural difficulties that attend a wound of the heart.

Considerable controversy has existed for the past 35 years regarding the best approach in managing penetrating heart trauma. In 1943, Blalock and Ravitch still advocated pericardiocentesis as a form of definitive treatment for cardiac tamponade secondary to penetrating wounds of the heart. The last five years have seen more medical centers favoring emergency operative intervention, pericardiocentesis being used for temporary decompression of cardiac tamponade, if indicated, prior to direct cardiac repair.

Emphasis must be placed on the severity of heart injuries, though recent records show that they are not appreciated as soon as they should be. The physician must also have a high index of suspicion for the possibility of cardiac injury in nonpenetrating trauma to the chest, though this is less obvious than an open wound.

SURGICAL ANATOMY

The heart lies within the thoracic cavity between the two lungs (Fig. 17–1). The walls of the thorax and the fibrous sac, the pericardium, help protect the heart. The pericardium is a fibroserous sac in which the heart and origins of the great vessels are contained. The heart lies behind the sternum and the cartilages of the third through the seventh ribs on the left side in the mediastinum. Only a small portion of the anterior surface comes in direct contact with the chest wall. The majority of the anterior surface is separated from the anterior wall of the thorax by the lungs and pleura. Posteriorly the bronchi, the esophagus, the descending thoracic aorta and the posterior part of the mediastinal surface of each lung lie adjacent to the heart. The heart is covered by pleura laterally.

The pericardium consists of an outer fibrous layer and an inner serous layer. The serous layer is continuous with the epicardium at the junction of the pericardium and the great vessels of the heart. The epicardium covers the heart and great vessels. The pericardial cavity is a potential space between the epicardium and the serous layer

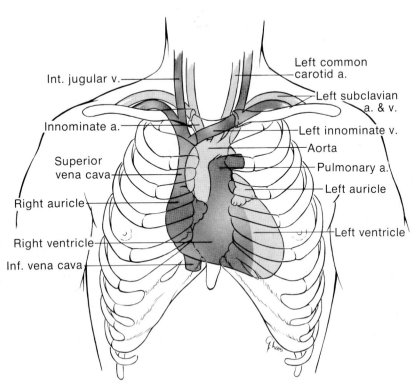

Figure 17–1. The heart and associated great vessels lie within the thoracic cavity between the two lungs. The heart lies in the mediastinum behind the sternum and the cartilages of the third through the seventh ribs on the left.

of the pericardium. The two layers are normally in contact, with a slight amount of serous fluid between the two surfaces. The fibrous layer forms a sac which is fused with the external coats of the great vessels; the base is attached to the central tendon and the muscular fibers of the left side of the diaphragm. There are also superior and inferior pericardiosternal ligaments. The heart is a conical, hollow muscular organ. In the adult it measures about 12 cm in length by 9 cm in width by 6 cm in depth. The

weight can vary between 230 and 340 grams, the heavier weights occurring in males. The heart is divided by a septum into right and left halves, and a constriction subdivides each half into two cavities — the atrium (upper) and the ventricle (lower). Therefore, the heart consists of four chambers: right and left atria and right and left ventricles (Fig. 17–2). The division of the heart into four cavities is indicated by grooves on its surface. The atria are separated from the ventricles by the coronary

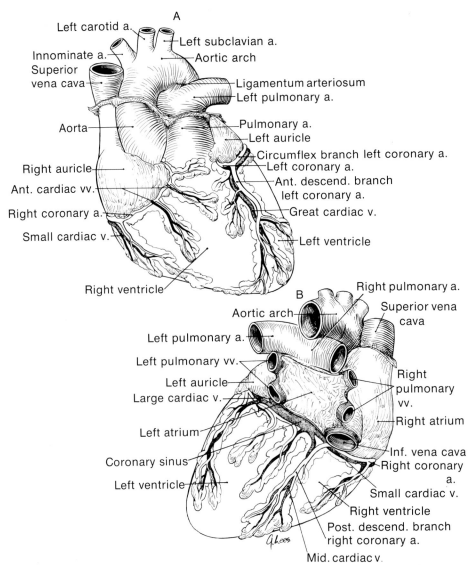

Figure 17–2.   The chambers of the heart, origins of the great vessels, and coronary arteries are shown from the sternocostal surface (A) and the dorsal surface and base of the heart (B).

sulcus, which contains the trunks of the nutrient coronary arteries to the wall of the heart. The interatrial groove separates the two atria. The ventricles are separated by two grooves. The base of the heart is directed upward, backward and to the right. It is formed mainly by the left atrium. Four pulmonary veins empty into the left atrium. The apex is directed downward, forward and to the left. The sternal costal surface of the heart is formed chiefly by the right ventricle. The diaphragmatic surface is formed by both ventricles.

The interested reader is referred to standard anatomical texts for additional details regarding the heart and great vessels.

INCIDENCE

In 1908, Matas noted that there had been a total of 160 reported cases of heart wounds after the operations of 1896. Since then, many series of heart wounds have been documented. Recent reports show an increasing incidence of recognized cardiac trauma. The greater number of gunshot wounds in many urban centers is associated with the rise in cases of penetrating heart wounds, while high speed transportation, mainly the automobile, is frequently associated with blunt cardiac trauma.

Even as early as 1941, Elkin had reported an increased incidence during the preceding ten years. Parmley and co-workers (1958A) evaluated 456 postmortem cases of penetrating wounds of the heart and aorta but stressed that the true incidence of cardiac trauma had not been established. Assessing numbers is complicated by the high mortality rate of heart wound victims. Isaacs (1959) reported, for instance, that from 1937 to 1959 more than 50 per cent of the 133 patients were dead on arrival at Johns Hopkins Hospital. Only 86 of the 459 patients analyzed by Sugg et al. (1968) arrived alive in the emergency room of Parkland Hospital in Dallas.

Other reports of note were those of Griswold and Drye (1954), who found 108 cardiac wounds at Louisville General Hospital in 20 years (1933–1953); Naclerio (1964), who recorded 249 penetrating wounds in 13 years (1950-1963); Wilson and Bassett

(1966), who saw 200 patients and a total of 205 wounds in 16½ years (1949–1965); and Beall and his co-workers (1972), who had 269 patients with penetrating cardiac injuries in Houston within 20 years (1951–1971). In 13 years, Lemos and his colleagues (1976) treated 121 patients with cardiac wounds at the University of São Paulo Medical School, or one out of each 10,000 patients admitted, about one case per month. Similarly, in Atlanta, Symbas and co-workers (1976) treated 102 patients with penetrating cardiac heart wounds, between 1964 and 1974.

The true incidence of cardiac trauma in the military experience is difficult to ascertain. On the battlefield many cardiac wounds are immediately fatal. This is emphasized by one of the typical case reports from World war I. Dixon and McEwan (1916) reported one wounded heart in a series of 123 wounds of the thorax. These authors proclaimed, "probably nearly all cardiac wounds produced death from haemorrhage too quickly to allow of the patients being removed alive even to a short distance from the battlefield." Interest in wounds of the heart increased greatly during World War II. Harken (1946) reported a unique experience in removing foreign bodies from the heart and adjacent major vessels in 134 patients. His diagram, shown in Figure 17–3, represents the area of wounding of 129 missiles.

There was one major report of injuries to the heart during the Korean conflict. Valle (1955) reported an incidence of 4.2 per cent of injuries to the heart and mediastinum: 117 injuries in a group of 2811 chest casualties treated at Tokyo Army Hospital from August, 1950, to March, 1953. In this group, however, there were only 19 cases of foreign bodies in the heart and 42 pericardial effusions. The remainder of the injuries were to the mediastinum and structures adjacent to the heart.

Cardiac trauma during the Vietnam War has not been completely documented. Gielchinsky and McNamara (1970) reported 10 heart injuries in a series of 353 intrathoracic combat injuries at the 24th Evacuation Hospital, an incidence of 2.8 per cent. The records of nearly 120 patients with cardiac wounds in Vietnam are included in the long term follow-up effort in the Vietnam Vas-

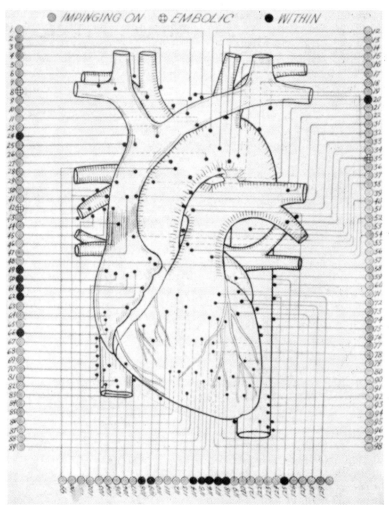

Figure 17–3. This diagram represents gross localization of foreign bodies in relationship to the heart and great vessels from the World War II experience at the 160th General Hospital. (Harken, D. E., Surg. Gynecol. Obstet., *83*:117, 1946.)

TABLE 17–1. CARDIAC WOUNDS: VIETNAM EXPERIENCE*

YEAR	NUMBER OF PATIENTS
1966	2
1967	4
1968	20
1969	31
1970	35
1971	2
Unknown	2
Total:	96

*From Geer, T. M., and Rich, N. M., Vietnam Vascular Registry, Unpublished data, 1972.

cular Registry. Specifically, details of 96 cardiac injuries have been evaluated (Geer and Rich, 1972). The majority of these injuries occurred between 1968 and 1970 (Table 17–1). At least 21 different surgical facilities participated in the care of patients with cardiac injuries (Table 17–2).

ETIOLOGY

The etiology of heart wounds is of extreme importance. Small pericardial and myocardial wounds with tamponade caused by ice picks or sharp instruments might be

TABLE 17–2. INITIAL
TREATMENT OF CARDIAC
TRAUMA: VIETNAM
EXPERIENCE*

LOCATION	NUMBER OF PATIENTS
24th Evac	19
27th Surg	12
3rd Field	7
NSA-DaNang	6
12th Evac	5
93rd Evac	5
3rd Surg	4
67th Evac	4
71st Evac	4
91st Evac	4
3rd Med (USMC)	4
2nd Surg	2
18th Surg	2
29th Evac	2
45th Surg	2
95th Evac	2
USS Sanctuary	2
1st Med (USMC)	1
36th Evac	1
85th Evac	1
Unknown	7
Total:	96

*From Geer, T. M., and Rich, N. M., Vietnam Vascular Registry, Unpublished data, 1972.

successfully treated by pericardiocentesis. On the other hand, larger wounds of the pericardium and myocardium caused by bullets, with which there is likely to be severe and progressive bleeding, should be managed by immediate thoracotomy and cardiorrhaphy. The following statistics reported in 1968 by Sugg and associates emphasize the relatively high mortality rate associated with gunshot wounds in contrast to stab wounds:

The instrument used to inflict the injury plays a major role in determining survival. Of 373 patients dead on arrival, 299, or 80 per cent, died because of gunshot wounds, whereas 74 deaths (20 per cent) followed stab wounds.... In contrast, of the 86 patients admitted alive, 48, or 56 per cent, were injured by stab wounds, and only 38 (44 per cent) by gunshot wounds. Thus, of 337 gunshot wounds, only 38 of the patients (11 per cent) were alive on arrival at the hospital. Of 122 stab wounds, 48 of the patients (39.3 per cent) were alive on admission to the hospital, again pointing out the greater lethality of gunshot wounds.

The high mortality rate of gunshot wounds has also been documented by others; gunshot wounds always represent less than 50 per cent of the cases in clinical reports, while they constitute a higher percentage in postmortem series (Beall et al., 1966B; Yao et al., 1968; Steichen et al., 1971; Bolanowski et al., 1973).

Stab wounds of the heart were most frequent in initial reports. The use of ice picks, as well as different types of knives, has been documented (Fig. 17–4 and Table 17–3). Among 38 cases of penetrating cardiac wounds reported in 1941 by Elkin, there were 27 knife wounds and 10 wounds caused by ice picks. There was only one gunshot wound. When Ransdell and Glass reviewed 20 cases of gunshot wounds of the heart in 1960, they noted that "A review of the literature does not reveal a single sizable series of gunshot wounds of the heart encountered in civilian practice." Other reports indicating the traditional predominance of stab wounds over gunshot wounds include those of Wilson and Basset (1966) (Table 17–4); Yao and colleagues (1968), who found about 88 per cent of cardiac wounds associated with stab wounds; Jones and Helmsworth (1968), who showed a stab wound incidence of 81.6 per cent between 1937 and 1967; Hewitt et al. (1970), who reported an incidence of 86 per cent in a 20 year series; and Steichen and associates (1971), who found an 83 per cent incidence.

However, the changing pattern in the etiology of civilian heart wounds was emphasized by Carrasquilla and associates (1972), who stated that gunshot wounds were increasing both relatively and absolutely to involve nearly 50 per cent of the heart wounds in their recent experience. Of 27 cases of gunshot wounds between 1957 and 1970, almost half occurred in the last three years. Beall and co-workers (1972) also documented an increase in gunshot wounds between 1966 and 1971 in relation to those encountered during the previous 14 years (Table 17–5). (Shotgun blasts were found to be the most lethal; seven were involved in the combined series, and three occurred in the latter period of the study. These patients died from massive trauma.) Thus, by 1974, Trinkle and associates found that one-third of their 45 patients with pene-

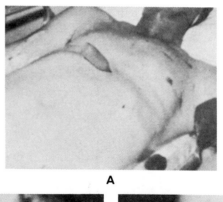

A

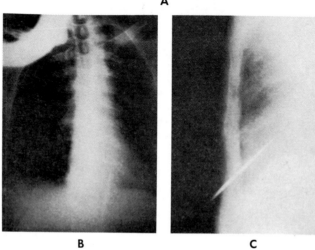

B   C

Figure 17-4. For many years, the ice pick has been a frequent wounding instrument in heart wounds. (A) An emergency room patient wounded with a six inch tapered ice pick that entered the heart. (B) and (C) Antero-posterior and lateral roentgenograms of the chest, respectively, demonstrating the ice pick wound of the heart. (Hart, T. J., Jr., and Gregoratos, G., Milit. Med., *139*:289, 1974.)

trating pericardial wounds had gunshot wounds. Meanwhile, stab wounds constituted only 55 per cent of the cardiac wounds treated at Grady Memorial Hospital in

Atlanta between 1964 and 1974 (Symbas et al., 1976). The civilian experience in São Paulo, Brazil, during a recent 13 year period (Lemos et al., 1976) is similar to that reported by many civilian centers in the United States. Again, gunshot wounds represent the majority of those treated (Table 17-6).

TABLE 17-3. STAB WOUNDS OF THE HEART CAUSED BY VARIOUS TYPES OF KNIVES: CIVILIAN EXPERIENCE IN CINCINNATI*

WEAPON	NUMBER OF PATIENTS	PER CENT
Knife (undefined)	53	72
Switchblade	7	8
Pocketknife	8	10
Ice Pick	3	4
Butcher knife	2	3
Paring knife	2	3
Total:	75	100

*Modified from Jones, E. W., and Helmsworth, J., Arch. Surg., *96*:1968.

TABLE 17-4. ETIOLOGY OF PENETRATING WOUNDS OF THE PERICARDIUM OR ITS CONTENTS: CIVILIAN EXPERIENCE IN DETROIT (January, 1949-July, 1965)*

INSTRUMENT	NUMBER	PER CENT
Knife	185	90.2
Ice pick	11	5.4
Gun	9	4.4
Total:	205	100.0

*From Wilson, R. F., and Bassett, J. S., J.A.M.A., *195*:513, 1966.

TABLE 17–5. CAUSES OF INJURY: CIVILIAN EXPERIENCE IN HOUSTON*

	NUMBER OF PATIENTS		NUMBER OF DEATHS		MORTALITY RATE (PER CENT)	
	1951–1965	1966–1971	1951–1965	1966–1971	1951–1965	1966–1971
Stab wounds	102	30	36	4	22	13
Gunshot wounds	35	42	14	13	40	31
Total:	197	72	50	17	25.4	23.6

*Modified from Beall, A. C., Jr., Patrick, T. A., Okies, J. B., Bricker, D. L., and DeBakey, M. E., J. Trauma, *12*: 468, 1972.

As evidenced in this table, blunt trauma is also a significant concern in cardiac wound treatment. The first surgical salvage of a blunt traumatic rupture of the heart was reported in 1955 by DesForges and co-workers. The increasing incidence of blunt trauma is probably related to a heightened awareness of these injuries and an increasing number of automobile accidents, in which contact with the steering wheel can often cause chest compression (Fig. 17–5). Jones and colleagues (1975) emphasized that cardiac contusion was associated most frequently with automobile accidents: 38 of 48 cases in their experience (Table 17–7). DeMuth and associates (1967) reported eight patients with contusion of the heart. Five were involved in automobile accidents, one sustained a compression injury from another source, one patient was struck by a

baseball bat and one by a fist. Yet another etiologic factor was reported by Hurwitt and Seidenberg (1953). They described a patient who experienced rupture of the heart during cardiac massage.

Representative series which show the relationship of blunt trauma to penetrating trauma include the report by Pomerantz and Hutchison (1969) from Denver (in which there were 11 stab wounds and three injuries secondary to blunt trauma) and that by Mattox and colleagues (1974) from Houston (in which there were 22 gunshot wounds, 11 stab wounds and four blunt injuries).

Other representative reports emphasize many unusual etiologies. Kleinsasser (1961) presented the case of a 30 year old man who felt a sudden pain in his chest while mowing his lawn with a rotary mower. A piece of

TABLE 17–6. ETIOLOGY OF CARDIAC WOUNDS: SÃO PAULO, BRAZIL*

AGENT	CAUSE	MALES	FEMALES	TOTAL
Stab 50 patients 41.32%	Suicide Aggression	9 (19.1%) 38	1 (33.33%) 2	10 40
Gunshot 67 patients 55.37%	Suicide Aggression Accident	4 (8.33%) 42 2	7 (36.84%) 12 –	11 54 2
Contusion 4 patients 3.31%	Accident	3	1	4
Total:		98	23	121

*From Lemos, P. C. P., Okumura, M., Azevedo, A. C., Paula, W. de, and Zerbini, E. J., J. Cardiovasc. Surg., *17*:1, 1976.

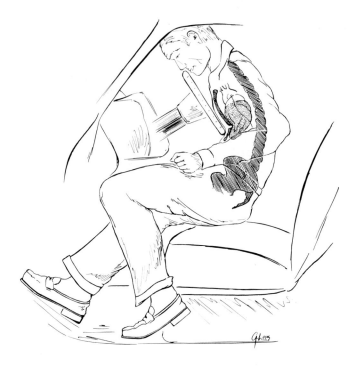

Figure 17–5. Myocardial contusion secondary to blunt trauma of the chest associated with steering wheel injuries in automobile accidents has been increasing. When examining automobile accident victims, a high index of suspicion must be maintained to prevent overlooking this important diagnostic possibility.

wire, set into motion by the rotary mower blade, penetrated the heart and lodged in the interventricular septum. A number of similar cases have been presented. One of the most recent was included in the series from the Medical College of Virginia, in which one young patient had an accidental injury from a flying nail while using a power lawn mower; this case was one of a series of 30 consecutive patients with penetrating cardiac wounds, including 17 gunshot wounds and 12 stab wounds (Szentpetery and Lower, 1977). Ben Hur and co-workers (1964) presented the unusual case of a

TABLE 17–7. CARDIAC CONTUSION: MODE OF INJURY—CIVILIAN EXPERIENCE IN NEW ORLEANS*

MODE	PATIENTS	PER CENT
Automobile accident	38	79
Pedestrian accident	4	9
Motorcycle accident	3	6
Fall	3	6
Total:	48	100

*Modified from Jones, J. W., Hewitt, R. L., and Drapanas, T., Ann. Surg., *181*:567, 1975.

perforating injury of the heart caused by a nail fired from a stud-gun (Fig. 17–6). The stud-gun is an instrument which resembles a pistol and functions according to a similar principle, its ejecting force being provided by gunpowder. It is used to insert nails and screws. A 26 year old fitter and turner felt a sudden sharp pain in his left upper chest while fixing nails with a stud-gun and he noticed blood oozing from a small wound in that region. A roentgenogram of the chest revealed a metal foreign body in the area overlying the left diaphragm. After a left anterior thoracotomy was performed, perforation of the apex of the heart by the nail was recognized. Both wounds of the heart were successfully closed by atraumatic cardiac sutures. An unusual injury involved a Hollywood actor who fell on his ski pole, the tip of which penetrated the heart (Handsaker, 1971). An Air Force Academy cadet accidentally ran a javelin through his heart (Hospital Tribune, 1969). The accident occurred when the cadet was running toward the Academy's intramural fields and did not see a fellow cadet ahead of him carrying a javelin. The javelin suddenly became impaled in the ground and the cadet ran into the end of the javelin. The cadet's heart was pierced and his vena cava

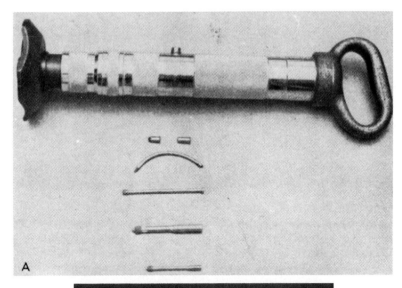

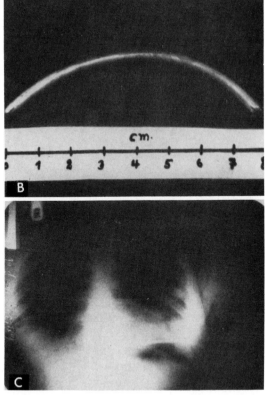

Figure 17–6. (A) A typical stud-gun, with the nails and screws often used with it. Although this is a useful instrument in industry, injuries, some fatal, have been caused by it. (B) An 8 cm nail that was successfully removed, (C) shown as perforating the apex of the heart in the anteroposterior chest roentgenogram of the patient. (Ben Hur, N., Gemer, M., and Milwidsky, H., J. Trauma, 4:850, 1964.)

punctured. Immediate resuscitative measures and emergency surgery contributed to his survival.

Cardiac perforation caused by catheters have been mentioned in a number of reports. Lawton and associates (1969) presented the problems of ventricular perforation associated with cardiac catheterization (Fig. 17–7). Thomas and associates (1969) presented the cases of two patients with pericardial tamponade from cardiac perforation of a central venous cannula. Other similar reports include those by Brandt and colleagues (1970), Fitts and colleagues (1970), Geis and associates (1970), Eshaghy and co-authors (1973) and Dosios and co-workers (1975). Kuiper (1974) documented fatal cardiac tamponade in a patient receiving total parenteral nutrition when the catheter which was being used per-

forated the right ventricle. Baek and co-workers (1973) presented an unusual case of cardiac tamponade following wound tract injection. A 20 year old man had a stab wound of the epigastrium 2 inches below the xiphoid and 1 inch medial to the left anterior costal margin. Contrast medium was injected into the sinus tract of the abdominal wound without realizing that there was also a coexistent pericardial injury. This experience points up the fact that all penetrating wounds of the upper abdomen and lower thorax should be considered as having coexistent pericardial injuries.

Missile emboli to the heart represent an unusual and fascinating type of injury. There are numerous case reports to attest to the professional interest and challenge in managing these types of injures. Morton and colleagues (1971) reported three cases

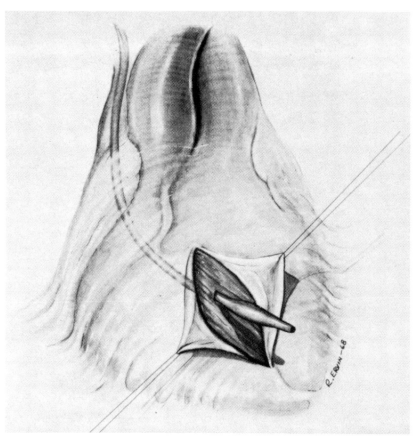

Figure 17–7. Intracardiac perforation has been caused by an assortment of catheters such as those used for coronary angiography, central venous pressure monitoring, and parenteral nutrition. This illustration shows the tip of a catheter protruding from the right ventricle with no associated bleeding. (Lawton, R. L., Rossi, N. P., and Funk, D. C., Arch. Surg., 98:213, 1969.)

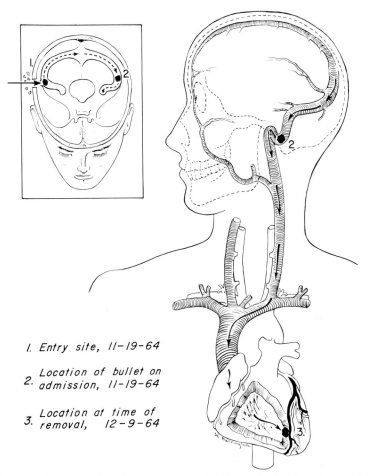

1. *Entry site, 11-19-64*

2. *Location of bullet on admission, 11-19-64*

3. *Location at time of removal, 12-9-64*

Figure 17–8. Presumed route of the missile in a case of bullet embolism from the head to the heart. Initially, an emergency craniotomy was necessary to stop hemorrhage, and 19 days later a cardiotomy was performed to retrieve the bullet. (Hiebert, C. A., and Gregory, F. J., J.A.M.A., *229*:442, 1974.)

in which a bullet embolized from a major vein of the lower extremity to the right ventricle. They noted that, since the first description of embolism of a foreign body from a peripheral vein to the heart by Davis in 1834, approximately 43 similar cases of venous embolization of foreign bodies to the heart had been reported in the English literature. Hiebert and Gregory (1974) reported an unusual case of a 17 year old male who was shot with a .22 caliber long rifle, soft-nose bullet. He had been hunting deer when a companion's gun accidentally discharged and the bullet struck the victim behind the right ear. The bullet entered the cranial vault and migrated via the transverse venous sinus to the opposite side of the skull, passing from there through the major

venous return to the right ventricle (Fig. 17–8). An emergency craniotomy was necessary to stop the initial hemorrhage, and the bullet was removed 19 days later by open cardiotomy. The authors stressed that the location of the bullet adjacent to the left anterior descending coronary artery justified removal of this foreign body from the heart.

The majority of heart wounds treated by military surgeons have resulted from fragment wounds. Gunshot wounds of the heart are usually fatal. In one major World War II series of 75 injuries of the heart and pericardium, 53 soldiers were wounded by shell fragments, 21 by small arms fire and one had a self-inflicted stab wound (Samson, 1948).

TABLE 17–8. CARDIAC WOUNDS AT A MILITARY EVACUATION HOSPITAL IN VIETNAM: CHARACTERISTICS OF CARDIAC MISSILE INJURY*

PATIENT	MODE OF INJURY	LOCATION OF INJURY	ASSOCIATED INJURY	OUTCOME
L.M.	Fragment	Right atrium	Right lung	Survived
L.L.	Fragment	Left atrium	Left lung, colon, jejunum, ileum, diaphragm, extremities	Survived
S.F.	Fléchette	Left ventricle, right atrium	Left lung	Survived
D.D.	Fléchette	Right ventricle	Left lung, colon, duodenum, diaphragm, spleen	Survived
L.D.	Fragment	Right ventricle	Left lung	Survived
W.D.	Fragment	Right atrium	Both lungs	Died
B.R.	Fragment	Right ventricle	Right lung, extremities, face	Survived
F.F.	Fléchette	Aortic-pulmonary outflow	Both lungs, extremities	Survived
I.W.	Gunshot AK–47	Right ventricle	Spinal cord, both lungs	Survived
M.T.	Fragment	Left ventricle	Both lungs	Survived

*From Gielchinsky, I., and McNamara, J. J., J. Thor. Cardiovasc. Surg., *60*:603, 1970.

Low velocity missiles, such as small fragments from anti-personnel and anti-tank mines, mortars, grenades, rockets and bombs, have been responsible for the majority of wounds in Vietnam which resulted in pericardial tamponade. In contrast to the more extensive damage to the heart and great vessels, due to high velocity wounds, which usually resulted in immediate exsanguination, pericardial tamponade from fragments could be treated more successfully, with an appreciable survival rate. Early diagnosis and prompt management were of paramount importance to achieve this goal. Tassi and Davies (1969) reported 10 patients who developed pericardial tamponade and who were treated for wounds of the heart and great vessels at the 27th Surgical Hospital in 1968. All patients had small fragment wounds. In the series reported by Gielchinsky and McNamara (1970), more than half of their 10 patients

had fragment wounds (Table 17–8). (Of particular interest were the three cardiac wounds caused by fléchettes [see Chap. 2].) In the review of cardiac cases included in the Vietnam Vascular Registry, nearly three-fourths of the injuries were caused by fragments (Table 17–9).

CLINICAL PATHOLOGY

Penetrating wounds of the pericardium and/or the myocardium due to sharp instruments or low velocity missiles are the most frequent types of injuries reported. The right ventricle in its anterior position is the cardiac chamber most frequently injured. One of the early civilian reports by Elkin in 1941 demonstrates the approximate location of heart wounds (Fig. 17–9). Recent reports emphasize the vulnerability of the right ventricle. Trinkle and

TABLE 17–9. ETIOLOGY OF CARDIAC TRAUMA IN VIETNAM*

WOUNDING AGENT	NUMBER OF PATIENTS	PER CENT	DEATHS
Fragment	71	74.0	7
Gunshot	11	11.5	1
Fléchette	3	3.1	0
Stab	3	3.1	0
Unknown	8	8.3	2
Total:	96	100.0	10

*From Geer, T. M., and Rich, N. M., Vietnam Vascular Registry, Unpublished data, 1972.

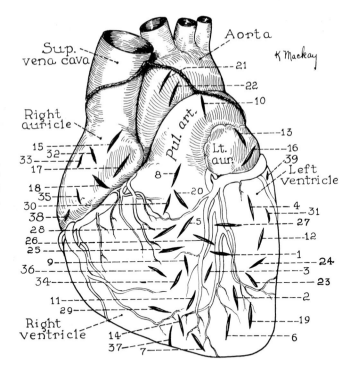

Figure 17-9. This composite drawing shows the approximate locations of heart wounds reported in the civilian experience in Atlanta. (Elkin, D. C., Ann. Surg., *114*:169, 1941.)

associates (1974) found that the site of injury among 45 patients with penetrating wounds of the pericardium was the right ventricle in 17 patients, the left ventricle in 13 patients, the right atrium in six and an assortment of other locations, identified in Figure 17–10, in the remaining 9. In three patients there was only violation of the pericardium without any direct cardiac injury. Fallah-Nejad and colleagues (1975) reported the sites of penetrating cardiac injuries in their series of 20 patients: (1) seven in the right ventricle; (2) six in the left ventricle; (3) five in the right atrium; (4) one in the left atrium; and (5) one in the pulmonary conus. Szentpetery and Lower (1977) found the right ventricle injured in 12, the left ventricle injured in 10 and an assortment of other injuries among 30 consecutive patients with penetrating cardiac wounds.

The World War II combat experience varies somewhat in that the left ventricle was involved more often than the right ventricle (Samson, 1948) (Table 17–10). This is the exception, however, because the location of cardiac wounds in the Vietnam experience again emphasizes the predominance of wounds of the right ventricle (Geer and Rich, 1972) (Table 17–11). As alluded to above, the majority of these wounds are penetrating wounds. In contrast, perforating wounds are often immediately fatal due to rapid exsanguination.

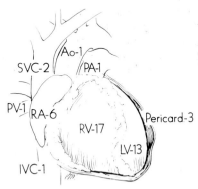

Figure 17–10. This illustration identifies the site of injury in 45 patients with penetrating pericardial wounds. This five year experience beginning in July, 1968, in San Antonio, Texas, is representative of civilian experience in a large urban center. Ao = aorta; SVC = superior vena cava; PA = pulmonary artery; PV = pulmonary vein; RA = right atrium; RV = right ventricle; LV = left ventricle; IVC = inferior vena cava. (Trinkle, J. K., Marcos, J., Grover, F. L., and Cuello, L. M., Ann. Thorac. Surg., *17*:230, 1974.)

TABLE 17–10. WORLD WAR II BATTLE WOUNDS:
TYPE OF CARDIAC WOUND, 57 CASES*

ANATOMICAL POSITION INVOLVED	Contusion	Pure Laceration	Laceration and Contusion	Perforated Chamber	Embolism to Heart	Total
Ventricle						
Left	7	7	5	7	0	26
Right	5	2	2	3	2	14
Both	3	0	2	0	0	5
Auricle						
Left	0	0	0	2	0	2
Right	1	1	0	7	0	9
Right auricle and right ventricle	0	0	1	0	0	1
Total lesions:	16	10	10	19	2	57
Deaths						
Total:	11	1	5	9	1	27
Due to heart (rate)	6(37.5%)	1(10%)	4(40%)	8(42.1%)	1(50%)	20(35.1%)

*Modified from Samson, P. C., Ann. Surg., *127*:1127, 1948.

Nonpenetrating blunt trauma usually results in diffuse contusion of the myocardium. However, the extent of cardiac injuries secondary to blunt trauma to the chest may range from minor subepicardial or subendocardial hemorrhage (Fig. 17–11) to actual rupture of the myocardium. When there is sufficient force involved in a nonpenetrating injury to cause actual cardiac laceration, a fatal outcome frequently occurs. Patients who have had blunt trauma to the chest with cardiac trauma of varying degrees may have electrocardiographic changes, arrhythmias, cardiac failure, car-

diac tamponade or hemothorax. Cardiac injuries from blunt trauma to the chest wall may or may not be associated with rib fractures or obvious chest wall deformity. Injuries have been reported with only apparently minor trauma (Parmley et al., 1958, B, C). When Parmley and associates (1958 B, C) reviewed 546 autopsies in patients who had nonpenetrating traumatic cardiac injuries, they found that 353 of the 546 patients died of rupture of the heart. Of these 353 patients, 106 had multiple chamber ruptures and 80 had associated aortic rupture. There were only 23 patients with cardiac rupture who survived the initial injury. Two of these survived seven days, and the remainder survived within a period ranging from 30 minutes to three days. Rupture of the ventricle, which occurred nearly twice as often as rupture of the atrium, was fatal immediately except for one patient with right ventricular rupture who survived several hours.

In addition to the penetrating wounds, contusions of the myocardium and cardiac lacerations, there can be other more unusual types of injuries to the valves of the heart, the interventricular or interatrial septum, the coronary vessels and the conduction system of the heart. Representative

TABLE 17–11. CARDIAC
TRAUMA IN VIETNAM:
LOCATION OF WOUNDS*

SITE	NUMBER	PER CENT
Right ventricle	40	44.9
Left ventricle	22	24.7
Right atrium	7	7.9
Left atrium	5	5.6
Unknown	15	16.9
Total:	89	100.0

*From Geer, T. M., and Rich, N. M., Vietnam Vascular Registry, Unpublished data, 1972.

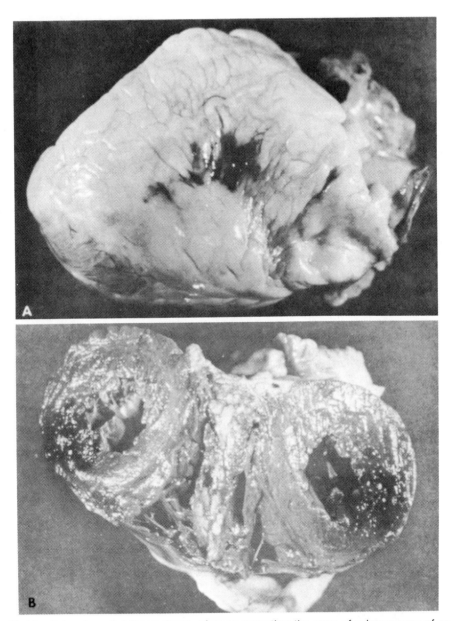

Figure 17–11. Subendocardial hemorrhage, often representing the apex of a larger area of myocardial damage, is usually found at autopsy. This abrupt transition from damaged tissue to normal myocardium contrasts with the more gradual transition seen in myocardial infarction secondary to coronary arterial occlusion. (A) This specimen shows a small area of injury evident on the external surface of the heart. (B) Transection of the specimen, however, shows a large subjacent area of mural damage. (DeMuth, W. E., Jr., Baue, A. E., and Odom, J. A., Jr., J. Trauma, 7:443, 1967.)

case reports of these unusual injuries include the removal of a wire lodged in the interventricular septum (Kleinsasser, 1961); two patients with penetrating wounds of cardiac valves, one with mitral insufficiency and the other with tricuspid insufficiency (Pate and Richardson, 1969) (Fig. 17–12); three patients with intracardiac lesions including an aortic–right ventricular fistula (Hardy and Timmis, 1969) (Fig. 17–13); and coronary arterial injuries (Tector et al., 1973) (Fig. 17–14). Patients have developed left ventricular aneurysms after penetrating wounds, as reported in the civilian experience by Kakos and colleagues (1971) and in the military experience by Aronstam and co-workers (1970) (Fig. 17–15).

Associated pathology frequently ac-

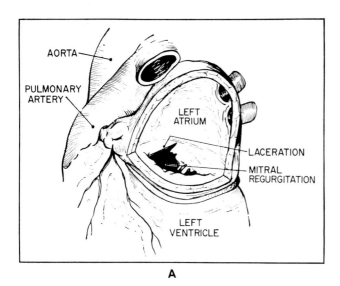

A

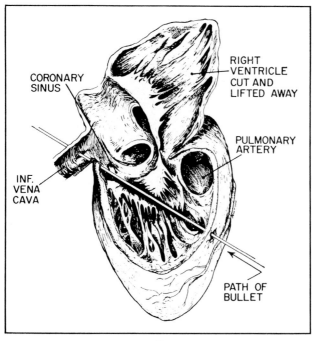

B

Figure 17–12. Wounds of the heart can involve the cardiac valves. (A) Shows laceration of the aortic leaflet of the mitral valve with resultant regurgitation. (B) In a second case, injuries occurred to the interventricular and interatrial septum, tricuspid valve and conduction mechanism. (Pate, J. W., and Richardson, R. L., Jr., J.A.M.A., *207*:309, 1969.)

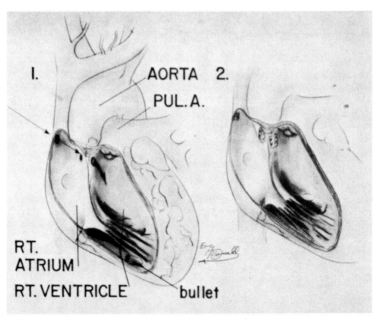

Figure 17–13. (1) A bullet passed through the right atrium, through the route of the aorta and then through the right ventricular outflow tract. (2) The aorto-right atrial fistula and the aorto-right ventricular fistula were closed with 000 mersilene sutures over Teflon felt backing. (Hardy, J. D., and Timmis, H. H., Ann. Surg., *169*:906, 1969.)

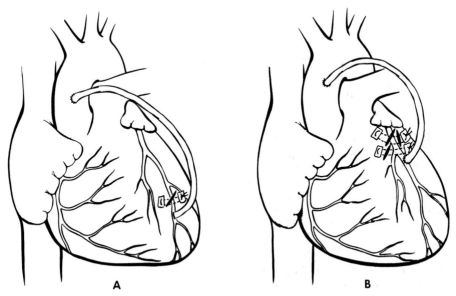

Figure 17–14. The coronary arteries may be involved in heart wounds. Successful management of these unusual wounds has improved in the past five years. (A) Repair of a cardiac laceration using sutures with felt patches and an aortocoronary saphenous vein bypass graft to supply the distal left anterior descending coronary arterial system. (B) Similar repair techniques of cardiac lacerations high on the left ventricular wall with an aortocoronary saphenous vein bypass graft to supply the proximal and distal left anterior descending coronary artery. (Tector, A. J., Reuben, C. F., Hoffman, J. F., Gelfand, E. T., Keelan, M., and Worman, K., J.A.M.A., *225*:282, 1973.)

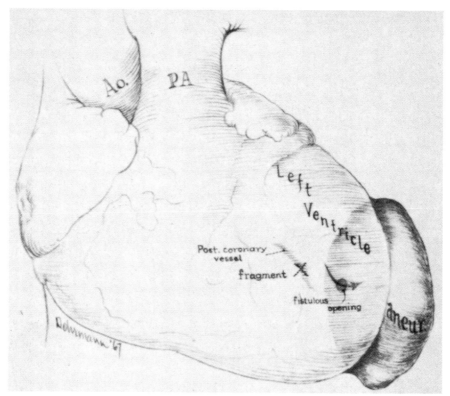

Figure 17–15. A traumatic left ventricular aneurysm, 4 × 10 cm, communicating with the left ventricle through a 1.5 cm defect. The preoperative anteroposterior roentgenogram demonstrated the aneurysm with the offending mortar fragment at the apex of the left ventricle. (Aronstam, E. M., Strader, L. D., Geiger, J. P., and Gomex, A. C., J. Thorac. Cardiovasc. Surg., 59:239, 1970.)

companies cardiac wounds. This is emphasized by the report of Ricks and associates (1965), who found that concomitant organ injury was associated with a striking rise in the mortality from 12 per cent when there was injury of one associated organ to 69 per cent with two or more associated organ injuries in their 31 patients with gunshot wounds of the heart. All but one of the 31 patients had one or both lungs injured together with the associated cardiac wound. Sugg and colleagues (1968) found that 30 survivors of penetrating heart wounds had no associated injuries. However, 33 patients who survived penetrating wounds of the heart had a total of 84 associated injuries (Table 17–12). Carrasquilla and associates (1972) emphasized the high percentage of associated injuries with gunshot wounds of the heart: 44 associated injuries occurred in 24 of 27 patients (Table 17–13). The organs most frequently involved included the lung (14), liver (8), esophagus (3), spleen (3), stomach (3) and inferior vena cava (3). Only 3 of

TABLE 17–12. ASSOCIATED INJURY OF SURVIVORS: PENETRATING WOUNDS OF THE HEART—DALLAS COUNTY*

Hemothorax	16
Pneumothorax	15
Stomach	8
Lung	7
Liver	7
Diaphragm	5
Arm	5
Pancreas	4
Internal mammary artery	3
Spleen	2
Kidney	2
Colon	2
Intercostal artery	2
Mandible	1
Pulmonary artery	1
Esophagus	1
Renal vein	1
Gallbladder	1
Mesentery	1
Total:	84

*From Sugg, W. L., Rea, W. J., Ecker, R. R., Webb, W. R., Rose, E. F., and Shaw, R. R., J Thor. Cardiovasc. Surg., 56:531, 1968.

TABLE 17–13. CLINICAL FINDINGS AND FATE OF 27
PATIENTS WITH GUNSHOT WOUNDS OF THE HEART:
DETROIT GENERAL HOSPITAL, 1957–1970*

PATIENT No.	INITIAL BP (mm Hg)	CARDIAC TAMPONADE	SITE OF CARDIAC INJURY	ASSOCIATED INJURIES	RESULTS
1	0	No	LA	Lu, V	Lived
2	75	No	RV	Lu, Spn	Lived
3	50	Yes	RV	Lu	Lived
4	60	No	RA, LV		Died
5	70	Yes	LV	Li	Lived
6	0	Yes	LA, RV	Lu, Li, St	Lived
7	0	Yes	LA, LV	Lu	Died
8	0	Yes	LV, RV	Lu, Li	Lived
9	60	Yes	LA	Lu, V, O	Lived
10	0	Yes	LV		Lived
11	0	Yes	LV, RV	Li, Pa, Du, V, Je	Lived
12	0	No	RA	Lu, JVC, O	Died
13	70	No	LA, RA	Es	Lived
14	60	No	RV	Lu	Lived
15	90	No	RA	Lu, O	Lived
16	0	Yes	LV	Es, IVC	Lived
17	80	No	RA, RV	St, Spl, IVC	Lived
18	90	Yes	LV	Lu, V	Lived
19	0	No	LV	Lu	Died
20	80	Yes	RA	Li	Lived
21	80	No	RV	Li, Je, O	Lived
22	50	No	LV	Lu	Lived
23	0	Yes	RA	Lu	Lived
24	130	No	RV	Li, St, Spl	Died
25	0	No	LV, RV		Died
26	0	Yes	RA, RV	Es, Ao	Died
27	0	Yes	RA	Li, Co, BN	Lived

BP = blood pressure; LA = left atrium; RV = right ventricle; RA = right atrium; LV = left ventricle; Lu = lung;
V = large vessel; Spn = spine; Li = liver; St = stomach; O = other (neck, arms, legs); Pa = pancreas; Du = duodenum;
Je = jejunum; IVC = inferior vena cava; Es = esophagus; Spl = spleen; Ao = aorta; Co = colon; BN = bones, spine.
*From Carrasquilla, C., Wilson, R. F., Walt, A. J., and Arbulu, A., Ann. Thor. Surg., *13*:208, 1972.

their 27 patients had an isolated gunshot
wound of the heart.

Retained foreign bodies within the
heart or the pericardium have been the
subject of long interest and discussion.
Harken (1946) outlined techniques for approaching and removing foreign bodies
from the cardiac chambers. Examples of the
intracardiac missiles that were removed
from World War II wounds are shown in
Figure 17–16. Bland and Beebe (1966)
reported a 20-year follow-up report of
World War II cases involving missiles in the
heart. There were 40 former soldiers in the
study, and all veterans survived the 20-year
follow-up period. An interesting example of
a complication that can be associated with
retained foreign bodies in the heart is
shown in Figure 17–17.

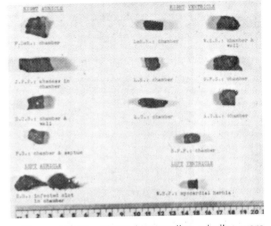

Figure 17–16. These intracardiac missiles were
removed from World War II casualties at the 160th
General Hospital. (Harken, D. E., Surg. Gynecol.
Obstet., *83*:117, 1946.)

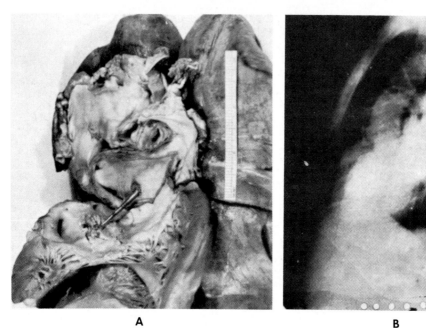

Figure 17-17. (A) This photograph shows the heart specimen opened with the tip of an ice pick projecting from the posterior wall of the left atrium. The mitral valve had been punctured, with associated endocarditis. (B) Lateral roentgenogram of the chest shows ice pick penetating the heart. Clinically, the patient had multiple peripheral emboli from this source of injury. (Lowen, H. J., Fink, S. A., and Helpern, M., Circulation, 2:426, 1950.)

PATHOPHYSIOLOGY

There are three primary physiologic disturbances associated with cardiac trauma: (1) hemorrhage, (2) pericardial tamponade and (3) cardiac failure. Every cardiac injury has some degree of hemorrhage, which may vary from hemorrhage into the myocardium associated with contusion to exsanguinating hemorrhage into the intrathoracic cavity, or outside the thoracic cavity, associated with penetrating or perforating wounds. The latter type of hemorrhage is frequently associated with early mortality. Impaired cardiac function from penetrating trauma is unusual and is seen only in the rare instances previously noted, such as trauma to a heart valve, the conduction bundle or a major coronary artery.

Frequently, the dominant physiologic injury in surviving patients is cardiac tamponade. Cardiac tamponade provides an early opportunity for survival; however, it also very rapidly contributes to mortality associated with cardiac wounds (Fig. 17–18). The tamponade can delay or stop bleeding from a cardiac laceration, allowing the patient to survive long enough for definitive therapy. Cardiac tamponade occurs quickly because the normal pericardium can accommodate only 100 to 250 ml of blood. There is a progressive fall in cardiac output as the intrapericardial pressure rises with expanding cardiac tamponade. Isaacs (1959) performed clinical studies on 60 patients with penetrating wounds of the heart and correlated his results with experimental observations. He found that elevation of the intrapericardial pressure to 17 cm of saline solution virtually stopped cardiac output unless additional infusion of fluid was given to elevate the venous pressure. Stein and associates (1973) emphasized that in the presence of associated blood loss, cardiac tamponade could occur with as little as 200 ml of blood in the pericardial sac because hemodynamic mechanisms of compensation and especially the increase in central venous pressure were preempted. The ultimate restriction of cardiac output results from the external compression to prevent diastolic filling of the ventricles. Alcohol, positive pressure anes-

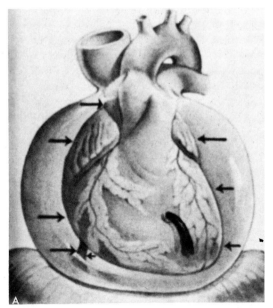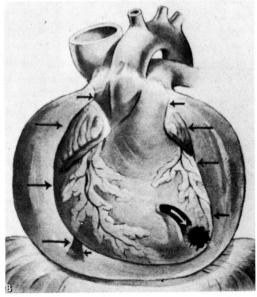

Figure 17–18. If the myocardial wound remains open and there is little or no decompression from the pericardial wound, cardiac tamponade results. Death may follow rapidly if pericardiocentesis or pericardotomy is not performed expeditiously. (A) Although pericardiocentesis may on occasion be effective as definitive therapy, thoracotomy, pericardotomy and cardiorraphy are frequently required and are the most effective procedures. If the myocardial wound closes with clot formation and bleeding stops temporarily, there may be early stabilization of the cardiac wound. (B) However, delayed tamponade with resultant death can occur if the clot retracts and dislodges with recurrent hemorrhage into the pericardial sac. This unpredictable situation adds additional support to the operative approach with cardiorrhaphy. (Naclerio, E. A., *Dis. Chest*, *46*:1, 1964.)

thesia and various anesthetic agents have been demonstrated to decrease the tolerance to cardiac tamponade in patients with penetrating wounds of the heart. The release of cardiac tamponade will increase cardiac output, help restore normal circulatory blood volume and alleviate anoxia.

CLINICAL FEATURES

As previously emphasized, cardiac trauma, particularly large penetrating wounds, may result in immediate death. Patients may collapse in profound shock, or they may develop shock more gradually over an ensuing period of several hours, the latter frequently associated with an expanding cardiac tamponade. A high index of suspicion for cardiac trauma is extremely important. Because pericardial tamponade is encountered frequently by the average physician, the diagnosis can often be overlooked, with a resultant tragic outcome

because tamponade is one of the true medical emergencies. Beck's triad, associated with cardiac tamponade, of decreased arterial pressure, elevated venous pressure manifested by distended neck veins, and muffled heart sounds has been helpful; however, not all of these signs may be apparent. The patient is frequently weak, restless and thirsty, with other signs frequently associated with a patient in shock. Chest pain is usually not severe.

Immediately upon admission to an emergency area, it is of paramount importance that all clothing be removed. All patients with wounds of the precordium, chest, back or upper abdomen should be examined for signs of cardiac tamponade. It must be remembered that with reduced blood volume, hypotension with pulsus paradoxus and jugular venous distension may appear only after the volume deficit has been corrected.

Representative statistics emphasize some of the problems in establishing the diagnosis of cardiac trauma. Ricks and associates (1965) found that 18 of the 31 patients had no recordable blood pressure on arrival in the emergency room; however, the classic signs of pericardial tamponade did not appear until partial restoration of blood volume by intravenous fluids was accomplished. Yao and associates (1968) found one or more of the triad of elevated central venous pressure, muffled heart sounds and paradoxical arterial pressure in 62 of 71 patients with stab wounds of the heart; however, only 25 of their patients had all three classic signs. Trinkle and associates (1974) noted that the classic triad was rarely present or helpful diagnostically in the 45 patients in their series. They emphasized that paradoxical pulse pressure was difficult to ascertain without continuous arterial monitoring, arterial and venous pressure were frequently altered by their injuries, and the intensity of the heart sounds varied with body build. Fallah-Nejad and co-workers (1975) noted that only 50 per cent of their 20 patients with penetrating cardiac injuries initially exhibited the classic triad.

Fallah-Nejad and co-workers (1975) emphasized that penetrating cardiac injuries can appear in an unusual and insidious manner, making diagnosis more difficult. In their series of 20 cases of cardiac injury, 10 cases had unusual and subtle symptoms, several of which were life-threatening. These authors chose to categorize the unusual manifestations as early, intermediate or late. Among the unusual early manifestations were sudden onset of shock during laparotomy performed for apparent abdominal trauma; cardiac arrest on arrival in the emergency room; and cerebral air embolus that mimicked symptoms of possible irreversible anoxic brain damage. The early manifestations were recognized in four patients. The unusual intermediate manifestations, which were recognized in two patients, included myocardial infarction with cardiogenic shock and peripheral bullet embolism, both discovered in the early recovery period. The remaining four patients had late complications that included pseudoaneurysm, ventricular septal defect, valvular damage and recurrent pericarditis. These late complications were observed between one month and 21 years after cardiac injury.

Various authors have cited specific signs and symptoms in their respective series of patients with cardiac trauma. Ricks and associates (1965) emphasized that many of their patients were delirious and required restraints at the time of initial evaluation. Trinkle and associates (1974) found that the systolic arterial pressure was below 90 mm Hg in 31 patients and was unobtainable in 10. Fallah-Nejad and associates (1975) emphasized that the biphasic clinical picture of initial hypotension with rapid response to volume replacement, which was then followed by secondary hypotension and cardiac arrest, could be another unusual pattern of the early appearance of cardiac tamponade for which immediate resuscitative thoracotomy could be a life-saving procedure.

DIAGNOSTIC CONSIDERATIONS

The physical diagnosis of penetrating cardiac trauma may be obvious. On the other hand, cardiac tamponade may be confused with pulmonary embolism, cardiac failure and overtransfusion.

Central Venous Pressure. Accurate measurement of the central venous pressure is an important early diagnostic maneuver. If the venous pressure is above 15 cm of saline solution, the test is essentially diagnostic. Trinkle and associates (1974), in recording central venous pressure preoperatively in 27 patients, found a reading above 20 cm of water in 18 patients and below 5 cm in only two patients. They felt that falsely elevated central venous pressure could be due to straining, shivering or a malpositioned catheter.

Chest Roentgenogram. A chest roentgenogram will usually not show cardiac enlargement with tamponade because the pericardium does not easily distend. On the other hand, even under battlefield conditions, there may be an increased cardiac diameter that can be appreciated (Fig. 17–19). Hemothorax is a common finding, particularly with concomitant injuries. Anteroposterior and lateral roentgenograms of the chest

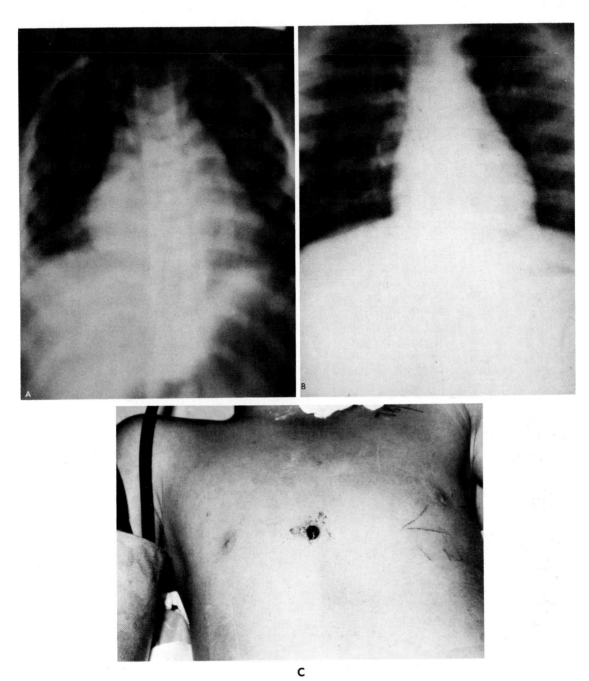

C

Figure 17–19. (A) This chest roentgenogram taken at the time of hospital admission shows increased cardiac diameter secondary to pericardial tamponade. (B) The postoperative chest roentgenogram shows a normal cardiac size. (C) The entry wound of the missile is obvious in this operating room photograph. (Courtesy Dr. Tassi.) This was one of ten patients treated at the 27th Surgical Hospital in 1968 in Vietnam. (Tassi, A. A., and Davies, A. L., Am. J. Surg., *118*:535, 1969.)

should be obtained to identify the location of foreign bodies. If a missile or fragment entered the heart and the point of exit cannot be found, peripheral embolization of the missile should be highly suspected. This is particularly true if a follow-up roentgenogram of the chest does not show the foreign body that was previously apparent in the area of the heart. Also, roentgenograms of other areas of anatomy should be performed if early peripheral embolization is suspected. A roentgenogram of the chest may appear normal in a patient who has had nonpenetrating chest trauma. There may be a generalized increase in the cardiac silhouette. If there is an associated pericardial tear, hemothorax may be obvious, which will obscure the cardiac borders. A pneumopericardium may only become obvious after tube thoracostomy (Fig. 17–20). Trinkle and associates (1974) found the chest roentgenogram to be of little diagnostic assistance in patients with heart wounds, except for two patients with intrapericardial air. These authors warned that roentgenograms, frequently taken in the recumbent anteroposterior position with partial expi-

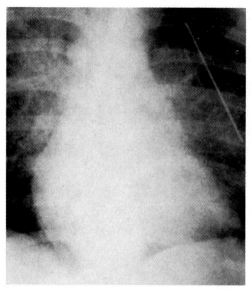

Figure 17–20. This roentgenogram demonstrates a pneumopericardium that may be present with a cardiac injury if there is a pericardial tear. There must be an associated pneumothorax, or the pneumothorax may occur after tube thoracostomy for hemothorax. (Noon, G. P., Boulafendis, D., and Beall, A. C., Jr., J. Trauma, *11*:122, 1971.)

ration, could give a false impression that there was widening of the mediastinum and the heart.

Electrocardiogram. The electrocardiogram has been of some assistance. Yao and co-workers (1968) emphasized that muffled heart sounds and elevation of the S-T segment in precordial electrocardiographic leads may support the diagnosis of pericardial penetration. As should be anticipated, specific wounds to the coronary arteries and conduction areas of the heart would be associated with specific changes on the electrocardiogram. Noth (1946) reviewed the electrocardiographic patterns in penetrating wounds of the heart.

Additional Methods. Other diagnostic techniques include echocardiography, angiocardiography and radioisotope scanning; however, there is usually little practical application of these techniques. Hemodynamic monitoring can be practically applied as outlined in Figure 17–21. Shoemaker and co-workers (1970) recently evaluated the details of hemodynamic alterations in acute cardiac tamponade following penetrating cardiac injuries.

Pericardiocentesis has been advocated for both diagnosis and treatment of penetrating wounds of the pericardium (Fig. 17–22). One of the reasons for false negative findings in pericardiocentesis is the high incidence of clot within the pericardium, with little or no free blood. The recent experience by Trinkle and associates (1974) emphasizes some of the limitations; they utilized pericardiocentesis in 18 patients and got seven false negative and three false positive results, establishing an error factor of greater than 50 per cent. Because of this experience, these authors used a preliminary subxyphoid pericardial window in 21 of 45 patients with penetrating wounds of the heart. Fallah-Nejad and colleagues (1975) also recently reported that easy diagnostic access to the pericardium could be obtained by the subxyphoid technique, as described by Sauerbruch in 1925, in any case in which there was a high index of suspicion of cardiac trauma.

The complex aspects of unusual wounds of the heart associated with trauma to heart valves, coronary arteries, conduction bundles and so forth are represented by the

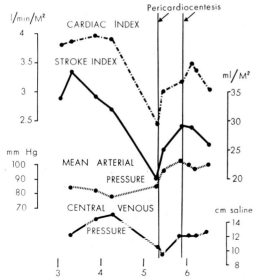

Figure 17–21. Data illustrate the hemodynamic alterations in a 30 year old man who sustained a stab wound of the precordium. His neck veins were distended on admission, heart sounds were clear but somewhat irregular, blood pressure was 115/78, pulse rate was 110 beats per minute and respiratory rate was 32 breaths per minute. The lungs were clear on auscultation except for some decrease in breath sounds at the right base. Electrocardiograms revealed atrial fibrillation and variations in QRS complexes. The diagram represents progressive deterioration of the cardiac index and stroke index, even though arterial pressures were stable. Pericardiocentesis performed at 5:15 and 5:50 P.M. reversed this trend. (Yao, S. T., Vanecko, R. M., Printen, K., and Shoemaker, W. C., Ann. Surg., *168:* 67, 1968.)

following case. Trauma to a heart valve is rarely diagnosed in an injured patient because the injury is usually so severe that death results before the patient can be transported to a definitive treatment center. Fallah-Nejad and associates (1975) presented the case of a 46 year old woman who sustained a stab wound of the anterior left chest in 1950. Although she was initially treated with an intercostal chest tube, she subsequently required an open thoracotomy on the left with decortication for a trapped lung. Six years later she developed chest pain and shortness of breath. At the time of hospital readmission in 1956 for full evaluation, a diagnosis of minimal mitral insufficiency was made and the patient was discharged. She remained essentially asymptomatic for the next 18 years until she was readmitted to the hospital in 1974, 24 years after the original stabbing, because of decreased tolerance for exercise, chest pain and a loud systolic murmur at the apex. Mitral insufficiency was confirmed by cardiac catheterization when contrast medium injected into the right ventricle also showed opacification of the left atrium. During open heart surgery, an opening was found in the pericardium from the original stab wound which also lacerated the base of the anterior leaflet of the mitral valve. Successful repair of the mitral valve was possible.

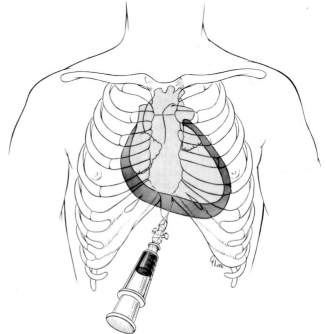

Figure 17–22. Pericardiocentesis has been utilized both for diagnosis and for treatment of pericardial tamponade associated with penetrating wounds of the pericardium. Aspiration should be accomplished by the perixyphoid route using a long thin-walled needle.

TREATMENT

There is nothing more disconcerting than to hold in one's hand a writhing, jumping heart and blindly attempt to find a wound deep in a gushing whirlpool of blood.

Griswold and Maguire, 1942

Management of patients with cardiac trauma has been outlined by numerous authors who have developed a series of logical methods of treatment. Reducing the time from injury to definitive treatment is of primary importance. As has previously been emphasized, many heart wounds are rapidly fatal because of exsanguinating hemorrhage which, for practical reasons, cannot be treated. On the other hand, cardiac tamponade, which can be treated, is also responsible for fatalities following cardiac trauma. Initially, a brief history which would note the time of injury may be possible. Of paramount importance would be information regarding the wounding agent, including specific identification of the weapon or other type of wounding agent. A complete and rapid physical examination with the patient disrobed should be carried out to specifically look for associated injuries. If any airway problems exist, an endotracheal tube should be inserted for ventilatory assist. At the same time, vital signs and central venous pressure monitoring should be obtained.

The treatment of shock remains a primary goal in managing most heart wounds. Multiple large bore intravenous catheters should be inserted for necessary fluid and blood replacement. Catecholamines, such as epinephrine and isoproterenol, may be useful for short periods of time to increase myocardial contractility. Despite the probable elevated intrapericardial pressure, appropriate fluids, 1 to 3 liters of electrolyte solution or whole blood, should be infused rapidly to elevate venous pressure in order to enhance cardiac filling. If the patient's condition is stable, upright and anteroposterior and lateral inspiratory chest roentgenograms should be obtained, as well as an electrocardiogram. If a massive hemothorax or pneumothorax is present, closed thoracotomy for chest tube drainage may be

indicated to allow rapid reexpansion of the lung.

If the patient is moribund and cardiac tamponade is a possibility, pericardial aspiration should be performed immediately (see Fig. 17–22). Varying amounts of blood may be obtained, ranging from as little as 10 ml to as much as 400 ml. However, the result may also be dramatic, with a prompt improvement in the patient's blood pressure from an imperceptible level and a return of consciousness. During the procedure, an electrocardiogram should be monitored to detect any arrhythmia that might develop. If allowed to persist, cardiac tamponade can be disastrous.

If the aspiration is ineffective and no blood is returned by pericardiocentesis but the diagnosis of cardiac tamponade still remains likely, a prompt subxyphoid digital exploration should be performed. A short incision is made in the linea alba, separating the diaphragm behind the xyphoid process and digitally entering the pericardium (Fig. 17–23).

Cardiac arrest may develop before the patient can be taken to the operating room. This has been particularly true of patients with gunshot wounds of the chest. External closed techniques have not been as effective as resuscitation performed with the chest open, especially if the patient has been hypovolemic. Moreover, closed massage may cause increased bleeding from a penetrating wound of the pericardium, with resultant increase in the cardiac tamponade. Open cardiac massage allows reduction of any existing cardiac tamponade, temporary digital control of hemorrhage from the myocardium and an opportunity to improve cardiac output. Immediate thoracotomy should also be considered with a penetrating cardiac injury if there is continued hemorrhage or rapidly progressing cardiac tamponade which does not respond to the previously mentioned procedures.

It may be necessary to continue resuscitation in the operating room for massive bleeding and hypotension. In addition to the procedures previously described, a nasogastric tube and Foley catheter should be inserted to decompress the stomach and to monitor the urinary output, respectively.

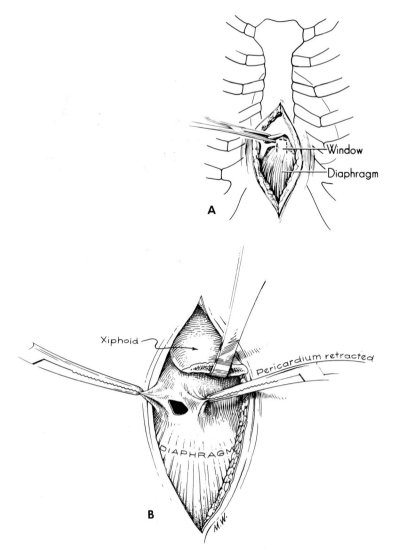

Figure 17–23. Technique for creating the pericardial window used in 21 of 45 patients. (A) A vertical midline incision is made over the lower sternum and upper abdomen. The tip of the xyphoid process is grasped with a clamp and elevated so that the attachment of the diaphragm to the posterior surface of the xyphoid can be severed. (Trinkle, J. K., Marcos, J., Grover, F. L., and Cuello, L. M., Ann. Thorac. Surg., *17:*230, 1974.) (B) An incision in the inferoanterior shelf of the diaphragm creates an extrapleural window in the pericardium for diagnosis and decompression. (Arom, K. V., Richardson, J. D., Webb, G., Grover, F. L., and Trinkle, J. K., Ann. Thorac. Surg., *23*:545, 1977.)

Anesthesia should be minimal for patients with cardiac injuries, particularly in the initial stages of the operation. High concentrations of oxygen should be maintained to provide adequate pulmonary ventilation. Immediate thoracotomy on the involved side may be indicated. There may be increased diagnostic problems in patients with cardiac tamponade, however. In addition to the diagnostic and therapeutic pericardiocentesis, the preliminary subxyphoid pericardial window might be accomplished in the operating room. If blood is encountered in the pericardium, the incision can be extended into a median sternotomy. Once

an area of bleeding from a wound in the myocardium has been established, temporary tamponade can be performed by pressure from the surgeon's finger until appropriate sutures can be applied.

There are varying opinions regarding the incision which will provide the most expeditious approach to the wounded heart. For specific situations, this may range from the anterolateral thoracotomy through the fourth intercostal space on the side of injury, to a lateral thoracotomy, to a median sternotomy. If open cardiac massage has been utilized through a left thoracotomy, temporary compression of the descending thoracic aorta can be accomplished to improve coronary and cerebral circulation. Precautions similar to those used in open intracardiac surgery may be instituted to prevent fatal complications of air embolus. Bleeding from a heart wound can usually be controlled temporarily by digital pressure without undue compression of the heart. Nonabsorbable suture, larger size 0 or 00, such as cardiovascular silk, wedged to a long, slender needle, should be utilized.

These sutures should be passed through a sufficient amount of the myocardium, approximately 5 mm from the edges of the wound, and the sutures tied just tightly enough to stop the bleeding without cutting through the myocardium or creating the ischemia of the myocardium (Fig. 17–24). Frequently, two or four sutures will be satisfactory. If a coronary artery is next to the laceration, it should be avoided with a U-shaped horizontal mattress suture. De-

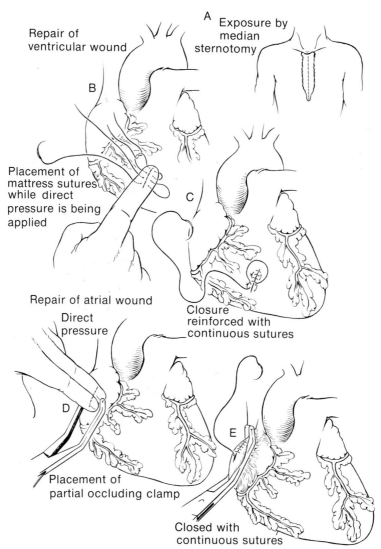

Figure 17–24. A number of techniques can be successful in approaching cardiac wounds, including exposure by median sternotomy (A). Temporary digital tamponade can be followed by placement of sutures beneath the finger (B). Hemostasis can be ensured and the closure reinforced with a second suture in a continuous fashion (C). Repair of an atrial wound can be accomplished by initial digital control with placement of a partial occluding clamp (D). Closure can then be accomplished with a continuous vascular suture (E).

tails regarding unusual and specific injuries will be found in other parts of this chapter, and the interested reader should be referred to standard texts on cardiac surgery for management of wounds of cardiac valves, coronary arterial wounds, septal injuries and wounds of the vena cava. Cardiopulmonary bypass may be of value in unusual situations; however, many patients with cardiac injuries are treated where cardiopulmonary bypass is not immediately available. Temporary balloon catheter contol may be of value. Autotransfusion of patients with cardiac wounds has been successful in some series; however, the true merit of this modality remains uncertain.

Treatment of patients with blunt chest trauma resulting in myocardial contusion differs greatly, in general, from that of patients sustaining penetrating cardiac injuries. Treatment of the former should be similar to that for patients with myocardial infarction, namely, bed rest and serial observations with electrocardiogram and blood enzyme determinations. There may be an unusual myocardial laceration with cardiac tamponade which should then be treated as previously outlined. The pump-oxygenator, however, should be available if operative intervention is required. Laceration of the myocardium secondary to blunt trauma may be too extensive to be able to obtain or maintain control of hemorrhage by digital pressure.

POSTOPERATIVE CARE

In addition to the usual postoperative measures, serial electrocardiograms should be obtained. Anteroposterior and lateral chest roentgenograms should also be obtained at regular intervals.

Physiotherapy plays an important role in the early rehabilitation of these patients.

RESULTS

Disagreement persists regarding early management of wounds of the heart. While some feel that pericardiocentesis should be the definitive treatment for virtually all penetrating wounds of the heart, thoracotomy being reserved only for patients who do not improve or who subsequently deteriorate after initial stabilization, others favor immediate thoracotomy and cardiorrhaphy using pericardiocentesis only as a diagnostic tool or as a temporizing expedient to keep the patient alive until thoracotomy can be performed. Sugg and associates (1968) reviewed the literature and documented the various mortality rates in the management of heart wounds treated by aspiration (Table 17–14) compared to those treated by thoracotomy (Table 17–15). Sugg and colleagues (1968) reported their own results, showing an improvement in the mortality rate when they changed their policy to

TABLE 17–14. MANAGEMENT OF HEART WOUNDS BY PERICARDIOCENTESIS*

AUTHOR	YEAR	NUMBER OF CASES	PER CENT MORTALITY
Bigger	1940	3	00.0
Blalock and Ravitch	1943	2	00.0
Blau	1945	3	00.0
Anderson and Starbuck	1946	4	00.0
Ravitch and Blalock	1949	9	11.0
Elkin and Campbell	1951	18	11.0
Menendez	1951	4	25.0
Cooley et al.	1955	28	10.7
Royster and Basher	1958	17	00.0
Isaacs	1959	40	10.0
Beall et al.	1961	78	5.5
Ricks et al.	1965	11	9.0
Beall et al.	1966	126	14.3

*From Sugg, W. L., Rea, W. J., Ecker, R. R., Webb, W. R., and Shaw, R. R., J. Thor. Cardiovasc. Surg., 56:531, 1968.

TABLE 17–15. HEART WOUNDS TREATED BY THORACOTOMY*

Author	Year	Number of Cases	Per Cent Mortality
Peck	1909	160	63.0
Pool	1912	77	45.5
Smith	1923	49	28.6
Schoenfeld	1926	25	36.0
Bigger	1932	53	36.5
Bigger	1939	141	50.0
Elkin	1941		
Griswold and Maguire			
Nelson	to	149	38.0
Linder and Hodo			
Blau	1945		
Maynard et al.	1952	81	42.7
Cooley et al.	1955	14	50.0
Farringer and Carr	1955	30	36.7
Maynard et al.	1956	32	25.0
Lyons and Perkins	1957	14	14.2
Isaacs	1959	20	30.0
Beall et al.	1961	12	33.0
Boyd and Streider	1965	16	25.0
Ricks et al.	1965	17	59.0
Maynard et al.	1965	58	8.6
Beall et al.	1966	17	47.0

*From Sugg, W. L., Rea, W. J., Ecker, R. R., Webb, W. R., and Shaw, R. R., J. Thor. Cardiovasc. Surg., 56:531, 1968.

immediate operation as a standard treatment of cardiac wounds (Table 17–16). They found that prior to 1966, 10 of 18 deaths in patients with cardiac wounds treated by pericardiocentesis were due to recurrent tamponade.

Ricks and associates (1965) advocated pericardiocentesis as the primary method of managing gunshot wounds of the heart based on their experience involving 19 of 31 patients who received pericardiocentesis either as definitive treatment or in preparation for operation; they had only three deaths, for a mortality rate of about 15 per cent. These authors advocated leaving the pericardiocentesis needle in place in pa-

tients requiring operative intervention to allow additional release of pericardial fluid and to prevent cardiac arrest during induction of anesthesia.

Beall and associates (1972) emphasized that there was a changing pattern of surgical management of penetrating wounds of the heart. They advocated a more aggressive approach toward early operative intervention. Fallah-Nejad and co-workers (1975) stated that they frequently encountered a large amount of clotted blood and hemorrhage; therefore, they adopted a similar policy of treating cardiac injuries primarily with thoracotomy, while reserving pericardiocentesis for use in selected cases as a

TABLE 17–16. MORTALITY BY METHOD OF TREATMENT: MANAGEMENT OF PENETRATING WOUNDS OF THE HEART*

Years	Alive on Arrival	Pericardiocentesis		Surgery	
		No. Treated	Died	No. Treated	Died
1959–1965	49	34	15(44%)	15	3(20%)
1966–1967	37	1	0(0%)	36	5(14%)
Total:	86	35	15(43%)	51	8(16%)

*Modified from Sugg, W. L., Rea, W. J., Ecker, R. R., Webb, W. R., and Shaw, R. R., J. Thor. Cardiovasc. Surg., 56:531, 1968.

temporary measure from the time of admission until the time of operative intervention. Trinkle and colleagues (1974) treated all 45 of their patients with penetrating wounds of the pericardium by immediate operation: none were merely observed or treated only by pericardiocentesis. These authors favored median sternotomy to allow a preliminary subxyphoid pericardial window to be performed in patients with cardiac tamponade and a thoracotomy if massive bleeding occurred into the pleura. They did not use cardiopulmonary bypass in operating on 45 patients with penetrating wounds of the pericardium. They did emphasize that technical adjuncts include in-flow occlusion, electrical fibrillation, partially occluding clamps and stabilizing traction sutures. Trinkle and associates (1974) outlined a series of technical maneuvers that they utilized in treating their patients with penetrating wounds of the pericardium (Fig. 17–25). In utilizing the preliminary subxyphoid pericardial window in 21 patients, blood or blood with clot was encountered in 18. The subsequent incision used by the San Antonio group included a left thoracotomy in 21 patients, a median sternotomy in 15, a right thoracotomy in 4, a pericardial window in 3, laparotomy with transdiaphragmatic pericardial window in 1 and a bilateral thoracotomy in 1 patient. Trinkle and co-workers (1974) reported five early deaths among 45 patients with penetrating pericardial injuries, for a mortality rate of about 11 per cent. Three deaths were due to uncontrolled bleeding from associated injuries, including a gunshot wound of the liver, another to the abdominal aorta and a severe stab wound to the subclavian artery and vein. One patient died of an arrhythmia on the fourth postoperative day, and another patient died from hypoxia during nasotracheal suctioning on the third postoperative day. There were two deaths more than 30 days postoperatively due to hypoxic brain damage and complications of tracheal stenosis. This represented a combined early and late mortality of 15.5 per cent.

Even among the most devastating cardiac wounds—those associated with gunshot wounds—there has been an improvement in the mortality rates. Ransdell and Glass (1960) reported 20 cases of gunshot wounds of the heart, with an overall mortality of approximately 65 per cent. In 15 patients who underwent cardiorrhaphy, there was an operative mortality rate of about 53 per cent. Of the five patients who received no specific treatment, all died. Carrasquilla and associates (1972) favored immediate thoracotomy in managing 27 patients with gunshot wounds of the heart. They were able to obtain a survival rate of approximately 74 per cent among 27 patients who sustained gunshot wounds of the heart, for a mortality rate of approximately 26 per cent, a significant reduction from the mortality rate of approximately 65 per cent reported 12 years earlier (Ransdell and Glass, 1960). Carrasquilla and colleagues (1972) reported survival of 20 of 27 patients with gunshot wounds of the heart because of their program of treatment, characterized by immediate respiratory support, blood volume expansion and thoracotomy with direct control of the cardiac injury. They felt that other factors favorably influencing the survival rate were an initial blood pressure of 50 mm Hg or higher, cardiac tamponade and injury to only one chamber; all nine patients with damage to only one chamber and tamponade survived (see Table 17–13). These authors found a surprising lack of correlation between the number of associated injuries and the mortality rate, a finding in sharp contrast to studies on trauma to other organs. They believed that this was related to the cardiac injury being the determining prognostic factor, with other injuries being relatively mild by comparison.

Carrasquilla and associates (1972) classified the deaths in their series by involvement of the cardiac chambers: in 4 of 11 patients the right ventricle was involved; in 3 of 11 patients the left ventricle; in 3 of 9 patients the right atrium; and in 1 of 5 patients the left atrium. Although there was no significant difference in mortality for the various chambers involved, there was an increased chance of death; four of nine patients died when there was simultaneous involvement of two chambers. There were two patients who survived and left the hospital in satisfactory condition after initially being pronounced dead on arrival in the emergency room. Both patients had no heartbeat, pulse, blood pressure or respira-

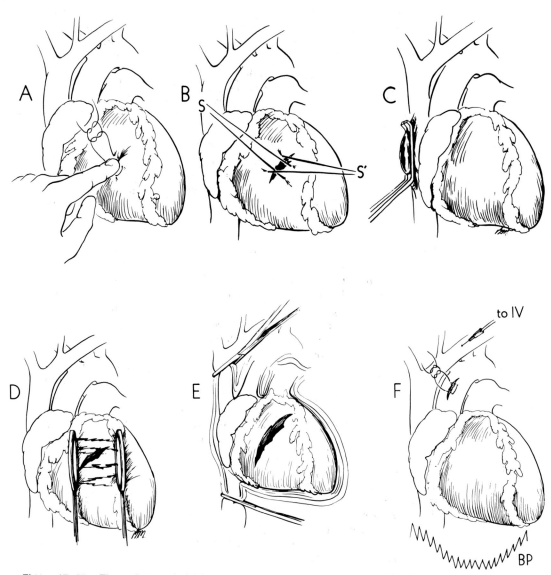

Figure 17–25. The various technical maneuvers used to repair lacerations of the heart and intrapericardial vessels. (A) Actively bleeding wounds of the right ventricle are tamponaded with the finger, a large mattress suture on a big needle is passed under the finger and tied, and a second layer of sutures can then be accurately placed in a dry incision. (B) Large wounds of the ventricle are treated by placing horizontal mattress sutures on either side of the lesion and crossing these to temporarily stop bleeding, followed by definitive suture placement. (C) Partially occluding clamps can be applied temporarily to the atrial appendage or great vessels to allow suture of the dry, decompressed structure. (D) Stilette wounds of the ventricle or great vessels were treated by electrically fibrillating the heart for decompression with intermittent massage while repairing the wound, placing the defibrillating paddles vertical to the surface of the heart, and discharging them at 20 watt-sec to produce fibrillation if standard fibrillating electrodes were not available. This technique has recently been discontinued because it is difficult to defibrillate the heart. Also, the heart enlarges somewhat, making it more difficult to repair the wound. The technique of inflow occlusion is preferred, since the same purpose is accomplished of arresting the heart but with a smaller, decompressed organ on which to work. (E) Intermittent inflow occlusion can be created quickly by placing vascular clamps on the venae cavae. The heart shrinks, and exsanguinating hemorrhage can be controlled for 60 to 90 sec while sutures are placed in the dry, decompressed laceration. (F) An intravenous drip of trimethaphan or high concentrations of halothane will temporarily decrease the aortic and left ventricular pressure to allow safe closure of a wound in the transiently decompressed chamber. (Trinkle, J. K., Marcos, J., Grover, F. L., and Cuello, L. M., Ann. Thorac. Surg., 17:230, 1974.)

TABLE 17–17. PENETRATING WOUNDS OF THE PERICARDIUM AND HEART: WAYNE STATE UNIVERSITY— DETROIT GENERAL HOSPITAL, 1957–1975*

	TOTAL NUMBER	NUMBER LIVED	NUMBER DIED
Stab and gunshot wounds	323	271 (80.5%)	52 (19.5%)
Stab wounds	265	227 (85%)	38 (15%)
Gunshot wounds	58	44 (76%)	14 (24%)

*From Asfaw, I., and Arbulu, A., Surg. Clin. N. Am., 57:37, 1977.

tion; however, because they were still warm, vigorous attempts at resuscitation, including open cardiac massage which was started in the emergency room to provide immediate control of the cardiac injury, was accomplished with restoration of a vigorous beat in the heart. There were 5 deaths among 13 patients who had no obtainable blood pressure on admission to the hospital. There were 2 deaths among 14 patients who had a systolic pressure of 50 mm Hg or higher. Cardiac tamponade appeared to improve the prognosis, with only 2 deaths in 14 patients who had tamponade, in contrast to 5 patients who died among 13 patients who did not have tamponade. Three of four patients with a combination of unobtainable blood pressure and no tamponade died.

Asfaw and Arbulu (1977) provided a recent update of the statistics from the extensive experience at the Detroit General Hospital in managing 323 patients with penetrating wounds of the heart (Table 17–17). These authors again emphasized the importance of a systematic approach to patients with penetrating cardiac injuries. They noted that many generations of surgi-

cal residents under staff supervision had been able to maintain consistently excellent results because of an organized plan. Szentpetery and Lower (1977) have reported one of the most recent series involving management of penetrating wounds of the heart. They, too, have noted the changing concepts and recommend immediate operation for all patients, with pericardiocentesis employed only as a diagnostic tool and/or for emergency relief of tamponade. They had an overall mortality rate of 13 per cent.

The necropsy findings reported by Naclerio (1964) emphasize the two major factors contributing to early death in patients sustaining penetrating heart wounds: exsanguination in the majority, and tamponade in a significant number (Table 17–18).

The results of managing severe cardiac trauma associated with blunt trauma can be found in scattered reports of individual cases or small series. An example is the report by Noon and co-workers (1971), who had two patients with rupture of the heart secondary to blunt trauma. Surgical repair of rupture of the left atrium was successful

TABLE 17–18. SALIENT NECROPSY FINDINGS IN A SERIES OF 35 PATIENTS DYING BEFORE SURGERY*

CAUSES	NUMBER OF PATIENTS
Exsanguination from cardiac wounds (without sufficient tamponade to control hemorrhage)	20
Exsanguination from associated injury (with varying degrees of tamponade)	
Internal jugular vein	1
Femoral vessels	1
Abdominal viscera	2
Tamponade (with minimal loss of blood)	10
Injury to common conduction bundles (without tamponade or exsanguination)	1
Total:	35

*Modified from Naclerio, E. A., Dis. Chest, 46:1, 1964.

TABLE 17–19. RUPTURE OF THE HEART SECONDARY TO BLUNT TRAUMA*

	BP ADM.	CYANOSIS	CVP	CHEST X-RAY	PERICARDIO-CENTESIS	TIME TO SURGERY	LOCATION OF TEAR	TYPE OF THORACOTOMY	ADDITIONAL INJURIES
Desforges, 1955	70/40	Yes	—	Right hemothorax	No Right chest	9 hours	Right atrium SVC	Right thoracotomy	Fractured left femur
Bogdain, 1966	0/0	Yes	—	Multiple rib fxs., enlarged heart	Yes	Not stated	Left atrial appendage	Left thoracotomy	RLL hematoma
Rotman, 1970	60/40	Yes	—	Not done	No	Not stated ? 1 hour	Right ventricle	Not known	Traumatic VSD 10 days postop., repaired 2 mos. later
Borja, 1970	60/40	Yes	—	Mediastinum wide, hazy RLL	No	2 hours	Right atrial appendage and lateral RA	Left thoracotomy extended across sternum	Lacerations of knees
Noon, 1971	0/0	Yes	20	Multiple rib fxs.	Yes	Not stated ? 1 hour	LAA	Left thoracotomy	Flail left chest
Siderys, 1971	Not known	Not known	—	Left hemothorax	No, left chest tube	2–3 hours	LAA	Left thoracotomy	Depressed skull fracture
SCVMC	0/0	Yes	35	Mediastinum wide	Yes	Not stated	Right atrial appendage	Median sternotomy	None
R.H.	0/0	Yes	25	Normal	Yes, bloody	1 hour	Right atrium IVC	Median sternotomy	Facial lacerations
T.A.	0/0	Yes	25–54	Normal	Trans. abd. bloody	4–5 hours	Right atrial appendage	Median sternotomy	Fx. left lobe of liver; compound fx. left tibia, fibula
J.S.	70/30	Yes	14–20	Normal heart, left hemothorax	Yes, bloody	1 hour	Right ventricle outflow	Median sternotomy	Facial laceration and Fx. zygoma; hematoma of mesocolon

*From Trueblood, H. W., Wuerflein, R. D., and Angell, W. W., Ann. Surg., 177:66, 1975.

TABLE 17–20. SUMMARY OF 10 PATIENTS TREATED WITH PERICARDIAL TAMPONADE, 27TH SURGICAL HOSPITAL, CHU LAI, REPUBLIC OF VIETNAM, APRIL 1968–DECEMBER 1968*

CASE	CONDITION ON ARRIVAL	PERI-CARDIO-CENTESIS	SYSTOLIC BLOOD PRESSURE AT OPERATION	ASSOCIATED INJURIES	INCISION	CARDIAC INJURY	OUTCOME
1	Mild shock	Yes	80 mm Hg	None	Sternal split	Outflow of right ventricle	Survived
2	Severe shock	Yes	Unobtainable	Perforations (20), small bowel	(L) Anterior thoractomy	Apex of right ventricle	Died
3	Stable	No	Under 80 mm Hg postinduction	Laceration, liver	Thoracoabdominal	None found	Survived
4	Severe shock	No	Under 80 mm Hg	Laceration, lingula, spleen	(L) Anterior thoracotomy	Transected coronary artery	Died
5	Mild shock	Yes	Under 80 mm Hg	Intracranial fragment	(L) Posterior lateral thoracotomy	Right ventricle	Died
6	Mild shock	Yes	Stable	Laceration of spleen	Thoracoabdominal	Right ventricle	Survived
7	Mild shock	Yes	Under 80 mm Hg	Bilateral leg amputations	(L) Anterior thoracotomy	Apex of right ventricle	Survived
8	Severe shock	No	Unobtainable	None	(R) Anterior thoracotomy	4 cm laceration post. (R) ventricle	Survived
9	Stable	No	80 mm Hg	None	(R) Posterolat. thoracotomy	Anterior right ventricle	Survived
10	Severe shock	Yes	80 mm Hg	Multiple wounds of extremities	(L) Anterior thoracotomy	Anterior right ventricle	Survived

*Modified from Tassi, A. A., and Davies, A. L., Am. J. Surg., *118*:535, 1969.

in both patients who had been involved in automobile accidents. Trueblood and colleagues (1973) reported their management of three patients with rupture of the heart secondary to blunt trauma and reviewed the previous literature (Table 17–19). Jones and co-workers (1975) documented their results in managing patients with cardiac contusions: a total of 48 patients with four deaths. Recent experience from one of the busy hospitals in Vietnam is documented in Table 17–20. There was a 30 per cent mortality among 10 patients with pericardial tamponade (Tassi and Davies, 1969). Two of the three deaths resulted from associated injuries. One patient died from septic complications of an abdominal injury, and another patient died from a head injury. The only patient who died as a direct result of the heart wound suffered injury to the anterior descending coronary artery.

Gielchinsky and McNamara (1970) recorded that in their series from the 24th Evacuation Hospital, all 10 patients who sustained heart wounds required a thoracotomy. This procedure was necessary in 80 per cent of the patients immediately following hospital admission. Seven of the eight required immediate thoracotomy because of acute tamponade and evidence of continued intrathoracic blood loss. Cardiorrhaphy was necessary for persistent bleeding in seven cardiac wounds, and the remaining patient died during the operation owing to bleeding from a large atrial tear with associated hypovolemic shock. Of the two remaining patients in this series of 10 cardiac injuries who were not operated upon immediately, one patient was operated upon three days after wounding because of the development

of a pericardial tamponade. It was felt that this tamponade resulted from indirect damage to the heart by the cavitational effect of a high velocity AK–47 bullet wound without direct injury from the missile itself. The last patient had multiple fléchette wounds. Because of the appearance of the position of the fléchette entirely within the myocardium determined by chest roentgenograms, the patient was evacuated to the United States where the fléchette was removed from the base of the heart near the aortic root with the use of cardiopulmonary bypass. The one patient who was admitted in profound shock out of the 10 patients with cardiac injury was the only patient in this series who died. These statistics in the Vietnam Vascular Registry reveal that more than 50 per cent of the patients required immediate operation following cardiac trauma in Vietnam (Table 17–21). Left thoracotomy was the incision of choice in about 59 per cent of the patients who had an operation (Table 17–22). The mortality rate among 96 patients was approximately 10 per cent, with four deaths directly due to cardiac injury (Table 17–23). Nearly 50 per

TABLE 17–22. CARDIAC TRAUMA IN VIETNAM: INCISIONS (51 Patients)*

	NUMBER	PER CENT
Left thoracotomy	30	58.8
Median sternotomy	11	21.6
Right thoracotomy	5	9.8
Bilateral anterior thoracotomy	4	7.8
Thoracoabdominal	1	2.0
Total:	51	100.0

*From Geer, T. M., and Rich, N. M., Vietnam Vascular Registry, Unpublished data, 1972.

TABLE 17–21. CARDIAC TRAUMA IN VIETNAM: TREATMENT*

	PATIENTS	PER CENT
Immediate operation	50	62.5
No operation	20	25.0
Pericardiocentesis only	2	2.5
Delayed operation	8	10.0
Total:	80	100.0

*From Geer, T. M., and Rich, N. M., Vietnam Vascular Registry, Unpublished data, 1972.

TABLE 17–23. CARDIAC TRAUMA IN VIETNAM: CAUSE OF DEATH*

Cardiac injury	4
Hemorrhage—shock	4
Head injury	1
Peritonitis	1
Total:	10

*From Geer, T. M., and Rich, N. M., Vietnam Vascular Registry, Unpublished data, 1972.

Four or five esophageal arteries arise from the front of the aorta, as well as small mediastinal arteries.

Anomalies may cause significant problems when encountered with trauma. Coarctation of the thoracic aorta and vascular rings, including a double aortic arch, are well-recognized major anomalies (Strandness, 1969). Occasionally, a small aberrant artery arises from the right side of the thoracic aorta and travels upward to the right behind the trachea and esophagus, representing the remnant of the first dorsal artery. It may enlarge to form the first portion of the right subclavian artery.

The most important physiologic characteristic of the thoracic aorta is that acute occlusion can be tolerated for only short periods of time, often no longer than 15 or 20 minutes. Occlusion longer than 20 minutes has a progressively increasing risk of paraplegia and may also precipitate acute left ventricular failure. Renal ischemia, progressing to renal shutdown, and hepatic ischemia develop with slightly longer periods of occlusion, 30 to 60 minutes.

PENETRATING INJURIES TO THE AORTA

INCIDENCE

In 1970 Symbas and Sehdeva reviewed reports and found a total of 43 patients who had been successfully treated for penetrating injuries of the thoracic aorta. Their review included patients who developed arteriovenous fistulas and were operated upon at a later time. In Table 18–1, experiences from 17 different reports from 1922 through 1970 are emphasized. The first successful repair of a stab wound is credited to a Russian surgeon, Dshanelidze, who in 1922 repaired an 8 mm puncture wound of the intrapericardial ascending aorta in a 20 year old man (Lilienthal, 1926). In the subsequent 30 years, four other successful repairs of stab wounds were reported, all of which involved the intrapericardial ascending aorta, most likely, with the intrapericardial location preventing exsanguination. A stab wound of the

TABLE 18–1. SUCCESSFUL REPAIR OF PENETRATING WOUNDS OF THE THORACIC AORTA: CASES OF HISTORICAL NOTE AND RECENT REPRESENTATIVE EXAMPLES

AUTHOR	AGE	WOUNDING AGENT	SIZE OF LACERATION	LOCATION	TYPE OF REPAIR
1. Dshanelidze (1922)	20	Not given	8 mm	Ascending	Suture
2. Blalock (1934)	18	Ice pick	Not stated	Ascending	Suture
3. Elkin (1941)	28	Ice pick	Not stated	Ascending	Suture
4. Elkin (1944)	44	Knife	Not stated	Ascending	Suture
5. Beattie and Greer (1952)	21	Penknife	14 mm	Ascending	Suture
6. Kleinert (1958)		Bullet	15 mm	Descending	Suture with patch
7. Baret et al. (1958)		Knife	15 mm	Descending	Suture
8. Perkins and Elchos (1958)	16	Knife	20 mm	Arch	Suture
9. Beall (1960)	17	Bullet	Not stated	Descending	Suture
10. Diveley et al. (1961)	28	Wire	2 mm	Ascending	Wire removed; suture
11. Beall et al.* (1962)	23	Knife	Not stated	Arch	Suture
12. Stelzner et al. (1963)		Bullet	Not stated	Ascending	
13. Overbeck et al. (1968)		Metal splinter	Not stated	Ascending	
14. Symbas and Sehdeva** (1970)	22	Sword	Not stated	Descending	Suture
15. Symbas and Sehdeva (1970)	25	Bullet	Not stated	Descending	Suture
16. Fromm et al. (1970)	17	Bullet (0.22 caliber)	10 mm	Descending	Suture
17. Fromm et al. (1970)	23	Bullet	Not stated	Descending	Suture

*Acute arteriovenous fistula.

**Two additional stab wounds mentioned in report.

TABLE 18–2. INCIDENCE OF INJURIES
OF THE THORACIC AORTA

	AUTHOR	TOTAL ARTERIES	AORTA	PER CENT
War Series				
WW I	Makins (1919)	1191	5*	—
WW II	De Bakey and Simeone (1946)	2471	3*	—
Korea	Hughes (1958)	304	0	0
Vietnam	Rich et al. (1970A)	1000	0	0
Civilian Series				
Houston	Morris et al. (1960)	220	23*	—
Atlanta	Ferguson et al. (1961)	200	0	0
Denver	Owens (1963)	70	0	0
Detroit	Smith et al. (1963)	61	2	3.3
Dallas	Patman et al. (1964)	271	6*	—
Los Angeles	Treiman et al. (1966)	287	11*	—
St. Louis	Dillard et al. (1968)	85	8	9.4
New Orleans	Drapanas et al. (1970)	226	11	4.9
Memphis	Cheek et al. (1975)	155	3	1.9
Jackson	Hardy et al. (1975)	360	14	3.9
New York	Bole et al. (1976)	126	2	1.6

*Abdominal and thoracic aortas.

aortic arch was not successfully repaired until 1958 (Perkins and Elchos). In Table 18–2, eight reports of experiences with civilian arterial injuries are tabulated, representing a total of over 1400 arterial injuries. In this large group there were a total of 61 injuries that involved either the abdominal or thoracic aorta. Dillard and colleagues (1968) reported eight patients who sustained trauma to the thoracic aorta among 85 patients with arterial injuries, an incidence of 9.4 per cent. In New Orleans Drapanas and co-workers (1970) included 11 patients with injuries of the thoracic aorta in their series of 226 arterial injuries for a 4.9 per cent incidence. The largest individual experience has been reported by Beall and co-authors (1967) from Houston, involving 15 patients with injuries from penetrating wounds.

Military experience with thoracic aortic injuries was negligible until the Vietnam Conflict. Only five cases are mentioned from World War I, three from World War II, and none from the Korean Conflict (see Table 18–2). There was no distinction made between trauma to the abdominal aorta as opposed to the thoracic aorta. In the interim report from the Vietnam Vascular Registry of 1000 acute major arterial injuries, the only three aortic injuries found all involved the abdominal aorta

(Rich et al., 1970A). A subsequent more extensive evaluation of the Vietnam experience was carried out by Billy and associates (1971). This study included a thorough review of the experience in Vietnam between 1965 and 1970 with more than 6500 patients' records from the Vietnam Vascular Registry and with the records of more than 7800 patients who had missile wounds evaluated by the Wound Data Ammunitions Effectiveness Team. There were a total of 138 aortic injuries. Among the total of 39 aortic wounds that were treated, 20 involved the thoracic aorta. However, among the autopsy cases, there was a much higher incidence of thoracic aorta involvement—85 cases compared to only 14 cases involving abdominal aortic injury (Fig. 18–2).

ETIOLOGY

Most of the first successful repairs of aortic injuries were for lacerations from a small stab wound, such as that produced by an ice pick (Fig. 18–3). An unusual injury was reported by Diveley and associates (1961) of a 28 year old man who had experienced a sharp pain in the anterior chest while pushing a rotary lawnmower. A chest

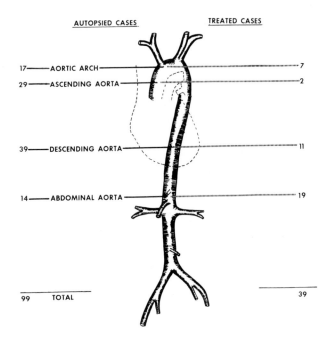

AUTOPSIED CASES		TREATED CASES

17——— AORTIC ARCH ———————————————— 7

29——— ASCENDING AORTA ———————————— 2

39——— DESCENDING AORTA ———————————— 11

14——— ABDOMINAL AORTA ———————————— 19

99   TOTAL   39

Figure 18–2. Distribution of aortic injuries in autopsied and treated cases among combat casualties in Vietnam. The largest number of injuries (50) involved the descending thoracic aorta. (Billy, L. J., Amato, J. J., and Rich, N. M., Surgery, 70:385, 1971.)

roentgenogram revealed a metallic foreign body adjacent to the ascending aorta (Fig. 18–4). At operation a heavy rusty wire 5 cm in length was removed. Overbeck and co-authors (1968) described laceration of the ascending aorta by a metal splinter. In recent years successful repairs following low velocity bullet wounds have been reported. Fromm and colleagues (1970) reported a case of a 17 year old male shot

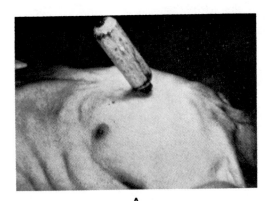

A

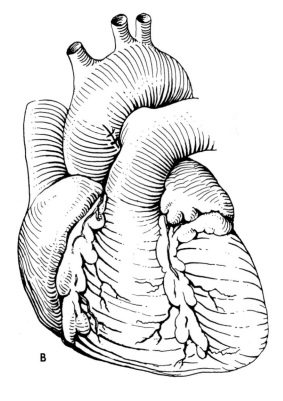

B

Figure 18–3. (A) Early successful repair of the thoracic aorta was possible following stab wounds, such as that with an ice pick shown in this photograph. In this case, lateral suture repair of a small laceration of the ascending aorta was performed. (B) Location and repair of stab wound. (McCann, W. J., N.Y. State J. Med., 58:3177, 1958.)

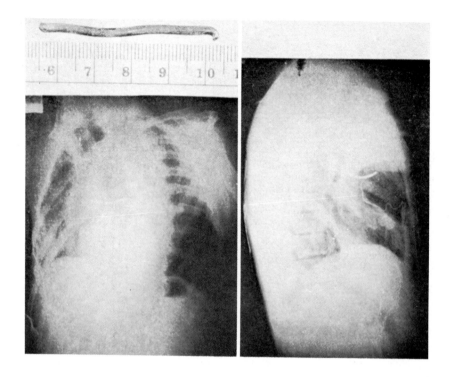

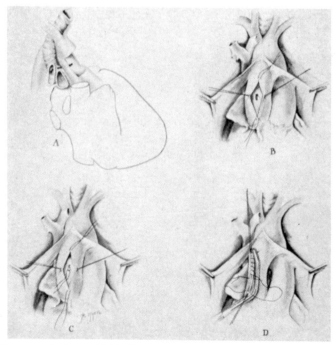

Figure 18–4. (A) Anteroposterior and lateral roentgenograms of the chest show a piece of wire (recovered wire above on left) which penetrated the chest of a 28 year old man who was pushing a rotary lawn mower. (B) Schematic drawing depicts the location of the wire and the method of removal from the ascending aorta. (Diveley, W. L., Rollin, A. D., Jr., and Scott, H. W., Jr., J. Thorac. and Cardiovasc. Surg., *41*:23, 1961.)

TABLE 18-3. ETIOLOGY OF THE WOUNDING AGENT IN VIETNAM

WOUNDING AGENT	NUMBER	PER CENT
Fragment	13	65
Bullet	6	30
Flechette	1	5
Total:	20	100

TABLE 18-4. EXTENT OF THE PENETRATING INJURY TO THE THORACIC AND ABDOMINAL AORTAS IN THE VIETNAM EXPERIENCE*

	AUTOPSIED CASES	TREATED CASES
Laceration	46 (46.5%)	23 (58.9%)
Perforation	15 (15.2%)	8 (20.5%)
Transection	34 (34.3%)	1 (2.6%)
Contusion	1 (1.0%)	0 (0.0%)
False aneurysm	0 (0.0%)	1 (2.6%)
Not stated	3 (3.0%)	6 (15.4%)
Total:	99 (100.0%)	39 (100.0%)

*Modified from Billy, L. J., Amato, J. J., and Rich, N. M., Surgery, 70:385, 1971.

with a 0.22 caliber pistol who survived despite a through-and-through perforation of the aorta just below the left subclavian artery. One similar case involving a gunshot wound perforating the aorta about 3 cm below the left subclavian artery was also reported.

With military injuries from high velocity bullets, survival is rare. Of the 20 injuries in Vietnam in surviving patients, 13 resulted from shell fragments, six from low velocity bullets and one from a flechette (Table 18-3).

One obscure case involving a penetrating wound of the thoracic aorta is worth noting for historical interest. Edmundson (1936) reported a patient who had been wounded by an arrow at close range. Despite the fact that the wounded man's friends tried to remove the arrow by cutting and pulling, the patient did survive 13 hours to reach a hospital. Unfortunately, the patient exsanguinated when the arrow was surgically removed. Another description of historical interest involves the legendary "Maltese twist" (Lindskog et al., 1962). This involved extending the victim's neck prior to thrusting a long knife into the thorax through the substernal notch. The knife was then twisted to sever the great vessels from the heart.

CLINICAL PATHOLOGY

Most injuries in surviving patients are small lacerations or perforations (Table 18-4). Transection was seen only once in a surviving patient. Usually injury involved either the ascending aorta or the descending aorta. Arch injuries are unusual, perhaps because of its short length and restricted location.

Survival can occur with fairly small lacerations of the thoracic aorta. This is emphasized in Table 18-1, in which nearly all reported lacerations were small enough to allow successful repair. The ice pick stab wounds reported by Blalock (1934) and Elkin (1941) were essentially no more than puncture wounds. Minimal tissue damage occurs with knife wounds, as demonstrated in the successful repair of lacerations of the thoracic aorta. Also, low velocity bullets cause minimal tissue damage. A 0.22 caliber gunshot wound of the descending aorta reported by Fromm and colleagues (1970) created only a 10 mm through-and-through perforation which was occluded by thrombus at the time of exploration.

Catheter perforations of the thoracic aorta have essentially been limited to small perforating injuries which might only be intramural (Hurwitt and Seidenberg, 1965). Atheromatous changes can potentiate the hazard of this type of injury. Nevertheless, this injury can occur in the normal aorta of a young adult (Fig. 18-5).

CLINICAL FEATURES

The dominant feature is a penetrating thoracic wound with intrathoracic hemorrhage and shock. If the intrapericardial ascending aorta is involved, signs of cardiac tamponade may dominate the clinical picture. In most instances there are no signs to

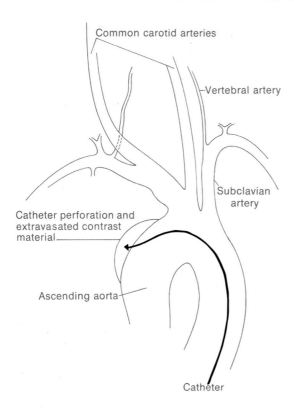

Figure 18–5. Extravasation of contrast media following perforation of the aortic arch by a catheter and guide used in performing an aortogram is obvious. Nonoperative management was successful. (W.R.G.H., 1968.)

distinguish aortic injuries from the usual penetrating wounds of the thorax with intrathoracic bleeding, shock and hemothorax. A continuous murmur has occasionally been detected with penetrating injuries which create an acute arteriovenous fistula.

Beall and co-workers (1962) described a case of a 23 year old man stabbed one hour earlier above the suprasternal notch (Fig. 18–6). A marked continuous thrill and bruit over the anterior chest was immediately detected.

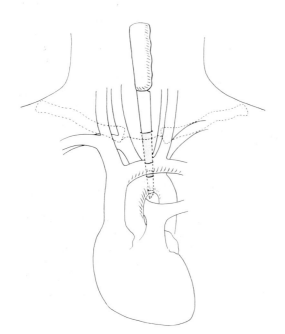

Figure 18–6. Diagram shows tract of knife wound through left innominate vein and aortic arch exiting from posteroinferior aspect of the arch. Lateral suture repair of all lacerations was successful. (Beall, A. C., Jr., Roof, W. R., and DeBakey, M. E., Ann. Surg., *156*: 823, 1962.)

DIAGNOSTIC CONSIDERATIONS

In some patients the possibility of aortic injury may be suggested by chest roentgenograms which demonstrate a missile near the aorta with a surrounding hematoma (Fig. 18–7).

SURGICAL MANAGEMENT

Thoracotomy is usually required promptly because of continued intrathoracic bleeding and shock. Initial resuscitation involves rapid transfusion of blood for correction of shock, soon followed by thoracotomy. For wounds possibly involving the ascending aorta or the aortic arch, a median sternotomy provides the best exposure (see Fig. 18–8). Otherwise, a left posterolateral thoracotomy should be used, which widely exposes the entire descending thoracic aorta. In almost all patients the injury is a small laceration which can be repaired by suture. In some instances hemorrhage has temporarily ceased because a blood clot has formed in and around the laceration. Before the pleura over the hematoma is incised, the possibility of aortic injury should be considered and the aorta isolated proximally and distally.

Two other possibilities should be considered. The first is the use of arterial autotransfusion by heparinizing the patient, aspirating blood from the thoracic cavity and reinfusing it through a cannula placed in the common femoral artery. This has been satisfactorily performed in a number of patients with penetrating thoracic injuries. The other consideration is temporary aortic bypass because occlusion of the aorta for longer than 20 minutes may cause permanent paraplegia in some patients. The simplest form of aortic bypass is establishment of a temporary shunt between the proximal and distal aorta, with either a plastic tube (Fig. 18–9), preferably heparinized, or a large, long, Dacron graft sutured to the aorta proximally and distally.

Once preliminary plans have been made, the mediastinal pleura can be incised and the hematoma evacuated. Temporary occlusion of the aorta is usually required. Of the 20 patients operated upon in Vietnam,

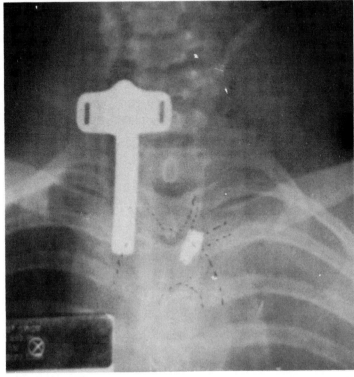

Figure 18–7. The presence of a missile near the aorta with or without an associated hematoma seen on a roentgenogram of the chest should alert one to the possibility of aortic injury. (Vietnam Vascular Registry #7,128. Courtesy Audiovisual Service, Walter Reed Army Institute of Research.)

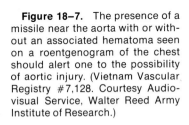

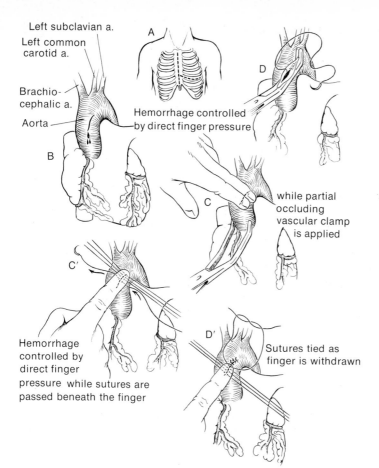

Left subclavian a.

Left common carotid a.

Brachio- cephalic a.

Aorta

A

Hemorrhage controlled by direct finger pressure

D

B

C

while partial occluding vascular clamp is applied

C′

Hemorrhage controlled by direct finger pressure while sutures are passed beneath the finger

D′

Sutures tied as finger is withdrawn

Figure 18–8. (A) Median sternotomy provides rapid access to expose wounds of the ascending aorta and the aortic arch. (B) Laceration of the ascending aorta. (C) Digital compression controls hemorrhage while a partial occluding clamp is applied. (D) Arteriorrhapy is then possible. (C′) Interrupted sutures can be passed under the finger. (D′) Hemostasis can be maintained by slowly withdrawing the finger as the sutures are tied in succession.

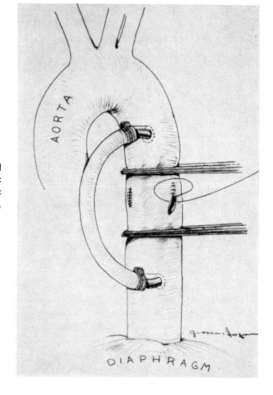

Figure 18–9. A heparinized plastic tube can be used as a temporary aortic bypass during repair of the thoracic aorta. This can help prevent distal ischemia during aortic occlusion. (Symbas, P. N., and Sehdeva, J. S., Ann. Surg., 171:441, 1970.)

TABLE 18–5. REPAIR OF THE THORACIC AORTA IN VIETNAM CASUALTIES

NUMBER	METHOD
16	Suture
2	Prosthesis
1	Dacron patch
1	Excision of fragment
Total: 20	

16 were repaired by suture, and only two required insertion of a prosthesis (Table 18–5). Neither of the patients requiring a prosthesis ultimately survived. One patient had the unusual condition of a fragment imbedded in the wall of the aortic arch (Fig. 18–10), which was successfully removed at operation.

The main hazard at operation, aside from exsanguination, is paraplegia from prolonged occlusion of the aorta. If these haz-

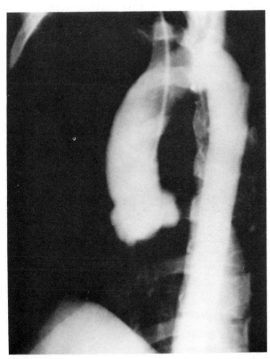

Figure 18–10. A small fragment is embedded in the adventitia of the inferior portion of the aortic arch in this Vietnam casualty. At the time of removal of the fragment at Walter Reed General Hospital, it was recognized that only the adventitia of the aorta had been penetrated. (Billy, L. J., Amato, J. J., and Rich, N. M., Surgery, 70:385, 1971.)

ards have been avoided at operation, postoperative care is similar to that for any thoracotomy for penetrating injury of the chest. Complications in surviving patients have fortunately not been significant. There have been no instances of infection with dehiscence of the vascular repair, thrombosis or late formation of an aneurysm.

NONPENETRATING INJURIES OF THE AORTA

INCIDENCE

The classic report by Parmley and coworkers in 1958 of 275 patients with rupture of the aorta from nonpenetrating causes focused clinical attention on this unusual injury. A subsequent extensive review of reported surgical experiences with this condition by one of the authors (FCS) in 1961 found only two instances in which thoracotomy had been successfully performed within the first few days after injury. With increasing familiarity with this lesion, combined with aortography and improved techniques of thoracic surgery, a decade later Paton and co-authors (1971) found reports of over 200 patients, 30 of whom had been operated upon within 48 hours of injury. Another comprehensive review of 110 patients was published by Rittenhouse and colleagues in 1969. In a recent review of the English literature, Symbas and colleagues (1973) found 204 case reports of surgical treatment of thoracic aortic rupture from blunt trauma, and they reviewed the case histories of six similar patients from their hospital.

ETIOLOGY

Rupture of the thoracic aorta usually occurs in an injury that produces acute horizontal deceleration. Apparently the aortic arch and the descending thoracic aorta decelerate at different velocities, resulting in transverse rupture either in the ascending aorta or in the aortic isthmus just beyond the left subclavian artery. Hence, such injuries most commonly result from

TABLE 18–6. TYPES OF ACCIDENTS IN WHICH NONPENETRATING TRAUMA PRODUCED AORTIC RUPTURE OR RUPTURE ASSOCIATED WITH CARDIAC INJURY IN 275 INDIVIDUALS*

CAUSE	ISOLATED AORTIC RUPTURE	COMBINED WITH CARDIAC INJURY	TOTAL
Automobile	114	42	156
Airplane	12	31	43
Vehicle vs. pedestrian	9	7	16
Fall (long distance)	12	12	24
Motorcycle	3	1	4
Automobile vs. train	0	2	2
Compression by heavy object	4	0	4
Buried by dirt	1	0	1
Direct blow by object	5	0	5
Unknown	11	9	20
Total:	171	104	275

*Modified from Parmley, L. F., Mattingly, T. W., and Manion, W. C., Circulation, *17*:953, 1958.

automobile or airplane accidents and rarely from a fall, compression by heavy objects or a direct blow to the chest (Table 18–6). In a total of 171 isolated ruptures studied by Parmley and co-workers (1958), the injury was sustained in an automobile, an airplane or some other type of motor vehicle in 138 of the 171. Mulder and Grollman (1969) reported a series of nine patients, eight injured in an automobile accident and one in an airplane accident. Paton and co-workers (1971) reported six patients, all injured in automobile accidents. Rupture of the thoracic aorta has occasionally been associated with external cardiac massage. Patterson and colleagues (1973) cited one case and added two of their own. Schwartz and associates (1975) reviewed 19 posttraumatic false aneurysms following automobile accidents in Minneapolis.

CLINICAL PATHOLOGY

About 80 per cent of patients exsanguinate immediately, but between 10 and 20 per cent live long enough for diagnosis and treatment. Injuries in almost all surviving patients are located just beyond the left subclavian artery, for transverse tears of the intrapericardial ascending aorta are virtually always fatal (Table 18–7). In surviving patients the hemorrhage is initially contained by the aortic adventitia and mediastinal adventitia (Fig. 18–11). The ability of the mediastinal pleura to contain hemorrhage is astonishing. Some patients have survived transection of the aorta with retraction of the ends for as much as 1 cm. The danger of fatal rupture into the left hemithorax is ever present after injury for as long as two months. If rupture has not occurred by this time, mediastinal fibrosis apparently has progressed to such an extent that subsequent acute rupture is almost unknown. Instead, a chronic aneurysm develops which enlarges at a very slow rate. Lesions have been recognized as late as 10 to 20 years after the initial injury. Such aneurysms enlarge much more slowly than other traumatic aneurysms, remaining stationary for long periods of time. When enlargement eventually occurs, symptoms first appear from compression of the left main bronchus. Many asymptomatic patients are first detected with a traumatic aneurysm when a chest roentgenogram made for other reasons discloses a calcified posterior mediastinal mass.

TABLE 18–7. SITES OF RUPTURE OF THE AORTA DUE TO NONPENETRATING TRAUMA TABULATED TO SHOW THE INCIDENCE OF RUPTURE OF A SPECIFIC SITE AND THE FREQUENCY OF ASSOCIATED CARDIAC INJURY IN 275 INDIVIDUALS*

SITE OF RUPTURE	ISOLATED AORTIC RUPTURE	COMBINED WITH CARDIAC INJURY	TOTAL
Ascending aorta	17	47	64
Arch	16	6	22
Isthmus	95	29	124
Thoracic aorta	27	8	35
Abdominal aorta	11	2	13
Multiple sites	5	12	17
Total:	171	104	275

*Modified from Parmley, L. F., Mattingly, T. W., and Manion, W. C., Circulation, *17*:953, 1958.

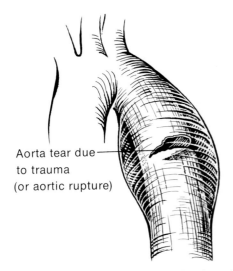

Figure 18–11. Survival of the injured patient with an injured thoracic aorta is possible. Hemorrhage can be contained in the aortic adventitia.

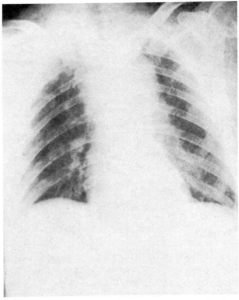

Figure 18–12. Widening of the mediastinum following trauma to the chest heralds the probability of aortic rupture. This roentgenogram shows mediastinal widening and multiple rib fractures on the right in a 41 year old man involved in an automobile accident. (Spencer, F. C., Guerin, P. F., Blake, H. A., and Bahnson, H. T., J. Thorac. Cardiovasc. Surg., 41:1, 1961.)

Most injuries have occurred in young adult males, probably because of the frequency with which they are involved in automobile accidents. A report by Meyer and colleagues in 1969 of repair of a traumatic rupture in an 8 year old boy was thought to be the first successful treatment of rupture of the aorta in a child.

CLINICAL FEATURES

Often there are no signs or symptoms in a patient with a crushing injury of the chest to indicate that rupture of the aorta has occurred. Usually there are multiple rib fractures with hemothorax, dyspnea and varying degrees of shock. However, peripheral pulses are normal, and murmurs, though reported, are rare. The hallmark of aortic rupture is the finding on chest roentgenogram of widening of the mediastinum (Fig. 18–12). This widening, resulting from hemorrhage within the mediastinum, has been found in virtually every case reported involving rupture of the aorta. Although such widening can be produced by hematoma due to factors other than aortic rupture, its presence must be interpreted with extreme gravity. In most patients the simple finding of widening of the mediastinum is an indication for immediate aortography. This is emphasized because asymptomatic

patients have been reported again and again who had no finding other than widening of the mediastinum until exsanguination abruptly occurred days or weeks after injury. Aortography was first used by one of the authors (FCS) with a case treated at Walter Reed General Hospital in 1960. It can promptly establish or exclude the diagnosis (Fig. 18–13).

Once the diagnosis has been established by aortography, thoracotomy should be promptly performed, using a posterolateral incision. Preparations should be made beforehand for bypass of the thoracic aorta, preferably keeping a pump-oxygenator on a standby basis. Probably the safest approach is to expose first the femoral artery and vein for cannulation in the event that bypass is needed. Once the patient has been heparinized, blood can be aspirated from the pleural cavity and reinfused. Left atrial-femoral bypass is another method, the first used historically, but is slightly more complicated, as the pericardium must be opened and the left atrium cannulated.

An attractive method of bypass, not requiring heparin, is the insertion of a

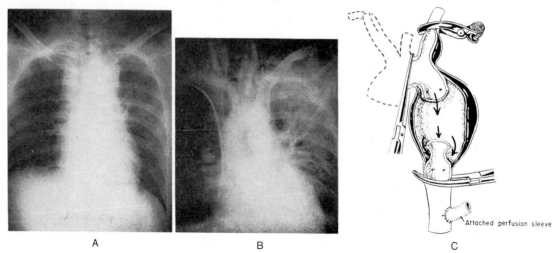

A   B   C

Figure 18–13. (A) Admission roentgenogram shows mediastinal widening. (B) Aortogram reveals the area of aortic rupture as a localized irregular enlargement of the aorta distal to the subclavian artery. (C) Drawing shows the operative findings. (Spencer, F. C., Guerin, P. F., Blake, H. A., and Bahnson, H. T., J. Thorac. Cardiovasc. Surg., *41*:1, 1961.)

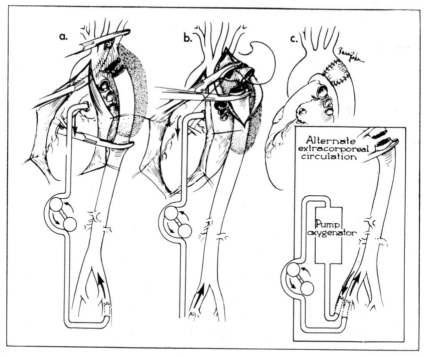

Figure 18–14. Cardiopulmonary bypass. (a) Left atrial to femoral artery pump bypass instituted, proximally aortic control obtained transpericardially, distal aortic and left subclavian artery control obtained outside of area of hematoma. (b) Hematoma entered, proximal and distal aortic clamps reapplied immediately above and below area of transection, and aortic continuity re-established with graft. (c) Completed operation. Insert: Alternate technique of extracorporeal circulation using partial cardiopulmonary bypass with pump oxygenator from femoral vein to femoral artery. (Beall, A. C., Jr., Arbegast, N. R., Ripepi, A. C., Bricker, D. L., Diethrich, E. B., Hallman, G. L., Cooley, D. A., and DeBakey, M. E., Arch. Surg., *98*:595, 1969.)

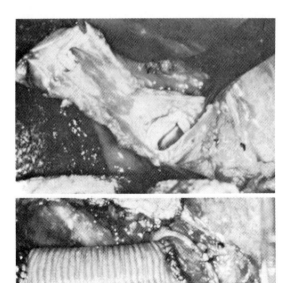

Figure 18–15. (A) The incised aneurysm shows the two ends of the aorta widely separated because of intimal retraction. (B) After resection of the aneurysm, arterial continuity was restored with a Dacron prosthesis. (Spencer, F. C., Guerin, P. F., Blake, H. A., and Bahnson, H. T., J. Thorac. Cardiovasc. Surg., *41*:1, 1961.)

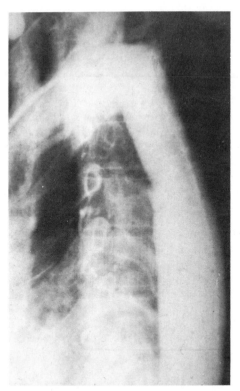

Figure 18–17. This angiogram shows patency of a Dacron prosthesis 12 years after repair of a posttraumatic false aneurysm performed at Walter Reed General Hospital in 1963. (N. M. R., 1976.)

large plastic tube between the aorta proximally and either the aorta distally or the common femoral artery. When circumstances permit, this type of bypass is ideal because of its simplicity and because heparin is not required. Preparations, when possible, should be made, however, for the more standard cardiopulmonary bypass because of the risk of abrupt intrathoracic

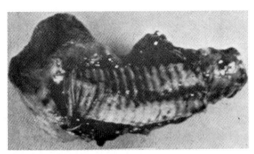

Figure 18–16. This infected Teflon prosthesis, with surrounding tissue, was removed six months after the initial operation on the thoracic aorta. This serious complication has not been frequently reported. (Rittenhouse, E. A., Dillard, D. H., Winterscheid, L. C., and Merendino, K. A., Ann. Surg., *170*: 87, 1969.)

hemorrhage once the thorax has been opened (Fig. 18–14).

The aorta proximal and distal to the site of injury should be isolated before the hematoma is explored. Proximal aortic control is usually best obtained by opening the

TABLE 18–8. MORTALITY OF 110 PATIENTS OPERATED UPON FOR TRAUMATIC AORTIC RUPTURE BETWEEN 1950 AND 1967*

CAUSE OF DEATH	NUMBER OF PATIENTS
Hemorrhagic shock	11
Esophageal rupture and mediastinitis	4
Ventricular fibrillation	2
Cardiac injury	1
Renal failure and pneumonia	1
Undetermined	1
Total:	20

*Adapted from Rittenhouse, E. A., Dillard, D. H., Winterschild, L. C., and Merendino, K. A., Ann. Surg., *170*:87, 1969.

pericardium and encircling the aorta between the left carotid and left subclavian arteries. Distal control can easily be obtained at a convenient level. If an aortic injury is strongly probable, temporary occlusion of the aorta proximally and distally with vascular clamps should be performed before the hematoma is opened. Once the hematoma has been explored and an aortic laceration found, insertion of a short prosthetic graft, usually Dacron, is usually necessary (Fig. 18–15). The approximation of the transected ends of the aorta and repair by direct suture have usually not been possible. Once repair has been done, the prognosis is good. Postoperative complications are infrequent. Trauma to the recurrent laryngeal nerve, coursing around the ligamentum arteriosum near the site of injury, has been reported, because the nerve is often concealed in adjacent hematoma. Usually recovery after operation has been complete with no significant late complications. The rare dreaded complication of infection of the prosthetic graft was reported in one patient by Rittenhouse and colleagues in 1969. Three months after operation infection of the graft became clinically apparent and did not respond to massive doses of antibiotics administered for several weeks. A repeat operation was performed six months after the initial operation, at which time the infected graft was replaced with a homograft (Fig. 18–16). Although the long term fate of the homograft is uncertain, 2½ years following operation the patient was asymptomatic.

Experiences with operations upon 110 patients for traumatic aortic rupture between 1950 and 1967 are summarized in Table 18–8. Twenty deaths occurred, usually from shock, ventricular fibrillation or associated injuries of the esophagus with infection. One long-term follow-up at Walter Reed General Hospital includes the angiographic demonstration of a patent prosthesis 12 years after repair of the thoracic aorta Fig. 18–17).

CHAPTER 19

INJURIES OF THE ABDOMINAL AORTA

Injuries of the abdominal aorta were of little clinical significance until recent years, because in most cases death resulted soon after the injury from exsanguinating hemorrhage. However, the possibilities of repair have increased substantially owing to more rapid methods of transportation of wounded patients and increased success with resuscitation and vascular repair. In addition, trauma to the abdominal aorta is now more important because of the increasing frequency of traumatic injuries in the civilian population.

Historically, the first successful repair was performed by Wildegans in 1926, who sutured a 1 cm stab wound of the abdominal aorta. However, 40 years later, Richards and colleagues (1966) were able to find a total of only 12 cases in which a successful repair had been done (Table 19–1). The first survivor after a penetrating missile wound of the abdominal aorta was reported by Dubinskiy in 1944, who sutured a 0.3 cm shrapnel wound. In 1948 Holzer reported two successful repairs of gunshot wounds.

Before the Vietnam Conflict, successful repair of aortic injuries in military casualties

TABLE 19–1. THE FIRST 40 YEARS OF SUCCESSFULLY REPAIRED PENETRATING WOUNDS OF THE ABDOMINAL AORTA*

AUTHORS	CAUSE OF INJURY	TYPE OF INJURY	TYPE OF REPAIR
Wildegans (1926)	Stab wound	1 cm laceration	Suture
Dubinskiy (1944)	Shrapnel wound	3 mm laceration	Suture
Holzer (1948)	Gunshot wound	5 mm laceration	Vitallium tube graft
Holzer (1948)	Gunshot wound	1 cm laceration	Suture
Beall (1960)	Stab wound	Laceration	Suture
Beall (1960)	Gunshot wound	Laceration	Suture
Beall (1960)	Gunshot wound	Laceration	Suture
Beall (1960)	Gunshot wound	Laceration	Suture
Manlove et al. (1960)	Gunshot wound	Laceration, 6 mm entrance, 20 mm exit	Suture
Bradham et al. (1962)	Gunshot wound	Laceration, 1.0 × 0.5 cm entrance and exit	Suture
Jensen (1963)	Gunshot wound	5 mm laceration	Suture
Love and Evans (1963)	Gunshot wound	8 mm laceration	Suture
Richards et al. (1966)	Gunshot wound	Laceration	Suture
Richards et al. (1966)	Gunshot wound	Laceration	Suture

*Adapted from Richards, A. J., Lamis, P. A., Rodgers, J. P., Jr., and Bradham, G. B., Ann. Surg., *164*:321, 1966.

TABLE 19–2. INCIDENCE OF INJURIES OF THE ABDOMINAL AORTA

	AUTHORS	TOTAL ARTERIES	AORTA	PER CENT
War Series				
WW I	Makins (1919)	1191	5*	0.4*
WW II	DeBakey and Simeone (1946)	2471	3*	0.1*
Korean	Hughes (1958)	304	0	0.0
Vietnam	Rich et al. (1970A)	1000	3	0.3
Civilian Series				
Houston	Morris et al. (1960)	220	23*	1.0*
Atlanta	Ferguson et al. (1961)	200	5*	0.3*
Denver	Owens (1963)	70	2	2.9
Detroit	Smith et al. (1963)	61	0	0.0
Dallas	Patman et al. (1964)†	271	6*	2.2*
Los Angeles	Treiman et al. (1966)	287	11*	3.8*
St. Louis	Dillard et al. (1968)	85	8‡	9.4‡
New Orleans	Drapanas et al. (1970)	226	12	5.3
Dallas	Perry et al. (1971)†	508	26*	5.1*
Jackson	Hardy et al. (1975)	360	22	6.1
Memphis	Cheek et al. (1975)	155	25	16.1
New York	Bole et al. (1976)	126	11	8.7

*Abdominal and thoracic aorta.
†This is a continuing series from the same center.
‡Abdominal aorta and branches.

was negligible (Table 19–2). DeBakey and Simeone in 1946 reported only three injuries among 2471 arterial injuries in World War II, while Hughes (1958) found no aortic injuries in a total of 304 arterial injuries in the Korean Conflict. In the Vietnam casualties, Billy and co-authors (1971) reported 33 patients with abdominal aortic trauma, some of whom were found at autopsy, but 14 of the 33 survived.

If patients with abdominal aortic injuries are to be successfully managed, immediate resuscitation is mandatory, with surgical repair of the aortic defects frequently playing a vital role in resuscitative attempts.

SURGICAL ANATOMY

After the descending aorta passes through the chest as the thoracic aorta, it continues in the median plane as the abdominal aorta. The aortic opening of the diaphragm in front of the lower border of the last thoracic vertebra marks the beginning of the abdominal aorta. Termination of the abdominal aorta occurs in front of the lower part of the body of the fourth lumbar vertebra when it divides into the two common iliac arteries. As the abdominal aorta passes downward, it pursues an oblique course, inclining slightly to the left. Feller and Woodburne (1961) made an extensive study of 100 abdominal aortas from fixed cadavers and found the average length of the abdominal aorta to be 13 cm.

The celiac and aortic plexuses are in intimate relationship with the abdominal aorta. Also in close proximity from above downward are the following: the pancreas and splenic vein; the left renal vein; the third portion of the duodenum; the root of the mesentery and the superior mesenteric vessels; and the peritoneum which separates the lower part of the aorta from the small intestine (Fig. 19–1). Posteriorly, the abdominal aorta rests on the bodies of the lumbar vertebra and the intravertebral discs. However, the aorta is separated from these structures by the anterior longitudinal ligament. On either side, the proximal abdominal aorta is related to the crus of the diaphragm. Distally, the sympathetic chain is in close relationship on each side. The inferior vena cava lies close to the aorta on the right side as high as the second lumbar vertebra, but above this the aorta is separated from the vena cava by the right

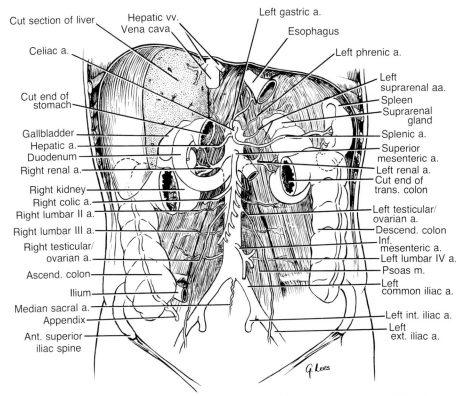

Figure 19–1. The surgical anatomy of the abdominal aorta with its major branches. The close proximity of numerous intra-abdominal organs is emphasized.

crus. On the left side, the fourth portion of the duodenum and coils of the jejunum are in close proximity below the level of the crus.

The branches of the abdominal aorta are classified under two headings, single and paired. Feller and Woodburne (1961) have evaluated the variation in the origin of the aortic branches. There are four single branches from the abdominal aorta. The highest branch is the celiac artery, closely followed by the superior mesenteric artery (Fig. 19–1). In the most distal portion, the inferior mesenteric artery originates. The last single branch is the median sacral artery which arises from the posterior and inferior portion of the aorta and runs into the pelvis.

The pelvic arteries are the first paired branches from the abdominal aorta, and these traverse the lower surface of the diaphragm. Occasionally, a small pair of middle suprarenal arteries may be iden-tified. The relatively wide renal arteries originate from the sides of the aorta less than one inch below the level of the superior mesenteric artery, opposite the second lumbar vertebra. Accessory renal arteries may also be present, especially on the left side. The testicular arteries in the male or the ovarian arteries in the female are a pair of long, slender arteries which arise from the anterior surface of the abdominal aorta a short distance below the renal arteries. Four pairs of lumbar arteries usual-ly originate from the posterior surface of the abdominal aorta in series with the inter-costal arteries of the thoracic aorta. Feller and Woodburne (1961) found five pairs of lumbar arteries in 26 per cent of the aortas in their study.

Pathways of potential collateral circula-tion include branches of the celiac as well as the superior and inferior mesenteric arteries, the lumbar arteries and the epi-gastric arteries in the abdominal wall.

INCIDENCE

The true incidence of aortic trauma is undoubtedly much higher than documented because many patients do not survive long enough to reach medical attention. The over-all frequency of injuries of the abdominal aorta in both military and civilian life is tabulated in Table 19–2.

Aortic injuries have comprised less than 1 per cent of all arterial trauma in past military experience. Rich and associates (1970A) recorded only three patients with abdominal aortic injuries; all three survived: 0.3 per cent of 1000 acute major arterial injuries in an interim Vietnam report. A subsequent, more detailed search of over 6000 records in the Vietnam Vascular Registry revealed that 20 patients with aortic injuries had arrived alive at military hospitals in Vietnam. These results were combined with those of a special study of wound ballistics which included an additional 14 autopsied cases with trauma to the abdominal aorta sustained in Vietnam (Billy et al., 1971). The over-all incidence remained approximately 0.3 per cent.

The incidence of abdominal trauma in civilian practice has not differed greatly from that in the military except in the past few years. Often when trauma to the thoracic and abdominal aortas has been included, with no separation of acute arterial injuries from those with delayed recognition, such as false aneurysms, the incidence of injuries has ranged from zero to approximately 5 per cent of all arterial injuries. Morris and colleagues (1960), in reviewing 220 arterial injuries in Houston, documented 23 aortic injuries, approximately 1 per cent of the arterial injuries in their series. Drapanas and colleagues (1970) documented 12 abdominal aortic injuries in New Orleans, 5.3 per cent of the 226 arterial injuries. Dillard and co-authors (1968) in St. Louis listed eight persons among their 85 patients with arterial injuries who had trauma to the abdominal aorta and its branches, but they did not specify how many involved only the abdominal aorta. As noted in Table 19–2, the recent large series by Perry and colleagues (1971) combines injuries of the thoracic and abdominal aortas: 26 injuries out of 508 arterial injuries, for an incidence of 5.1 per cent. Three series reported in 1975 and 1976 showed an increase in the number of injuries of the abdominal aorta. In a series of 360 arterial injuries in Jackson, Hardy and co-authors (1975) found 22 wounds of the abdominal aorta for an incidence of 6.1 per cent. Bole and associates (1976) found an incidence of 8.7 per cent in New York City. The highest incidence of injuries of the abdominal aorta in civilian series of arterial injuries was reported in 1975 by Cheek and colleagues from Memphis.

Emphasizing the increase in the number of patients seen in urban centers with trauma to the aorta, Fromm and colleagues (1970) reported that ten patients arrived alive in their emergency room in a 2½-year period starting in July, 1967. Allen and co-workers (1972) expanded the Houston series to 91 patients with traumatic injuries of the aorta, including 63 injuries of the abdominal aorta. Stone and associates (1973) reported 51 patients with penetrating wounds of the abdominal aorta in Atlanta. Lim and colleagues (1974) treated 32 acute abdominal aortic injuries during a five year period in San Francisco.

ETIOLOGY

The majority of the injuries have been lacerations from knife wounds or low velocity missile wounds. It might be predicted that most survivors from missile wounds would be from low velocity missiles, because more destructive high velocity missiles usually produce exsanguination. Holzer (1948) reported two of the earliest cases of successful management of gunshot wounds of the abdominal aorta. One patient was a 26 year old woman shot with a .32 caliber revolver, and the second patient was a 28 year old man shot with a .22 caliber rifle. Beall (1960) reported the first large series of injuries of the aorta. There were 10 patients who sustained gunshot wounds and four patients who had been stabbed in the abdominal aorta. In his series all were males, and the majority were in the second and third decades of life, except for one 47 year old female who received a gunshot wound. Perdue and Smith (1968) mentioned that two of their patients had combined aortic–vena caval injuries caused by shotgun blasts; both injuries proved fatal following massive blood loss. Fromm and

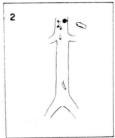
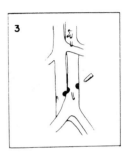
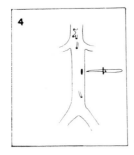
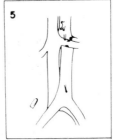
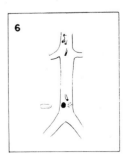

Figure 19–2. These diagrams represent six survivors sustaining penetrating abdominal injuries. Two were stabbed with knives and four received gunshot wounds. (Drapanas, T., Hewitt, R. L., Weichert, R. F., and Smith, A. D., Ann. Surg., *172*:351, 1970.)

associates (1970) reported that all ten aortic injuries, the majority involving the abdominal aorta, were caused by gunshot wounds. In a recent civilian series of 226 acute arterial injuries, Drapanas and co-workers (1970) reported 12 patients with abdominal aortic injuries, including six survivors. Four of their patients sustained gunshot wounds and two were stabbed (Fig. 19–2). Stone and associates (1973) reported 41 of 51 wounds of the abdominal aorta were gunshot. Lim and co-workers (1974) found 19 gunshot wounds, 11 stab wounds and two injuries by blunt trauma.

Two of the three survivors in the Vietnam experience sustained high velocity gunshot wounds to the abdominal aorta (Rich et al., 1970A). Trauma to the abdominal aorta in 20 patients in Vietnam was caused by eight gunshot wounds (Table 19–3).

Nonpenetrating injuries of the abdominal aorta are infrequent. In the classic review by Parmley and associated (1958) of nonpenetrating aortic trauma, only 13 cases of abdominal aortic injury were found among a total of 275 cases. Several unusual cases of blunt trauma to the abdominal aorta may be cited. Walker and Walker (1961) described a 50 year old patient injured in an automobile accident who developed severe claudication soon thereafter. Two years later a 3 cm segmental occlusion of the abdominal aorta by a partially calcified thrombus was found below the renal arteries and removed. It was felt that the previous injury had lacerated the intima of the aorta at the site of an atheromatous plaque. Tomatis and co-workers (1968) described a patient who sustained an abdominal aortic injury when the car she was driving at about 25 miles per hour struck the rear of a parked car. Welborn and Sawyers (1969) described a 33 year old patient and Borja and Lansing (1970) described a 45 year old patient, both of whom developed traumatic aortic thrombosis after automobile accidents. Finally, Hewitt and Grablowsky (1970) reported development of a traumatic dissecting aneurysm in a 65 year old patient after blunt trauma. A similar injury was de-

TABLE 19–3. ETIOLOGY OF THE WOUND AGENT IN ABDOMINAL AORTIC INJURIES IN VIETNAM

ETIOLOGY	NUMBER	PER CENT
Fragment wounds	9	45
Gunshot wounds	8	40
Iatrogenic	1	5
Fléchette	1	5
Undetermined	1	5
Totals	20	100

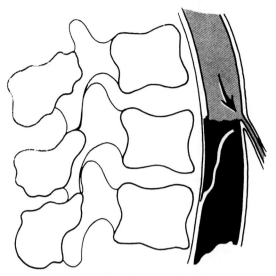

Figure 19–3. The mechanism of production of a traumatic dissecting aneurysm of the abdominal aorta. The aorta was struck against a lumbar vertebra by blunt trauma sustained in a surf board accident. This produced a tear in the intima and media of the posterior wall with resultant dissection and occlusion of the aorta. (Ngu, V. A., and Konstam, P. G., Brit. J. Surg., 52:981, 1965.)

scribed by Ngu and Konstam (1965) in a 37 year old woman who was injured when her surf board unexpectedly grounded on a sandy beach, causing a traumatic dissecting aneurysm of the abdominal aorta (Fig. 19–3). Wilson (1974) reported rupture of the distal aorta in a 12 year old caused by a saddle horn.

Although iatrogenic injuries of the abdominal aorta are infrequent, they do occur. This can be particularly true in the arteriosclerotic aorta when a translumbar aortogram is attempted. Similar to the more frequent injury of the common iliac artery, injury of the abdominal aorta also has occurred as a complication of intervertebral disc surgery which was initially

emphasized by Harbison (1954). Unusual events have also been recorded as the cause of injury to the abdominal aorta. Occlusion of the aortic bifurcation has occurred following migration of the ball from an aortic valve prosthesis (Krosnick, 1965).

CLINICAL PATHOLOGY

The usual pathologic finding in a patient surviving an abdominal aortic injury is a small laceration, because extensive lacerations or transections are usually fatal. All the surviving patients described in the review by Richards and associates (1966) had lacerations which were usually smaller than 1 cm (Table 19–1). In Vietnam a few patients have survived with more extensive wounds. Figure 19–4 illustrates a case in Vietnam in which a soldier sustained a high velocity gunshot wound of the abdomen. In addition to the trauma to the abdominal aorta, there were lacerations of the left hemidiaphragm, spleen, left kidney and transverse colon with contusion of the fundus of the stomach. The bullet which was lying in the aorta severed the left renal artery at its origin in entering the aorta and also lacerated the posterior wall of the aorta.

Blunt trauma to the abdominal aorta has been recognized and treated occasionally in the past 10 years. The blunt trauma usually results in intimal lacerations with intimal flaps or subintimal hematomas which result in thrombosis of the aorta. Figure 19–5 is an operative photograph of a subintimal hematoma of the aortic bifurcation with occlusion of the distal aorta in a 27 year old female injured in an automobile accident (Tomatis et al., 1968). The drawing in Figure 19–6 shows the mechanism of

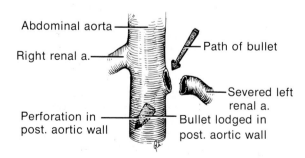

Abdominal aorta
Right renal a.
Path of bullet
Severed left renal a.
Perforation in post. aortic wall
Bullet lodged in post. aortic wall

Figure 19–4. Gunshot wound of the abdominal aorta with the missile remaining in the aorta. The left renal artery was severed at its origin as the bullet entered the aorta. (Courtesy of Dr. W. Y. Walker. Redrawn from original operation report at 67th evacuation hospital March 19, 1967.) (See also Figure 20–12.)

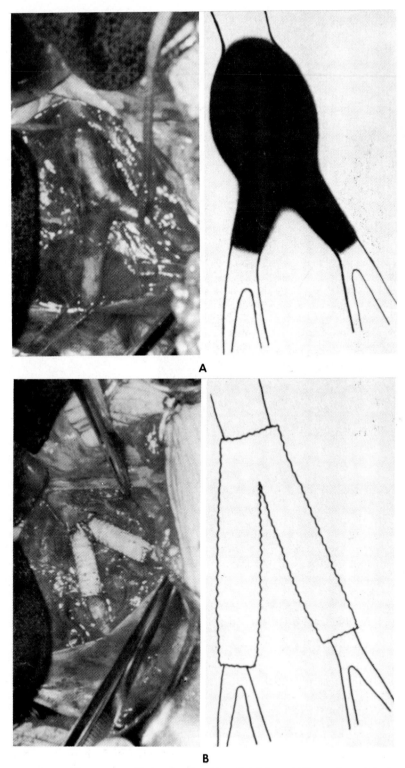

A

B

Figure 19–5. Subintimal hematoma (A) that involved the distal 5 cm of the aorta and the proximal portion of both common iliac arteries. It was necessary to replace this injured area with a Dacron prosthesis (B). (Tomatis, L. A., Doornobs, F. A., and Beard, J. A., J. Trauma, 8:1096, 1968. Copyright 1968, The Williams and Wilkins Co., Baltimore.)

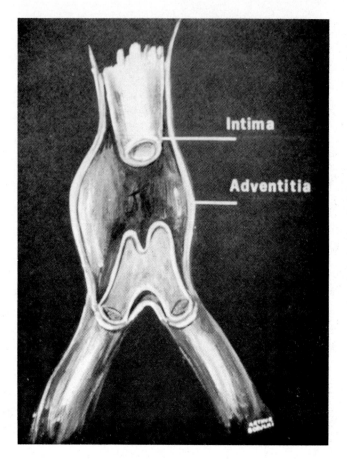

Figure 19-6. Mechanism of aortic occlusion presented in Fig. 19-5. The dissected intima and adjacent tissue had rolled into an obstructing ball which completely occluded the lumen. (Tomatis, L. A., Doornobs, F. A., and Beard, J. A., J. Trauma, 8:1096, 1968. Copyright 1968, The Williams and Wilkins Co., Baltimore.)

aortic obstruction that can occur with blunt trauma to the abdominal aorta. Sloop and Robertson (1975) reported two rare cases of laceration of the intima of the abdominal aorta by blunt trauma with resultant partial vessel occlusion. Pennington and Drapanas (1975) described an unusual case of acute post-traumatic coarctation of the abdominal aorta associated with hypertension.

The involvement of a diseased aorta often potentiates the problems associated with aortic trauma. This has been particularly notable in some patients with blunt trauma to the abdominal aorta. Ngu and Konstam (1965) documented that the aorta was moderately atheromatous in their 37 year old female patient. Borja and Lansing (1970) described advanced changes of arteriosclerosis in their 45 year old male patient. Hewitt and Grablowsky (1970) also reported severe atheromatous disease in their 65 year old male patient.

Concomitant injuries of the abdominal

viscera are common. Figure 19-7 is a sketch used by Manlove and associates (1960) to demonstrate the path of a bullet through other intra-abdominal organs prior to perforating the aorta. Beall (1960) found associated injuries, usually multiple, in all but one of 14 patients with trauma to the abdominal aorta (Table 19-4). The large and small bowel, liver and vena cava were most frequently involved, but the spleen, pancreas and kidney were also injured. Similar involvement of other organs near the aorta has been found in soldiers injured in Vietnam (Billy et al., 1971). Mattox and colleagues (1975) reported 29 cases of acute combined injuries to the aorta and inferior vena cava. An unusual concomitant injury was recently reported which resulted in a fistula between the thoracic duct and the abdominal aorta (Fig. 19-8); the fistula spontaneously closed in less than one month (Nguyen and Lewin, 1970).

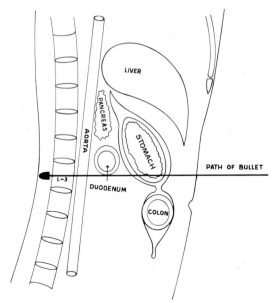

Figure 19-7. Path of a bullet as it passed through the stomach, mesenteries of the transverse colon and small bowel, and aorta to lodge beneath the skin to the left of the vertebral column. This illustrates the frequency of concomitant visceral injuries associated with penetrating wounds of the aorta. (Manlove, G. H., Quattlebaum, F. W., Flom, R. S., and LaFave, J. W., Amer. J. Surg., *99*:941, 1960.)

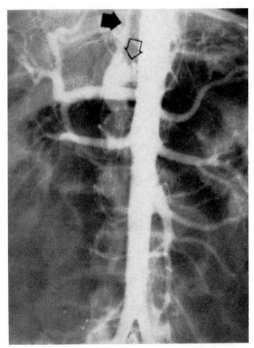

Figure 19-8. An abdominal aortogram that reveals an irregular fistulous tract between the upper abdominal aorta and the thoracic duct in the area of the cisterna chyli. (Nguyen, L. Q., and Lewin, J. R., J.A.M.A., *211*:499, 1970.)

CLINICAL FEATURES

Severe shock from massive intraperitoneal hemorrhage usually dominates the clinical picture. This was emphasized by

TABLE 19-4. CONCOMITANT INJURIES ASSOCIATED WITH PENETRATING ABDOMINAL TRAUMA

	BEALL, 1960	DRAPANAS ET AL., 1970	BILLY ET AL., 1971
Abdominal Aortic Injuries	14	12	19
Concomitant Injuries			
Small bowel	9	3	7
Large bowel	4	2	5
Vena cava	3	4	6
Liver	5	5	5
Kidney	1	1	5
Diaphragm	0	0	2
Stomach	0	6	3
Spleen	1	2	3
Pancreas	1	5	3
Renal vein	0	4	0

Bole and associates (1976). Thirteen of 14 patients with aortic injury, including 11 of the abdominal aorta, arrived at their hospital with no recordable blood pressure. All but three of 32 patients with acute abdominal aortic injury reported by Lim and coworkers (1974) were in profound shock on admission. Nevertheless, absence of shock does not preclude injury to the abdominal aorta. Peritoneal irritation from concomitant multiple intestinal injuries is usually present. Often the severe shock with imminent death requires laparotomy before a definitive diagnosis can be made. Roberson (1967) described a 38 year old male who had combined stab wounds of the abdominal aorta and vena cava without the formation of an arteriovenous fistula which were discovered at the time of an exploratory celiotomy.

In the unusual instance of traumatic thrombosis, the findings are those of acute aortic occlusion, as with a saddle embolus. Distal pulses are absent, and the lower extremities are cold, often anesthetic and paralyzed. In the rare instance of an acute arteriovenous fistula, an abdominal bruit may appear. Williams and Robinson (1961) reported on this problem, which was managed by immediate repair. Buscaglia and co-workers (1969) documented the formation of an arteriovenous fistula between the aorta and the portal vein in a 13 year old boy who was shot in the epigastrium. Yajko and Trimble (1974) presented two patients and reviewed the literature of arterial bullet embolization following abdominal gunshot wounds involving the aorta.

DIAGNOSTIC CONSIDERATIONS

If the patient is stable, roentgenograms of the abdomen may be of assistance. A large, soft-tissue density might represent a retroperitoneal hematoma. The presence of a bullet in the area of the aorta or the

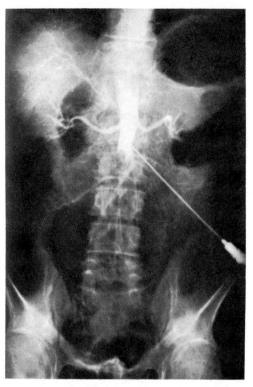

Figure 19–10. This translumbar aortogram demonstrates a traumatic dissection of the abdominal aorta, which was secondary to blunt trauma from an automobile accident. There is complete occlusion of the abdominal aorta near the level of the origin of the inferior mesenteric artery. (Hewitt, R. L., and Grablowsky, O. M., Ann. Surg., *171*:160, 1970.)

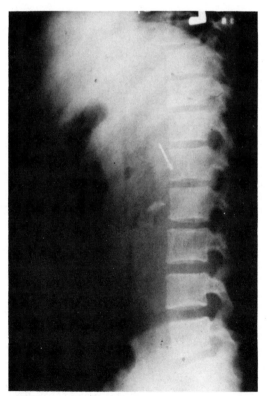

Figure 19–9. This patient sustained a fléchette wound of the abdomen. The missile is visualized in the vicinity of the abdominal aorta. Successful repair of the laceration of the abdominal aorta was possible. (Courtesy Dr. Harold Snyder, 36th Evacuation Hospital, 1967.)

demonstration that the aorta was in the path of a missile should arouse suspicion of an aortic injury. In Figure 19–9, a fléchette is seen which traumatized the aorta in a soldier in Vietnam. Aortography may provide assistance when there is some question, particularly in nonpenetrating abdominal trauma, and may substantiate the clinical impression of aortic trauma. Occlusion of the abdominal aorta just below the origin of the inferior mesenteric artery is demonstrated by the translumbar aortogram in Figure 19–10.

SURGICAL TREATMENT

Of historical interest in the repair of abdominal aortic trauma is the management of one of the first reported gunshot wounds of the abdominal aorta by Holzer (1948). He mentioned that an unsuccessful

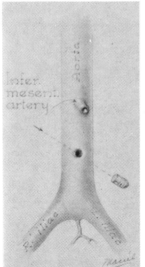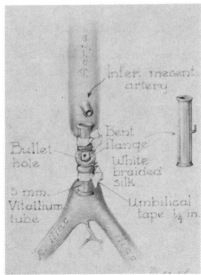

Figure 19–11. Course of a bullet through the abdominal aorta. Because of ragged wound edges and because it was impossible to suture the lacerations of the entrance and exit wounds to preserve continuity of the aorta, it was necessary to utilize a Vitallium tube within the lumen of the aorta. This procedure of historical interest was performed prior to the general acceptance of what we now consider to be proper methods of arterial repair. (Holzer, C. E., Jr., Surgery, *23*:645, 1948.)

attempt was made to close a through-and-through perforation of the aorta with silk sutures. The edges of the wounds were ragged, and there was considerable loss of substance in the damaged segment. He felt that ligation of the vessel was inadvisable because of the possibility of secondary hemorrhage or gangrene of the lower extremities, and he decided to re-establish the continuity of the aorta by means of a Vitallium tube (Fig. 19–11).

Immediate resuscitation and laparotomy clearly provide the only chance for survival from trauma to the abdominal aorta. Whether it is in the combat zone, such as in Vietnam, where rapid helicopter evacuation has frequently brought severely wounded patients to a definitive surgical center within minutes after wounding, or whether it is in a large metropolitan area, where the system of transportation of the injured is functioning at peak performance, rapid transportation of patients sustaining injuries of the abdominal aorta will provide the surgeon with more challenging opportunities. Fromm and associates (1970) reported that, in the preceding 2½ years, a vigorous transportation policy by the Police Department brought 10 patients with gunshot wounds of the aorta to the Detroit General Hospital alive. Similarly, in 1970, Drapanas and colleagues stated that the average time interval between injury and arrival in their operating room was least for survivors with abdominal aortic trauma, and this time interval was only 36

minutes. Jensen (1963) documented that team work and prompt aggressive treatment can make it possible to repair successfully a bullet wound of the abdominal aorta, even in a small community hospital.

Beall and associates (1969) diagrammed the evaluation and preparation of patients for the operating room who had major intra-abdominal vascular injuries (Fig. 19–12). A team effort in the emergency room will increase the possibility of survival of the injured patient. Immediate ventilatory support, usually by endotracheal intubation, should be a prime consideration. Circulatory support is of equal importance and should be carried out by rapid intravenous infusion of a balanced electrolyte solution through one or more large caliber venous cannulas in upper extremity venotomies. Whole blood replacement should be available as soon as possible. If the patient's condition is stable, additional evaluation, such as routine roentgenograms and selective abdominal arteriography, might be considered. There has been some interest in the possible use of external counterpressure by using the Gardner and Storer G-suit, and Ludewig and Wangensteen (1969) demonstrated in experimental models the value of external pressure in delaying death from exsanguinating hemorrhage due to lacerated arteries. Rutherford (1969) recently stated that he felt the G-suit, in selected instances, might be helpful to allow time to transport the patient to the operating room to prepare him for the

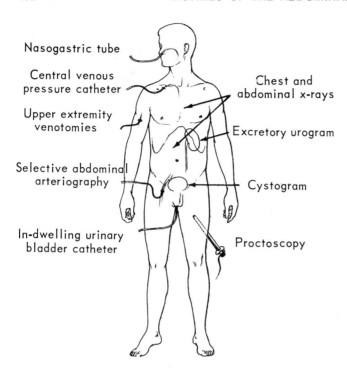

Nasogastric tube

Central venous
pressure catheter

Upper extremity
venotomies

Selective abdominal
arteriography

In-dwelling urinary
bladder catheter

Chest and
abdominal x-rays

Excretory urogram

Cystogram

Proctoscopy

Figure 19–12. This diagram outlines the preparation and evaluation of a patient with major abdominal vascular injuries. (Beall, A. C. and co-authors, Surgical Management of Cardiovascular Trauma. Exhibit Brochure, Houston, Texas, Baylor College of Medicine and Ben Taub General Hospital, 1969.)

surgical procedure and set up the necessary blood for transfusions. Blaisdell (1969), however, remarked that, in the same period of time that it would take to get the patient into the G-suit, it would be possible to take the patient to the operating room and obtain definitive control of the injured artery. Although use of the G-suit was considered in Vietnam, no known successful clinical application of the G-suit in patients with aortic trauma has been reported.

At operation adequate exposure can be obtained best through a long midline incision (Fig. 19–13). After rapid evacuation of the blood to improve evaluation of the injury, apply direct digital pressure over the laceration of the aorta to control the hemorrhage until noncrushing vascular clamps can be applied proximally and distally to the injured site. Attempts to accomplish extensive dissection without digital tamponade of the wound may result in exsanguinating hemorrhage. Intraluminal balloon control of hemorrhage can be effective with the temporary use of a large Fogarty balloon catheter or a large-bag Foley catheter. Temporary occlusion of the proximal abdominal aorta can be accomplished by use of an aortic com-

pressor which avoids extensive dissection of the upper abdomen (Conn et al., 1968) (Fig. 19–14). If a retroperitoneal hematoma is present, this should not be disturbed until adequate personnel, vascular instruments and blood are available to manage the aortic injury with its potential rapid blood loss. The aorta can be approached by reflecting the right colon and small bowel mesentery. Buscaglia and co-workers (1969) illustrated both the right-sided approach, displacing the right colon and duodenum to the left (Fig. 19–13), and an alternate approach, displacing the left colon and pancreas to the right; the latter is particularly useful for injuries near the renal artery.

In most patients, after appropriate débridement of the edges of the laceration of the aorta, lateral suture can be carried out. Fortunately, a prosthesis is rarely necessary, but this may be the only available material for more extensive injuries. Cheek and associates (1975) recommended soaking the prosthesis in cephalosporin solution before implanting. Wrapping the prosthesis in omentum has also been suggested.

Major concomitant venous injuries are frequent, particularly those involving the

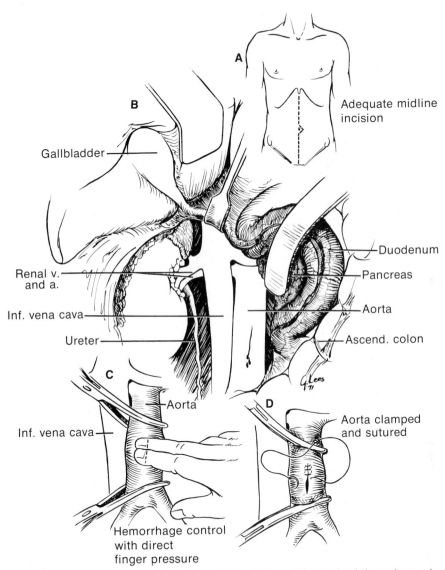

Figure 19–13.   Adequate exposure of the abdominal aorta is rapidly obtained through an adequate midline incision. Digital compression of the laceration will control hemorrhage prior to repair, which is frequently possible by suture of the laceration. Additional exposure can be obtained as illustrated from the right side.

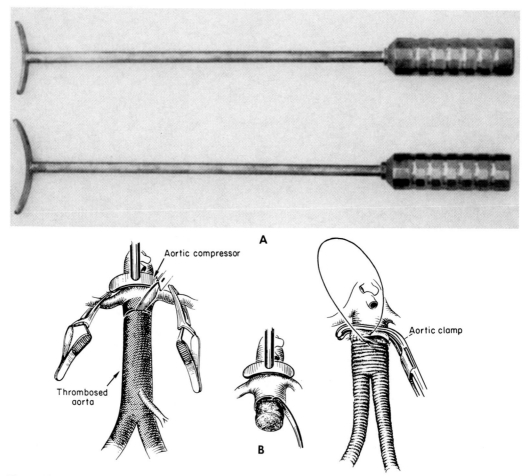

Figure 19–14. Aortic compression clamp (A) designed to allow the curved end of the occluder to compress atraumatically the aorta above the celiac axis against the vertebral bodies, (B) thus eliminating time required for dissection and application of vascular clamps. (Conn, J., Jr., Trippel, O. H., and Bergan, J. J., Surgery, *64*:1158, 1968.)

inferior vena cava or the common iliac veins. Repair of the venous injuries should be carried out; this is frequently possible by lateral repair. The safest management of a concomitant colon injury would include the performance of a colostomy. Copious irrigation of the peritoneal cavity may help eliminate the possibility of infection.

POSTOPERATIVE CARE

The maintenance of an adequate blood pressure by adequate fluid and blood replacement throughout the operative procedure and into the early postoperative period and continuing antibiotic therapy

are mandatory. Peripheral pulses, particularly the femoral and pedal pulses, should be easily palpable following repair of the injured abdominal aorta. If these are not present or if they disappear in the early postoperative period, arteriography may be indicated to help identify the etiology of the problem. In contrast to the situation in many injuries of major arteries of the extremities where collateral circulation may be adequate if the primary arterial repair fails, it is more important in this case to insure restoration of flow through the aorta rather than to give any thought to the possible development of collateral circulation.

If Dacron has been utilized to restore the

integrity of the abdominal aorta and this becomes infected, it must be removed and the aorta ligated. Serious consideration must then be given to the possibility of an extra-anatomical bypass to maintain lower extremity viability.

RESULTS

The 1966 review by Richards and colleagues of 12 reported cases of successful repair of penetrating wounds of the abdominal aorta by lateral suture emphasizes that patients with minor lacerations of the abdominal aorta have the greatest chance for survival, because of being alive upon arrival at the hospital and because of operative management which allows closure of small lacerations with a few sutures.

In the series of penetrating wounds of the abdominal aorta presented by Beall (1960), there were only four of 14 patients, approximately 29 per cent, who survived. Beall emphasized that the major cause of death was irreversible shock. Owens (1963) reported the cases of two patients with fatal wounds of the abdominal aorta. One patient, a 30 year old man, was shot through the abdominal aorta, superior mesenteric artery and inferior vena cava. All three vessels were repaired, but a perforation of the third portion of the duodenum was missed. In spite of two subsequent operations, the patient died on the twelfth postoperative day from peritonitis. Drapanas and co-authors (1970) reported a 50 per cent survival of 12 patients with abdominal aortic trauma (Fig. 19–2). Allen and co-authors (1972) expanded Beall's Houston series to 63 patients and the mortality rate remained high at 70 per cent. Lim and co-workers (1974) found their mortality rate to be 63 per cent for 33 patients in San Francisco.

Surprisingly enough, in the few patients who have required insertion of a prosthesis, infection has not occurred despite the presence of associated abdominal injuries. However, the total experience with the use of prostheses for abdominal aortic injuries is quite small. Methods of repair used by various groups are summarized in Table 19–5. In a group of 42 patients in whom repair was accomplished, a suture repair was used in 33 and a prosthesis in eight. Cheek and colleagues (1975) used nine Dacron prostheses in repair of aortoiliac gunshot wounds without any suture line complications despite heavy contamination from associated perforations of the small bowel and/or colon. In contrast, there were five suture line distruptions in primary repairs in their series. Hardy and associates (1975) reported a 58 per cent mortality rate for 36 aortic injuries (thoracic and abdominal). They emphasized that sepsis was responsible for five of seven postoperative deaths.

Mattox and co-workers (1975) emphasized specific problems associated with penetrating injuries of the suprarenal aorta. Among 28 patients, 16 died either in the operating room or within 24 hours. There were ten survivors.

In nonpenetrating trauma of the abdominal aorta, several methods of management have been successful. Ngu and Konstam (1965) performed a thrombectomy through an aortotomy with suture of the displaced intima and media back to the proximal edge of the tear from the adventitia. Borja and Lansing (1970) performed a longitudinal aortotomy with extraction of fresh thrombus. After they performed an endarterectomy in addition, it was possible to perform a successful arteriorrhaphy. On the other

TABLE 19–5. METHOD OF REPAIR OF ABDOMINAL AORTIC TRAUMA: REPRESENTATIVE SERIES

AUTHORS	AORTA	SUTURE	PROSTHESIS	MISCEL-LANEOUS	NONE
Beall (1960)	14	9	1	0	4
Richards et al. (1966)*	10	9	0	1	0
Fromm et al. (1970)	6	0	5	0	1
Billy et al. (1971)	19	15	2	0	2

*Literature review of successful repairs (Beall's four patients listed under his name) plus two by the authors.

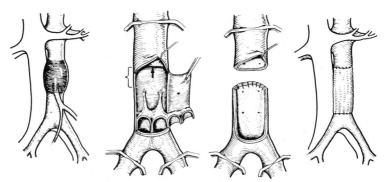

Figure 19–15. Periadventitial hemorrhage at the time of the operation following blunt trauma of the abdominal aorta. When the aorta was opened, the intima and media were seen rolled into an occluding ball-shaped mass at the aortic bifurcation. The intima and media were reattached and continuity was re-established by a Dacron prosthesis. (Welborn, M. B., Jr., and Sawyers, J. L., Amer. J. Surg., *118*:112, 1969.)

hand, Tomatis and associates (1968) found that the blunt trauma had caused a significant subintimal hematoma of the aortic bifurcation, and they elected to replace this with a bifurcated Dacron prosthesis. Welborn and Sawyers (1969) successfully combined reattachment of the torn intima and media with the utilization of a prosthesis to restore continuity of the aorta (Fig. 19–15). Hewitt and Grablowsky (1970)

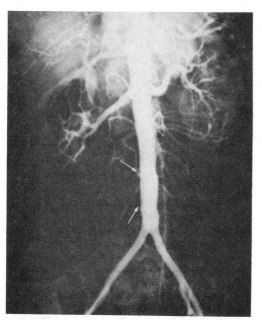

Figure 19–16. This aortogram was performed two months after the operative procedure described in Fig. 19–15. Restoration of normal blood flow past the area of the prosthesis is demonstrated. (Welborn, M. B., Jr., and Sawyers, J. L., Amer. J. Surg., *118*: 112, 1969.)

utilized a Dacron aortofemoral bypass for an acute traumatic dissecting aneurysm of the abdominal aorta secondary to blunt trauma.

There is a total of 20 patients included in the Vietnam Vascular Registry who have had surgical management of their abdominal aortic injuries. It was possible to perform a suture closure of lacerations in 75 per cent of these wounds, or in 15 patients. Two patients required the use of Dacron prostheses, and three patients did not survive long enough for the surgeon to complete a definitive surgical procedure. The six patients who expired (30 per cent mortality rate) included one patient with a Dacron prosthesis and two patients who had lateral suture of their abdominal aortic lacerations.

FOLLOW-UP

Complications in patients who survive repair of an aortic injury have been infrequent; however, the number of follow-ups has also been small. Welborn and Sawyers (1969) reported a one-year follow-up of their patient with blunt trauma (Fig. 19–15). An aortogram two months after operation confirmed adequate restoration of blood flow (Fig. 19–16).

None of the patients injured in Vietnam is known to have developed any complications. Five of these patients have been seen for detailed delayed evaluation at Walter Reed General Hospital. Two patients were injured nearly ten years earlier.

CHAPTER 20

INJURIES OF MISCELLANEOUS INTRA-ABDOMINAL ARTERIES

> Repair, or replacement by graft, of major vessels, such as the ...superior mesenteric artery...must be considered.
>
> **G. V. Pontius, B. C. Kilbourne, and E. G. Paul, Chicago, 1957**

Injuries of the major branches of the abdominal aorta are fortunately uncommon. There is even less frequent documentation of successful reconstruction of injured visceral arteries. The six major branches most frequently involved are the celiac artery and its two major tributaries, the hepatic and splenic, the superior and inferior mesenteric arteries and the renal arteries. Injuries of the abdominal aorta itself and of the iliac arteries are separately considered in Chapters 19 and 21, respectively.

Almost all such injuries result from penetrating wounds, usually with multiple injuries of adjacent organs. Nonpenetrating abdominal trauma with injury to blood vessels may be more difficult to diagnose than penetrating trauma. The clinical picture is predominately that of shock from intra-abdominal hemorrhage. If this does not occur and there is tamponade by adjacent structures, the trauma to the visceral artery may be difficult to identify. This injury may not be apparent, then, for a delayed period of time until a diagnosis of an arteriovenous fistula or false aneurysm is made. Only rarely are symptoms of regional organ ischemia present. The diagnosis is often first made during emergency laparotomy to control hemorrhage. Some injuries to visceral arteries, such as trauma to the renal artery, may be extremely important for organ viability. However, viability of the kidney may already be lost by the time a patient reaches a definitive surgical center. On the other hand, injuries to other branches, such as the superior mesenteric or the inferior mesenteric arteries, may have minimal significance because of the rich collateral circulation that usually exists if only one of the three major branches supplying the bowel is not functioning.

457

TABLE 20–1. INCIDENCE OF INJURIES TO INTRA-ABDOMINAL ARTERIES

	AUTHOR	TOTAL ARTERIES	VISCERAL	PER CENT
War Series				
WW I	Makins (1919)	1191	0	0
WW II	DeBakey and Simeone (1946)	2471	2	0.01
Korean	Hughes (1958)	304	0	0
Vietnam	Rich et al. (1970A)	1000	0	0
Civilian Series				
Houston	Morris et al. (1960)	220	0	0.0
Atlanta	Ferguson et al. (1961)	200	15	7.5
Denver	Owens (1963)	70	3	4.3
Detroit	Smith et al. (1963)	61	2	3.3
Dallas	Patman et al. (1964)	271	18	6.6
Los Angeles	Treiman et al. (1966)	159	11	6.9
Houston	Beall et al. (1967)	343	16	4.7
New Orleans	Drapanas et al. (1970)	226	10	4.4
Dallas	Perry et al. (1971)	508	24	4.7
Memphis	Cheek et al. (1975)	155	0	0.0
Denver	Kelly and Eiseman (1975)	116	8	6.9
Jackson	Hardy et al. (1975)	353	26	7.4

Also, ligation of the traumatized splenic artery is an acceptable procedure, and this injury may be regarded as so insignificant that it is not documented.

Only meager information has been published from reports of military vascular injuries, but several reports of injuries of visceral arteries following civilian trauma have been recorded. These articles have been analyzed in detail in preparing this chapter. The 1975 report by Hardy and co-workers from the University of Mississippi documenting 26 visceral arterial injuries among 353 arterial injuries, an incidence of 7.4 per cent, represents recent increased recognition of these injuries (Table 20–1).

SURGICAL ANATOMY

The largest branch of the abdominal aorta is the celiac artery. It originates from the aorta between the medial crura of the diaphragm and passes anteriorly above the pancreas where its major tributaries originate. In nearly 90 per cent of patients there are three major branches: the left gastric, the splenic and the hepatic arteries (Strandness, 1969). Numerous variations exist in the remaining 10 per cent. Strandness (1969) has emphasized the great variation in blood supply beyond the

division of the celiac artery, stating that "variation is constant." The representative anatomy is shown in Figure 20–1. The left gastric and splenic arteries, when injured, can be best managed by ligation. The hepatic artery is surgically the most significant, because ligation carries the grave risk of fatal hepatic ischemia. One of the major collateral pathways for the hepatic artery is through the superior pancreaticoduodenal artery, which anastomoses with the inferior pancreaticoduodenal from the superior mesenteric.

The superior mesenteric artery arises from the anterior surface of the aorta beneath the pancreas, slightly distal to the origin of the celiac artery and slightly proximal to the origin of the renal arteries (Fig. 20–2). The middle colic artery is the first branch. Tributaries of the middle colic connect with similar tributaries of the inferior mesenteric artery via the marginal artery of the colon. The inferior mesenteric artery arises at a relatively constant anterior position from the abdominal aorta near the body of the third lumbar vertebra.

The paired renal arteries arise from the lateral aspects of the aorta, the left usually arising slightly higher than the right, near the upper portion of the second lumbar vertebra. Accessory renal arteries are frequent, and in some patients focal in-

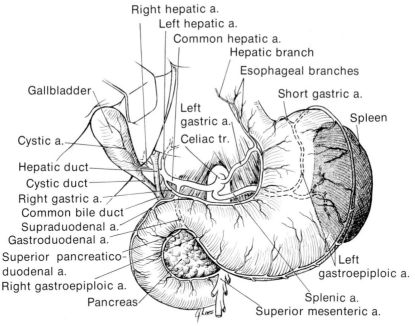

Figure 20–1. Artist's conception of the surgical anatomy of the celiac axis and its three major branches. Some detail of collateral circulation and adjacent viscera is included.

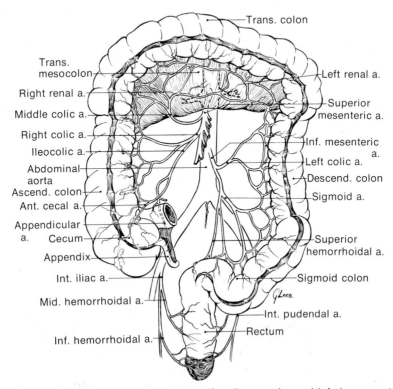

Figure 20–2. A second artist's conception representing the superior and inferior mesenteric arteries as well as the renal arteries with adjacent viscera.

farcts of the kidney are produced if such arteries are ligated.

INCIDENCE

Virtually no information concerning visceral arterial injuries has been reported from the four major military conflicts of this century (Table 20–1). Only in the World War II series by DeBakey and Simeone (1946) were two renal arterial injuries mentioned. No documented injuries were found in the 1970 Interim Vietnam Report by Rich and colleagues of 1000 injuries; subsequently, however, several repairs of injuries of the superior mesenteric and hepatic arteries have been documented in the Vietnam Vascular Registry.

Killen (1964) reviewed a number of reported series of intra-abdominal visceral injuries secondary to nonpenetrating abdominal trauma. He found that there was a 1.2 per cent incidence of vascular involvement in 1320 patients. There are relatively few studies that deal specifically with intra-abdominal vascular trauma. Reports of several series of visceral arterial injuries in civilian life are tabulated in Table 20–1. In a review of 200 arterial injuries, Ferguson and co-workers (1961) found five injuries of the abdominal aorta, four of the superior mesenteric, three splenic injuries, two renal, two hepatic, one inferior mesenteric, one left gastric, one celiac axis and one middle colic (Fig. 20–3). The most comprehensive review of intra-abdominal vascular trauma was published by Perdue and Smith in 1968, who analyzed 126 injuries in 90 patients (Fig. 20–4). Their series included injuries of the abdominal aorta and iliac artery, as well as of the vena cava and large veins. The renal artery was injured in six patients, the superior mesenteric in four, the hepatic in four, the splenic in three and the inferior mesenteric in one.

Buscaglia and associates (1969) described 46 intra-abdominal vascular injuries, eight of which involved the visceral branches. The group of 226 arterial injuries reported by Drapanas and co-workers in 1970 included six injuries of the renal artery, three of the superior mesenteric and one of the hepatic. Similarly, in the report by Perry and colleagues in 1971 of 508 arterial inju-

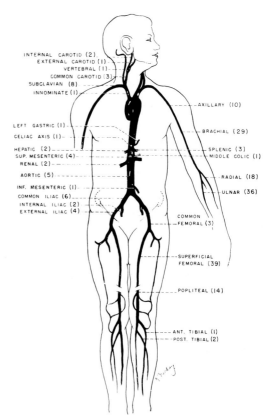

Figure 20–3. The incidence of trauma to intra-abdominal branches of the aorta are outlined and compared with other arterial injuries in an early large civilian report. (Ferguson, I. A., Byrd, W. M., and McAfee, D. K., Ann. Surg., *153*:980, 1961.)

ries, the renal artery was most frequently injured, a total of nine cases. Among the 24 visceral arterial injuries, there were also seven injuries of the superior mesenteric, four hepatic, two celiac and two splenic injuries. The report by Beall and co-workers (1967) of 16 visceral arterial injuries included nine of the superior mesenteric, five renal and two inferior mesenteric among 343 arterial injuries.

A recent increase in the incidence of recognized and reported visceral arterial injuries is emphasized by two 1975 reports (Table 20–1). The incidence was approximately 7 per cent of civilian arterial injuries in Denver, 8 of 116 according to Kelly and Eiseman (1975), and in Jackson, 26 of 353, as reported by Hardy and colleagues (1975).

Other reports in the past five years have concentrated on small series and reviews of

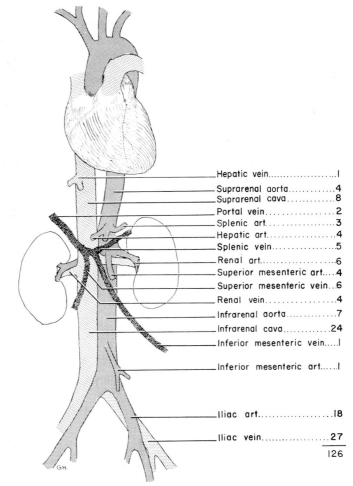

Figure 20–4. This illustration cites the location of injury of 126 vessels in 90 patients. This is the most comprehensive review of intra-abdominal vascular trauma involving branches of the abdominal aorta. (Perdue, G. D., and Smith, R. B., Surgery, *64*:562, 1968.)

Hepatic vein....................1
Suprarenal aorta............4
Suprarenal cava............8
Portal vein.................2
Splenic art.................3
Hepatic art.................4
Splenic vein...............5
Renal art....................6
Superior mesenteric art....4
Superior mesenteric vein..6
Renal vein.................4
Infrarenal aorta............7
Infrarenal cava............24
Inferior mesenteric vein.....1
Inferior mesenteric art.....1

Iliac art...................18
Iliac vein.................27
126

specific visceral arteries. Fullen and associates (1972) presented details in managing eight injuries of the superior mesenteric arterial circulation during a 16-year period ending in 1970 in Cincinnati. From a series of over 700 patients, injuries to the superior mesenteric artery occurred in about 1 per cent of penetrating wounds of the abdomen. Sturm and co-workers (1975) documented 14 cases of blunt renal vascular trauma, with the renal artery involved in 10. These cases were found in a series of 466 patients treated for renal injuries.

ETIOLOGY

Injuries to the visceral arteries have been caused most frequently by penetrating abdominal trauma (Fig. 20–5). Many of the reported series, however, do not indicate the etiology of the injury for the specific artery. In their series of 90 patients with 126 intra-abdominal vascular injuries, Perdue and Smith (1968) found that the majority of the injuries (in 65 patients) were caused by low and high velocity missiles. They noted that 14 patients had stab wounds, 5 patients had nonpenetrating trauma, and 5 patients had shotgun wounds.

Since Ulvestad's report in 1954 of a 22 year old patient sustaining nonpenetrating trauma to the abdomen when he was caught between the tail gate of a truck and a loading platform, there have been a number of reports of blunt trauma causing visceral arterial trauma. Shuck and Trump (1961) reviewed nonpenetrating abdominal trauma with injury to the blood vessels and reported six of their own cases; however, the majority of these were venous injuries.

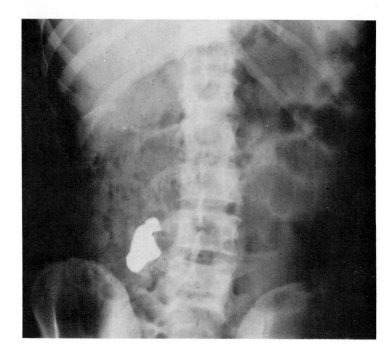

Figure 20–5. Penetrating abdominal trauma has caused the majority of visceral arterial injuries. (N. M. R., 2nd Surgical Hospital, Vietnam, 1966.)

Renal arterial thrombosis following blunt trauma has been reported with increasing frequency. One example of thrombosis of the left renal artery is shown in Figure 20–6. In 1970 Grablowsky and colleagues reported 4 such cases and found a total of 10 similar cases reported by others. An extensive report of renal pedicle injuries was published by Guerriero and co-workers in 1971, which described 43 injuries of the renal artery or vein in 33 patients (Table 20–2). Most patients had penetrating injuries, but six had blunt trauma. Sullivan and associates (1972) described six patients with renal arterial occlusion following blunt trauma (Fig. 20–7). Sturm and co-authors

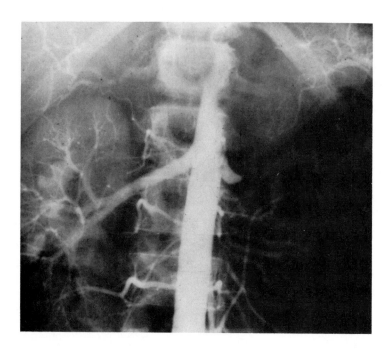

Figure 20–6. Thrombosis of the left renal artery caused by blunt trauma in a 35 foot fall demonstrated by aortography three months after injury. The patient was being evaluated for hypertension. (N.M.R., W.R.G.H., 1973.)

TABLE 20–2. RENAL PEDICLE INJURIES: TYPE OF INJURY*

	NUMBER OF PATIENTS	DEATHS	PER CENT
Penetrating	27	10	37
Large caliber or high velocity	12	5	41
Small caliber or low velocity	9	3	33
Stab wounds, single	2	0	0
Stab wounds, multiple	1	1	100
Shotgun	3	1	33
Blunt	6	2	33
TOTAL:	33	12	36

*From Guerriero, W. G., Carlton, C. E., Jr., Scott, R., and Beall, A. C., Jr., J. Trauma, *11*:53, 1971. Copyright 1971, The Williams & Wilkins Company, Baltimore.

(1975) evaluated and treated 10 renal arterial lesions secondary to blunt trauma.

Although the specific number of cases is not known, in Vietnam an interesting problem existed involving blunt trauma to the branches of the abdominal aorta in patients who had been involved in helicopter accidents. Five patients treated at the 2nd Surgical Hospital in 1966 had significant intraperitoneal hemorrhage secondary to lacerations of branches of the mesenteric arteries as a result of this mode of injury.

Occasionally, iatrogenic injuries have occurred to the visceral arteries. Trauma to the hepatic artery during cholecystectomy has been of particular concern. Details involving the effect of accidental hepatic artery ligation and humans have been removed by Brittain and associates (1964). Lucas and co-workers (1971) found hepatic arterial thrombosis in 18 patients from a series of 119 hepatic artery catheterizations which were performed for infusion chemotherapy of malignant lesions of the liver (Fig. 20–8). Ikard and Merendino (1970) reported accidental excision of the superior mesenteric artery during radical cancer surgery. Two similar cases have been treated at Walter Reed General Hospital in the past five years.

CLINICAL PATHOLOGY

Laceration or complete transection of one of the major branches of the abdominal aorta is often as rapidly fatal owing to exsanguinating hemorrhage as trauma to the aorta itself. Therefore, many patients will not survive long enough to reach a definitive surgical center. On the other hand, tamponade of the injured vessel may occur from the surrounding extraperitoneal hematoma, as described by May and co-authors (1965) (Fig. 20–9).

Blunt trauma to the visceral arteries has

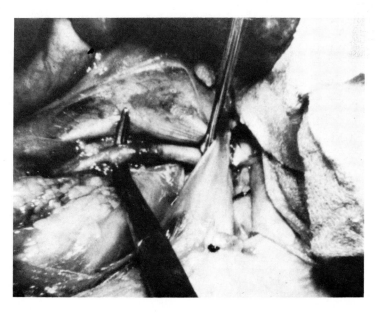

Figure 20–7. The right renal artery, beneath the clamp, has an obvious area of contusion proximal to the clamp which was caused by blunt trauma. The aorta is to the right and the vena cava is retracted with a vein retractor. Excision of the contused segment with reanastomosis of the renal arterial ends was performed. (Sullivan, M. J., Smalley, R., and Banowsky, L. H., J. Trauma, *12*:509, 1972.)

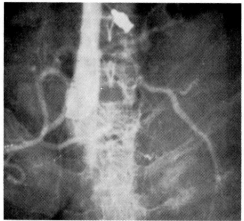

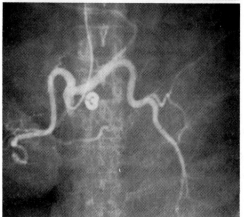

Figure 20–8. The precatheterization celiac angiogram demonstrates a normal hepatic artery. The postcatheterization (three months) bottom celiac angiogram demonstrates hepatic artery thrombosis. (Lucas, R. J., Tumacder, O., and Wilson, G. S., Ann. Surg., *173*:238, 1971.)

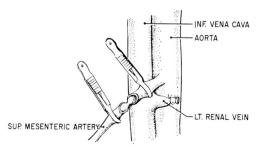

Figure 20–9. Diagrammatic representation of the superior mesenteric artery almost completely transected by a .22 caliber bullet 2 cm from the aorta. There was a large retroperitoneal hematoma with little free blood in the peritoneal cavity. (May, A. G., Lipchik, E. O., and DeWeese, J. A., Ann. Surg., *162*: 869, 1965.)

recently been noted in renal arterial trauma. Intimal lacerations with resultant intimal flaps or subintimal hematomas have caused thrombosis (Fig. 20–10). Grablowsky and co-workers (1970) reported the case of a 16 year old patient who was injured in a motorcycle accident three days prior to admission to their hospital. Bilateral renal arterial intimal tears with subintimal hematomas occurred (Fig. 20–11). Fullen and associates (1972) correlated the anatomical location of superior mesenteric arterial trauma with the extent of resultant ischemic bowel (Table 20–3).

CLINICAL FEATURES

In contrast to extremity vessel injuries in which external hemorrhage is usually ap-

TABLE 20–3. SUPERIOR MESENTERIC ARTERIAL INJURY*

Zone	ANATOMICAL CLASSIFICATION Segment of SMA Involved
I	Trunk proximal to first major branch
II	Trunk between pancreaticoduodenal and middle colic
III	Trunk distal to middle colic
IV	Segmental branches, jejunal, ileal or colic

	CLASSIFICATION BY ISCHEMIC EXTENT	
	Ischemic Category	Bowel Segments Affected
Grade 1.	Maximal	Jejunum, ileum, right colon
Grade 2.	Moderate	Major segment, small bowel and/or right colon
Grade 3.	Minimal	Minor segment or segments, small bowel or right colon
Grade 4.	None	No ischemic bowel

*Modified from Fullen, W. D., Hunt, J., and Altemeier, W. A., J. Trauma, *12*:656, 1972. Copyright 1972, The Williams & Wilkins Company, Baltimore.

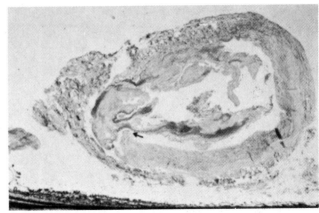

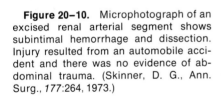

Figure 20–10. Microphotograph of an excised renal arterial segment shows subintimal hemorrhage and dissection. Injury resulted from an automobile accident and there was no evidence of abdominal trauma. (Skinner, D. G., Ann. Surg., *177*:264, 1973.)

parent with penetrating wounds and in which hemorrhage can be readily controlled by compression, intra-abdominal vascular injuries are more inaccessible to examination, and bleeding cannot be readily controlled by external compression. Resultant hemorrhage is often massive, and the severity of the condition may be suspected by the degree of associated shock. Confirmation can be made by laparotomy. Perdue and Smith (1968) emphasized that in all of their 90 patients with intra-abdominal vascular injuries, it was obvious that there was

a possibility of vascular injury, although the definitive diagnosis was not made prior to an exploratory celiotomy. The presence of a bruit should alert the examiner to the possibility of an acute arteriovenous fistula between one of the visceral arteries and its accompanying vein. Hematuria may be present with renal pedicle trauma.

Roentgenograms of the abdomen can provide some assistance. A large soft tissue density might represent a retroperitoneal hematoma. The presence of an intraperitoneal missile with associated physical find-

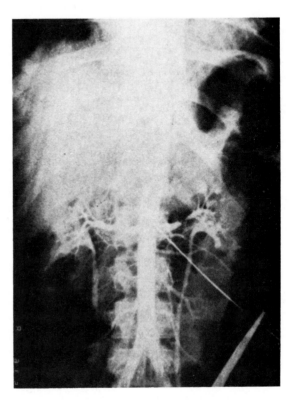

Figure 20–11. Aortogram revealing high-grade stenosis of both renal arteries secondary to subintimal hematomas. Retained radiopaque medium from a previous retrograde pyelogram is noted in the pelvis of both kidneys. (Grablowsky, O. M., Weichert, R. F., Goff, J. B., and Schlegel, J. U., Surgery, *67*:895, 1970.)

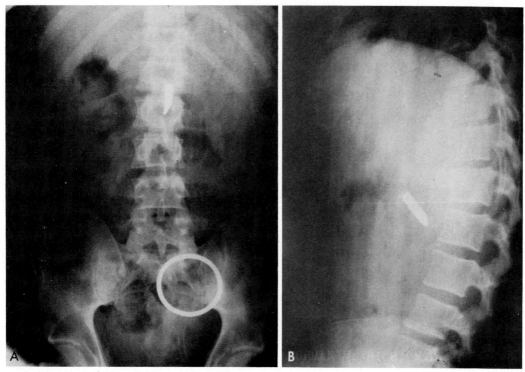

Figure 20–12. (A) A missile in the abdomen demonstrated on roentgenogram should arouse suspicion of possible intra-abdominal vascular trauma. (B) This bullet from an AK–47 rifle severed the left renal artery in an American casualty in Vietnam. (Courtesy of Dr. Walter Y. Walker from the 67th Evacuation Hospital, 1967.) (See also Figure 19–4.)

ings should arouse suspicion of possible vascular injury (Fig. 20–12). An excretory urogram may demonstrate nonfunction of the kidney or extravasation of contrast medium with injuries to the renal pedicle; however, false-negative studies have been as high as 30 per cent (Guerriero et al., 1971). Aortography may provide assistance when there is some question, particularly in nonpenetrating abdominal trauma, and it may substantiate the clinical impression of an arterial injury. The value of arteriography at a delayed time after the initial trauma is demonstrated in Figure 20–11, in which a nearly total occlusion of both renal arteries is demonstrated.

Concomitant injuries of adjacent structures are the rule rather than the exception with intra-abdominal vascular injury. This is emphasized in Table 20–4; only 6 of 90 patients had an isolated vascular injury (Perdue and Smith, 1968). In addition to

TABLE 20–4. INJURIES OF MAJOR ABDOMINAL VESSELS: ASSOCIATED INJURIES (1956–1965)*

ASSOCIATED INJURIES	NO. OF PATIENTS	NO. OF DEATHS	PER CENT DEATHS
Isolated vascular injury	6	1	17
One other organ system	25	10	40
Two other organ systems	23	6	26
Three other organ systems	24	12	50
Four or more organ systems	12	6	50
Total:	90	35	39

*From Perdue, G. D., and Smith, R. B., Surgery, *64*:562, 1968.

concomitant venous injuries, injuries to the bowel, liver, spleen, pancreas and kidney are also common.

SURGICAL TREATMENT

Because of resultant hemorrhage associated with intra-abdominal vascular injury, resuscitation in the emergency room by plasma volume expansion with balanced solutions and dextran, followed by whole blood transfusion when available, is mandatory. However, the bleeding may have to be controlled by an operative procedure. Exploratory celiotomy should not be delayed in an attempt to achieve stability of the patient. In 90 patients with intra-abdominal vascular injury, the average delay between admission and operation was about 2 hours in the survivors and about 1½ hours in the fatalities (Perdue and Smith, 1968).

General preoperative preparation and supportive care similar to those given the patient with injury to the abdominal aorta are necessary and should be part of the team effort to increase salvage of these patients. Adequate exposure through a long midline incision will provide the best access for rapid control of hemorrhage and repair of the vascular trauma (Fig. 20–13). A drop in blood pressure can be anticipated with the release of the peritoneal tamponade when the abdomen is opened. Direct digital control over the arterial laceration or simple squeezing of the severed arterial end between the surgeon's fingers can be effective until noncrushing vascular clamps are applied. Evacuation of the intra-abdominal blood will expedite this maneuver. If a retroperitoneal hematoma is present, this should not be disturbed until adequate personnel, vascular instruments, and blood are available to manage the potential rapid blood loss from the arterial injury. Dissection may then be undertaken more safely. In some instances isolation and temporary occlusion of the abdominal aorta at the diaphragm may be helpful, though occlusion of the aorta for longer than 20 to 30 minutes can cause serious ischemic injury of the visceral organ.

Débridement of all devitalized tissue and foreign material is of paramount importance. This is necessitated by the fact that there is usually associated visceral trauma. Débridement of the artery should include all grossly traumatized tissue. Areas of in-

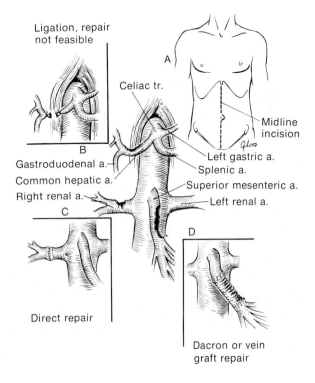

Figure 20–13. (A) Midline incision provides rapid exposure of the intra-abdominal vessels. (B, C, D) Various arterial injuries and method of management.

timal fracture with subintimal hematoma are usually managed most satisfactorily by resection. Vascular clamps should be alternately released both proximal and distal to allow flow of blood, and a Fogarty catheter passed distally will help insure that there is no remaining local thrombus. Heparinization will help minimize thrombus formation during this operative procedure.

A range of acceptable procedures exists in managing visceral arterial injuries (Fig. 20–14). Ligation of the splenic artery with splenectomy might be the most expeditious, and this is a perfectly acceptable procedure. However, loss of a kidney is certainly more significant if the same approach is used in managing renal arterial injuries. Unfortunately, organ viability may have already been lost if arterial flow to the kidney has been interrupted more than 90 minutes. Either end-to-end anastomosis or autogenous venous grafts provide the best repair of traumatized visceral arteries. Because of the usual associated contamination from concomitant organ injury, prosthetic material should be avoided.

Ulvestad (1954) was able to repair successfully a 6-mm longitudinal laceration of the superior mesenteric artery with three interrupted 00000 arterial silk sutures. He noted that within a few seconds the color and peristalsis of the small bowel and colon improved markedly. There was also an injury to the jejunum and a concomitant superior mesenteric venous injury. Killen (1964) noticed the same improvement in the appearance of the bowel after lateral repair of three small defects in the anterior wall of the superior mesenteric artery with 00000 arterial silk sutures. Ulvestad was also able to perform a lateral repair of a 10-mm longitudinal rent in the anterior wall of the superior mesenteric vein. May and co-authors (1965) were able to perform an end-to-end anastomosis of the superior mesenteric artery approximately five hours after the patient had been shot with a .22 caliber bullet. Twelve days after repair, an aortogram demonstrated patency of the superior mesenteric artery (Fig. 20–15). Repair of concomitant venous injuries should be accomplished if at all feasible. Because of loss of viability of the bowel, it might be necessary to resect a portion of the bowel prior to completion of the operative procedure.

With injuries of the renal artery, the choice of arterial repair or nephrectomy depends upon several factors. Obviously one must always be certain that the opposite kidney is present and intact. The duration of renal ischemia is another important consideration. Complete ischemia beyond 60 to 90 minutes jeopardizes renal function almost to an irreversible degree. The remarkable case described by Morton and Crawford (1972), however, is worthy of

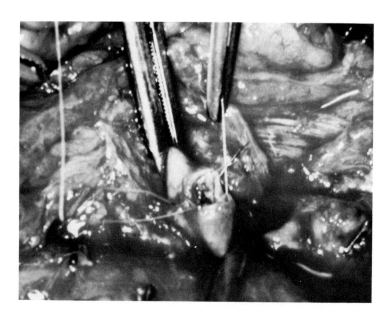

Figure 20–14. Visceral arterial injuries can be managed by a variety of methods. Successful end-to-end anastomosis of this severed superior mesenteric artery was possible. (N.M.R., W.R.G.H., 1974.)

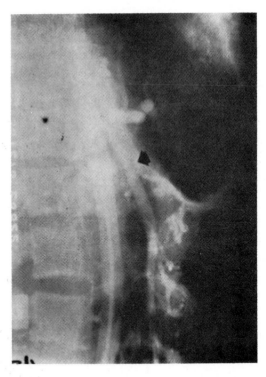

Figure 20-15. Aortogram showing the superior mesenteric artery 12 days after reconstruction. Arrow indicates a slight constriction at the site of anastomosis. (See Figure 20-9.) (May, A. G., Lipchik, E. O., and DeWeese, J. A., Ann. Surg., *162*:869, 1965.)

study in this regard; it demonstrated the ultimate partial recovery of kidneys that seemed almost certainly nonviable at operation. When a renal arterial injury is repaired in the presence of advanced ischemia, a long term possibility of inducing renal vascular hypertension must be considered. This may be the result of stenosis of the arterial repair or irreversible ischemic injury in the kidney. One such instance was reported by Guerriero and co-workers in 1971. A 17 year old patient with thrombosis of both renal arteries was operated upon following blunt trauma. Repair was completed 19 hours after injury, yet it was initially successful. Three months later aortography was performed because of hypertension, and stenosis of an inferior mesenteric vein graft to the left renal artery was found (Fig. 20-16). At a subsequent operation this area was resected and reconstructed, but the hypertension persisted.

Although repair of the hepatic artery may be as important as that of the renal artery to preserve organ viability, the celiac artery may be ligated if necessary, with the realization that collateral circulation will be sufficient.

Antibiotics should be started in the preoperative period and continued throughout the operation into the postoperative period. Intraoperative arteriography may be beneficial in insuring patency of the repair and in identifying residual distal thrombus.

POSTOPERATIVE CARE

Because it is impossible to evaluate the quality of peripheral pulses and other possible associated findings such as edema, general supportive care is most significant in the postoperative period. A postoperative arteriogram will delineate the patency of the repair if this becomes questionable. Also, following renal arterial repair, an intravenous pyelogram will provide information with which to evaluate renal function. Hypertension in the postoperative period following renal artery reconstruction should arouse suspicion of renal arterial stenosis. This might be accompanied by the presence of a bruit along the course of the renal artery. Albuminuria may herald renal vein thrombosis. The presence of a postoperative fever and changes in the polymorphonuclear cells indicating the possibility of an infection should also alert one to the possibility of nonviability of tissue, such as bowel, kidney or liver.

A significant complication posing a

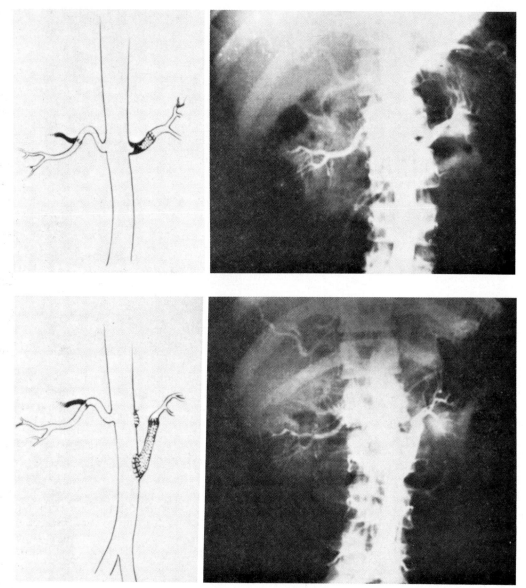

Figure 20–16. The artist's drawing and the aortogram (above) revealed stenosis of the inferior mesenteric vein graft utilized to reconstruct the left renal artery. Additional evaluation (below) revealed repair of the left renal artery stenosis with a saphenous vein bypass graft. (Guerriero, W. G., Carlton, C. E., Jr., Scott, R., and Beall, A. C., Jr., J. Trauma, *11*:53, 1971. Copyright 1971, The Williams & Wilkins Co., Baltimore.)

serious threat to the patient's life would be wound infection with subsequent disruption of the anastomosis, causing acute hemorrhage.

RESULTS

With the application of the accepted principles of vascular surgery, successful results can be anticipated following repair of even relatively small visceral arteries. Al-though limited in number, repair of both the hepatic and superior mesenteric arteries with successful results has been reported, as well as similar success in managing trauma to the larger renal arteries.

Considering all intra-abdominal vascular trauma, Perdue and Smith (1968) reported a 39 per cent mortality rate with 35 deaths among their 90 patients. Fifteen of their patients exsanguinated in the operating room before resuscitation had been com-

TABLE 20–5. INJURIES OF VISCERAL VESSELS: MORTALITY (1956–1965)*

VISCERAL VESSELS	No. INJURED	DEATHS
Splenic		
Artery only	1	1
Artery and vein	2	0
Vein only	3	2
Hepatic		
Artery	4	2
Vein	1	0
Portal vein	2	1
Renal		
Artery only	5	3
Artery and vein	1	0
Vein only	3	0
Superior mesenteric		
Artery only	3	1
Artery and vein	1	0
Vein only	5	1
Inferior mesenteric		
Artery only	1	1
Vein only	1	0

*From Perdue, G. D., and Smith, R. B., Surgery, *64*:562, 1968.

pleted. An additional 10 patients underwent a complete operative procedure but died within the first 24 hours. The final 10 delayed postoperative deaths included infection as the most significant complication. Among the 55 survivors, it is important to emphasize that major complications developed in 30 patients. Table 20–5 outlines the injuries to visceral vessels with the corresponding mortality rates in their series. Guerriero and co-authors (1971) described the details in managing 33 patients with renal pedicle injuries. There were 12 deaths in their series for a mortality of 36 per cent (Table 20–2). Morton and Crawford (1972) added a case of a patient with bilateral traumatic renal arterial thrombosis to a review of similar cases and concluded that nephrectomy would probably be required in unilateral thrombosis to prevent hypertension, while vascular reconstruction should be attempted in bilateral injuries. In their case revascularization was performed 18 hours after injury (Table 20–6). Sturm and associates (1975) recently

TABLE 20–6. MANAGEMENT AND RESULTS OF RENAL VESSEL INJURY*

SEX, AGE	SITE AND TYPE OF INJURY	ASSOCIATED INJURIES	DELAY IN DIAGNOSIS	MANAGEMENT	FOLLOW-UP IVP ON SIDE OF INJURY
M, 35	Rt. vein laceration	Fractured femur, tibia, ankle, pelvis	None	Repair	Normal 7 mos
F, 17	Rt. artery laceration	Ruptured liver	None	Repair	Nonfunction 1 yr
M, 23	Lt. artery laceration	Ruptured colon	None	Repair	Died from assoc. inj.
F, 17	Rt. vein laceration	Ruptured diaphragm, liver, colon; hemothorax; fractured tibia, radius; head injury	None	Repair	Died from assoc. inj.
F, 52	Lt. vein laceration	Ruptured spleen; subdural hematoma	None	Nephrectomy	——
F, 74	Rt. artery thrombosis	Ruptured diaphragm, spleen, small bowel	None	Nephrectomy	Died from assoc. inj.
M, 16	Rt. artery thrombosis	Abdominal wall avulsion	12 hrs	Conservative	Nonfunction 8 yrs
M, 2	Rt. artery laceration	Abdominal bowel infarction	12 hrs	Delayed Nephrectomy	Died from assoc. inj.
F, 19	Rt. artery thrombosis	Ruptured liver	24 hrs	Conservative	Nonfunction 5 yrs
M, 36	Lt. artery thrombosis	Ruptured liver, spleen	24 hrs	Conservative Delayed Nephrectomy	——
M, 21	Lt. artery thrombosis	Fractured lumbar vert.	3 yrs	Conservative	Nonfunction 6 yrs
M, 48	Rt. artery and vein laceration	Ruptured aorta, bowel, liver, spleen, ureter; subdural hematoma	D.O.A.	——	——
M, 57	Rt. vein laceration	Ruptured liver, colon, iliac artery; head injury	D.O.A.	——	——
M, 17	Rt. artery laceration	Ruptured liver, spleen; head injury	Died in O.R.	——	——

*From Sturm, J. T., Perry, J. F., Jr., and Cass, A. S., Ann. Surg., *182*:696, 1975.

TABLE 20–7. CLINICAL FEATURES OF 10 REPORTED CASES OF TRAUMATIC RENAL ARTERY THROMBOSIS*

Reference	Age	Sex	Cause of Injury	Associated Injuries	Involved Kidney	Signs	Diagnostic Studies	Diagnosis Confirmed By	Surgical Treatment	Result
Von Recklinghausen (1861)	13	M	Fall from building	Fractures of skull, arm, leg	Left	?	None	Autopsy	None	Died 8 days
Barney and Mintz (1933)	?	M	Fall from car	?	Left	Microscopic hematuria	None	Autopsy	None	Died 8 days
Beck (1951)	23	M	Motocycle accident	Liver laceration	Right	?	None	Autopsy	None	Died 4 mos
Hirschberg and Soll (1942)	48	M	Fall from truck	None	Left	Microscopic hematuria, flank pain	IVP	Operation	Nephrectomy	Recovered
Owan and Pearlman (1952)	36	F	Auto accident	Multiple fractures	Right	?	IVP	Operation 3 mos later	Nephrectomy for hypertension	Recovered (normotensive)
Collins and Jacobs (1961)	?	?	Fall from tree	?	Left	Microscopic hematuria, flank pain, swelling	Aortogram 4 days after trauma	Operations 4 days after trauma	Nephrectomy	Recovered
Lichtenheld (1961)	20	M	Auto accident	Fracture of spine	Left	Microscopic hematuria	IVP 2 days after trauma, aortogram	Operation (remote)	Nephrectomy for hypertension	Recovered (normotensive)
Hemley and Finby (1962)	12	M	Fall from sledge	None	Left	Microscopic hematuria	IVP, aortogram 3 mos	Operation 4 mos	Nephrectomy for hypertension	Recovered (normotensive)
Steiness and Thayson (1965)	18	M	Motorcycle accident	None	Bilateral	Microscopic hematuria	IVP, aortogram	Operation (57 hrs)	Lt. nephrectomy, rt. arterial reconstruction	Prolonged renal failure, hypertension, died 256 days
Present case	17	M	Auto-pedestrian accident	Bilateral fractured tibias	Bilateral	Microscopic hematuria, anuria	IVP, retrograde pyelogram, aortogram	Operation (18 hrs)	Bilateral arterial reconstruction	Living with asymptomatic hypertension 4 years

*Morton, J. R., and Crawford, E. S., Ann. Surg., 176:62, 1972.

emphasized the low salvage rate with blunt renal pedicle injuries (Table 20–7). They reported a 50 per cent mortality among 14 patients.

Results obtained by Fullen and co-workers (1972) in managing eight superior mesenteric arterial injuries (Fig. 20–17) are outlined in Table 20–8. Mattox and associates (1974) reported 46 patients with critical injuries of the suprarenal aorta, suprarenal vena cava or proximal few centimeters of the celiac axis or superior mesenteric artery at the Ben Tabu General Hospital between January, 1969, and December, 1973. There were 14 patients with superior mesenteric artery or celiac axis injury. Nine of these 14 patients also had concomitant injuries to the aorta, vena cava or portal vein. These injuries were often encountered during exposure of the aorta and vena cava. Ligation of the proximal celiac axis was accomplished in four patients, and adequate collateral circulation was evident at the time of ligation. A Dacron prosthetic replacement was utilized in one patient with proximal superior mesenteric arterial injury. One patient had replantation of the superior mesenteric artery into the aorta, and another had the superior mesenteric artery implanted into an aortic Dacron prosthesis. Two of the four patients who had ligation of the celiac axis survived, and the one patient who had replantation of the superior mesenteric artery survived. None of these

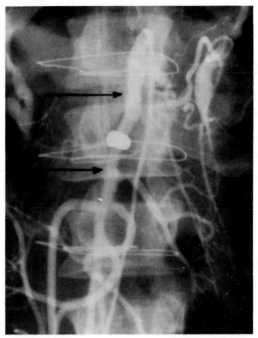

Figure 20–17. This postoperative arteriogram shows a patent 3.5 cm saphenous vein graft repair of the superior mesenteric artery without any constriction at the anastomotic sites (arrows). (Fullen, W. D., Hunt, J., and Altemeier, W. A., J. Trauma, *12*:656, 1972. Copyright 1972, The Williams & Wilkins Co., Baltimore.)

patients showed evidence of mesenteric or hepatic insufficiency.

Ikard and Merendino (1970) presented the case of a 20 year old female who had

TABLE 20–8. SUPERIOR MESENTERIC ARTERIAL INJURY*

Case No.	Classification	Management	Associated Injury	Complications	Result
1	Grade 1, Zone IV	Ligation and major resection	Liver, small bowel	Malabsorption	Late death
2	Grade 2, Zone III	Arteriorrhaphy	Stomach, liver, jejunum, renal artery and vein	– – –	Operative death
3	Grade 4, Zone IV	Ligation	Small bowel	None	Good
4	Grade 4, Zone IV	Ligation	Small bowel, IVC, ureter	Wound infection	Good
5	Grade 4, Zone IV	Ligation	Liver, stomach, lung	None	Good
6	Grade 3, Zone IV	Ligation and minor resection	Small bowel	None	Good
7	Grade 1, Zone III	Vein patch angioplasty	Spleen, colon, duodenum, IVC, pancreas	Enterocutaneous fistula and sepsis	Hospital death
8	Grade 1, Zone III	Distal SMA perfusion and vein graft	Pancreas, duodenum, spinal cord	None	Good

*Modified from Fullen, W. D., Hunt, J., and Altemeier, W. A., J. Trauma, *12*:656, 1972. Copyright 1972, The Williams & Wilkins Company, Baltimore.

resection of a large intra-abdominal mass by a standard Whipple procedure. During the dissection there was arterial bleeding from what was thought to represent the large superior branch of the superior mesenteric artery. This was clamped. However, the entire small bowel and right colon became dusky and pulseless. Obviously, the superior mesenteric artery itself, rather than a large first branch, had been clamped and ligated. Approximately two hours after division of the superior mesenteric artery, a Dacron aortosuperior mesenteric bypass was performed. There was immediate change of color of the involved bowel, and pulsations were felt throughout. Based on experimental (Wright and Hobson, 1975) and clinical (Hobson et al., 1976) experience, the ultrasound device (Doppler) can be of value in determining intestinal viability.

The limited number of visceral arteries which have been repaired in Vietnam have not been associated with any recognized complication. Two asymptomatic patients seen at Walter Reed General Hospital had audible bruits, indicating probable patency of saphenous vein grafts in the superior mesenteric artery. Arteriograms would be needed for these patients as well as several other patients with renal arterial and hepatic arterial repairs to definitely establish patency without stenosis of the repair site.

FOLLOW-UP

There is limited follow-up of patients who have had repair of visceral arteries. Because there are relatively few patients with this type of injury and even a smaller number who have had repairs of their injuries, it is paramount that an effort be made to provide follow-up evaluation.

If the patient survives the immediate

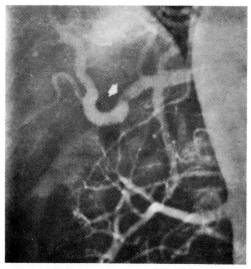

Figure 20–18. This retrograde aortogram was obtained 1 year after reconstruction of the hepatic artery by end-to-end anastomosis (arrow). (May, A. G., Lipchik, E. O., and DeWeese, J. A., Ann. Surg., *162*:869, 1965.)

postoperative period and organ function is maintained, there should be no additional significant problems. Patients with stenosis of a renal arterial repair and hypertension must be observed more carefully. Also, if a prosthesis was utilized in the repair, careful observation should be insured because of the potential for late complications of thrombosis and false aneurysm formation at the suture line.

If any possible symptomatology develops, arteriography can be helpful in delineating the status of the repair site. In Figure 20–18 a patent end-to-end anastomosis of the hepatic artery is demonstrated one year after reconstruction.

There have been no known problems in survivors with visceral arterial injuries who have been followed in the Vietnam Vascular Registry.

CHAPTER 21

ILIAC ARTERY INJURIES

Trauma to the common, external and internal iliac arteries has been relatively infrequent as compared to major extremity arterial injuries. Among the injuries incurred during major wars in this century—World War I (Makins, 1919), World War II (DeBakey and Simeone, 1946), Korea (Hughes, 1958) and Vietnam (Rich et al., 1970A)—the incidence of iliac artery injury has been less than 3 per cent (Table 21–1). In several major civilian series, however, the incidence has been over twice as great. In some series, iliac artery injuries are grouped together without specifying the exact anatomical site of injury. Injury to the internal iliac (hypogastric) artery is relatively insignificant. Associated intra-abdominal injuries may greatly complicate the management of iliac artery injuries, especially when there is contamination by bowel content.

The critical nature of both the common and external iliac arteries is indicated by the fact that about 50 per cent of extremities become gangrenous if the injured artery is ligated or if there is immediate failure of arterial repair. Certain anatomical features may complicate arterial reconstruction. With extensive soft tissue injuries which destroy much of the peritoneum, coverage of the arterial repair with soft tissues may be difficult. Associated intra-abdominal injuries may further complicate reconstruction. If there is contamination of the wound with intestinal contents, insertion of a prosthesis is most hazardous because of the serious risk of infection, possibly with fatal secondary hemorrhage. Finally, in all surgical procedures involving the iliac artery, proximity of the ureter, normally crossing near the bifurcation of the common iliac artery, must be remembered. In secondary operations complicated by extensive scar tissue in the area, identification and protection of the ureter can be difficult.

SURGICAL ANATOMY

The two common iliac arteries are the terminal branches of the aorta arising on the front of the body of the fourth lumbar vertebra to the left of the midline. Each is about 5 cm in length. As they diverge they pass downward and laterally over the psoas muscle in a course roughly parallel to the pelvic brim (Fig. 21–1). The right common iliac artery is usually somewhat longer than the left and passes more obliquely across the last lumbar vertebra.

Both common iliac arteries are covered anteriorly by peritoneum. Also, the ureter crosses over the division of each common iliac artery (Fig. 21–2). On the right side the inferior vena cava and the right common iliac vein are lateral to the artery. The common iliac vein lies medial to and partly behind the left common iliac artery.

The common iliac arteries divide into the internal and external iliac arteries opposite the fibrocartilaginous area between the last lumbar vertebra and the sacrum. Normally there are no major branches of the

475

TABLE 21–1.   INCIDENCE OF ILIAC ARTERY INJURIES

AUTHORS	TOTAL ARTERIES	COMMON ILIAC	PER CENT	EXTERNAL ILIAC	PER CENT	TOTAL ILIACS	PER CENT
War Series							
WW I Makins (1919)	1202	1	0.1	4	0.3	5	0.4
WW II DeBakey and Simeone (1946)	2471	13	0.5	30	1.2	43	1.7
Korean Hughes (1958)	304	—	—	—	—	7	2.3
Vietnam Rich et al. (1970A)	1000	9	0.9	17	1.7	26	2.6
Civilian Series							
Houston Morris et al. (1960)	220	—	—	—	—	17	7.7
Atlanta Ferguson et al. (1961)	200	6	3.0	4	2.0	10	5.0
Denver Owens (1963)	70	3	4.3	5	7.1	8	11.4
Detroit Smith et al. (1963)	61	—	—	5	8.2	5	8.2
Dallas Patman et al. (1964)	271	8	3.0	4	1.5	12	4.4
Los Angeles Treiman et al. (1966)	159	—	—	—	—	11	6.9
St. Louis Dillard et al. (1968)	85	—	—	—	—	2	2.4
New Orleans Drapanas et al. (1970)	226	3	1.3	—	—	9	4.0
Dallas Perry et al. (1971)*	508	20	3.9	6	2.7	31	6.1
Memphis Cheek et al. (1975)	155	—	—	11	2.2	14	9.0
Denver Kelly and Eiseman (1975)	116	—	—	—	—	8	6.9
New York Bole et al. (1976)	126	9	7.1	4	3.2	13	10.3

*This is a sequential study including the earlier report.

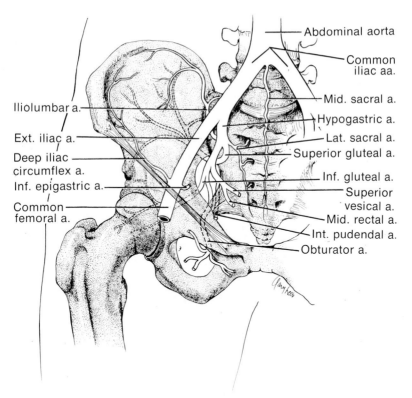

Figure 21–1. The common iliac arteries arise at the bifurcation of the abdominal aorta. The two major divisions are the external and internal (hypogastric) iliac arteries. The major branches are also shown.

common iliac arteries. In some patients, however, there may be small vessels to the neighboring ureter and other surrounding structures. The iliolumbar artery occasionally originates from the common iliac artery. Rarely, accessory renal arteries have originated from the common iliac arteries.

At the common iliac artery bifurcation, the external iliac artery is the larger of the two and is the continuation of the main trunk of the abdominal portion of the major arterial supply to the lower extremity. The external iliac artery passes obliquely downward and laterally along the medial border of the psoas major muscle to terminate midway between the anterior superior spine of the ileum and symphysis beneath the inguinal ligament, where it becomes the common femoral artery. Peritoneum covers the external iliac arteries on the anterior and medial surfaces; the ileum on the right and the sigmoid colon on the left are in close proximity.

Because the only two branches of the external iliac artery are both near its termi-

nation, the external iliac is primarily a conduit between the common iliac and the common femoral arteries and does not supply an abundant source of collateral vessels. The two major branches, however, the inferior epigastric artery and deep iliac circumflex artery, can become important re-entry points for collateral supply to the common femoral artery. The inferior epigastric (deep epigastric) artery arises medially immediately above the inguinal ligament and extends superiorly beneath the rectus abdominus muscle. It has an important anastomosis with the thoracic artery and may also communicate with the obturator artery. The deep iliac circumflex artery also arises just above the inguinal ligament from the lateral aspect of the external iliac artery opposite the origin of the inferior epigastric artery. It ascends obliquely and laterally under the inguinal ligament toward the anterior superior iliac spine. The extensive anastomosis about the iliac crest provides an important collateral blood supply to the femoral arteries via the

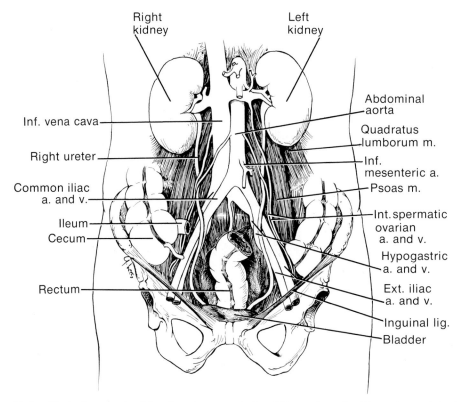

Figure 21–2. Illustration emphasizing the close proximity of the ureters, the iliac veins and the intestine to the iliac arteries.

ascending branch of the lateral femoral circumflex artery (Fig. 21–3). Although the collateral circulation through the major parietal pathways and the major visceral pathways shown in Figure 21–3 are more significant in aortoiliofemoral occlusive disease, these collateral pathways may also be important in iliac artery trauma. They are responsible for the near 50 per cent extremity viability after acute occlusion of the common or external iliac arteries.

The external iliac veins are a continuation of the corresponding common femoral veins and begin beneath the inguinal ligament. Initially they are on the medial side of the external iliac artery and then behind it.

The internal iliac (hypogastric) artery is a short, thick vessel which is smaller than the external iliac and is about 4 cm in length. There is considerable variation in the branching of the hypogastric artery, but it usually bifurcates into anterior and posterior divisions to supply the pelvic girdle and the pelvic viscera. Some of the

major branches include the superior gluteal, internal pudendal and obturator arteries. There is an extensive collateral bypass between the majority of the branches, forming a transpelvic collateral circulation.

INCIDENCE

Table 21–1 outlines the representative military and civilian experience with iliac artery injuries. In civilian series, the average incidence has been about 5 per cent, and in military experience, 2 to 3 per cent. In a number of series there is no difference between common and external iliac artery injuries, and rare mention of internal iliac artery injuries.

Makins (1919) reported on the British experience with arterial trauma in World War I, finding only five iliac artery injuries, four of which involved the external iliac artery, for a 0.4 per cent of the 1202 total arterial injuries. DeBakey and Simeone (1946) found 13 common iliac artery injuries

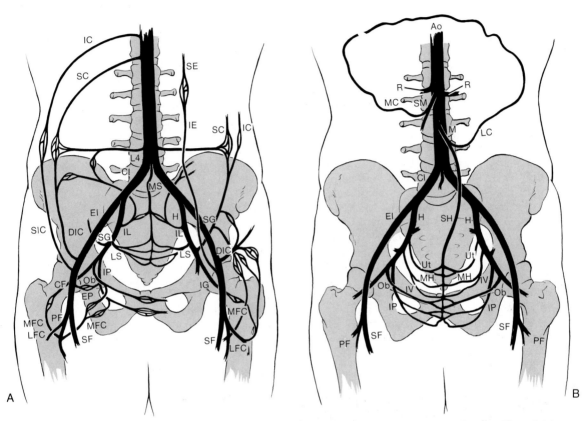

Figure 21–3. Branches of the iliac arteries form important potential collateral pathways: (A) parietal pathways and (B) visceral pathways. (Drawn after Strandness, D. E., Jr., Collateral Circulation in Clinical Surgery. Philadelphia, W. B. Saunders Co., 1969.)

Ao	Aorta	LFC	Lateral femoral circumflex
Asc	Ascending branch	LS	Lateral sacral
CF	Common femoral	MFC	Medial femoral circumflex
CI	Common iliac		
Des	Descending branch	MS	Middle sacral
DIC	Deep iliac circumflex	Ob	Obturator
EI	External iliac	PF	Profunda femoris
EP	External pudendal	SC	Subcostal
H	Hypogastric	SE	Superior epigastric
IC	Intercostal	SF	Superior femoral
IE	Inferior epigastric	SG	Superior gluteal
IG	Inferior gluteal	SIC	Superficial iliac circumflex
IL	Iliolumbar		
IP	Internal pudendal		
L	Lumbar		

Ao	Aorta	MC	Middle colic
CI	Common iliac	MH	Middle hemorrhoidal
EI	External iliac	Ob	Obturator
H	Hypogastric	PF	Profunda femoris
IH	Inferior hemorrhoidal	R	Renal
IM	Inferior mesenteric	SF	Superficial femoral
IP	Internal pudendal	SH	Superior hemorrhoidal
IV	Inferior vesical	SM	Superior mesenteric
LC	Left colic	Ut	Uterine

and 30 external iliac artery injuries among 2471 injuries in World War II, for a frequency of 1.7 per cent. In the Korean Conflict, Hughes (1958) found seven iliac injuries among 304 cases: an incidence of 2.3 per cent. In the interim report from Vietnam (Rich et al., 1970A), of 1000 arterial injuries, there were 17 injuries of the external iliac, and nine of the common iliac (Fig. 21–4).

In a total of 12 reports of civilian arterial injuries, the frequency of iliac artery involvement varied from as low as 2.4 per cent, with two injuries among 85 total arterial injuries in St. Louis (Dillard et al., 1968), to 11.4 per cent, with eight iliac injuries among 70 total arterial injuries in Denver (Owens, 1963). The majority of the series, however, cited an incidence of approximately 5 per cent. In the largest series reported by Perry and co-authors (1971) from Dallas, there were 31 iliac artery injuries among a total of 508 arterial injuries, for a 6.1 per cent incidence. Trauma to the external iliac artery was usually reported more frequently than involvement of the common iliac artery, except for the notable exception of the Dallas series, in which Perry and co-workers (1971) documented 20 common iliac artery

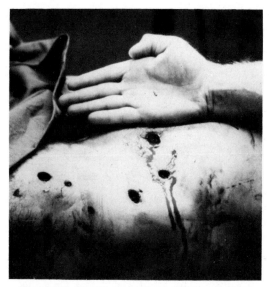

Figure 21–4. Although the multiple small fragment wounds from an M-26 fragmentation grenade did not appear severe, there were two lacerations of the left external and common iliac arteries. (Rich, N. M., Milit. Med., *133*:9, 1968.)

injuries compared to only 11 external iliac artery injuries and the New York series in which there were nine common iliac artery injuries and only four external iliac artery injuries (Bole et al., 1976).

In specifically considering internal abdominal vascular injuries, Perdue and Smith (1968) reported that 19 of their 90 patients from Atlanta with 126 intra-abdominal vascular injuries had involvement of the iliac artery: an incidence of about 21 per cent.

The internal iliac artery (hypogastric) has been specifically mentioned briefly in several series. From the Atlanta study, Ferguson and associates (1961) mentioned trauma to two hypogastric arteries among their 200 arterial injuries: an incidence of 1 per cent. Smith and co-workers (1963) from Detroit included one hypogastric injury among their 61 arterial injuries. In the Dallas study, Patman and co-authors (1964) documented three hypogastric artery injuries in their series of 271 arterial injuries. In the subsequent study from that same city, Perry and co-workers (1971) stated this number had increased to seven hypogastric artery injuries among 508 arterial injuries: an incidence of approximately 1.4 per cent. In the military experience, Makins (1919) mentioned only one hypogastric artery injury in the British World War I experience, and DeBakey and Simeone (1946) mentioned only one hypogastric injury among 2471 acute arterial injuries among Americans in their World War II study.

ETIOLOGY

Among the 28 iliac artery injuries reported from Vietnam (Rich et al., 1970A), the majority of wounds were caused by fragments from different exploding devices. Only five injuries resulted from gunshot wounds. In civilian reports, the specific wounding agents are seldom mentioned; however, there is nothing to suggest that they differ from the usual causes of arterial injuries—knives and low velocity missiles.

In recent years blunt trauma and iatrogenic injuries have increased in importance as causes of iliac artery injuries. Lord and associates (1968) reported 11 cases of major vascular injury during elective abdominal operations and included two injuries of the common iliac artery. One occurred as a result of hemorrhage during hysterectomy, and the other in association with an anterior resection of the colon. The most dramatic iatrogenic injury is that of iliac artery injury during removal of a herniated nucleus pulposus. The resultant acute arterial injury has resulted either in massive blood loss or in the formation of an arteriovenous fistula. A recent review by Boyd and Farha (1965) reported two cases and reviewed 23 from the literature. The majority have involved the common iliac arteries (Table 21–2). The right common iliac artery was involved in 11 cases, and the left common iliac artery was involved almost as frequently—in nine cases. There was one additional injury between the common iliac artery and vein, but the side was not identified.

Birkeland and Taylor (1969) presented an extensive review of major vascular injuries associated with lumbar disc surgery. A brief review of the cases that they listed as acute iliac artery trauma is outlined in Table 21–3. Arteriovenous fistulas involving the iliac vessels, as well as other vascular trauma to the aorta and vena cava, are excluded. These authors also emphasized that several large series, including 25 cases reported by Harbison (1954), 106 cases reported by DeSaussure (1959) and 59 cases reviewed by Hohf (1963), did not specifically outline the nature and location of the vascular trauma from the information obtained by sending out questionnaires to orthopedic surgeons and neurosurgeons. Data from the collected series by Birkeland and Taylor (1969) combined with the report by DeSaussure (1959) included four arterial injuries. By far the most common vascular injury was a laceration of the left common iliac artery, which is particularly vulnerable, immediately anterior to the fourth lumbar intervertebral disc. Out of the total of 74 arterial injuries, there were 41 left common iliac artery lacerations: 55.4 per cent. In the most recent review by Jarstfer and Rich (1976), statistical problems were emphasized from an analysis of previous reports. Five additional cases were added to 68 cases from a literature review, and the right common iliac artery was found to be involved most frequently.

Ouchi and colleagues (1965) reported a patient who developed acute occlusion of the external iliac artery from blunt trauma in the region of the inguinal ligament (Fig. 21–5). Thomford and co-workers (1969) reported five patients with iliac and femoral artery injuries associated with blunt skeletal trauma. One patient was crushed between a steel pole and a machine, with resulting fractures of the right ischium and separation of the pubic symphysis. Another patient sustained multiple fractures of the left pubis and ilium with separation of the left sacroiliac joint when struck by an automobile. Arteriography demonstrated occlusion of the left external iliac artery (Fig. 21–6). A third patient had extensive fractures of the right pubis, transverse processes of the lumbar vertebra and separation of the left sacroiliac joint after being crushed by falling logs. Arteriography showed an obstruction of the right common iliac artery immediately beyond the bifurcation of the aorta (Fig. 21–7).

An unusual complication of open heart surgery with retrograde perfusion through the femoral or iliac artery is a retrograde dissection. Kay and associates (1966) reported 14 such dissections over a period of eight years, during which almost 1100 operations were performed. All dissections occurred among 378 patients who were over 40 years of age, a frequency of 3 per cent. Additional studies found unrecognized dissections in other patients. They concluded that retrograde perfusion of the common femoral artery in patients over 40 years of age would be associated with a 3 per cent incidence of clinically obvious retrograde dissection, and an additional 3 per cent would have a dissection that would not be recognized (Fig. 21–8).

Smith and associates (1963) reported four injuries of the external iliac artery during inguinal herniorrhaphy. This injury has undoubtedly occurred much more frequently than previously reported in the surgical literature.

There are few reports of injury to the internal iliac artery from blunt trauma. Such an injury can occur with pelvic fracture or operative procedures in the area. Smith and co-workers (1963) reported one case of laceration of the internal iliac artery during removal of a ruptured intervertebral disc.

Text continued on page 485

TABLE 21–2. REPORTED CASES OF ARTERIOVENOUS FISTULA FOLLOWING DISC SURGERY*

Authors	Operative Signs			Location		Duration (Mos.)	Cardiac Status	Treatment and Results
	Change in Bl. Pres. and Pulse	Bleeding in Joint Space	Injury Recognized at Operation	Disc	Fistula			
Linton and White (1945)	Yes	No	No	L-4-5	Right common iliac artery and inferior vena cava	9	Cardiomegaly	Sympathectomy and ligation right common iliac artery and right external iliac vein; good
Holscher (1948)	Yes	Yes	Yes	L-4-5	Right common iliac artery and vein	6	Normal	Quadruple ligation; good
Von Kaenel (1954)	Unknown	Unknown	No	Unknown	Left common iliac artery and vein	18	Unknown	Attempted repair; died
Rasmussen (1954)	Unknown	Unknown	No	Unknown	Iliac artery and vein	¾	Unknown	Sympathectomy and ligation; fair; loss of anterior half of foot
Cooper (1954)	Unknown	Unknown	No	L-4-5	Left common iliac artery and vein	2	Unknown	Sympathectomy and ligation; fair; claudication
Harbison (1954)	No	Yes	No	L-4-5	Left common iliac artery and vein	6	Cardiomegaly, failure	Arteriorrhaphy and venorrhaphy; good
Glass and Ilgenfritz (1954)	Yes	No	Yes	L-4-5	Right common iliac artery and inferior vena cava	1¼	Cardiomegaly, failure	Quadruple ligation and excision; good
Kirklin (1954)	Unknown	Unknown	Unknown	Unknown	Aorta and inferior vena cava	Unknown	Cardiomegaly, failure	Resection and graft; venorrhaphy; good
Mack (1956)	No	No	No	L-4-5	Right common iliac artery and inferior vena cava	1⅔	Cardiomegaly, failure	Ligation and division right common iliac artery; good
Fortune (1956)	No	No	No	L-5, S-1	Left common iliac artery and vein	3	Cardiomegaly, failure	Died during investigation; postmortem diagnosis
Smith et al. (1957)	Yes	Yes	No	L-4-5	Right common iliac artery and vein	1	Cardiomegaly, failure	Arteriorrhaphy and venorrhaphy; good
Smith et al. (1957)	Yes	No	No	L-4-5	Left common iliac artery and vein	1¼	Cardiomegaly, failure	Arteriorrhaphy and venorrhaphy; good
DeBakey et al. (1958)	Unknown	Unknown	No	Unknown	Aorta and inferior vena cava	24	Normal	Aortorrhaphy; venorrhaphy; good
DeBakey et al. (1958)	Unknown	Unknown	No	Unknown	Aorta and inferior vena cava	8	Normal	Resection and graft; venorrhaphy; good
Grimson (1958)	Unknown	Unknown	No	Unknown	Aorta and inferior vena cava	Unknown	Cardiomegaly, failure	Resection and graft; venorrhaphy; good
Hardin and Allen (1958)	Unknown	Yes	No	Unknown	Left common iliac artery and vein	6	Cardiomegaly, failure	Resection and graft; venorrhaphy; good
Sze et al. (1960)	No	No	No	L-4-5	Right common iliac artery and vein	22	Normal	Arteriorrhaphy; venorrhaphy; good
Steinberg et al. (1961)	Unknown	Unknown	No	L-4-5	Right common iliac artery and inferior vena cava	9½	Cardiomegaly, failure	Arteriorrhaphy; venorrhaphy; good
Horton (1961)	Yes	No	No	L-4-5	Right common iliac artery and vein	¼	Shock; 6 days	Resection and graft; venorrhaphy; good
Horton (1961)	Unknown	Yes	No	Unknown	Left common iliac artery are vein	84	Cardiomegaly, failure	Arteriorrhaphy; venorrhaphy; good
Hufnagel et al. (1961)	No	No	No	L-4-5; L-5, S-1	Right common iliac artery and inferior vena cava	8	Normal	Arteriorrhaphy; venorrhaphy; good
Taylor and Williams (1962)	Yes	Yes	No	L-4-5	Left common iliac artery and vein	96	Cardiomegaly, failure	Ligation and division left common iliac artery; venorrhaphy; good
Taylor and Williams (1962)	Unknown	Unknown	No	Unknown	Right common iliac artery and vein	30	Cardiomegaly, failure	Transarterial repair; good
Boyd and Farha (1963)	No	No	No	L-5, S-1	Left common iliac artery and vein	7½	Cardiomegaly	Sympathectomy and quadruple ligation; good
Boyd and Farha (1963)	No	No	No	L-4-5	Right common iliac artery and vein	44	Normal	Arteriorrhaphy; venorrhaphy; good

*From Boyd, D. P., and Farha, G. J., Ann. Surg., *161*:524, 1965.

TABLE 21–3. ACUTE ILIAC ARTERY INJURIES IN LUMBAR DISC SURGERY*

Authors	Number of Cases	Disc Level	Type of Injury	Vessels Involved	Diagnosis Early 1st 24 Hours	Diagnosis Late After 24 Hours	Treatment	Results and Remarks
Seeley et al. (1954)	2	L-4-5	Tear	Left common iliac	+	–	Primary repair	Recovery
		L-4-5	Tear	Right common iliac	–	–	Arterial homograft, unsuccessful ligation	Delayed recovery
Mack (1956)	2	L-4-5	Tear	Left common iliac	+	–	Ligation	Recovery
		L-5-S1	Tear	Right internal iliac	+	–	Attempted primary repair	Died
Shumacker et al. (1961)	1	L-4-5	Tear	Left common iliac	+	3 days	Primary anastomosis	Recovery
Freeman (1961)	1	L-4-5	Tear	Left common iliac	+	–	Primary repair	Died 36 hours after operation
Mayfield (1961)	1	–	Tear	Iliac artery	+	–	Repair	Recovery
Boyd and Farha (1965)	1	L-4-5	Tear	Right common iliac artery	+	–	Primary anastomosis	Recovery
Birkeland and Taylor (1969)	1	L-4-5	Tear	Left common iliac artery	+	–	Primary repair	Recovery

*Modified from Birkeland, I. W., and Taylor, T. K. F., J. Bone Joint Surg., 51B:4, 1969. Arteriovenous fistulas are excluded from this table, which emphasizes acute arterial injuries. Also, some series, including the large reports by Harbison (1954), DeSaussure (1969) and Hohf (1967), did not specify the nature and location of the arterial injury.

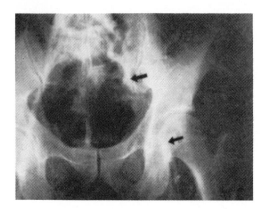

Figure 21–5. Preoperative translumbar aortogram shows occlusion of the left external iliac artery (top arrow) with reconstitution of the superficial and deep femoral arteries (bottom arrow). (Ouchi, H., Ohara, I., and Kijima, M., Surgery, 57:220, 1965.)

Figure 21–6. After a patient sustained multiple fractures of the left pubis and ilium, with separation of the left sacroiliac joint, the above arteriogram was obtained. The left lower extremity was cold, pale, pulseless, and flaccid. Occlusion of the left external iliac artery is demonstrated. (Thomford, N. R., Curtiss, P. H., and Marable, S. A., J. Trauma, 9:126, 1969. Copyright 1969, The Williams & Wilkins Co., Baltimore.)

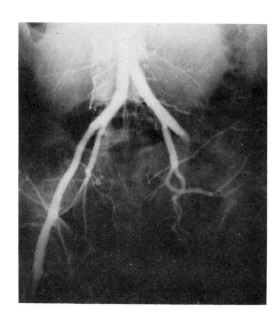

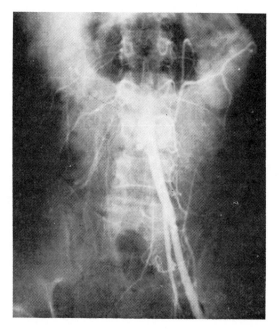

Figure 21–7. Arteriogram demonstrating occlusion of the right common iliac artery at its origin. The patient sustained fractures of the right pubis and left transverse processes of the lumbar vertebra, with separation of the left sacroiliac joint, when he was crushed by a falling log. The right lower extremity was pale, cold, pulseless, and flaccid. (Thomford, M. R., Curtiss, P. H., and Marable, S. A., J. Trauma, 9:126, 1969. Copyright 1969, The Williams & Wilkins Co., Baltimore.)

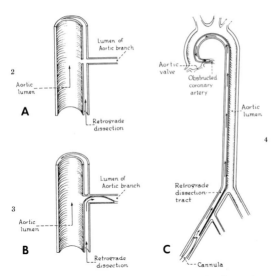

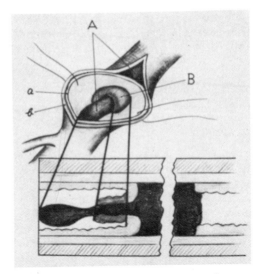

Figure 21-8. (A) Retrograde ilioaortic dissection shows shearing off of the intramural portion of the aortic branch from the outer portion with luminal patency maintained. (B) Retrograde ilioaortic dissection extends into and along the wall of an aortic branch, with compression and occlusion of the lumen of the branch. (C) Blood enters the wall of the right iliac artery just above the site of perfusion in a retrograde ilioaortic dissection. The dissection extends along the entire length of the aorta and into the wall of a coronary artery, producing obstruction of the lumen with resulting myocardial ischemia. (Kay, J. H., Dykstra, P. C., and Tsuji, H. K., Amer. J. Surg., *111*:464, 1966.)

Figure 21-9. Intraluminal protrusion of completely dissected intima. The lower half of the picture shows a longitudinal section of the injured artery. (A) Thrombus. (B) Intraluminally protruded intima. (a) Intima. (b) Media. (Ouchi, H., Ohara, I., and Kijima, M., Surgery, *57*:220, 1965.)

Among the bizarre examples of iliac artery injuries is the case reported by Smith and colleagues (1963), in which a butcher accidentally stabbed himself in the left groin with a 10-inch knife which transected the external iliac artery.

Thomford and co-workers (1969) reported similar findings following blunt skeletal trauma; in one patient only, the adventitia was intact. The intima and media had been disrupted, and the lumen was filled with thrombus.

In the retrograde ilioaortic dissections reported by Kay and associates (1966), the dissection began above the site of cannulation in eight of the 14 cases. A moderate degree of atherosclerosis was regularly present in the dissected vessels. The extent of the dissection varied from localization to the iliac artery to complete dissection of the

CLINICAL PATHOLOGY

Laceration was the most frequent type of injury among the 26 iliac artery injuries reported from Vietnam (Rich et al., 1970A). In only three injuries was the artery severed.

There are few data concerning the pathologic changes following blunt trauma to the iliac artery. In cases reported by Morris and associates (1957) and Ouchi and co-workers (1965), there was an intraluminal protrusion of the circumferentially fractured intima, with subintimal dissection and thrombus formation (Figs. 21-9 and 21-10).

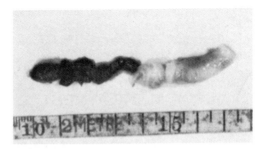

Figure 21-10. This segment of the external iliac artery with thrombus was removed following blunt trauma. At the trauma site there was an intraluminal protrusion of completely disrupted intima which caused the thrombosis. (Ouchi, H., Ohara, I., and Kijima, M., Surgery, 57:220, 1965.)

abdominal and thoracic aorta, even up to the carotid arteries. This extensive dissection occurred in about half the group.

CLINICAL FEATURES AND DIAGNOSTIC CONSIDERATIONS

With penetrating injuries the diagnosis is often obvious, because there is an open wound spurting bright red blood, associated with absence of distal pulses and a cold, pale, numb, immobile extremity. With blunt injuries diagnosis may be less obvious, especially if pulses are initially present following trauma, only to disappear as the torn intima prolapses into the lumen and becomes occluded with a thrombus or an enlarging intraluminal hematoma. In such instances, arteriography may be needed. Suspicion of an iliac artery injury may be raised by roentgenograms of the pelvis which disclose a fracture or a foreign body.

In iliac injuries associated with disc surgery, the classical finding is a machinery-type bruit over the lower abdomen following operation. Relatively few of the patients described in the review by Boyd and Farha (1965) had significant bleeding into the joint space at the time of disc removal. Only two of the 25 injuries described were recognized at the time of operation.

The possibility of concomitant injury of the iliac veins or the ureter always exists. Moore and Cohen (1968) reported an arteriovenous and ureteral injury complicating lumbar disc surgery in one patient. Perdue and Smith (1968), reporting 126 intra-abdominal vascular injuries among 90 patients, found that 12 of the 19 patients with iliac artery injuries had associated venous injuries.

SURGICAL TREATMENT

Severe shock from hemorrhage is common with iliac artery injuries. Transfusion of adequate amounts of blood and electrolyte solutions is the first important step in resuscitation. Even without massive external bleeding, there is often extensive blood loss into the retroperitoneal spaces. Antibiotics should be started promptly, especially if there is associated trauma to the intestines.

Control of hemorrhage may be difficult because a tourniquet is not applicable and direct pressure is similarly difficult. Packing with a large amount of gauze may be a satisfactory temporary expedient, but in some patients rapid surgical exposure is the only method for stopping bleeding. A midline abdominal incision is the preferred approach because of its simplicity and the access it affords to injuries of the intra-abdominal organs (Fig. 21–11). In less urgent instances when the distal external iliac artery is involved, an extraperitoneal approach can be made. This is usually performed with an incision a short distance above and parallel to the inguinal ligament, which splits the external oblique aponeurosis, then caudally detaches the internal oblique from the inguinal ligament to enter the retroperitoneal space.

Once hemorrhage has been controlled, with isolation of the artery both proximally and distally, the injury can be evaluated and adequate debridement performed. Concomitant venous injuries usually require repair initially to control bleeding. Copious irrigation with saline should be performed if intestinal contamination has occurred. A Fogarty balloon catheter should be routinely advanced into the distal arterial tree as far as possible, often below the knee,

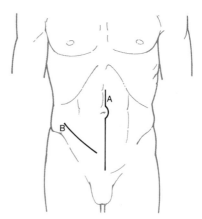

Figure 21–11. Incisions which can be utilized to approach the iliac arteries. (A) The midline incision is the most rapid approach. (B) An accepted alternate incision is the extraperitoneal approach.

because the extent and location of distal thrombi are notoriously unpredictable. Twenty-five milligrams of heparin in a dilute solution may be instilled later into the distal artery to retard subsequent development of thrombosis during arterial repair.

Methods of arterial reconstruction employed in 26 iliac artery injuries in the Vietnam Conflict are shown in Table 21–4. Lateral suture was possible in only two patients, but end-to-end anastomosis could be performed in 13. An autogenous vein graft was used in eight patients, an arterial graft in one and a Dacron prothesis in two. As mentioned earlier, a Dacron prosthesis is particularly hazardous in the presence of contamination of the wound by intestinal contents.

In the report of civilian arterial injuries from Houston, Morris and co-workers (1960) stated that most injuries could be repaired by suture (13 cases); grafts were required in only two instances.

With blunt injuries, a variety of techniques has been employed. Lord and associates (1958) described an unusual method of reconstruction following avulsion of the left common iliac artery during operative ligation of the internal iliac arteries for persistent hemorrhage two weeks after hysterectomy. Direct reconstruction was not feasible. The aortic end of the lacerated left common iliac artery was sutured, after which the distal left common iliac was anastomosed in an end-to-side fashion to the medial side of the right common iliac artery, 1 cm below the aortic bifurcation (Fig. 21–12). Good peripheral

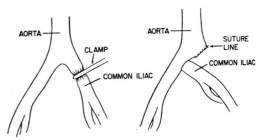

Figure 21–12. A more unusual method of reconstruction following avulsion of the left common iliac artery. After the lacerated left common iliac artery was sutured at its origin from the aorta, the distal left common iliac was anastomosed in an end-to-side fashion to the medial side of the right common iliac artery 1 cm below the aortic bifurcation. (Lord, J. W., Jr., Stone, P. W., Clouthier, W. A., and Breidenbach, L., Arch. Surg., 77:282, 1958. Copyright 1958, American Medical Association.)

pulses resulted and were still present 27 months later. If blunt trauma has caused extensive disruption of the intima with subintimal dissection, a bypass graft may be necessary (Beall et al., 1967).

Moore and Cohen (1968) described the management of a combined arterial, venous and ureteral injury complicating lumbar disc surgery. A Dacron prosthesis was used to repair the iliac artery defect (Fig. 21–13).

As with other arterial reconstruction, if distal pulses are not readily palpable after reconstruction, an operative arteriogram should be performed. The usual causes of failure of reconstruction are either undetected thrombus in the distal arterial tree or an intimal flap at the site of anastomosis.

POSTOPERATIVE CARE

Frequent observation of distal pulses following iliac artery reconstruction is the most important feature of postoperative care. Distal pulses should become palpable immediately, and should remain so. Absence of pulses may be due to thrombosis of the anastomosis or residual thrombi in the distal arterial tree. Vasospasm of sufficient intensity to obliterate distal pulses is very unusual.

If pulses are absent and viability of the extremity is in doubt, arteriography and re-operation should be performed. In some patients, exploration of the distal arterial tree with a Fogarty catheter may

TABLE 21–4. ILIAC ARTERY REPAIRS IN VIETNAM*

TYPE OF REPAIR	COMMON ILIAC	EXTERNAL ILIAC
Lateral suture	1	1
End-to-end anastomosis	3	10
Autogenous vein graft	3	5
Dacron prothesis	2	0
Autogenous artery graft	0	1
Totals:	9	17

*From Rich, N. M., Baugh, J. H., and Hughes, C. W., J. Trauma, *10*:359. 1970. Copyright 1970, The Williams & Wilkins Co., Baltimore.

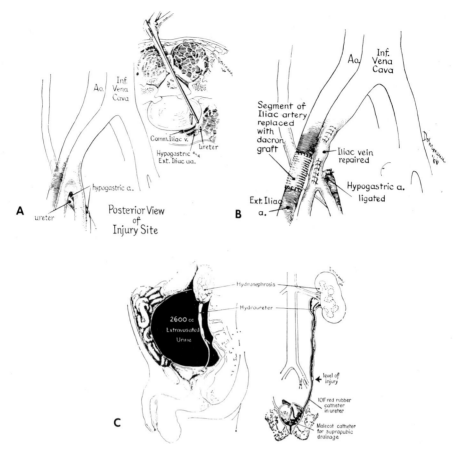

Figure 21–13. (A) The mechanism of vascular and ureteral injury with a pituitary rongeur, and the posterior view of the traumatized iliac vessels. (B) Posterior view of the surgical correction of the vascular defects. (C) The ureteral injury (identified at a second operation, 45 days after the laminectomy), retroperitoneal urinoma and surgical correction. (Moore, C. A., and Cohen, A., Amer. J. Surg., *115*:574, 1968.)

remove significant thrombi undetected at the previous operation. If the condition of the patient is precarious, especially in the presence of multiple injuries, re-operation may be avoided if motor and sensory function are intact in the extremity. An arterial reconstruction can be attempted at a later date.

With prolonged preoperative ischemia, the muscles of the lower extremity should be observed for the appearance of progressive rigidity, swelling or associated neuropathy, indicating the need for fasciotomy. However, fasciotomy is less frequently required for iliac artery injuries than for injuries to the femoral and popliteal arteries.

General supportive care includes the administration of antibiotics and ambulation as soon as possible. Heparinization is usually contraindicated because of its limited value in this situation and the hazard of bleeding into the wound. Sympathetic blocks are similarly of dubious value. Contaminated wounds that have initially been left open can be sutured within four to seven days in most patients.

COMPLICATIONS

Wound infection with secondary hemorrhage from disruption of the arterial repair is the most serious postoperative complication. This can be a life-threatening catastrophe, because massive hemorrhage can occur into the retroperitoneal spaces without external bleeding. Local pressure is often ineffective in controlling bleeding, and emergency operation may be necessary.

Several examples of these complications have been seen at Walter Reed General Hospital. One patient developed massive hemorrhage from a disrupted anastomosis in the right common iliac artery. Although he was a patient on the recovery ward, massive blood loss occurred before he could be moved to the operating room during a rather dramatic series of events. Ligation of the affected artery was performed, fortunately with sufficient collateral circulation available to maintain vitality of the extremity. If the patient's general condition is satisfactory, an extra-anatomic bypass may be considered, utilizing a greater saphenous vein bypass graft through the obturator foramen.

Several patients have been treated at Walter Reed General Hospital for infection of a Dacron prosthesis originally used to repair a major artery. One 20 year old patient had an injury of the right common femoral artery repaired with a 5 cm segment of knitted Dacron in Vietnam. A wound infection developed and three months following the initial injury it was necessary to excise the infected prosthesis at Walter Reed General Hospital. Fearing the loss of viability of the extremity, an extra-anatomic bypass with a saphenous vein graft brought through the obturator foramen was performed. Unfortunately, this graft also became infected, and the right common iliac artery was finally ligated to control hemorrhage. Fortunately there was enough collateral circulation to maintain viability of the extremity, although it

was marginal. The plethysmographic tracing from the ischemic extremity is shown in Figure 21–14. A few months later, the patient was able to walk at least two blocks without developing intermittent claudication.

Wound infection is particularly common if there is a concomitant injury to the bowel, especially with an intestinal fistula. One casualty from Vietnam was seen at Walter Reed General Hospital with infection surrounding a Dacron prosthesis used to reconstruct the left external iliac artery. Intensive topical therapy with antibiotics was attempted (Fig. 21–15); however, removal of the prosthesis was necessary before wound healing could be obtained. Another patient with an infected Dacron prosthesis in the common iliac artery, adjacent to an intestinal fistula, similarly required removal of the infected Dacron before healing could be obtained. Contrast media injected into the opening of the fistula not only outlined the communication with the small intestine but also showed the Dacron prosthesis surrounded with contrast material (Fig. 21–16).

In the absence of infection, thrombosis of a repaired iliac artery is usually due to avoidable technical errors or complications of a hematoma. Several such patients have required late arterial reconstruction because of significant claudication on ambulation (Fig. 21–17). Reconstruction with a saphenous vein graft was successful. A bizarre example of a traumatic false aneurysm causing distal embolization was

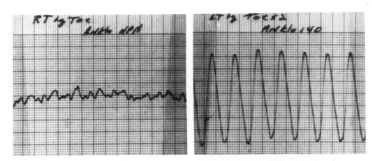

Figure 21–14. Although the plethysmographic tracing emphasizes the severe degree of ischemia in the right lower extremity, compared to the more normal tracing on the left, viability of the right lower extremity was maintained through collateral circulation which improved over a period of several months following right common iliac artery ligation. (Rich, N. M., Baugh, J. H., and Hughes, C. W., Arch. Surg.,*100*:646, 1970. Copyright 1970, American Medical Association.)

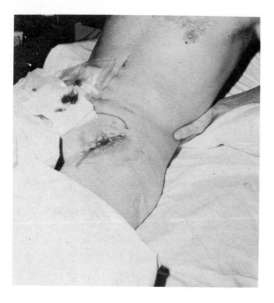

Figure 21–15. This Vietnam casualty developed a wound infection in the area of a left external iliac artery repair with a Dacron prosthesis. The small polyethylene catheter was placed to allow a dilute solution of topical antibiotics to be instilled every two hours. (Rich, N. M., and Hughes, C. W., J. Trauma, *12*:459, 1972. Copyright 1972, The Williams & Wilkins Co., Baltimore.)

reported by Waibel and Ludin (1966). A 40 year old male injured in an automobile accident had a posterior dislocation of the head of the femur with fracture of the acetabulum. The acetabulum was repaired with screws and steel wires. Ischemic pain appeared in the left foot six months later, and an arteriogram demonstrated occlusion of the right popliteal artery. Another ischemic episode appeared three days later, which was found to be due to acute occlusion of the common femoral artery. Emergency embolectomy was performed. Two months later a false aneurysm was detected in the external iliac artery developing because of injury from the tips of the two steel pins formerly used to repair the acetabulum (Fig. 21–18). It was impressive that embolic episodes preceded recognition of the false aneurysm by over two months.

Drapanas and co-authors (1970) found that slightly more than 50 per cent of the

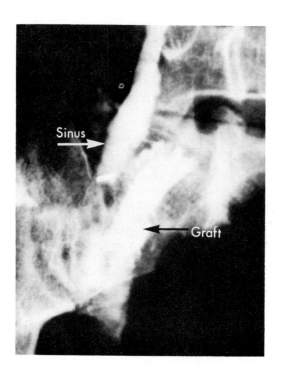

Figure 21–16. Contrast media injected into the opening of a fistula outlines not only the communication with the small intestines but also an infected Dacron prosthesis which had been used to bypass a right iliac artery injury. (W.R.G.H.)

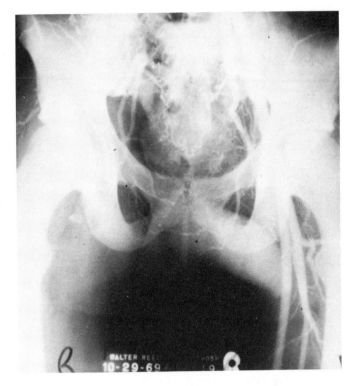

Figure 21–17. Abdominal aortogram with runoff demonstrates thrombosis of the right external iliac artery which had been repaired in Vietnam. There is also thrombosis of the right common iliac artery, with reconstitution of the right hypogastric through collaterals. Because the patient was limited in his daily activities by intermittent claudication, a greater saphenous vein graft was utilized to restore direct flow to the right lower extremity through the common femoral artery. (W.R.G.H.)

16 patients in their series who were evaluated following iliac and common femoral artery trauma had distal extremity edema following repair: nine patients with edema out of 16.

RESULTS

The most extensive experience with repair of injuries to the iliac arteries has come from the Vietnam Conflict. The interim Vietnam survey of 1000 major acute arterial injuries found 26 patients in whom an injured iliac artery had been repaired (Rich et al., 1970A) (Table 21–4). Among 17 repairs of the external iliac artery, direct anastomosis was possible in 10, while vein grafts were needed in five. There was one repair by lateral suture and one with an autogenous hypogastric arterial

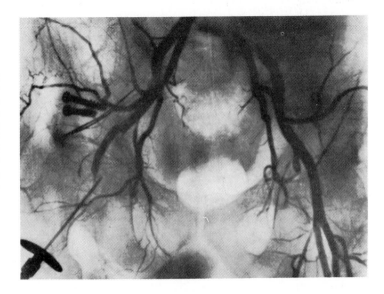

Figure 21–18. Arteriogram shows displacement of the right iliac artery in the area of the tip of two steel pins, which were responsible for the formation of a false aneurysm. Embolic episodes with ischemic changes occurred in the distal extremity prior to making the diagnosis of the iliac artery false aneurysm. (Waibel, P. P., and Ludin, H., Arch. Surg., 92:105, 1966.)

graft. In this group there were no amputations, although thrombosis occurred in three patients, and a postoperative hemorrhage in two patients ultimately required ligation of the external iliac artery in one. Among nine repairs of the common iliac artery, there were three direct anastomoses, three vein grafts, one lateral suture and two repairs of Dacron prostheses. There were three fatalities in this group, one of whom also required amputation of the injured extremity. Hence, the amputation rate for common iliac artery injuries was 11 per cent.

In the Korean Conflict, Hughes (1958) reported one amputation following a total of seven iliac artery reconstructions, an amputation rate of 14 per cent. Direct anastomosis was possible in four of the seven patients; transverse suture repair was possible in one, while two required vascular grafts. The World War II experience reviewed by DeBakey and Simeone (1946) found seven amputations required after 13 common iliac artery ligations (54 per cent), and 14 amputations following 30 external iliac artery ligations (47 per cent).

In most reports of civilian injuries, no differentiation is made between common and external iliac artery injuries. In 1960, Morris and associates reported experiences with 15 iliac artery injuries, with four deaths, two amputations and restoration of a peripheral pulse in nine patients. Two of the patients required reconstruction of the vascular graft. Patman and co-workers (1964) also reported a high fatality rate following iliac artery injuries. Drapanas and co-workers (1970) described experiences with 24 patients with iliac injuries, four of whom died. Similarly, Perry reported eight deaths in a group of 27 patients with injuries of the iliac artery, with all eight of the fatal cases having associated intra-abdominal injuries.

According to the review by DeSaussure in 1959, there was a high mortality rate of 42 per cent associated with left common iliac artery lacerations which occurred in lumbar disc surgery: 16 deaths among 38 patients. Birkeland and Taylor (1969), however, pointed out that DeSaussure's analysis did not indicate whether repair had been attempted.

FOLLOW-UP

In civilian series there are few long term follow-up data available concerning results after trauma to the iliac artery. An unusual experience that illustrates the extensive development of collateral circulation was reported by Lord and associates (1958), who described their experience with a 48 year old woman who had ligation of the common iliac artery following injury during excision of an extensive carcinoma of the colon. Severe ischemic signs were present initially but improved with anticoagulant therapy and sympathetic blocks. At the time of discharge from the hospital, claudication appeared upon walking two blocks, but two years later the patient was able to walk unlimited distances without claudication.

More than 10 patients have been evaluated at Walter Reed General Hospital following iliac artery injuries in Vietnam.

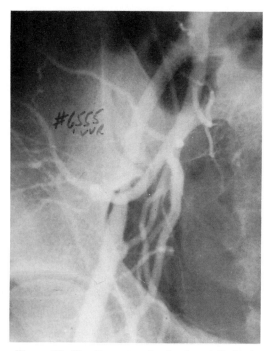

Figure 21–19. Because of a loud systolic bruit, this arteriogram was performed to rule out the formation of a false aneurysm or an arteriovenous fistula. Mild stenosis of the right external iliac artery approximately 8 cm from its origin was seen at the site of the end-to-end anastomosis which had been performed three weeks earlier in Vietnam. (Courtesy Dr. William Buhrow, Camp Zama, Japan.)

Although these represent a selected group, the complicated course and prolonged morbidity is impressive. Several have not had additional reconstruction. Associated neuropathy has greatly limited the function of the extremity in several patients. One 20 year old soldier sustained multiple fragment wounds from a booby trap in Vietnam and a laceration of the right external iliac artery on November 9, 1970. An end-to-end anastomosis of the right external iliac artery, as well as a cholecystectomy and suture of the lacerations, was performed at the 91st Evacuation Hospital. His postoperative course was uncomplicated. However, a loud systolic bruit was heard in the right femoral area several weeks later after transfer to the military hospital in Japan. There were good distal pulses. A question arose regarding the etiology of the bruit: was it a false aneurysm or an arteriovenous fistula? An arteriogram was performed, and this showed stenosis at the site of the arterial repair (Fig. 21–19). With additional follow-up through the Registry, the patient has had no additional problems.

CHAPTER 22

COMMON AND PROFUNDA FEMORAL ARTERY INJURIES

Injuries of the common femoral artery are of historical significance because repair of such an injury by Murphy in 1896 in Chicago is recognized as the first successful end-to-end anastomosis of an artery in man (see Chap. 1). The patient had developed a false aneurysm from a penetrating gunshot wound of the common femoral artery several days before (Fig. 1–4). At Murphy's historic operation, which was preceded by several months of experimental studies, the injured segment was excised and an end-to-end anastomosis performed by the invagination technique developed by Murphy.

Injuries of the common femoral and profunda femoral arteries are presented in this chapter, while those involving the superficial femoral artery are discussed in Chapter 23. The two groups are separated because of considerable difference in frequency of involvement and clinical characteristics. Injuries of the superficial femoral artery are among the most common peripheral artery injuries, while injuries of the common or profunda femoral are comparatively rare. In several reports the three different arteries are reported under the common heading, "femoral injuries"; therefore, the exact frequency of injury is un-

certain (Makins, 1919; Hughes, 1958). In general, however, common femoral injuries occur in approximately 5 per cent of all peripheral arterial injuries, and profunda femoris (deep femoral) injuries in about 1 per cent (Table 22–1). This low rate of injury is probably due to both the short length of the two arteries and their proximal location in the thigh. The importance of common femoral injuries, however, is clearly indicated by the grim fact that in World War II the amputation rate was over 80 per cent for common femoral injuries treated by ligation, making this the most critical of all arteries supplying the extremities (DeBakey and Simeone, 1946). This point is of some significance in the management of civilian vascular trauma because of the increasing popularity of retrograde femoral catheterization for angiographic purposes. Kelly and Eiseman (1975) in Denver reported 17 common femoral arterial injuries contrasted by only 7 injuries of the superficial femoral artery.

Isolated injuries of the profunda femoris artery are relatively innocuous, but final decision concerning the importance of such injuries must be deferred for several years, because this artery is seldom occluded by

494

TABLE 22-1. INCIDENCE OF COMMON AND DEEP FEMORAL ARTERY INJURIES

	AUTHORS	TOTAL ARTERIES	COMMON FEMORAL	PER CENT	DEEP FEMORAL	PER CENT
War Series						
WW I	Makins (1919)	1202	*	–	*	–
WW II	DeBakey and Simeone (1946)	2471	106	4.3	27	1.1
Korean	Hughes (1958)	304	*	–	*	–
Vietnam	Rich et al. (1970A)	1000	46	4.6	–	–
Civilian Series						
Houston	Morris et al. (1960)	220	*	–	*	–
Atlanta	Ferguson et al. (1961)	200	3	1.5	–	–
Denver	Owens (1963)	70	*	–	*	–
Detroit	Smith et al. (1963)	61	1	1.6	–	–
Dallas	Patman et al. (1964)	271	5	1.8	3	1.1
Los Angeles	Treiman et al. (1966)	159	*	–	*	–
St. Louis	Dillard et al. (1968)	85	7	8.2	–	–
New Orleans	Drapanas et al. (1970)	226	7	3.1	8	3.5
Dallas	Perry et al. (1971)†	508	11	2.2	–	–
Detroit‡	Smith et al. (1974)	127	8	6.3	–	–
Memphis	Cheek et al. (1975)	155	*	–	*	–
Denver	Kelly and Eiseman (1975)	116	17	14.7	3	2.6
Jackson	Hardy et al. (1975)	360	22	6.1	4	1.1
New York	Bole et al. (1976)	126	8	6.3	5	4.0

*Listed with superficial femoral arteries as "femoral" arteries.
†This is a sequential study including the earlier report.
‡This report covers 1968–1973.

atherosclerosis and often is the most important route of collateral circulation following occlusion of the superficial femoral, iliac or common femoral arteries.

SURGICAL ANATOMY

As a direct continuation of the external iliac artery, the common femoral artery carries the main blood supply to the lower extremity. The common femoral artery begins immediately behind the inguinal ligament midway between the anterior superior spine of the ilium and the symphysis pubis and passes from the anterior toward the medial side of the thigh overlying the hip joint. Approximately 4 cm beyond its origin under the inguinal ligament, it bifurcates into the superficial and deep femoral arteries (Fig. 22–1).

Contained in the femoral (Scarpa's) triangle, the common femoral artery is enclosed, together with the femoral vein, in the fibrous femoral sheath.

The common femoral artery lies in a fairly superficial position, covered mainly by skin, fascia and subcutaneous tissue. The femoral vein is on the medial side of the artery, and the femoral nerve is on the lateral side in a protected position covered with fibers of the iliopsoas muscle and fascia (Fig. 22–2).

There are several superficial branches which arise from the common femoral artery. The superficial circumflex iliac and the superficial epigastric arteries arise approximately 1 cm below the middle of the inguinal ligament (Fig. 22–1). There are also small superficial and deep external pudendal arteries which pass in front of and behind the femoral vein, respectively.

Although the profunda femoris artery usually arises from the posterolateral aspect of the common femoral artery approximately 4 cm below the inguinal ligament, this can vary from 2 to 5 cm. There can be some variation, with the profunda femoris artery arising from the medial side or, more rarely, from the posterior aspect of the common femoral artery. Occasionally, the profunda femoris artery may arise at a distance exceeding 5 cm from the inguinal ligament, adjacent to the inguinal ligament or, rarely from the

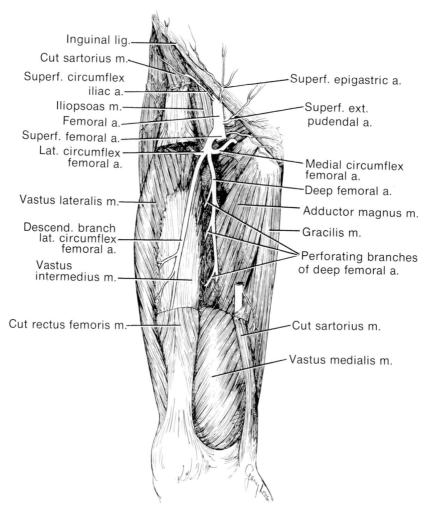

Figure 22–1. Origin of the common femoral artery under the inguinal ligament and its bifurcation into the superficial and deep femoral arteries which occurs within approximately 4 cm. Collateral branches include the superficial circumflex iliac, superficial epigastric and superficial and deep external pudendal arteries.

external iliac artery above the inguinal ligament. The profunda femoris artery can be nearly as large as the superficial artery at the level of bifurcation of the common femoral artery. As the profunda femoris artery leaves the femoral triangle, it passes behind the adductor longus muscle, continues down the thigh on the adductor magnus muscle and ends as the fourth perforating artery.

Within the first 2 cm beyond the origin, the profunda femoris artery usually has two major branches, the medial and lateral circumflex femoral arteries. There are also four perforating arteries included in its major branches, and the total length of the profunda femoris artery can be approximately 12 inches. Strandness (1969) stated that the major branches of the femoral system of the thigh may be regarded as independent units: the medial circumflex femoral artery to the upper adductors, the lateral circumflex femoral artery to the quadriceps, the profunda femoris and its perforating branches to the posterior musculature and adductors, and the highest (supreme) genicular artery from the superficial femoral artery to the vastus medialis muscle. He also emphasized, however, that the entire thigh has a rich, communicating,

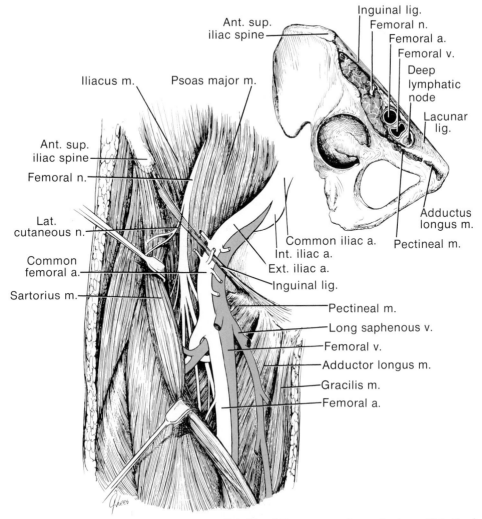

Figure 22–2. The femoral vein lies on the medial side of the common femoral artery within the femoral sheath. The femoral nerve is on the lateral side of the artery in a protected position covered by fibers of the iliopsoas muscle and fascia. The common femoral artery lies in a fairly superficial position in the femoral triangle covered mainly by skin, fascia and subcutaneous tissue.

large artery network among the large muscles. Although both the medial and lateral circumflex femoral arteries usually arise from the profunda femoris, as mentioned above, within 1 to 2 cm from its origin, one or both of these circumflex femoral branches can originate separately from the superficial or common femoral arteries. The lateral circumflex femoral artery is an extremely important collateral pathway with ascending, transverse and descending branches. The medial circumflex femoral artery passes medially and posteriorly with numerous small branches which can establish important collateral pathways.

There are numerous collateral pathways surrounding the hip (Fig. 22–3). The internal pudendal from the hypogastric artery anastomoses with the superficial and deep external pudendal branches of the common femoral artery; the superior and inferior gluteal branches of the hypogastric artery anastomose with the medial and lateral circumflex femoral and the perforating branches of the profunda femoris artery; the obturator branches of

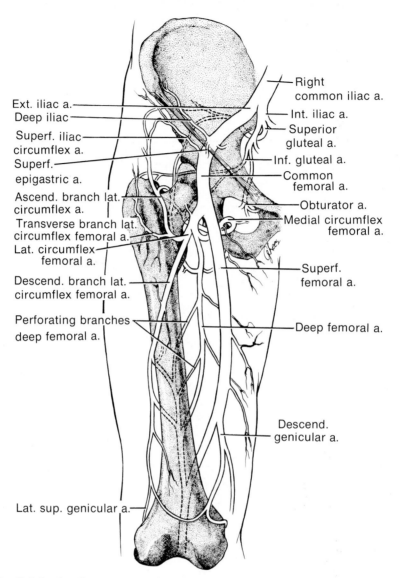

Figure 22–3. Collateral pathways surrounding the hip, emphasizing the numerous collaterals. The deep femoral artery provides an extremely important collateral pathway when there are superficial femoral artery obstructions.

the hypogastric anastomose with the medial circumflex femoral of the profunda femoris artery; the deep iliac circumflex of the external iliac anastomoses with the lateral circumflex femoral of the profunda femoris and the superficial femoral circumflex of the common femoral artery; and the inferior gluteal and the hypogastric anastomose with the perforating branches of the profunda femoris artery. The superficial epigastric arteries have a cross-anastomosis and also anastomose with branches of the inferior epigastric artery.

INCIDENCE

The frequency of common and profunda femoral artery injuries in four major military conflicts of this century (World Wars I and II, Korea and Vietnam) and nine separate reports of vascular trauma among civilians are shown in Table 22–1. In the military conflicts, common femoral injuries were reported separately only from World War II (106 such injuries) and Vietnam (46 injuries): a frequency near 5 per cent. In trauma among civilians, common femoral artery injuries have ranged from 2 to 8 per cent; however, the comparative rarity is indicated by the fact that a total of only 34 injuries is included in the civilian reports reviewed. Dillard and associates (1968) reported one of the highest incidences of common femoral artery injuries at 8.2 per cent when they documented trauma to seven common femoral arteries among 85 arterial injuries. Kelly and Eiseman (1975) documented 17 common femoral artery injuries among 116 arterial injuries for the highest incidence percentage. On the other hand, Perry and co-workers (1971), in reporting the largest number of arterial injuries (508), found only 11 common femoral artery injuries, for an incidence of 2.2 per cent.

In World War II 27 profunda femoris artery injuries were recognized, a frequency near 1 per cent of the total 2471 acute arterial injuries. In only five of the 14 civilian series tabulated are profunda femoris injuries mentioned—three by Patman and associates (1964) from Dallas, eight by Drapanas and co-authors (1970) from New Orleans, three by Kelly and Eiseman (1975) from Denver, four by Hardy and associates (1975) from Jackson, and five by Bole and co-workers (1976) in New York City. Commenting upon this low frequency rate, Saletta and Freeark (1972) recently suggested that such injuries had often been overlooked. They described six patients with profunda femoris artery injuries treated between 1966 and 1971 at Cook County Hospital.

ETIOLOGY

One hundred years ago Pick (1873) documented his thoughts regarding the etiology of common femoral artery trauma in a patient who developed an aneurysm without an external wound.

Among the 46 common femoral artery injuries in Vietnam (Table 22–2), 32 resulted from fragments from exploding missiles, ten from gunshot wounds and only one from blunt trauma. Three were of uncertain origin. The one instance of blunt trauma resulted from a motorbike accident, which involved traumatic contusion and

TABLE 22–2. ETIOLOGY OF COMMON FEMORAL ARTERY INJURIES: INTERIM VIETNAM REPORT OF 1000 ACUTE MAJOR ARTERIAL INJURIES*

WOUNDING AGENT	ARTERIAL INJURIES	PER CENT
Multiple fragment wounds	32	69.6
Gunshot wounds	10	21.7
Blunt trauma	1	2.2
Undetermined	3	6.5
Total	46	100.0

*From Rich, N. M., Baugh, J. H., and Hughes, C. W.: J. Trauma, *10*:359, 1970. Copyright 1970, The Williams & Wilkins Co., Baltimore.

thrombosis of the common femoral artery from the handle bar (Fig. 22–4). In the most recent and comprehensive review from the Vietnam experience involving 109 common femoral artery injuries, the percentages for etiological factors remained essentially the same as above (Rich et al., 1975B).

In the reports of civilian injuries of the common femoral artery, there are no distinctive characteristics except for the unusual examples of isolated cases resulting from blunt trauma, catheterization or surgical operations. Individual instances of blunt trauma include the report by Gryska (1962) of a 19 year old male struck in the groin by the tail-light of an automobile (Fig. 22–5); a report by Hershey and Spencer of transection of the common femoral artery following a groin laceration from a wooden stick (1963); and the report of Fraser (1965), who described a 54 year old man with a glancing injury from a heavy metallic casting, weighing about 60 pounds, dislodged from a rapidly rotating machine. Injuries have occurred during herniorrhaphy (Smith et al., 1963) and during operations for varicose veins (Owens, 1963). At Walter Reed General Hospital in the past 10 years, five patients have been treated for common femoral occlusion that developed after cannulation of the common femoral artery during open heart operations (Fig. 22–6). Four additional patients have developed femoral thrombosis after retrograde arterial catheterization for angiography (Fig. 22–7). An unusual example of rupture of the

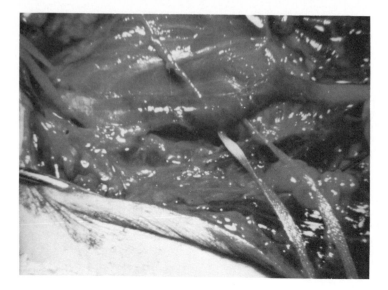

Figure 22–4. Marked contusion of the common femoral artery following blunt trauma during a motor bike accident in Vietnam. There was periadventitial hemorrhage and a subintimal hematoma with thrombosis; however, the intima remained intact. (Rich, N. M., *in* Dale, W. A. (Ed.), Management of Arterial Occlusive Disease. Year Book Medical Publishers, Inc., Chicago, 1971.)

Figure 22–5. Profuse contusion of the common femoral and external iliac arteries (the inguinal ligament was divided) with local thrombosis caused by blunt trauma from the tail-light of an automobile. It was possible to perform an adequate thrombectomy through the lower arteriotomy site below the area of injury. (Gryska, P. F., New Eng. J. Med., *266*:381, 1962.)

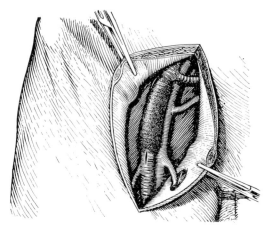

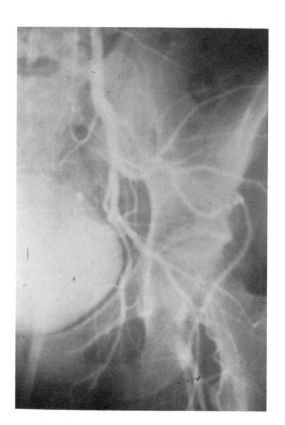

Figure 22–6. Angiogram demonstrates occlusion of the common femoral artery following canalization during an open heart procedure. Because the patient developed intermittent claudication, it was necessary to perform a saphenous vein graft approximately one year following the initial operation. (W.R.G.H.)

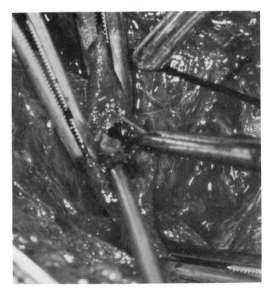

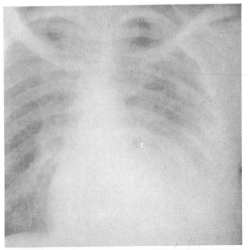

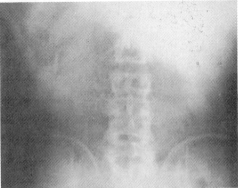

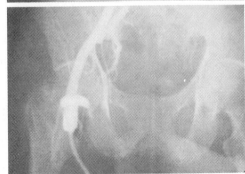

Figure 22–7. Appearance of a common femoral artery filled with thrombus following femoral artery catheterization for angiographic purposes. Either intimal disruption or the accumulation of thrombus on the catheter while it is in place can contribute to the thrombosis (Rich, N. M., Hobson, R. W. II, Fedde, C. W., and Collins, G. J., Jr., J. Trauma, *15*:628, 1975. Copyright 1975, The Williams & Wilkins Co., Baltimore.)

femoral artery following pelvic irradiation was described by Moore and associates (1971). A particularly unusual example of femoral injury was documented by Drapanas and colleagues (1970), who reported a bullet embolus to the common femoral artery in a patient who had sustained a gunshot wound of the thoracic aorta (Fig. 22–8).

The profunda femoris artery is particularly vulnerable to injury during orthopedic operations following fracture of the hip. Hohf (1963), in a survey in which approximately 1200 members of the Academy of Orthopedic Surgery responded, found 16 instances of profunda femoris artery trauma, 13 during hip operations and three during operations upon the femur. Similarly, Linton (1964) cited three separate reports of false aneurysms following orthopedic operations in which excessive lengths of the metallic screws used to fix prostheses in place had resulted in perforation of the profunda femoris artery (Dameron, 1964; Mayer and Slager, 1964; Bassett and Houck, 1964) (Fig. 22–9). A similar example was reported by Saletta and Freeark (1970), in which a tender swelling developing in the

Figure 22–8. At the time of obtaining this femoral arteriogram, a bullet embolus to the common femoral artery was demonstrated following a gunshot wound of the thoracic aorta. (Drapanas, T., Hewitt, R. L., Weichert, R. F., and Smith, A. D., Ann. Surg., *172*:351, 1970.)

upper thigh five days after immobilization of a fracture of the femur with a nail-plate was initially suspected of being an abscess until a bruit was recognized, after which an angiogram revealed a false aneurysm arising from the profunda femoris artery.

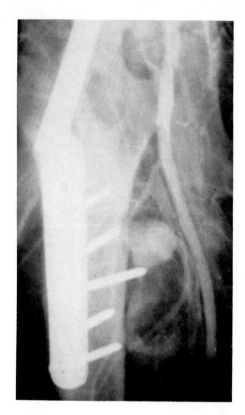

Figure 22–9. Trauma to the deep femoral artery during internal fixation of a subtrochanteric fracture or during subtrochanteric osteotomy and nail-fixation, as shown here, can be caused by a screw of excessive length. The right femoral arteriogram shows a false aneurysm of the deep femoral artery at the tip of a fixation screw. (Bassett, F. H., and Houck, W., Jr., J. Bone Joint Surg., *46-A*:583, 1964.)

Figure 22–10. This right femoral angiogram, in addition to showing arteriosclerotic occlusive disease in the superficial femoral artery, demonstrates a point of partial occlusion (arrow) of the deep femoral artery by the lesser trochanteric spike following internal fixation of an intertrochanteric fracture. (Aufranc, O. E., Jones, W. N., and Stewart, W. G., Jr., J.A.M.A., *191*:1073, 1965.)

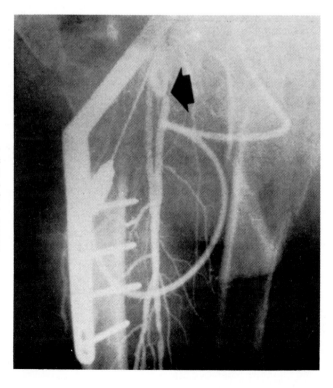

TABLE 22–3. CLINICAL FEATURES OF PROFUNDA FEMORIS ARTERY INJURIES CHICAGO, 1966–1971*

INJURING AGENT	SITE (DISTAL TO TAKEOFF)	BLOOD LOSS	BRUITS	PULSES	ANGIOGRAM
Buckshot	Right leg (1 cm)	Shock (4 units W.B. preop.)	0	Intact	Not performed
Drill point	Right leg (10 cm)	Large hematoma	Systolic	Intact	Positive (false aneurysm)
Gunshot wound	Left leg (10 cm)	Large hematoma	0	Intact	Positive (complete cutoff)
Gunshot wound	Left leg (#1, at origin; #2, 15 cm)	Moderate hematoma	0	Diminished	Positive (complete cutoff)
Stab	Left leg (10 cm)	Small hematoma	Systolic and diastolic	Intact	Positive (AV fistula)
Stab	Left leg (10 cm)	Recurrent hemorrhage (8 units W.B. preop.)	0	Intact	Positive (free extravasation of dye)

*Modified from Saletta, J. D., and Freeark, R. J., J. Trauma, 12:778, 1972. Copyright 1972, The Williams & Wilkins Co., Baltimore.

A different mode of injury was reported by Aufranc and associates (1965), who described three older patients in whom reduction of an intertrochanteric fracture of the femur had resulted in compression of the profunda femoris artery by the lesser trochanter. Symptoms of vascular insufficiency appeared because arteriosclerotic occlusion of the superficial femoral artery was already present (Fig. 22–10). Re-operation and excision of the trochanter corrected the problem.

The etiology of profunda femoris artery trauma in the urban trauma victim includes both characteristic gunshot wounds and stab wounds, as reported by Saletta and Freeark (1972) (Table 22–3).

CLINICAL PATHOLOGY

Laceration was the most frequent type of injury among 46 femoral injuries in Vietnam. There were only seven instances of transection of the artery, and three of contusion. In two of the three instances of contusion, the intima was ruptured. The third patient with the arterial contusion had a subintimal hematoma (Fig. 22–4). In the subsequent evaluation of 109 common femoral artery injuries, more than 50 per cent were lacerations (59 or 54.1 per cent), and 22 per cent (24) were transections (Rich et al., 1975B).

Similarly, among civilian injuries, lacerations are the most common. The most important clinical problem occurs with blunt injuries in recognizing fracture and prolapse of the intima with subsequent throm-

bosis and arterial occlusion. At the time of surgical exploration of a blunt injury, if the lumen is not directly examined, rupture and prolapse may be overlooked with the subsequent development of thrombosis and gangrene.

Injuries of the profunda femoris artery almost always occur within the first few centimeters of the origin of the artery from the common femoral. The degree of ischemia produced, if the superficial femoral artery is intact, is minimal; therefore, hemorrhage and the development of a false aneurysm are the principal considerations.

As the femoral artery, nerve and vein lie parallel to one another within the femoral fascial sheath, near the anterior surface of the femur, concomitant injuries of these structures would be anticipated with injuries of the common femoral artery. In the 46 femoral artery injuries in Vietnam, the femoral vein was injured in 46 per cent of the cases, the femoral nerve in 24 per cent, and the femur was fractured in 22 per cent (Table 22–4). Among 109 common femoral

TABLE 22–4. CONCOMITANT INJURIES WITH 46 COMMON FEMORAL ARTERY INJURIES: INTERIM REPORT FROM VIETNAM*

INJURY	NUMBER	PER CENT
Femoral vein	21	46
Femoral nerve	11	24
Femoral fracture	10	22

*From Rich, N. M., Baugh, J. H., and Hughes, C. W., J. Trauma, 10:359, 1970. Copyright 1970, The Williams & Wilkins Co., Baltimore.

artery injuries, 58.7 per cent had associated venous injuries (Rich et al., 1975B).

CLINICAL FEATURES

In most patients the diagnosis of injury of the common femoral artery is obvious, because blood loss is excessive causing profound shock. There is usually bright red blood spurting from an open wound, in association with a cold, pale, pulseless, paralyzed extremity. With blunt trauma, however, the diagnosis can be less obvious, because peripheral pulses may initially be intact, only to later disappear as the torn intima prolapses into the lumen and causes thrombosis. Consistent findings include excessive blood loss and shock associated with an unusually large hematoma or a pulsatile hematoma in the femoral region.

With isolated lacerations of the profunda femoris artery, as emphasized by Saletta and Freeark (1972), the diagnosis is less obvious. The clinical features are those of significant hemorrhage but intact distal pulses. This combination of findings in the presence of a penetrating wound of the upper thigh should alert the physician to the possibility of laceration of the profunda femoris. There are no abnormal physical findings other than those of a penetrating wound with surrounding hematoma, but the diagnosis may be established by either surgical exploration or angiography.

DIAGNOSTIC CONSIDERATIONS

The finding of a lowered hematocrit may support the clinical diagnosis of femoral artery injury. Also, roentgenograms of the hip and thigh may help establish the clinical diagnosis of an associated fracture or a metallic foreign body which alerts the investigator to the possibility of femoral artery injuries.

Nevertheless, in blunt trauma to the common femoral artery and in the majority of profunda femoris artery injuries, angiography may provide the best diagnostic aid. The diagnosis in five of the six cases of profunda femoris artery injury reported by Saletta and Freeark (1972) was established by percutaneous femoral angiography.

SURGICAL TREATMENT

Severe hemorrhage and shock are frequent with common femoral injuries because of the large size of the artery. These findings may also be present with profunda femoris artery trauma. In addition to obvious external blood loss, there may be significant loss into the soft tissues of the thigh; therefore, transfusion of large volumes of blood is necessary. Control of hemorrhage can be difficult in some instances because a tourniquet cannot easily be employed. Direct pressure, often combined with temporary packing of the wound, will usually suffice. In unusual instances, complete control of hemorrhage cannot be obtained until surgical exploration is performed.

A particularly useful incision for surgical exploration is a longitudinal incision in the thigh placed directly over the femoral vessels (Fig. 22–11). If necessary, an extension superiorly above the inguinal ligament can then be curved outward parallel to the inguinal ligament. Hemorrhage from concomitant injuries of the femoral artery and vein may be particularly troublesome to control because bleeding can originate from six vessels: the proximal femoral artery and vein, the superficial femoral artery and vein and the profunda femoris artery and vein. Ineffectual attempts to control hemorrhage through limited incisions have led to isolated instances of astonishing degrees of blood loss, exceeding 10 liters, with resulting renal failure. If the injury is located so far proximally that the femoral vessels cannot be isolated beyond the inguinal ligament, the preferable approach is to incise the external oblique fascia above and parallel to the inguinal ligament, as in a conventional herniorrhaphy, and then detach part of the origin of the internal oblique muscle from the inguinal ligament, entering the extraperitoneal plane just above the inguinal ligament by dividing the

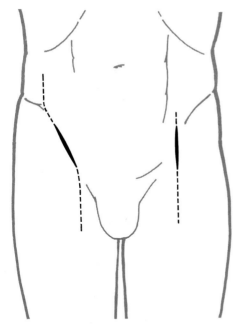

Figure 22–11. Surgical approach to the common femoral artery and its bifurcation. This longitudinal incision in the thigh can be extended in either direction. If the incision is carried laterally, the inguinal ligament can be temporarily detached from the anterior superior spine.

femoris can best be approached through a posterior incision made down to the level of the adductor magnus muscle after retracting the medial and lateral hamstring muscles with appropriate protection of the adjacent sciatic nerve.

Once the injury to the common femoral artery has been identified, a standard arterial reconstruction can usually be done without difficulty because of the large size of the artery. Reconstruction includes debridement and insertion of a distal Fogarty catheter to remove distal thrombi, followed by regional instillation of heparin, then appropriate arterial reconstruction. Small lacerations may be treated by lateral suture, including a vein patch graft if there is any sign of constriction. Most injuries following retrograde catheterization for angiography can be reconstructed in this manner, and nearly one-fourth of the 46 common femoral injuries in Vietnam were repaired by lateral suture (Table 22–5). Somewhat surprising is the fact that a saphenous vein graft was necessary in 25 of the 46 Vietnam injuries (54 per cent), perhaps because the

transversalis fascia (Fig. 22–12). This extraperitoneal approach, a standard one during the open heart procedures when the external iliac artery is cannulated for arterial perfusion, can be quickly performed and readily provides proximal control of both the artery and vein. An alternate, less preferable approach is simple division of the inguinal ligament through the previously placed longitudinal incision in the thigh.

With more distal injuries, the sartorius muscle may require mobilization or even transection where the superficial femoral artery passes under the sartorius into Hunter's canal.

Surgical exposure of the profunda femoris is more difficult as it courses posteriorly to the superficial femoral artery toward the femur and is traversed by several tributaries of the profunda femoris vein. The distal exposure of the profunda femoris artery requires partial division of the insertion of the adductor longus muscle onto the femur. In unusual instances the posterior tributaries of the profunda

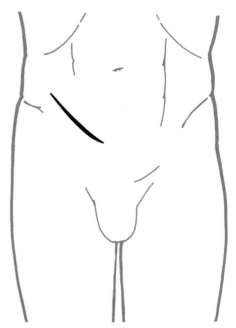

Figure 22–12. A separate incision utilizing the extraperitoneal approach to the external iliac vessels can be employed if proximal control of the femoral vessels cannot be easily obtained beyond the inguinal ligament.

TABLE 22–5. MANAGEMENT OF COMMON FEMORAL ARTERY INJURIES: INTERIM REPORT FROM VIETNAM*

Method	Number	Per Cent
Saphenous vein graft	25	54.3
Lateral suture	11	23.9
End-to-end anastomosis	8	17.4
Prosthesis	1	2.2
Ligation	1	2.2
Total	46	100.0

*From Rich, N. M., Baugh, J. H., and Hughes, C. W., J. Trauma, *10*:359, 1970. Copyright 1970, The Williams & Wilkins Company, Baltimore.

short common femoral artery is relatively inelastic. End-to-end anastomosis was employed in eight instances, a Dacron prosthesis in one; in one patient with a massive crush injury the artery was ligated.

Reconstruction of the profunda femoris artery should be considered if the vessel is large and reconstruction is simple. Although the risk of gangrene is negligible following ligation of the profunda femoris, instances of thigh claudication have been reported following ligation, and the vessel is a valuable source of collateral blood supply in future years if atherosclerotic occlusion of the superficial femoral artery develops.

POSTOPERATIVE CARE

Postoperative care is similar to that with other peripheral arterial injuries: both the presence of distal pulses and the neurologic function of the extremity should be carefully observed. Because of the large size of the common femoral artery, peripheral pulses should be palpable immediately after reconstruction. Otherwise, angiography and frequently re-operation should be done promptly because of the high frequency of gangrene with occlusion of the common femoral artery. Only if motor and sensory function are intact, indicating adequate blood flow to the extremity, is it safe to delay. Surgical exploration may be combined with operative angiography because the two most frequent findings of postoperative femoral occlusion are technical complications at the site of reconstruction and an unrecognized thrombus in the distal arterial tree.

With the degree of muscle ischemia produced by common femoral injuries, fasciotomy may be necessary if several hours elapse between the time of injury and reconstruction (see Chap. 5). As with peripheral arterial injuries in other areas, common femoral injuries with significant wound contamination are best treated by reconstruction, coverage of the site of reconstruction with surrounding soft tissues and delayed primary closure of the wound four to seven days later if there are no signs of infection.

COMPLICATIONS

The gravity of common femoral artery injuries is indicated by the fact that thrombosis or hemorrhage complicated the postoperative course in nearly one-fourth of the 46 femoral artery injuries treated in Vietnam (Table 22–6). Seven of these 11 complications eventually led to amputation, an over-all rate of 15 per cent. Complications most frequently developed when there was extensive soft tissue loss at the time of injury. Inadequate debridement often leads to infection and secondary hemorrhage, while extensive debridement may create the different problem of soft tissue coverage of the site of vascular reconstruction. Cohen and associates (1969) described one such example of a 22 year old patient with a high velocity gunshot wound of the right femoral triangle, which produced extensive destruction of all soft tissues, the femoral artery and vein. A saphenous vein graft was inserted between the common and superficial femoral arteries, but no venous re-

TABLE 22–6. COMPLICATIONS ASSOCIATED WITH 46 COMMON FEMORAL ARTERY INJURIES: INTERIM REPORT FROM VIETNAM*

Complications	Number	Per Cent
Thrombosis	6	13
Hemorrhage	5	11
Total complication rate	11	24
Amputation rate	7	15

*From Rich, N. M., Baugh, J. H., and Hughes, C. W., J. Trauma, *10*:359, 1970. Copyright 1970. The Williams & Wilkins Co., Baltimore.

pair was possible, and soft tissue coverage could not be obtained. Application of split thickness skin grafts was planned, but additional muscle necrosis prevented their prompt application, resulting in the vein graft remaining uncovered over a distance of 6 cm. The inevitable disruption of the distal suture line occurred two weeks later, requiring ligation of the artery, resulting in gangrene and a high thigh amputation. The patient died two days later from sudden massive pulmonary embolization.

At Walter Reed General Hospital a Vietnam casualty similarly required emergency treatment when hemorrhage began from disruption of an infected Dacron prosthesis used to repair the right common femoral artery (Fig. 22–13). Severe ischemia developed following ligation of the common femoral; as a result, the extremity was preserved with a saphenous vein graft inserted through the obturator canal.

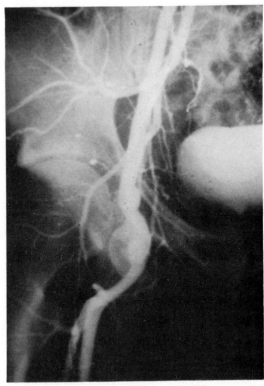

Figure 22–14. Angiogram demonstrates a false aneurysm formation with an unsuspected partial disruption of the distal anastomosis of a saphenous vein graft placed in the common femoral artery. This was discovered three weeks following the repair. (Courtesy Dr. Kenneth E. Thomas.)

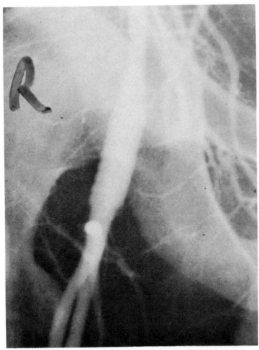

Figure 22–13. Angiogram demonstrating a patent Dacron prosthesis used in Vietnam to repair the right common femoral artery. Unfortunately, infection and subsequent disruption of one of the suture lines necessitated removal of the prosthesis and ligation of the common femoral artery at Walter Reed General Hospital approximately one month following injury. (Rich, N. M., Baugh, J. H., and Hughes, C. W., Arch. Surg., *100*:646, 1970.)

A final example of the hazard of complications with common femoral reconstruction was seen with a Vietnam casualty who had a common femoral reconstruction with a saphenous vein graft. Three weeks later a routine angiogram was performed although the wound appeared satisfactory and distal pulses were present. An unsuspected partial disruption of the distal anastomosis with a false aneurysm was found (Fig. 22–14). At re-operation the disrupted anastomosis, fortunately not infected, was successfully re-anastomosed.

Complications following attempted profunda femoris artery repair are rarely documented. One Vietnam casualty seen in follow-up at Walter Reed General Hospital had a thrombosis of an attempted proximal right profunda femoris artery repair using an autogenous saphenous vein graft (Fig. 22–15).

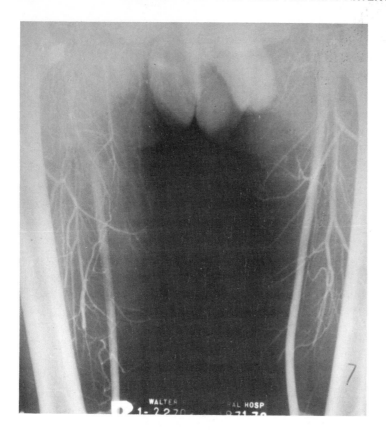

Figure 22–15. Angiogram demonstrates thrombosis of the right deep femoral artery which had previously been repaired in Vietnam using an autogenous saphenous vein graft. (W.R.G.H.)

RESULTS

When injuries of the common femoral were treated by ligation, the frequency of gangrene exceeded 80 per cent. In World War II, ligation of 106 common femoral arteries was followed by amputation in 86 (DeBakey and Simeone, 1946). In the Korean Conflict, Hughes (1958) reported the over-all amputation rate for femoral injuries as 12 per cent (11 amputations following 88 injuries), but the percentage of common femoral artery injuries among the total is not known. Among the 46 patients treated in Vietnam, amputation was eventually necessary in seven, a frequency of 15 per cent. This high frequency of amputation, exceeded only by popliteal injuries with a rate of 30 per cent, is partly due to the critical nature of the artery and partly to the frequency of subsequent wound complications. There were also three deaths among the 46 patients, one of which occurred on the sixth postoperative day from a pulmonary embolus. The subsequent Vietnam report (Rich et al., 1975B) expanded to 109 common femoral artery injuries. Table 22–7 outlines the method of management. Autogenous vein grafts were required in slightly more than one-half of the repairs. The total deaths remained at three for an overall mortality rate of 2.8 per cent. The amputation rate for 106 survivors was 13.2 per cent with 14 amputations.

TABLE 22–7. MANAGEMENT OF COMMON FEMORAL ARTERIAL INJURIES*

METHOD	NUMBER	PER CENT
Autogenous vein graft	62	56.9
End-to-end anastomosis	27	24.8
Lateral suture	11	10.1
Venous patch graft	3	2.75
Prosthesis	3	2.75
Thrombectomy	2	1.8
Exploration	1	0.9
Total	109	100.0

*From Rich, N. M., Hobson, R. W., II, Fedde, C. W., and Collins, G. J., Jr., J. Trauma, *15*:628, 1975. Copyright 1975, The Williams & Wilkins Co., Baltimore.

The gravity of common femoral injuries is similarly indicated in reports of civilian trauma. Patman and associates (1964) reported two amputations following five common femoral artery injuries among a group of 271 arterial injuries in Dallas. Drapanas and co-workers (1970) reported four deaths (25 per cent) in a combined series of 16 iliac and common femoral artery injuries.

FOLLOW-UP

Late results of common femoral artery repair up to a five year follow-up have been good. Eighteen of the 46 patients operated upon in Vietnam were subsequently evaluated at Walter Reed General Hospital. Only two of these required additional operative procedures. One patient with a systolic bruit from a localized constriction was asymptomatic and was not operated upon.

An interesting 15 year follow-up of a femoral vein graft in the femoral artery was reported by Murray in 1952. The patient had transection of the common femoral artery and vein, initially treated by ligation. Re-operation was performed within a few hours because of severe ischemia, at which time an 8 cm segment of the adjacent femoral vein was used to reconstruct the common femoral artery. This was functioning approximately 15 years later with no signs of dilatation or calcification on angiography.

Finally, some concern is indicated over the long term course in patients who have had ligation of the profunda femoris artery. The critical nature of this artery when atherosclerosis of the peripheral vessels occurs has been demonstrated hundreds of times during aortoiliac reconstructions. It similarly is the principal collateral pathway when atherosclerosis obstructs the superficial femoral artery. For this reason, the possibility exists that patients with ligations of the profunda femoris may develop unusually severe ischemia in later years if they are unfortunate enough to develop atherosclerotic occlusion of the superficial femoral artery.

CHAPTER 23

SUPERFICIAL FEMORAL ARTERY INJURIES

The superficial femoral artery is one of the most frequently injured arteries because of both its length and its relatively superficial location. In some reports the exact frequency is uncertain, because injuries of both the common femoral and superficial femoral arteries are collectively reported as "femoral artery injuries." This occurred in reports from both World War I (Makins, 1919) and the Korean Conflict (Hughes, 1958) (Table 23–1). In both groups the total femoral artery injuries accounted for nearly one-third of all arterial injuries seen. Similarly, in the interim Vietnam report (Rich et al., 1970A), nearly one-third of the injuries involved the superficial femoral artery.

Among civilian injuries, the frequency is less, but the importance may be even greater because such injuries often occur

TABLE 23–1. INCIDENCE OF SUPERFICIAL FEMORAL ARTERY INJURIES

	AUTHOR	TOTAL ARTERIES	SUPERFICIAL FEMORAL	PER CENT
WAR SERIES				
WW I	Makins (1919)	1202	366*	30.5*
WW II	DeBakey and Simeone (1946)	2471	177	7.2
			517*	20.9*
Korea	Hughes (1958)	304	95*	31.3*
Vietnam	Rich et al. (1970A)	1000	305	30.5
CIVILIAN SERIES				
Houston	Morris et al. (1960)	220	36*	16.4*
Atlanta	Ferguson et al. (1961)	200	39	19.5
Denver	Owens (1963)	70	12*	17.1*
Detroit	Smith et al. (1963)	61	9	14.8
Dallas	Patman et al. (1964)	271	41	15.1
Los Angeles	Treiman et al. (1966)	159	39*	24.5*
St. Louis	Dillard et al. (1968)	85	14	16.5
New Orleans	Drapanas et al. (1970)	226	31	13.7
Dallas	Perry et al. (1971)†	508	93	18.3
Denver	Kelly and Eiseman (1975)	116	7	6.0
Memphis	Cheek et al. (1975)	155	34*	21.9*
Jackson	Hardy et al. (1975)	360	51	14.2
New York	Bole et al. (1976)	126	21	16.7

*Listed only as "femoral arteries," including some common femoral and profunda femoris arteries.
†This is a sequential study including the earlier report by Patman et al. (1964).

with fracture of the femur. In such instances a delay in diagnosis and surgical correction may result in gangrene.

When superficial femoral arterial injuries were treated by ligation, slightly more than one-half of the extremities were lost from gangrene (DeBakey and Simeone, 1946). With arterial repair, the amputation rate has been greatly reduced to less than 10 per cent in several civilian reports and to approximately 12 per cent in Vietnam (Rich et al., 1970A).

SURGICAL ANATOMY

The superficial femoral artery is one of the two major branches of the common femoral (see Chap. 22). It extends from the common femoral artery proximally to the popliteal artery distally (Fig. 23–1). The course is a straight one, changing from an anterior location proximally to a posteromedial position distally. Proximally its position is relatively superficial, but terminally it lies deeper near the femur. In most of its

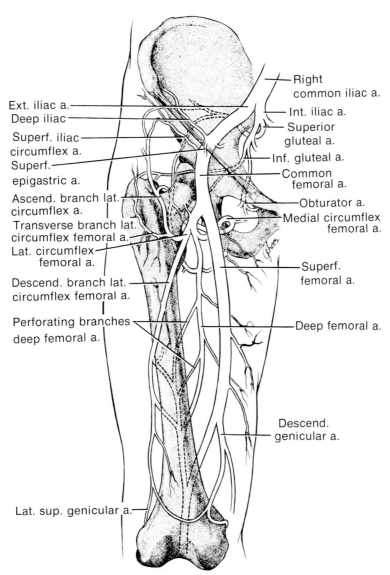

Figure 23–1. This anatomical drawing traces the course of the superficial femoral artery, the main conduit between the common femoral and popliteal arteries. In addition to numerous muscular branches, the supreme genicular (descending genicular) is an important collateral to the rich anastomosis around the knee.

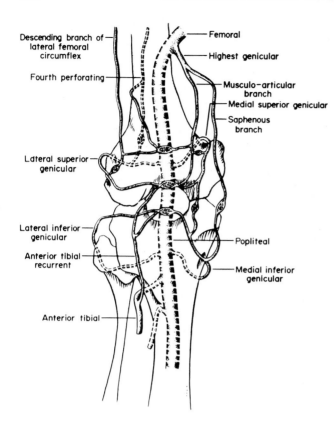

Descending branch of lateral femoral circumflex

Fourth perforating

Lateral superior genicular

Lateral inferior genicular

Anterior tibial recurrent

Anterior tibial

Femoral

Highest genicular

Musculo-articular branch

Medial superior genicular

Saphenous branch

Popliteal

Medial inferior genicular

Figure 23–2. This drawing illustrates collateral circulation in the region of the knee. Important collateral vessels are the highest (supreme) genicular, the medial and lateral superior genicular, and the medial and lateral inferior genicular arteries. (Levin, P. M., Rich, N. M., and Hutton, J. E., Jr., Arch. Surg., *102*:392, 1971, Copyright 1971, American Medical Association.)

course it is covered by the sartorius muscle. This subsartorial location is usually termed the adductor or Hunter's canal, an eponym originating from the approach used by John Hunter to ligate the artery in the treatment of popliteal aneurysms.

Several small muscular branches contribute little to collateral circulation, but the supreme genicular is most important. This originates from the distal superficial femoral in the lower part of the adductor canal (see Chap. 24) (Fig. 23–2). It divides into a superficial branch and a more important articular branch. This in turn descends to form a rich anastomosis around the knee joint.

The relationships of the artery to the femur are important, especially because of the frequency of arterial injuries combined with fracture of the femur. Proximally, in the femoral triangle near its apex, the artery lies near the medial surface of the shaft of the femur, separated only by the thin posterior portion of the vastus medialis muscle. Distally, the artery actually

lies behind the femur because of the obliquity of the medial surface of the femur. The superficial femoral vein, often bifid or even existing as more than two separate channels, lies in a posterolateral position behind the artery (Fig. 23–3). The femoral nerve and its divisions are lateral to the superficial femoral artery.

INCIDENCE

During World War I Makins (1919) found approximately a 30 per cent incidence of femoral artery injuries among British troops (Table 23–1). Almost 40 years later Hughes (1958) found a similar frequency during the Korean Conflict. In their review of the American World War II experience in the European theater, DeBakey and Simeone (1949) found a lower frequency of only about 7 per cent, 177 superficial femoral artery injuries among 2471 acute arterial injuries analyzed. In the interim Vietnam review of 1000 acute

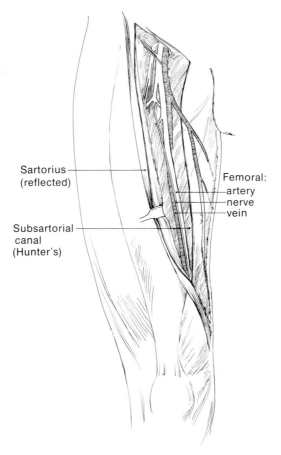

Figure 23–3. The major portion of the superficial femoral artery lies in the subsartorial adductor (Hunter's) canal. The superficial vein is in a posterolateral position, and the femoral nerve and its branches are found lateral to the superficial femoral artery.

major arterial injuries, there were 305 superficial femoral injuries, a frequency of 30.5 per cent (Rich et al., 1970A).

In civilian injuries, frequency ranges from about 14 to 20 per cent. There were 31 injuries in a group of 226 arterial injuries reported by Drapanas and colleagues (1970) and 39 among 200 arterial injuries reported by Ferguson and co-workers (1961) (Table 23–1). In the reports by Morris and associates (1960), Owens (1963) and Treiman and colleagues (1966), all femoral artery injuries were grouped together. The largest civilian series was reported by Perry and associates (1971), describing experiences with 93 such injuries among a total of 508 analyzed, a frequency of 18.3 per cent. The highest frequency was reported by Cheek and associates (1975) from Memphis, an incidence of 21.9 per cent, 34 superficial arte-

rial injuries among a total of 155 arterial injuries. The civilian reports, similar to those of military injuries, found frequent involvement of the brachial and femoral vessels because of their length and vulnerable location.

ETIOLOGY

There is a considerable difference in etiology between military and civilian injuries. Most military injuries result from fragment and high velocity gunshot wounds. Civilian injuries, however, are usually from low velocity gunshot wounds, stab wounds, fractures or other forms of blunt trauma.

Among 305 superficial femoral artery injuries in Vietnam, 173 (56.7 per cent) were caused by fragments from different exploding devices, while 113 were from gunshot wounds (37.1 per cent) (Table 23–2). Direct

TABLE 23–2. ETIOLOGY OF SUPERFICIAL FEMORAL ARTERY TRAUMA: INTERIM VIETNAM VASCULAR REGISTRY REPORT

AGENT	NUMBER	PER CENT
Fragment	173	56.7
Gunshot	113	37.1
Punji stick	3	1.0
Blunt	1	0.3
Stab	1	0.3
Propeller	1	0.3
Undetermined	13	4.3
Total:	305	100.0

*Modified from Rich, N.M., Baugh, J.H., and Hughes, C.W., J. Trauma, *10*:359, 1970. Copyright 1970, The Williams & Wilkins Company, Baltimore.

puncture by the primitive punji stick lacerated the superficial femoral artery in three patients (see Chap. 2). Only one instance of blunt trauma, a result of a helicopter crash, was found.

Among civilian injuries, Hershey and Spencer (1963) described seven cases—five from bullets, one from a shotgun and one from a stab wound. There has been considerable interest in recent years in the earlier detection of trauma of the superficial femoral artery in association with fracture of the femur. Kirkup (1963) emphasized that such injuries were particularly prone to occur with fractures of the femur in its mid or lower portion, probably due to closer proximity of the artery and bone in this area.

Other experiences have been reported by Couves and co-authors (1958), Klingensmith and co-workers (1965) and Morton and associates (1966). All emphasized the ease of overlooking a concomitant arterial injury with a severe fracture of the femur associated with massive swelling and discoloration. A typical case is that of a patient with a closed fracture of the femoral shaft who was placed in skeletal traction (Morton et al., 1966). Gradually during the day the pulses disappeared, sensory loss developed over the dorsum of the foot and ankle and dorsiflexion of the toes and ankles disappeared. Exploration of the artery, however, was postponed for an additional 24 hours because epidural anesthesia seemed to improve the situation. At the time of exploration, a thrombosed superficial femoral ar-

tery was found and replaced with a graft to restore distal circulation. Interest has been further heightened in cases such as this by the availability of arteriography, permitting a decision about patency of the superficial femoral artery without surgical exploration. Kootstra and colleagues (1976) reported the cases of eight patients with fractures of the shaft of the femur and concomitant lesions of the superficial femoral artery in civilian accidents treated in the Netherlands.

With fractures of the femur, injuries of the artery have also occurred during reduction of the fracture or during internal fixation. Stein (1956) reported an instance of erosion of a superficial femoral artery by a Steinmann pin. Bassett and Silver (1966) reported an instance of thrombosis of the artery following a third operation for nonunion of a fracture of the femur.

The superficial femoral artery has also occasionally been injured during operations such as ligation and stripping of the greater saphenous vein and during angiographic procedures using the percutaneous femoral approach. Eger and co-workers (1973) reported the case of inadvertent stripping of the superficial femoral popliteal and posterior tibial arteries during treatment of varicose veins.

White and associates (1968), in documenting a number of peripheral arterial injuries in infants and children, noted that one type of injury occurred with intramuscular drug injections. They presented the case of a 3 month old girl with pneumococcal pneumonia who was injected with 600,000 units of procaine penicillin in the muscles of the left mid-lateral thigh. The mother returned the baby to the Outpatient Department 20 hours later with a painful and cyanotic lower extremity. There was obvious arterial insufficiency, and an angiogram demonstrated a complete occlusion of the mid-superficial femoral artery (Fig. 23–4). Thrombectomy of an occluded 1-cm segment restored arterial flow; however, amputation of four toes was necessary two weeks later because of irreversible changes in the distal arterial blood supply.

Unusual cases of shark bite involve the superficial femoral artery, as shown in Figure 23–5.

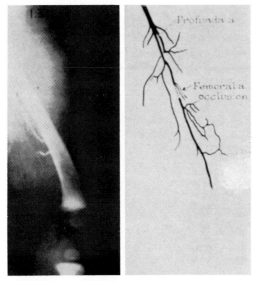

Figure 23–4. Complete occlusion of the superficial femoral artery in the adductor canal following a penicillin injection in the muscles of the left midlateral thigh of a three month old girl. This is one of the examples of peripheral arterial trauma associated with needling of an extremity that were treated at the Johns Hopkins Hospital. (White, J. J., Talbert, J. L., and Haller, J. A., Jr., Ann. Surg., *167*:757, 1968.)

CLINICAL PATHOLOGY

Most injuries of the superficial femoral artery are lacerations (Fig. 23–6), although transection, even with avulsion of a segment, has occurred from high velocity gunshot wounds in Vietnam. In an analysis of 169 injuries in Vietnam, there were 108 lacerations, 48 transections and 11 contusions with thrombosis associated with high velocity missiles (Table 23–3). Curiously enough, there were only two arteriovenous fistulas.

Contusion and thrombosis are produced by the temporary cavitational effect of a high velocity missile passing near the artery. This may fracture the intima with subsequent formation of a subintimal hematoma, prolapse of the intima into the lumen and eventual thrombosis (see Chaps. 2 and 3). Among civilian injuries, such a case was reported by Gryska in 1962. A patient sustained a gunshot wound of the thigh in which the bullet traversed the thigh some distance away from the superficial femoral artery. Because of distal ischemia, the artery was explored with the tentative diagnosis of "spasm." Intimal laceration with an occluding thrombus was found.

Morton and associates (1966) postulated that dissection of the intima of the artery occurred more frequently than was recognized. They cited experimental studies by Bergan in 1963, who found that stretching or crushing of the normal femoral artery injured the intima before the adventitia was damaged. With a circumferential injury of the intima, the dissection of the distal intima progressed to prolapse and eventual thrombosis.

Histologic changes found on microscopic examination of arterial injuries are similar

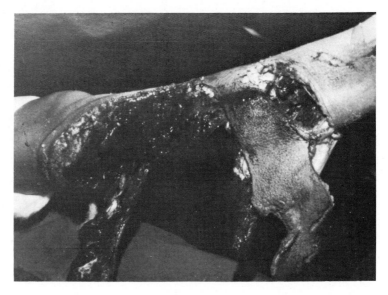

Figure 23–5. Shark bites have been associated with major vascular injuries in the extremities, with injury of the superficial femoral artery. This photograph shows the extent of associated massive soft tissue loss that frequently accompanies shark bites. (Courtesy Mr. J. A. M. White, Durban, South Africa.)

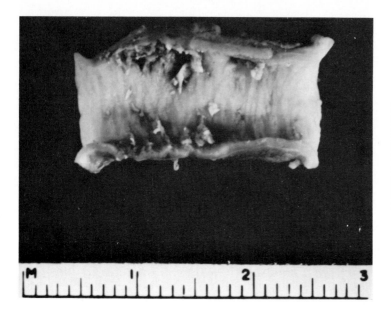

Figure 23–6. Multiple small fragment perforations were found in the superficial femoral artery in this Vietnam casualty. The margins of resection were normal. An autogenous saphenous vein graft was utilized in a successful repair. (Rich, N. M., Manion, W. C., and Hughes, C. W., J. Trauma, 9:279, 1969.)

to those found in other arteries. They range from loss of the intima and media with adventitial hemorrhage to simple rupture of the internal elastic membrane and small lacerations of the media, infiltrated with polymorphonuclear cells. Small areas of thrombin deposition may be seen overlying the fractures of the intima.

An arteriovenous fistula can easily result following penetrating injury, especially one of low velocity such as a stab wound, because the superficial femoral artery and vein lie close to one another. Among the 31 arteriovenous fistulas reported in a series of arterial injuries by Drapanas and co-workers (1970), there were two superficial femoral arteriovenous fistulas (Fig. 23–7).

Among 290 superficial femoral artery in-

TABLE 23–3. EXTENT OF ARTERIAL TRAUMA IN 169 SUPERFICIAL FEMORAL ARTERY INJURIES: INTERIM VIETNAM VASCULAR REGISTRY REPORT*

INJURY	NUMBER	PER CENT
Laceration	108	63.9
Transection	48	28.4
Contusion	11	6.5
Acute AVF	2	1.2
Total:	169	100.0

*Modified from Rich, N.M., Baugh, J.H., and Hughes, C.W., J. Trauma, *10*:359, 1970. Copyright 1970, The Williams & Wilkins Company, Baltimore.

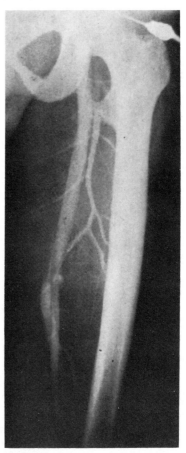

Figure 23–7. This femoral angiogram demonstrates acute arteriovenous fistula of the superficial femoral artery and vein following a stab wound. (Drapanas, T., Hewitt, R. L., Weichert, R. F., and Smith, A. D.: Ann. Surg., *172*:351, 1970.)

TABLE 23-4. CONCOMITANT TRAUMA ASSOCIATED WITH 290 SUPERFICIAL FEMORAL ARTERY INJURIES: INTERIM VIETNAM VASCULAR REGISTRY REPORT*

INJURY	NUMBER	PER CENT
Bone	72	24.8
Nerve	61	21.0
Vein	140	48.3

*Modified from Rich, N.M., Baugh, J.H., and Hughes, C.W., J. Trauma, *10*:359, 1970. Copyright 1970, The Williams & Wilkins Company, Baltimore.

juries analyzed in Vietnam (Rich et al., 1970A), the superficial femoral vein was also injured in nearly 50 per cent of the cases (Table 23-4). Fractures occurred in about one-fourth of the cases and injury to adjacent nerves in about one-fifth. In 12 injuries, only 4 per cent of the total evaluated, it was specifically mentioned that there was unusually extensive soft tissue destruction as well.

CLINICAL FEATURES

A wide spectrum of clinical findings occurs, ranging from those which make the diagnosis obvious to some which give little clue. The simple presence of a wound near the femoral vessels should alert the physician to the possibility of arterial injury. With bright red spurting blood, the diagnosis is obvious. Similarly it is quickly suspected if the hematoma is unusually large, often containing as much as 1000 to 1500 ml of blood. Such a large hematoma may be pulsatile, with an audible bruit. In the unusual injury which produces an acute arteriovenous fistula, the mass surrounding the wound may be small, but the classic continuous bruit and thrill can be detected.

The classic picture of a cold, pale extremity, often numb and partly paralyzed, quickly suggests an arterial injury. The diagnosis becomes more difficult, however, if distal pulses are palpable (see Chap. 5). In such instances the simple awareness of the possibility of arterial injury whenever a penetrating wound is near the femoral artery is of much value. An arteriogram or, alternatively, surgical exploration, is usually required to establish diagnosis.

Because blood loss is often severe with profound shock, the possibility of an arterial injury cannot be explored well until transfusion of blood has corrected the hypotension. Severe shock was common in Vietnam, often requiring rapid transfusion of 1500 to 2000 ml of unmatched O-negative blood before any pulses could be palpated.

With blunt trauma, such as fracture of the femur, the diagnosis is often obscure. This especially occurs when distal pulses are initially present, only to disappear later as disrupted intima prolapses into the lumen and causes thrombosis. Thus the importance of serial examination of peripheral pulses following fracture of the femur is clear. When a pulse is not palpable, the neurologic findings of decreased sensory and motor function are the best indicators of the urgency of operation. Loss of cutaneous sensation is the most sensitive indicator, usually beginning distally and extending in a stocking or glove distribution.

DIAGNOSTIC CONSIDERATIONS

In Vietnam the diagnosis was usually obvious and was confirmed by surgical exploration as soon as the patient was resuscitated from shock. Roentgenograms of the thigh were useful to identify metallic foreign bodies or detect a fracture (Fig. 23-8). Angiography was infrequently needed in Vietnam but is of particular value with civilian injuries from blunt trauma or closed fractures of the femur. It is also indicated when the missile has passed near an artery but distal pulses remain. Several characteristic angiographic abnormalities seen with arterial injury were described by Saletta and Freeark in 1970 (Fig. 23-9).

SURGICAL TREATMENT

Hemorrhage is often severe and must be quickly controlled. This can usually be done by direct pressure, often supplemented with a pressure dressing. Manual compression of the common femoral artery can secure proximal control. A tourniquet

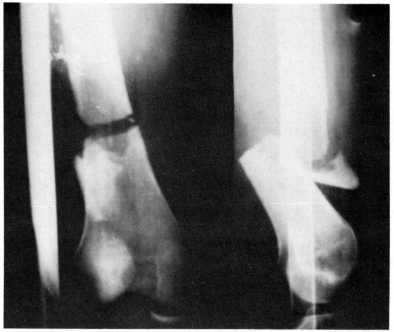

Figure 23–8. Roentgenograms of the thigh can be valuable in identifying metallic foreign bodies and femoral fractures, both of which may be responsible for superficial femoral arterial trauma. These anteroposterior and lateral views show a femoral fracture. (Rich, N. M., Baugh, J. H., and Hughes, C. W., Am. J. Surg., *118:* 531, 1969.)

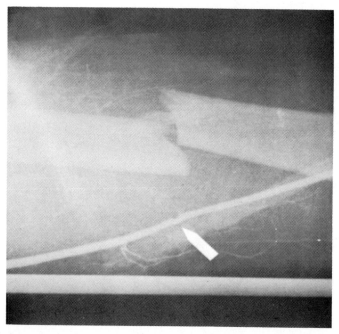

Figure 23–9. This femoral arteriogram in a patient with a closed fracture of the femur demonstrates a filling defect at the site of partial severance of the superficial femoral artery. This irregularity in the contour of a portion of the artery is considered to be one of five angiographic findings diagnostic for arterial injury. (Saletta, J. B., and Freeark, R. J., Orthop. Clin. North Am., *1:*93, 1970).

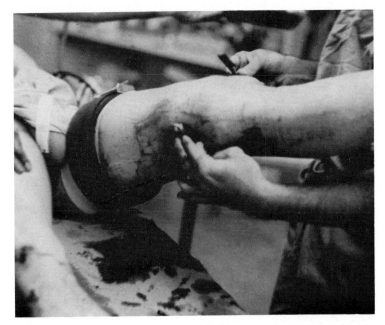

Figure 23-10. Temporary control of hemorrhage from an injured superficial femoral artery can be obtained with a pneumatic tourniquet in the operating room. (Rich, N. M., J. Cardiovasc. Surg., *11*:368, 1970.)

should normally be avoided because the potential complications far outweigh its usefulness (see Chap. 5). In the operating room a pneumatic tourniquet may be helpful at the beginning of the operation. As soon as the artery has been isolated proximal and distal to the point of injury, often requiring less than 15 to 20 minutes, the tourniquet can be released (Fig. 23–10). The usual resuscitative measures for traumatic shock are necessary. These include rapid administration of whole blood, adequate fluid replacement and administration of broad spectrum antibiotics.

At operation the superficial femoral artery is best approached along the anterior border of the sartorius muscle (Fig. 23–11). The exposure is facilitated if the patient is in a supine position with the extremity externally rotated and slightly flexed. Once

the incision is deepened through the deep fascia near the anterior border of the sartorius muscle, the femoral vessels can easily be found.

A longitudinal incision greatly simplifies isolation of the femoral artery proximal and distal to the point of injury. The exposure should not be compromised by attempting too large an exit or entrance wound in a different location in the thigh (Fig. 23–12). Usually the sartorius muscle can be mobilized sufficiently to permit adequate exposure, but it can be transected if necessary. Distally, near the femoral-popliteal junction, transection of part of the adductor magnus tendon may be necessary.

Once the artery has been occluded proximal and distal to the site of injury, the wound and the lacerated vessel can be debrided. Following debridement and irri-

Figure 23-11. This artist's conception of the surgical approach to the superficial femoral artery demonstrates the longitudinal incision along the anterior border of the sartorius muscle. The incision can be made over the suspected site of injury and then extended in either direction.

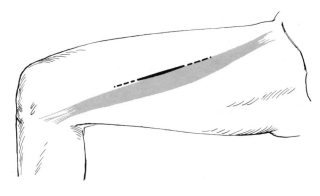

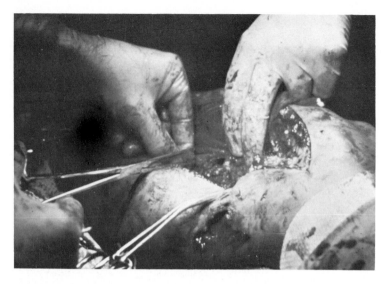

Figure 23–12. An elective incision along the anterior border of the sartorius muscle provided optimal anatomic exposure with a superficial femoral artery injury. Note the high velocity exit wound below the incision. Proximal and distal control of the severed artery were accomplished by the use of atraumatic vascular clamps. (Rich, N. M., J. Cardiovasc. Surg., *11*:368, 1970.)

gation, the distal artery should be explored with a Fogarty catheter to remove any distal thrombi. A dilute solution of heparin should then be instilled, and this can be repeated periodically until arterial repair is completed. Arterial repair is usually accomplished by an end-to-end anastomosis, or with a short autogenous vein graft, preferably the greater saphenous vein (Fig. 23–13). Autogenous vein grafts have been used most frequently in Vietnam (Table 23–5). Rarely, a lateral suture repair can be em-

ployed, usually with a tiny puncture wound. An autogenous vein patch graft can be used to eliminate constriction at the repair site. With the availability of autogenous vein grafts, there is essentially no indication for use of arterial prostheses of Dacron or Teflon. This is especially true in contaminated wounds because of the susceptibility of a prosthesis to infection. An infected prosthesis often leads to loss of the extremity or even death of the patient. A fine synthetic vascular suture is preferable,

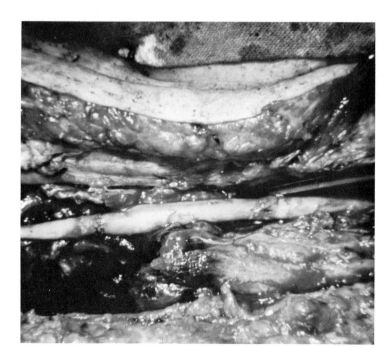

Figure 23–13. Autogenous greater saphenous vein grafts were used most frequently in Vietnam to replace arterial defects. Here a vein graft repair of the superficial femoral artery is demonstrated. (Rich, N. M., Baugh, J. H., and Hughes, C. W., J. Trauma, *10*:359, 1970.)

*Modified from Rich, N.M., Baugh, J.H., and Hughes, C.W., J. Trauma, *10*:359, 1970. Copyright 1970, The Williams & Wilkins Company, Baltimore.

TABLE 23–5. METHOD OF MANAGEMENT IN SUPERFICIAL FEMORAL ARTERY TRAUMA: INTERIM VIETNAM VASCULAR REGISTRY REPORT*

PROCEDURE	NUMBER	PER CENT
Autogenous vein graft	153	50.2
End-to-end anastomosis	121	39.7
Lateral suture	15	4.9
Autogenous artery	1	0.3
Prosthesis	0	0.0
Ligation	1	0.3
Undetermined	14	4.6
Total:	305	100.0

using a continuous over-and-over technique (see Chap. 5). Before the final sutures are tightened, the artery should be flushed both proximally and distally to expel any residual thrombi.

If distal pulses are not readily palpable after repair, intraoperative angiography is of great value in identifying distal thrombi, additional arterial lesions or technical mishaps in the arterial repair. As the superficial femoral artery is a large artery and such injuries usually occur in patients with normal arteries, a successful repair should almost always be obtained.

After arterial repair is completed, the area must be covered with adjacent soft tissue. Usually the sartorius muscle is available and provides an excellent cover. With massive soft tissue destruction, muscle flaps or even split thickness skin grafts may be necessary.

If edema of the leg is extensive, fasciotomy of the compartments below the knee is of particular value. Such edema occurs when a long period of time, six or more hours, elapses between injury and arterial reconstruction. It also is extensive when vein injuries have required ligation of the femoral vein or when soft tissue injuries have been unusually extensive (see Chap. 5).

A concomitant injury to the femoral vein should be repaired if possible. Fractures of the femur can usually be stabilized with external fixation prior to performance of the arterial repair. Internal fixation of fractures of the femur should be avoided (Rich et al., 1971A). It is recognized, however, that civilian experience continues to utilize internal fixation devices for many patients (Smith et al., 1974; Rosenthal et al., 1975; Sher, 1975). Repair of injuries of the femoral nerves should be delayed until a later time.

Delayed primary closure of the wound four to seven days after arterial reconstruction, if there are no signs of infection, is usually the best method of management.

POSTOPERATIVE CARE

Following operation the extremity should be observed closely for adequacy of distal pulses, return of sensory and motor function and edema in the leg and foot. If pulses disappear with recurrence of signs of ischemia, especially with loss of neurologic function, reoperation should be prompt. The two usual causes are a technical fault in the arterial reconstruction and an undetected distal thrombus. Angiography is particularly useful in these circumstances. It may be done before operation or in the operating room. The urgency of reoperation is best indicated by the degree of ischemia of the foot. If signs are severe, operation should be performed quickly to avoid muscle necrosis. The urgency is reinforced by the fact that almost all such cases are retrievable if the cause is quickly detected and found.

If thrombosis of the arterial reconstruction occurs but the extremity is not in jeopardy, as manifested by normal neurologic function, reoperation may be delayed if the patient's general condition is not satisfactory. In these instances the ultrasonic sounding device (Doppler) was of considerable value in Vietnam to confirm the presence of adequate arterial flow through collateral circulation, even though pulses were not palpable (Lavenson et al., 1971). Experience at Walter Reed Army Medical Center has also been corroborative with the use of the Doppler in determining adequate arterial flow through collaterals for extremity viability.

As mentioned earlier, if edema progresses to a significant degree, appropriate fasciotomy should be done over the muscle compartments in the leg.

In the subsequent days, the operative wound should be periodically inspected for signs of muscle necrosis or infection. If signs of infection are not present, delayed primary closure of the wound can be done in four to seven days after the initial arterial reconstruction.

COMPLICATIONS

The two most frequent complications following arterial repair are thrombosis and hemorrhage, the latter usually resulting from infection.

In the interim Vietnam Vascular Registry report, complications were found in 63 of 290 patients undergoing arterial repair, about one-fifth of the group. Seventeen had multiple complications. Approximately 63 per cent of the complications were thrombosis and about 37 per cent hemorrhage. The nature of many high velocity wounds with massive tissue destruction, some technical problems and severe contamination of the wound leading to infection all contributed to these complications.

The problem of repeated attempts to perform a vascular repair in the presence of infection is emphasized in the following case review in which a "second look" at the vascular repair was carried out. The patient initially sustained multiple fragment wounds with a transection of the right superficial artery and vein. Among the procedures performed was an end-to-end anastomosis of the greater saphenous vein proximal in the thigh near the saphenofemoral junction to the superficial femoral vein, which was more distal in the thigh, and a saphenous vein interposition graft repair of the superficial femoral artery. The following day a tri-compartment fasciotomy was carried out, and the vascular repairs were explored. On the fifth postinjury day when a delayed primary closure of the wound was carried out, there was one episode of brisk bleeding from the artery; however, it was stated that no further suture was necessary. Ten days following injury there was a disruption of the arterial anastomosis. Although it was mentioned that there was edematous tissue with necrosis surrounding the disrupted vein graft, a second greater saphenous interposition vein graft which was obtained from the opposite extremity was used to reconstitute the arterial flow. Three days following this second vein graft repair, there was another disruption of the repair at the proximal anastomosis, and minimal local resection and reanastomosis were carried out. At this time, which was nearly two weeks following the initial injury, a knee disarticulation was also necessary because of an infected leg. Approximately 16 days from the initial repair, a third major disruption occurred, and ligation of the superficial femoral artery was carried out. Five days subsequent to this last procedure, disruption of the proximal superficial femoral artery again occurred, and it was necessary to ligate the common femoral artery.

In 1971 Perry and colleagues reported the frequency of complications following repair of 63 civilian arterial injuries. There were three instances of bleeding, five of thrombosis and three of infection. Four of the five patients developing thrombosis were successfully reoperated upon. Technical faults at the initial operation were the usual cause.

Edema may be significant following arterial repair, probably from a combination of both venous and lymphatic obstruction. In a group of 31 patients reported by Drapanas and co-workers (1970), significant edema appeared in 11. Other complications, usually a result of an erroneous initial diagnosis, include arteriovenous fistula, development of a false aneurysm or thrombosis of the artery. The following two case reports illustrate some of these complications: (1) After being wounded by multiple grenade fragments in 1967, one patient reached the operating room of an evacuation hospital six hours after injury. The superficial femoral artery in the right thigh was exposed with a longitudinal incision. The operative note describes "artery in severe spasm but no injury . . . blocked with Xylocaine . . . entire right femoral artery exposed and found to be in severe spasm, but without direct injury . . . Xylocaine local block done." The patient was subsequently transferred to Japan without any comment about distal pulses. Three weeks after the initial injury, a pulsating, painful, swollen mass was noted in the right thigh. Distal pulses were palpable, and a bruit was audible over the mass. An arteriogram outlined a false aneurysm at the site where the superficial femoral artery had previously been described as being in spasm. At operation the aneurysm was excised and the artery reconstructed with an autogenous saphenous vein graft. After a complete recovery, the patient returned to military duty. On later examination, strong pedal pulses were found. There was, however, a moderate bruit over the mid-portion of the superficial femoral artery in the thigh. (2) A 25 year old officer sustained a through-and-through fragment wound to the right thigh in Vietnam in 1969. The operation began about two hours after injury, and an end-to-end anastomosis of the superficial femoral artery combined with ligation of the superficial femoral vein was completed within 4½ hours after injury. The early postoperative course was uncomplicated. Antibiotic therapy included penicillin and kanamycin. He was subsequently transferred to Japan and was being prepared for evacuation to the United States when bright bleeding began from the wound. Distal pulses were maintained, however, despite mild hypotension. The bleeding stopped following pressure for five minutes. Over the next six days there were several episodes of oozing of blood from the wound, although no bruit or thrill could be found. Approximately one month after operation, bleeding became more brisk, with bright red blood. At exploration a false aneurysm at the site of repair, with a small arteriovenous communication, was found. A subintimal tear was also found both proximal and distal to the area of anastomosis, suggesting either trauma or inadequate debridement at the initial operation. This area was resected and the arterial repair completed with an au-

togenous saphenous vein graft. Convalescence was uneventful with no signs of infection. A subsequent arteriogram showed a patent anastomosis, and evaluation four months later found strong pedal pulses.

RESULTS

As mentioned earlier, treatment of superficial femoral artery injuries by ligation results in an amputation rate slightly higher than 50 per cent. The World War II series analyzed by DeBakey and Simeone (1946) reported 97 amputations following ligation of 177 superficial femoral artery injuries (Table 23–6). In the Korean Conflict, one report described repair of 29 injuries with 18 vascular grafts (the majority being arterial homografts), seven lateral suture repairs and four end-to-end anastomoses (Spencer and Grewe, 1955). There were six amputations, for an amputation rate of 21 per cent. In the Vietnam experience from the interim report, there were 37 amputations following 305 reconstructions of the superficial femoral artery, for an amputation rate of 12.1 per cent (Rich et al., 1970A).

Among civilian series, Perry and coworkers (1971) reported no amputations after repair of 63 superficial femoral artery injuries. Drapanas and colleagues (1970) described three amputations after 31 arterial repairs, for an amputation rate of about 10 per cent. Two patients with arterial injury from blunt trauma were reported by Treiman and associates (1966); both later required amputation because of failure of repair. Patman and co-workers (1964) also described two amputations after repair of 41 superficial femoral artery injuries. There have been at least two reports

TABLE 23–6. SUPERFICIAL FEMORAL ARTERY TRAUMA: AMPUTATION RATE*

	SERIES	ARTERIES	AMPUTATIONS	PER CENT
Following ligation	World War II DeBakey and Simeone (1946)	177	97	54.8
Following repair	Vietnam Rich et al. (1970A)	305	37	12.1

*In the review of the Korean experience, Hughes (1958) did not separate the results of superficial femoral artery repair from those of common femoral and profunda femoris artery repairs.

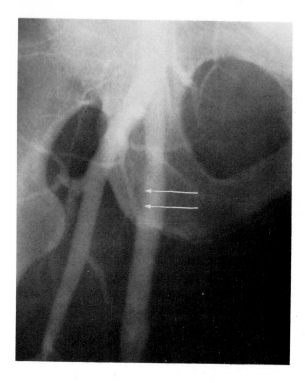

Figure 23–14. In the long-term follow-up of a Korean War casualty victim, there was angiographic evidence of a small arteriosclerotic plaque in the wall of the greater saphenous vein used about 20 years earlier as an interposition graft to repair the injured proximal superficial femoral artery. (W.R.G.H., 1972.)

of successful repair performed long after the arterial injury. Edwards and Lyons (1954) reported the case of a 7 year old boy successfully operated upon 24 hours after injury. Before operation the toes were black, with bullae over the foot and pre-

tibial region. At operation a 4-cm contused, thrombosed segment of the femoral artery was excised and replaced with a vein graft. Subsequently, only the toes required amputation. Roper and Provan (1965) described successful restoration of flow 17 days after

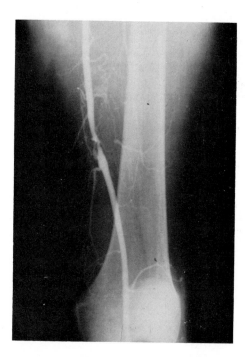

Figure 23–15. Eleven years after a lateral suture repair of the superficial femoral artery, severe stenosis was demonstrated angiographically at the original repair site. (W.R.G.H., 1968.)

internal fixation of a concomitant femoral fracture, when there was the first evidence of arterial insufficiency, and 27 days after the initial injury. Representative reports of recent civilian experience include those of Smith and associates (1974), Hermreck and colleagues (1974), Rosental and co-workers (1975) and Sher (1975).

Death following superficial femoral artery trauma has not been frequently noted. Drapanas and co-workers (1970) reported a mortality of 6.4 per cent among their 31 patients with superficial femoral artery trauma. Perry and co-workers (1971) documented three deaths in patients with superficial femoral artery injuries; however, all of their patients had multiple traumas involving the chest and head.

FOLLOW-UP

An unusual follow-up of 20 years' duration has been possible on one of the patients originally injured during the Korean Conflict. The patient has remained well, but there is laboratory evidence of hyperlipemia. An angiogram revealed a small arteriosclerotic plaque in the wall of the saphenous vein graft originally used to repair the superficial femoral artery (Fig. 23–14). Another patient was seen at Walter Reed Army Medical Center 11 years after a lateral suture repair of a puncture wound of the distal femoral artery. Angiography performed because of increasing claudication showed marked local stenosis (Fig. 23–15). Operation had a successful result obtained by excision of the stenotic area and performance of an end-to-end anastomosis.

Nearly one-third of the 305 patients with superficial femoral arterial injuries treated in Vietnam have subsequently been evaluated in the Peripheral Vascular Clinic at Walter Reed Army Medical Center. Evaluation has included plethysmography and Doppler tracings before and after exercise. Very few additional problems have been found in this follow-up. The majority of the complications occurred within the first two weeks. Nevertheless, in spite of successful arterial repair, significant disability has been seen in some patients due to chronic venous insufficiency and residual neurologic deficits. Routine angiography has not been performed, particularly in asymptomatic patients with strong distal pulses.

CHAPTER 24

POPLITEAL ARTERY INJURIES

At present, injuries of the popliteal artery have the highest amputation rate of all injuries to peripheral arteries, and accordingly they remain one of the most significant unsolved problems in the treatment of acute arterial injuries. Although Makins (1919) reported an amputation rate in World War I of only 41 per cent after ligation of the popliteal artery, in World War II Ogilvie (1944) reported that in the North African campaign the frequency of gangrene following ligation approached 100 per cent. The lower frequency of amputation in World War I was probably due to the fact that many seriously injured patients did not live to reach the operating room because evacuation frequently took 24 hours or longer. Ligation remained the usual form of treatment in World War II, with an overall amputation rate of nearly 73 per cent in the 502 patients reported in the collective review by DeBakey and Simeone in 1946.

Despite the introduction of techniques of vascular repair during the Korean Conflict, the rate of amputation remained nearly 32 per cent (Hughes, 1958). However, this constituted a vast improvement over the nearly 73 per cent amputation rate in World War II. In the Vietnam Conflict the amputation rate has remained virtually unchanged — about 32 per cent (Rich et al., 1969A). In a civilian series, Treiman and associates (1966) reported eight amputations following 18 popliteal injuries, repre-

senting about a 44 per cent amputation rate. Drapanas and associates (1970) reported that approximately 43 per cent — six injuries — of 14 popliteal artery injuries ended in amputation. Conkle and colleagues (1975) documented an amputation rate of about 44 per cent — 12 of 27 patients.

SURGICAL ANATOMY

The popliteal artery begins at the hiatus of the adductor magnus muscle as the distal continuation of the superficial femoral artery (Fig. 24-1). The proximal portion lies behind the distal one-third of the femur. More distally it is located behind the capsule of the knee joint, and a short distance beyond it terminates at the distal border of the popliteus muscle, dividing it into the anterior and posterior tibial arteries. Morris and associates (1960B) emphasized the many variations in the anatomy of the popliteal artery through an analysis of the arteriograms of 246 patients (Fig. 24-2). "Trifurcation" of the popliteal artery, with the peroneal artery originating at the same level as the anterior tibial artery, is frequently mentioned but is statistically unusual.

In addition to the terminal branches, normally there are genicular branches at different levels behind the knee joint, with excellent vascular anastomoses proximally

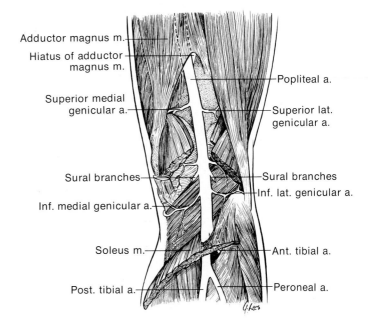

Figure 24–1. Posterior view of the popliteal artery and its major branches. The genicular branches are responsible for a rich collateral blood supply around the knee.

with the descending branch of the lateral femoral circumflex artery and distally with the anterior recurrent tibial artery.

Throughout its entire course the popliteal artery lies deep in the popliteal fossa, consecutively crossing the posterior surface of the femur, the capsule of the knee joint and the fascia of the popliteus muscle. Proximally, the artery is covered by the semimembranosus muscle, but at the level of the condyles of the femur it is covered mostly by subcutaneous tissue and fat. Distally, the plantaris muscle and nerves to the lateral head of the gastrocnemius muscle cross over the artery. At its termination it is covered by the triceps surae, composed of the two heads of the gastrocnemius muscle and the soleus muscle.

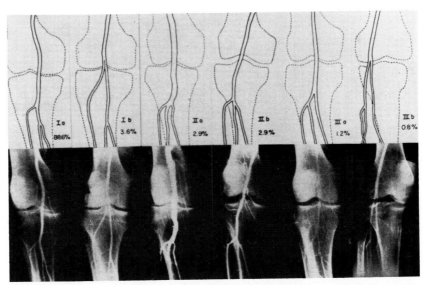

Figure 24–2. Multiple variations in the anatomy of the distal popliteal artery and its major branches. The most common configuration, as noted in *Ia,* was found in 88.6 per cent of the cases in this study. (Morris, G. C., Jr., Beall, A. C., Jr., Berry, W. B., Feste, J., and De Bakey, M. E., Surg. Forum, *10:*498, 1970.

The popliteal vein crosses from the lateral to the medial side of the artery in its mid-portion; often two popliteal veins are found. The vein and artery are closely adherent within a fascial sheath, explaining the frequency with which both structures are injured. The median popliteal nerve enters the popliteal fossa on the lateral side of the artery and crosses superficially to a medial location in the distal part of the popliteal space (Fig. 24–3).

There is some disagreement in the nomenclature regarding the segment of artery found between the origin of the anterior tibial artery and the origin of the peroneal artery. Occasionally this is termed "distal popliteal artery" but is probably more correctly described as "proximal posterior tibial artery." The need for precise nomenclature was clearly seen during the registration of several hundred popliteal artery injuries in the Vietnam Vascular Registry, in which a wide variety of terminology was found.

INCIDENCE

Popliteal artery trauma has been more frequent in military experience than in the civilian situation (Table 24–1).

Although Makins (1919) reported about a 12 per cent incidence, with 144 popliteal injuries among 1191 arterial injuries, the incidence has been generally higher in more recent conflicts. The World War II experience reported by DeBakey and Simeone (1946) revealed about a 20 per cent incidence — 502 popliteal injuries among 2741 acute arterial injuries. The incidence was nearly 26 per cent — 79 popliteal injuries among 304 arterial injuries — in the Korean Conflict (Hughes, 1958). It was also

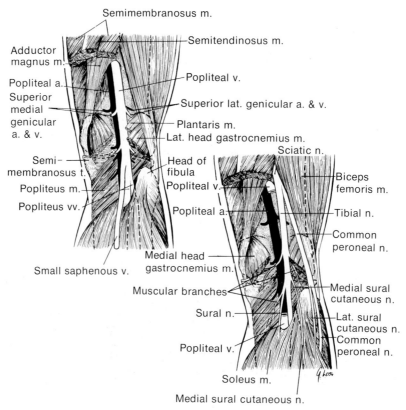

Figure 24–3. The close association of the structures in the neurovascular bundle found within the popliteal fossa is demonstrated in the above drawings.

TABLE 24–1. INCIDENCE OF POPLITEAL ARTERY INJURIES

	AUTHOR	TOTAL ARTERIES	POPLITEAL	PER CENT
	War Series			
WW I	Makins (1919)	1202	144	12.1
WW II	DeBakey and Simeone (1946)	2471	502	20.3
Korean	Hughes (1958)	304	79	25.9
Vietnam	Rich et al. (1970)	1000	217	21.7
	Civilian Series			
Houston	Morris et al. (1960A)	220	14	6.4
Atlanta	Ferguson et al. (1961)	200	14	7.0
Denver	Owens (1963)	70	14	20.0
Detroit	Smith et al. (1963)	61	6	9.9
Dallas	Patman et al. (1964)	271	7	2.6
Los Angeles	Treiman et al. (1966)	159	18	11.3
St. Louis	Dillard et al. (1968)	85	10	11.8
New Orleans	Drapanas et al. (1970)	226	14	6.2
Dallas	Perry et al. (1971)*	508	17	3.3
Denver	Kelly and Eiseman (1975)	116	6	5.2
Memphis	Cheek et al. (1975)	155	15	9.7
Jackson	Hardy et al. (1975)	360	20	5.6
New York	Bole et al. (1976)	126	12	9.5
Little Rock	Burnett et al. (1976)	94	8	8.5

*This is a sequential study including the earlier report.

higher in Vietnam, according to the interim reported by Rich and co-authors (1970A), which described about a 22 per cent incidence—217 popliteal injuries among 1000 acute major arterial injuries.

Brewer and associates (1969) reviewed several large series of civilian arterial injuries and found that popliteal injuries constituted about 12 per cent of the total group. There is considerable variation in the individual series, as demonstrated in Table 24–1. Owens (1963) reported the only incidence—14 popliteal injuries among 70 arterial injuries, or 20 per cent—which approached that of recent military experience. Morris and co-workers (1960A) reported 14 popliteal injuries among 220 arterial injuries—6.4 per cent in Houston. Ferguson and co-workers (1961) found a similar incidence of 7 per cent, representing 14 popliteal injuries among 200 arterial injuries. Smith and associates (1963) reported 6 popliteal injuries in a series of 61 arterial injuries—approximately 10 per cent. In Los Angeles Treiman and co-authors (1966) reported 18 popliteal injuries among 159 arterial injuries—about 11 per cent. There was approximately a 12 per cent incidence in St. Louis (Dillard et al., 1968), where 10 popliteal injuries were found among 85 arterial

injuries. Drapanas and associates (1970) reported 14 popliteal injuries in a series of 226 arterial injuries in New Orleans—approximately 6 per cent. Hermreck and co-workers (1974) reported a relatively high incidence of popliteal artery injuries at the University of Kansas Medical Center over a three year period, 1971 to 1973, with 6 of 36 arterial injuries involving the popliteal artery—an incidence of approximately 17 per cent. However, five recent series, 1975 to 1976, from Denver, Memphis, Jackson, New York and Little Rock show a range from 5 to 10 per cent (Table 24–1). Figure 24–4 shows a representative number of popliteal arterial injuries compared to injuries of other arteries in a recent civilian series. The lowest percentage in a major series is reported from Dallas, where Patman and associates (1964) recorded only 7 popliteal injuries among 271 arterial injuries—about 3 per cent. In the sequential study by Perry and co-workers (1971), the incidence remained approximately 3 per cent—17 popliteal injuries among 508 arterial injuries.

The young age of most patients in both military and civilian trauma is significant. In the Vietnam Vascular Registry the average age was 22, and an identical average age of 22 years was reported by

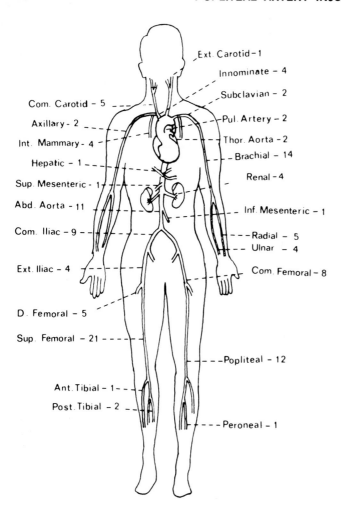

Ext. Carotid – 1
Innominate – 4
Subclavian – 2
Com. Carotid – 5
Axillary – 2
Pul. Artery – 2
Int. Mammary – 4
Thor. Aorta – 2
Hepatic – 1
Brachial – 14
Sup. Mesenteric – 1
Renal – 4
Abd. Aorta – 11
Com. Iliac – 9
Inf. Mesenteric – 1
Radial – 5
Ulnar – 4
Ext. Iliac – 4
Com. Femoral – 8
D. Femoral – 5
Sup. Femoral – 21
Popliteal – 12
Ant. Tibial – 1
Post. Tibial – 2
Peroneal – 1

Figure 24–4. Among 126 arterial injuries in 122 patients in the civilian experience in New York City, there were 12 injuries to the popliteal artery, as illustrated. (Bole, P. V., Purdy, R. T., Munda, R. T., Moallem, S., Devanesan, J., and Clauss, R. H., Ann. Surg., *183*:13, 1976.)

Brewer and co-workers (1969). A somber fact evolves from this frequency, because popliteal trauma is a major cause of amputation of the leg in young adults.

ETIOLOGY

Pick (1873) provided an early description of rupture of the popliteal artery and stated that it was a frequent type of arterial rupture, usually being caused by a violent blow on the front of the thigh with the foot fixed or by a similar type of force that would bend the knee backwards and violently stretch the popliteal vessels.

Representative differences in the causative factors in civilian and military trauma are shown in Table 24–2. In the group of 16 patients reported by Brewer and co-

workers (1969), nine injuries resulted from penetrating missiles, and there were seven fractures of the distal femur or dislocation of the knee. Similar types of closed trauma have occurred with less frequency in Vietnam. One helicopter crewman had a posterior displacement of a distal closed fracture of the femur which thrombosed the popliteal artery (Fig. 24–5). Amputation has frequently resulted from this type of injury, especially if the diagnosis was delayed. All 18 patients in Gorman's series (1969) incurred trauma to the popliteal artery as a result of a missile from an assortment of fragmenting devices. Of 150 popliteal injuries reported from Vietnam (Rich et al., 1969A), about 63 per cent were caused by fragments from a variety of exploding devices. Thirty-three per cent were caused by gunshot wounds, often with massive tissue

TABLE 24–2. ETIOLOGY OF WOUNDING AGENT

REPORT	ARTERIES INJURED	GUNSHOT WOUNDS	FRAGMENT WOUNDS	BLUNT TRAUMA	STAB WOUNDS AND MISCELLANEOUS
Civilian					
Brewer et al. (1969)	16	9 (56.3%)	0	7 (43.7%)	0
Conkle et al. (1975)	27	11 (40.7%)	0	14 (51.8%)	2 (7.5%)
Military					
Gorman (1969)	18	0	18 (100.0%)	0	0
Rich et al. (1969A)	150	33 (22.0%)	95 (63.3%)	7 (4.7%)	15 (10.0%)

destruction from the high velocity impact. Two injuries resulted from a punji stick, one of the primitive weapons widely used.

Conkle and associates (1975), in their recent series from Nashville, reported that slightly more than one-half of their 27 patients with popliteal arterial injuries had blunt trauma (Table 24–2). In contrast, Hardy and colleagues (1975) found that the majority of the popliteal arterial injuries in their series resulted from gunshot wounds (including three due to shotgun blasts)—11 of 20 cases. Among the remaining 9 cases were 7 which resulted from blunt trauma and 2 from stab wounds.

Additional detail regarding popliteal arterial trauma associated with femoral and tibial fractures and/or dislocation of the knee can be found in Chapter 7. Arterial injuries with associated fractures are more common than those with dislocations. Taylor and Wardill (1964) emphasized the difficulty in determining the true incidence of trauma to the popliteal artery with knee dislocations when they reported two cases.

Unusual types of popliteal injury include accidental lacerations during operation on the knee joint, especially from a meniscectomy. Dillard and associates (1968) reported an injury to the popliteal artery in a patient who had a Kirschner wire placed through the artery while skeletal traction for a femoral fracture was being applied. Vascular injuries have occurred with orthopedic procedures other than those in the management of fractures. Ferguson (1914)

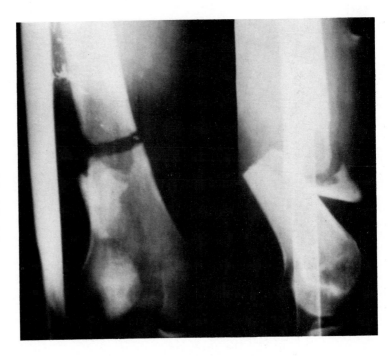

Figure 24–5. This displaced distal femoral fracture caused thrombosis of the popliteal artery, which was not recognized initially. Despite an attempted end-to-end anastomosis, after resection and thrombectomy of the distal popliteal artery, irreversible ischemia necessitated an amputation. (Rich, N. M., Baugh, J. H., and Hughes, C. W., Am. J. Surg., *118*:531, 1969.)

presented an infant who developed an arteriovenous fistula following an osteotomy
of the femur for genu valgum. Ligation of
both the popliteal artery and vein was carried out to obliterate the communication.
Dillard and Staple (1969) reported a case of
bullet embolization from the aortic arch to
the left popliteal artery (Fig. 24–6). Fish
and Hochhauser (1967) reported an injury
to the popliteal artery due to blunt trauma
in a 15 year old boy when he was tackled
from behind immediately after catching a
pass in a high school football game. They
speculated that constricting rubber bands
might have contributed to the causation of
this injury. There is nothing in the history
or clinical findings to suggest temporary
subluxation, and there were no fractures.
They also cited only one additional injury
of the popliteal artery due to blunt trauma
in their search through the literature. That
injury had been caused by a piece of steel.
Dainko (1972) reported the case of perforation of a popliteal artery with a Fogarty
balloon catheter (Fig. 24–7).

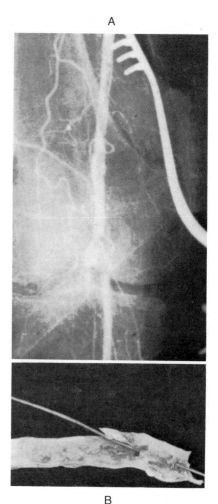

A

B

Figure 24–7. Trauma to the popliteal artery has
been caused by perforation secondary to passage of
a balloon catheter. This operative arteriogram reveals
extravasation of contrast material from the mid-
popliteal artery (A). Filling defects in the arteriogram
were caused by elevated intima. The specimen of the
popliteal artery which was removed at the time of
above-the-knee amputation shows the intimal
damage, with a probe demonstrating the area of
dissection in the vessel wall (B). (Dainko, E. A.,
Arch. Surg., *105*:79, 1972.)

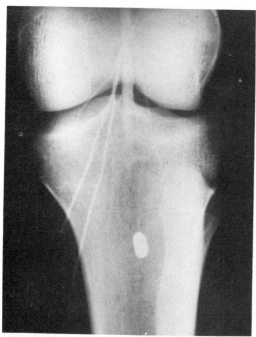

Figure 24–6. Occlusion of the distal popliteal artery is demonstrated in this angiogram; the bullet
embolus may be seen within the lumen of the popliteal artery. (Dillard, B. M., and Staple, T. W., Arch.
Surg., *98*:326, 1969.)

CLINICAL PATHOLOGY

Popliteal arterial injuries may involve
transection, laceration, or contusion and
thrombosis, or an acute arteriovenous fistula may be produced as a result of injury
to the concomitant vein. Gorman (1969)
reported nine transections, five contusions
with thrombosis and four lacerations in his
Vietnam experience. An arterial lesion is a
particularly deceptive lesion because frac-

ture of the intima with prolapse of the distal intimal flap into the lumen, with resulting thrombosis, may not be detectable from external examination of the artery, requiring an arteriotomy for inspection of the lumen (see Chap. 7, particularly Figs. 7–12 and 7–13).

With arterial injuries from high velocity missiles, a recurrent question is the amount of normal-appearing artery proximal and distal to the site of injury that should be sacrificed because of the velocity of impact. This is a crucial question in the popliteal fossa because of the limited mobility of the artery. Although adequate debridement is obviously necessary, sacrifice of grossly normal-appearing artery is unnecessary. Figure 24–8 demonstrates the resected portion of a popliteal artery injured by a fragment in Vietnam. In Figures 24–9 and 24–10, histologic sections from this representative popliteal artery injury are shown. Although the arteries may grossly appear normal, microscopic examination regularly discloses focal areas of laceration of the intima and media, disruption of the internal elastic membrane, localized areas of loss of the intima, infiltration of polymorphonuclear cells and scattered small fibrin plugs. Such changes may be found even 1 cm or more from the site of injury. Clearly, total excision of these areas is impractical, and fortunately the surgical results are not jeopardized by leaving these areas of focal microscopic trauma in situ. Rich and associates (1969C) revealed that the ultimate success of the arterial repair could not be correlated with the amount of normal artery sacrificed.

Surprisingly enough, arteriosclerotic plaques may be found even in persons injured in the second decade and may seriously complicate repair. Rich and co-workers (1969C) found three such patients, in one of whom an arteriosclerotic plaque led to thrombosis of an arterial anastomosis, which was fortunately salvaged with a second reconstructive procedure.

With the proximity of many structures in the popliteal fossa, the frequency of associated injuries is great. Rich and Hughes (1969), in the preliminary report from the Vietnam Vascular Registry, reported that popliteal artery injuries were accompanied by associated trauma more than injuries in any other group of major arteries. As shown in Table 24–3, in a group of 150 arterial injuries, the popliteal vein was injured in nearly 60 per cent of the patients; a fracture occurred in 50 per cent and a nerve injury in 47 per cent (Rich et al., 1969C). Conkle and colleagues (1975)

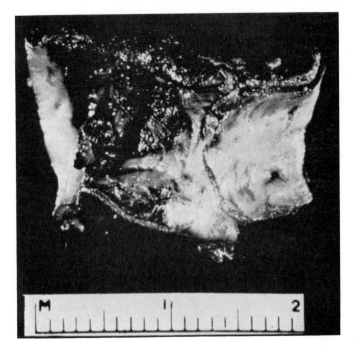

Figure 24–8. This resected segment of popliteal artery shows evidence of gross trauma caused by a fragment from an exploding device. A segment 2 to 3 mm distal to the gross trauma and more than 1 cm proximal to it was excised. (Rich, N. M., Manion, W. C., and Hughes, C. W., J. Trauma, 9:279, 1969. Copyright 1969, The Williams & Wilkins Company, Baltimore.)

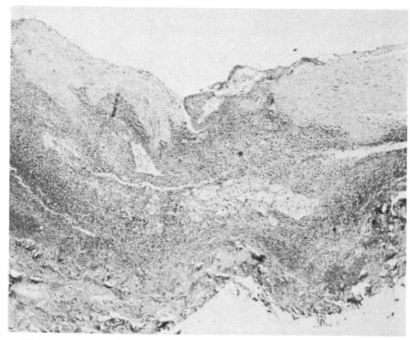

Figure 24–9. This photomicrograph of a hematoxylin and eosin–stained cross section of the popliteal artery (× 90) shows multiple disruptions, with hemorrhage and fibrin thrombus on the intimal surface. There is focal disruption of the media and marked perivascular hemorrhage with some disruption of the perivascular tissue. This section was taken from the smaller normal-appearing margin of the popliteal artery shown in Figure 24–8. (Rich, N. M., Manion, W. C., and Hughes, C. W., J. Trauma, 9:279, 1969. Copyright 1969, The Williams & Wilkins Company, Baltimore.)

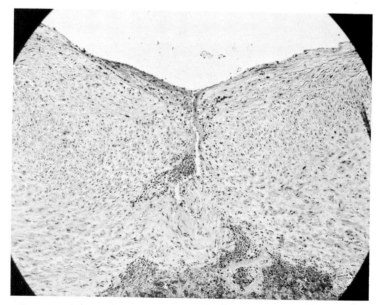

Figure 24–10. This photomicrograph of a hematoxylin and eosin–stained cross section of the popliteal arterial wall (× 275) shows partial laceration involving the intima and media. A fibrin plug is present over the site of injury. There is evident loss of intima, but the adventitia has minimal damage. This represents the larger area of normal-appearing margin of the popliteal artery shown in Figure 24–8. (Rich, N. M., Manion, W. C., and Hughes, C. W., J. Trauma, 9:279, 1969. Copyright 1969, The Williams & Wilkins Company, Baltimore.)

TABLE 24–3. CONCOMITANT INJURIES ASSOCIATED WITH POPLITEAL ARTERY TRAUMA IN VIETNAM*

150 POPLITEAL ARTERY INJURIES		
Popliteal vein injuries	88	58.7%
Concomitant fractures	74	49.3%
Associated nerve trauma	71	47.3%

*Rich, N. M., Baugh, J. H., and Hughes, C. W., Am. J. Surg., *118*:531, 1969.

TABLE 24–4. INJURIES ASSOCIATED WITH POPLITEAL ARTERY TRAUMA— CIVILIAN EXPERIENCE IN NASHVILLE*

Popliteal vein	26/27
Peroneal or sciatic nerve	19/27
Concomitant fracture	8/27
Knee dislocation	5/27
Massive soft tissue injury	4/27

*Modified from Conkle, D. M., Richie, R. E., Sawyers, J. L., and Scott, H. W., Jr., Arch. Surg., *110*:1351, 1975. Copyright 1975, American Medical Association.

noted associated injuries in 26 of 27 patients with popliteal arterial trauma (Table 24–4). Hardy and co-workers found four posterior knee dislocations and four fractures associated with 20 popliteal arterial injuries.

CLINICAL FEATURES

Massive soft tissue injuries, fractures, neurologic injuries and venous injuries all frequently occur with popliteal artery injuries and significantly influence the resulting disability and methods of surgical repair. As mentioned earlier, the frequency of associated injuries is shown in Table 24–3.

The diagnosis may be obvious, with a gaping wound of the popliteal fossa associated with a cold, numb, pale leg. In other injuries, however, such as dislocation of the knee or a closed fracture of the femur, signs of arterial injury may be minimal and easily overlooked. This is particularly true if a dislocation of the knee has spontaneously reduced. A difficult diagnostic problem arises if pedal pulses are present. This may be true for a few hours with contusion of the popliteal artery, a distal flap of intima prolapsing into the lumen, which eventually leads to thrombosis. In Figure 24–11 the discovery of a wound in the popliteal fossa from a penetrating fragment alerted observers to an underlying arterial injury, although the distal extremity was warm and had a palpable dorsalis pedis pulse.

DIAGNOSTIC CONSIDERATIONS

A high index of suspicion of arterial injury is the keynote for early diagnosis. The possibility should be automatically considered with any penetrating or blunt trauma in the vicinity of the knee joint. Usually the diagnosis is easily made from the presence of a cold, pale, pulseless extremity, often with the absence of sensation and motor paralysis. If pedal pulses are present, however, clinical findings of ischemia are ab-

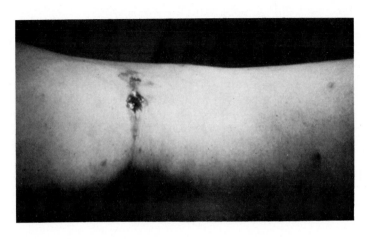

Figure 24–11. This penetrating fragment wound of the popliteal fossa was caused by an irregular piece of metal from a Viet Cong bobby trap. An injury in this location should alert one to the probability of trauma to the neurovascular bundle in the popliteal fossa, and exploration of the wound is mandatory (NMR, 2nd Surgical Hospital, An Khe, 1966). (Rich, N. M., *in* Dale, W. A. (ed.), *Management of Arterial Occlusive Disease.* Year Book Medical Publishers, Inc., Chicago, 1971.)

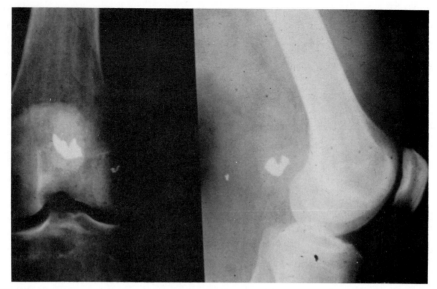

Figure 24–12.   The anteroposterior and lateral roentgenographic views of the popliteal fossa can be helpful in determining the presence of trauma to the popliteal artery. The large irregular fragment wound seen in the area of the neurovascular bundle above heralds the probability of popliteal vascular trauma. Both the large fragment and the adjacent small fragment came from an exploding booby trap (NMR, 2nd Surgical Hospital, 1966). (Rich, N. M., *in* Dale, W. A. (Ed.), Management of Arterial Occlusive Disease. Year Book Medical Publishers, Inc., Chicago, 1971.)

sent, and an injury may be detected only by arteriography or surgical exploration.

Lateral and anteroposterior radiographic views of the knee may provide valuable information. A displaced fracture immediately cautions that a popliteal injury may be present (see Fig. 24–5). Similarly, the location of a penetrating fragment near the artery warns that the injury may exist (Fig. 24–12).

Arteriography is superfluous and wastes valuable time if the diagnosis is obvious. However, with blunt trauma associated with swelling and contusion of an extremity, arteriography may be necessary to differentiate absent pulses due to vasospasm and edema from those due to an arterial injury. This is particularly true if a peripheral nerve injury is also present. A diagnosis of "arterial spasm" following a closed fracture of the femur is always dangerous and uncertain. Often the correct diagnosis will belatedly be found to be an arterial contusion with prolapse of the fractured intima into the lumen.

If neurologic function is absent in an extremity, with numbness and motor paralysis, the presence or absence of an arterial injury must usually be determined within four to six hours if muscle necrosis and gangrene are to be avoided. Such absence of neurologic function indicates a severe degree of ischemia. However, if neurologic function is present even though pulses are absent, there is less urgency in determining the exact diagnosis because gangrene is not impending. The ultrasonic sounding device (Doppler) can provide graphic documentation to substantiate the clinical impression of adequate collateral blood supply in an injury to the popliteal artery. A difficult diagnostic problem is determining whether loss of neurologic function is due to ischemia from an arterial injury or damage to a peripheral nerve.

SURGICAL TREATMENT

A posterior approach to the injured popliteal artery, with the patient in a prone position, is frequently best. This permits wide exposure both proximally and distally (Fig. 24–13). A modified "S"-shaped incision is made to avoid contracture across the knee joint, the superior limb of the incision being placed on the medial side of the thigh to expose the proximal popliteal artery. Through this incision a section of the greater saphenous vein can be obtained if a

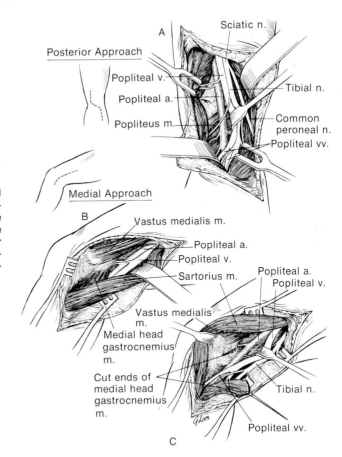

Figure 24–13. The posterior and medial approaches to the popliteal artery. A modified "S"-shaped incision is used in the posterior approach to avoid contracture across the knee joint. Either the medial or the posterior approach can be successfully utilized in exposing the popliteal artery.

vein graft is needed. Distally the skin incision can be extended as far as necessary, the two heads of the gastrocnemius being separated in the midline, a landmark readily located by the "blue and white stripe" of the lesser saphenous vein and sural nerve. A medial approach has been used for lesions in the proximal popliteal artery where exposure of the distal femoral artery is also needed. With this approach, the skin incision is made parallel to the distal portion of the sartorius muscle, the muscle being retracted posteriorly. The saphenous nerve should be identified and protected. Dissection is then carried through the fascia into Hunter's canal, the adductor tendon being isolated with the femoral artery passing through the adductor hiatus to become the popliteal artery. The adductor tendon beyond the adductor hiatus is usually divided to facilitate exposure. If necessary, additional distal exposure can be obtained by extending the original incision or by

making a separate incision on the medial aspect of the leg below the knee joint.

Initially, proximal control of the popliteal artery is needed to avoid hemorrhage. A pneumatic tourniquet may be used if a large hematoma is present or if there is difficulty in controlling the hemorrhage by pressure, but usually this is unnecessary. Following proximal control of the artery, distal control should also be obtained, as well as exposure of the popliteal vein. Adequate debridement of all devitalized tissue is crucial to arterial repair, to prevent the development of infection. This should be combined with extensive irrigation of the wound with saline. Antibiotics are normally given in large amounts before, during and after the operation.

Once the arterial injury has been isolated with appropriate mobilization of the artery proximally and distally, a decision can be made about the type of repair indicated. Debridement of the injured artery should be limited to arterial wall that has been grossly lacerated and contused. Following debridement the ends of the artery can be gently dilated and inspected for lacerations of the intima or thrombi in the lumen. Vascular occlusion clamps should be alternately released proximally and distally to note the flow of blood. Routine insertion of a Fogarty catheter distally, with advancement to the level of the ankle if possible, has been found to be particularly useful in Vietnam, often revealing unsuspected thrombi. The quality of the back bleeding may be misleading because distal clot can be present, associated with what appears to be adequate back bleeding.

A few tangential lacerations caused by sharp instruments may be repaired by lateral suture or a patch graft, but most injuries are best treated by resection of the injured segment followed by an end-to-end anastomosis or by insertion of a short segment of autogenous vein graft. A representative series detailing the types of reconstruction employed in Vietnam is shown in Table 24–5. The apparent simplicity of lateral suture is deceptive, since it often results in stenosis and thrombosis because the intima is usually fractured over a wider extent than can be determined by external inspection. With mobilization of the ends of the injured artery followed by flexion of the knee joint to about 15 degrees, end-to-end anastomosis can often be performed with minimal tension on the artery and with preservation of major branches (Fig. 24–14). Otherwise, a short graft of reversed autogenous greater saphenous vein should be inserted. Other possible donor sites, which are usually less desirable, include the lesser saphenous vein and the

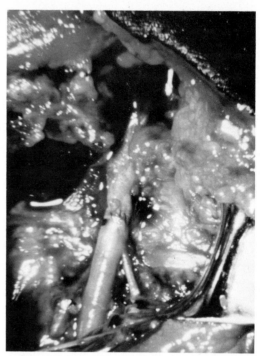

Figure 24–14. After minimal arterial debridement in this low velocity wound, successful end-to-end anastomosis of the popliteal artery was possible. This was performed without sacrifice of major branches or without creating undue tension on the suture line (NMR, 2nd Surgical Hospital, An Khe, 1966). (Rich, N. M., Baugh, J. H., and Hughes, C. W., J. Trauma, 10:359, 1970. Copyright 1970, The Williams & Wilkins Company, Baltimore.)

cephalic vein. Prosthetic grafts such as Dacron should be avoided in most patients because of the risk of infection in contaminated wounds, as well as the long term hazard of a prosthetic graft subject to recurrent flexion behind the knee joint.

An arteriogram at completion of the repair will outline the patency, or potential complications such as residual thrombus (Fig. 24–15). Following operation, an arteriogram should be made if pedal pulses are not palpable. Inability to detect a pulse may be due to edema or residual vasospasm, but this can be differentiated from thrombosis of the anastomosis or thrombi in the artery distal to the site of repair only by arteriography. Also, with multiple injuries, an additional distal arterial injury may be present. The decision regarding patency of the repair is particularly urgent if the foot remains anesthetic or paralyzed; otherwise, irreversible muscle ischemia may result within a few hours.

TABLE 24–5. INITIAL ARTERIAL REPAIR IN VIETNAM*

TYPE OF REPAIR	No.	PER CENT
Vein graft	64	51.6
End-to-end anastomosis	46	37.1
Lateral suture	11	8.9
Thrombectomy	2	1.6
Patch graft	1	0.8
Total:	124	100.0

*Rich, N. M., Baugh, J. H., and Hughes, C. W., Am. J. Surg., 118:531, 1969.

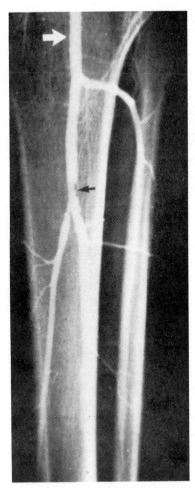

Figure 24–15. This angiogram shows retained thrombus in the tibial-peroneal trunk (black arrow) after initial thrombectomy. The white arrow indicates the level of end-to-end anastomosis of the popliteal artery. Angiography performed in the operating room can define potential complications, such as residual thrombus. (Bole, P. V., Purdy, R. T., Munda, R. T., Moallem, S., Devanesan, J., and Clauss, R. H., Ann. Surg., *183*:13, 1976.)

Injury of a popliteal vein, if not extensive, should surely be repaired. With extensive loss of soft tissue, often involving injury to both the popliteal and saphenous veins, repair of the popliteal vein may be mandatory, even to the extent of using an autogenous vein graft, to prevent loss of the extremity from massive acute venous occlusion, despite a successful arterial repair (see Chap. 8).

Concomitant fractures are usually adequately managed by external methods. Internal fixation is dangerous in contaminated wounds. Associated nerve injuries

should be recorded but not primarily repaired.

The site of arterial reconstruction must be covered by adjacent soft tissues, either fascia or muscles. Subsequently the skin and subcutaneous tissues can be left open for a delayed primary closure in three to six days. This is mandatory in military injuries where contaminated wounds with massive tissue injuries predominate. It is by far the safest method in avoiding serious infection with its disastrous complications.

Fasciotomy should be seriously considered if the extremity has been ischemic for several hours (Fig. 24–16), especially if swelling is marked or if there has been extensive venous injury as well. Experiences with fasciotomy have been described by many authors, including a recent review by Patman and Thompson (1970). Ernst and Kaufer (1971) have documented additional thoughts on the use of fibulectomy-fasciotomy as an important adjunct in the management of lower extremity arterial trauma (see Chap. 5). The use of fasciotomy can

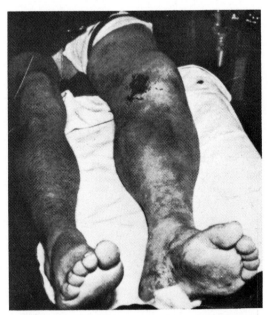

Figure 24–16. Tense swelling of the muscles of the left calf, without significant subcutaneous edema, was noted 12 hours after transection of the popliteal artery in this World War II combat casualty. Fasciotomy was considered to be a possible aid to the capillary circulation in this type of case, and this remains true at this time. (DeBakey, M. E., and Simeone, F. A., Ann. Surg., *123*:534, 1946.)

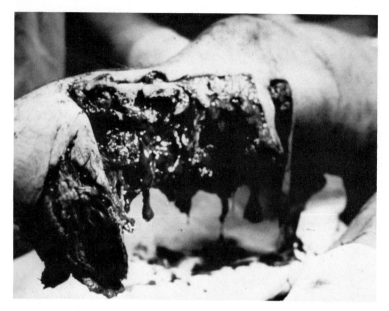

Figure 24–17. Massive soft tissue injury of the right lower extremity caused by fragments from an exploding 105 mm artillery round is illustrated in this operating room photograph. In addition to the destruction of the popliteal artery, there was also osseous loss, nerve deficits and venous insufficiency (NMR, 2nd Surgical Hospital, An Khe, 1966). (Rich, N. M., Baugh, J. H., and Hughes, C. W., Am. J. Surg., *118*:531, 1969.)

usually be determined by palpation of the distal muscles. Muscles which are soft to palpation after operation but which become turgid and hard within a few hours benefit greatly from fasciotomy; otherwise, gangrene or extensive fibrosis with contractures may result.

Ligation of the popliteal artery may be necessary in some unusual situations but should be avoided if at all possible. Perhaps a major instance in which ligation is indicated is when infection has occurred with secondary hemorrhage. Gangrene usually results.

There is still a place for primary amputation, particularly in wounds with massive tissue destruction, such as that demonstrated in Figure 24–17.

Extensive trauma involving fractures of long bones and tissues in and around the popliteal area create particular extremity salvage problems. Although primary amputation may be considered the wisest choice in some of these injuries, Evans and Bernhard (1971) have emphasized the value of tibial artery bypass for ischemia resulting from fractures. In presenting the case reports of four of their patients, they have demonstrated the value of extended vein bypass grafts similar to those to the distal tibial and peroneal arteries in patients with arteriosclerotic occlusive disease.

POSTOPERATIVE CARE

Pedal pulses should be palpable soon after reconstruction. Detecting a pulse is a critical point, because this is the only certain guarantee that the arterial reconstruction is patent. Recent studies have found that the ultrasonic sounding device (Doppler) may be useful in edematous extremities, indicating that a pulse is present though not palpable. This has been particularly helpful in determining in Vietnam casualties which extremity will remain viable despite the decreased arterial flow (Lavenson et al., 1970, 1971).

If a pulse cannot be felt, possible causes include thrombosis of the arterial repair, vasospasm and edema. As repeatedly stated, the safest guideline for determining the circulation in an extremity without a palpable pulse is neurologic function. If sensation and motor function are intact, there is little risk of gangrene, and clinical observation may be safely continued. However, with a numb, paralyzed extremity, the presence of adequate blood flow must quickly be determined, usually by arteriography, to prevent irreversible ischemic injury. If peripheral nerve injuries are present, however, this valuable clinical guide of neurologic function cannot be used.

Similarly, if a previously palpable pulse disappears following operation, the urgency of determining whether the arterial repair has thrombosed or not can be judged by the neurologic function. An arteriogram should be performed immediately if neurologic function is impaired; otherwise, observation may be continued, especially if multiple injuries contraindicate additional diagnostic studies.

Heparin, sympathetic blocks or lumbar sympathectomy have little role in the postoperative care. In the presence of other injuries, the risk of bleeding contraindicates the use of heparin. There is little or no evidence that lumbar sympathectomy will salvage a seriously ischemic extremity, and in extremities with adequate blood flow, a sympathectomy is superfluous.

The muscles in an extremity should be palpated frequently for signs of edema developing in the fascial compartments, especially the anterolateral and posterior compartments, composed principally of the gastrocnemius and soleus muscles. Extensive fasciotomy should be done promptly if the muscles become indurated.

A particularly difficult problem arises when arterial repair has been performed several hours after injury, following which pulses return to the foot but the leg muscles become progressively hard and indurated, despite wide fasciotomies. Such patients quickly become critically ill with high fever, tachycardia and signs of systemic toxicity. The basic pathology includes areas of ischemic necrosis in the muscles in the leg, with the problem of a "viable foot" but extensive necrosis of tissues in the leg. Some extremities can be salvaged by very radical debridement of the devitalized muscle, with closure of the skin at a later date. Surprisingly good function may remain in the leg after widespread removal of most of the gastrocnemius-soleus muscle group. Unless there is prompt recognition of the clinical problem followed by radical debridement, however, systemic absorption from the gangrenous tissues, with high fever, tachycardia, renal failure and shock, can seriously jeopardize the life of the patient.

Most contaminated wounds are left open for delayed primary suture. Immobilization is usually done with a posterior splint or a bivalved long leg cast, the knee joint often being kept in slight flexion with the extremity elevated to minimize formation of edema. Quadricep strengthening exercises should be instituted to avoid loss of strength and motion at the knee. Periodic inspection of the wound is necessary to be certain that all devitalized tissues were adequately debrided and infection is not developing. If no signs of infection are present, the skin can be sutured four to five days after the initial operation. Despite extensive contamination of the wound at the time of injury, the combination of adequate debridement, antibiotic therapy and delayed primary suture is highly effective in preventing serious infection in almost all patients. Hence, concern about the risk of infection is rarely a valid cause for not performing arterial reconstruction.

COMPLICATIONS

Postoperative thrombosis is one of the most frequent serious complications. It is almost always due to error in surgical technique, such as inadequate resection of the injured artery, stenosis of the anastomosis or excessive tension. Residual thrombi in the distal arterial tree may also result in thrombosis from inadequate flow. The realization that failure of an arterial anastomosis is almost always due to surgical technique is critical; otherwise, the erroneous decision may be reached that reoperation should not be justified because reconstructive failure would probably occur again. Actually, the only contraindication to reoperation is a critically ill patient whose life would be jeopardized. As arterial injuries usually occur in arteries which were previously normal, a patency rate approaching 100 per cent following reconstruction should be routinely obtained. If the initial repair fails in the combat zone and extremity viability is maintained through collateral circulation, a reoperation can be postponed until after the patient has been evacuated to a more stable situation.

A puzzling syndrome of gangrene from massive acute venous occlusion may develop after a successful arterial repair if there has been concomitant extensive tissue injury with loss of both the popliteal and saphenous veins. Although a pedal pulse is

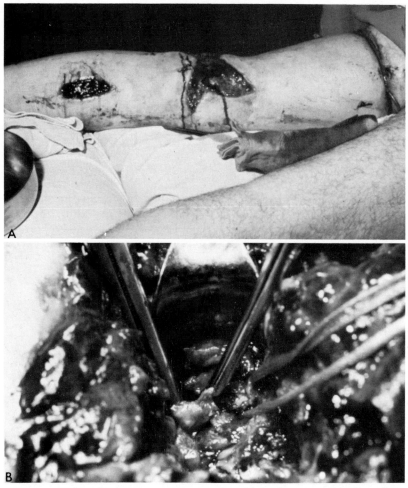

Figure 24–18. Acute hemorrhage from an infected end-to-end anastomosis of the popliteal artery necessitated ligation of the artery at Walter Reed Army Medical Center 33 days after injury in Vietnam (A). (Rich, N. M., Baugh, J. H., and Hughes, C. W., J. Trauma, *10*:359, 1970. Copyright 1970, The Williams & Wilkins Company, Baltimore.) This close-up view of the popliteal fossa illustrates disruption of one-half of the popliteal arterial suture line (B). (Vietnam Vascular Registry #31, NMR.)

present, the extremity gradually becomes swollen and cyanotic from progressive engorgement with blood, a condition resembling phlegmasia cerulea dolens. Amputation is usually inevitable, although fasciotomy should be used to decompress the extremity. Prevention of this complication is the main indication for reconstruction of the popliteal vein when possible (see Chap. 8).

Postoperative hematoma is a frequent complication in wounds which have been sutured primarily. The hematoma should be promptly evacuated, usually in the operating room, because of the risk of superimposed infection.

The most disastrous complication after arterial reconstruction is infection followed by disruption of the suture line and hemorrhage (Fig. 24–18). This complication was so frequent in both World War I and World War II that attempts at arterial reconstruction were abandoned. Only with the advent of rapid evacuation of casualties, antibiotics, widespread debridement followed by delayed primary closure and modern techniques of vascular repair did arterial reconstruction become feasible without constituting a threat to the patient's life. Of these several features, debridement and delayed primary closure are the most important because the infection which develops is almost always due to inadequate debridement.

When secondary hemorrhage develops, ligation of the popliteal artery is usually indicated. One patient's case history emphasizes the problem associated with infected vascular repair. A greater saphenous vein segment was used to reconstruct the popliteal artery. Approximately two weeks later there was massive arterial bleeding from the wound. An attempt was made to repair a hole in the vein graft; however, three days later there was recurrent massive arterial hemorrhage, and it was necessary to ligate the distal superficial femoral artery. Attempts at reconstruction by complicated bypass procedures are difficult, are often unsuccessful and should be attempted only if the patient's life is not jeopardized. Ligation of the popliteal artery several days or

weeks after injury may not necessarily result in gangrene if adequate collateral circulation has developed. This can be determined within hours after ligation because neurologic function is immediately lost. If the extremity has normal motor and sensory function, it will remain viable even though claudication is usually present.

In some patients an initially successful arterial reconstruction will gradually fail, with progressive weakening and eventual disappearance of pedal pulses, at times months or years after the original repair (Fig. 24–19). Such late occlusions are usually due to progressive stenosis from fibrous tissue in the area of anastomosis. If claudication is disabling, a secondary reconstruction with an autogenous vein graft is usually successful.

RESULTS

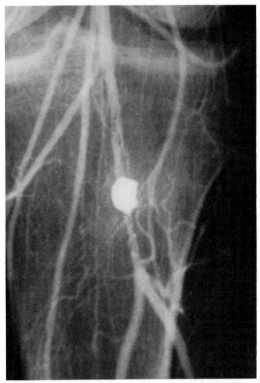

Figure 24–19. This angiogram performed at Walter Reed Army Medical Center demonstrates thrombosis of the popliteal artery 1½ years after an initial lateral suture repair in Vietnam. The adjacent offending fragment overlies the artery. Additional reconstruction using a saphenous vein graft replacement was successful. (Vietnam Vascular Registry #57, NMR.)

As stated earlier, the amputation rate following popliteal injuries remains higher than that after any other peripheral arterial injury, primarily because injuries of the popliteal artery result in such a severe degree of ischemia. The amputation rate has remained nearly 30 per cent in both the Korean Conflict (Hughes, 1958) and the Vietnam War (Rich et al., 1970A) (Table 24–6). The gravity of popliteal injuries is similarly indicated by the fact that nearly 60 per cent of all amputations in military casualties in the initial Vietnam experience resulted from injuries involving the popliteal artery (Rich and Hughes, 1969). In this overall analysis of amputation after peripheral arterial injuries, the amputation rate was 12.7 per cent, but if injuries to the popliteal artery were excluded, the amputation rate for all other arterial injuries considered collectively would be only 6.7 per cent. The frequency of amputations derived from a total of 217 popliteal artery injuries studied in Vietnam remains at approximately 30 per cent (Rich et al., 1970A). Ligation of an injuried popliteal artery results in gangrene in most patients, the incidence varying from 70 to 100 per cent, depending on the associated soft tissue injury and massive destruction of the collateral circulation. The combination of

TABLE 24–6. AMPUTATION RATES FOLLOWING POPLITEAL ARTERY TRAUMA*

SERIES	AUTHOR	INJURIES	AMPUTATIONS	PER CENT
After Ligation				
WW I	Makins (1919)	144	62	43.1
WW II	DeBakey and Simeone (1946)	502	364	72.5
Korean	Hughes (1958)	11	8	72.7
After Repair				
Korean	Hughes (1958)	68	22	32.4
Vietnam	Rich et al. (1970)	217	64	29.5
Houston	Morris et al. (1960A)	11	2	18.2
Denver	Owens (1963)	14	2	14.3
New Orleans	Treiman et al. (1966)	18	8	44.4
New Orleans	Brewer et al. (1969)	16	6	38.0
Los Angeles	Drapanas et al. (1970)	14	6	42.8
Dallas	Perry et al. (1971)	12	1	8.3
Israel	Eger et al. (1972)	10	1	10.0

*Modified from Rich, N. M., Jarstfer, B. S., and Geer, T. M., J. Cardiovasc. Surg., *15*:340, 1974.

fracture of the femur and ligation of the popliteal artery makes gangrene a virtual certainty.

The complexity of determining the factors responsible for poor results following popliteal artery reconstruction is obvious in the following representative case. One patient in Vietnam had an extensive soft tissue wound of the left lower extremity. A greater saphenous vein graft was used to repair the popliteal artery, and the popliteal vein was repaired end-to-end. The initial vascular repair was successful; during the second procedure done five hours later, some distal thrombus was retrieved with a Fogarty balloon catheter and fasciotomies were performed. There was considerable swelling in the extremity following the vascular reconstructions. At the time that an above-the-knee amputation was necessary on the third postoperative day, the vein graft in the popliteal artery appeared to be functioning well. It was felt that there were multiple contributing factors, including the massive soft tissue injury, the distal thrombus and the acute venous hypertension.

Rich and associates (1974B) evaluated the causes and possible prevention of amputation for popliteal arterial repair failure. A review of 125 popliteal artery injuries which resulted in amputation revealed that technical problems and prolonged ischemic time contributed to many failures. Associated injuries were more frequent (Table 24–7) than in reported series previously outlined that included successful cases. The following measures were recommended to reduce popliteal artery repair failure:

1. Early recognition with prompt repair.

2. Adequate resuscitation and support: blood, fluids, antibiotics, etc.

3. Adequate wound and arterial debridement.

4. Removal of distal thrombus with Fogarty catheter: heparinization.

5. Repair without tension: end-to-end anastomosis or autogenous saphenous vein graft (contralateral).

6. Early and adequate fasciotomy, if indicated.

7. Repair of concomitant popliteal vein injuries: including autogenous vein grafts.

TABLE 24–7. CONCOMITANT INJURIES ASSOCIATED WITH POPLITEAL ARTERY TRAUMA RESULTING IN AMPUTATION— VIETNAM EXPERIENCE*

Popliteal vein	98 (78.4%)
Fracture/dislocation	79 (63.2%)
Nerve	67 (53.6%)
Soft tissue	64 (51.2%)

*Rich, N. M., Jarstfer, B. J., and Geer, T. M., J. Cardiovasc. Surg., *15*:340, 1974.

8. External immobilization of associated fractures.

9. Provide soft tissue coverage of arterial repair.

10. Rule out additional arterial trauma: intraoperative angiography.

11. Accept primary amputation in select cases with massive trauma.

The development of an adequate collateral circulation, not only for extremity viability but also for adequate flow to give moderate pain-free ambulation in daily activity, is always a possibility (Fig. 24–20). Often the function of an extremity is determined principally by the associated bone and nerve injuries. Through the Vietnam Vascular Registry, more than 500 patients sustaining popliteal artery injuries in Vietnam are being followed. Late complications requiring reconstructions have been infrequent. One late complication after re-

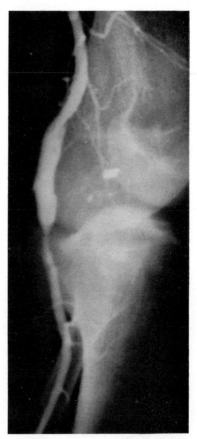

Figure 24–21. This angiogram demonstrates severe stenosis at the distal anastomosis of a saphenous vein graft repair of the popliteal artery. Clinically, there was a high-pitched bruit over the repair site. (Rich, N. M., Baugh, J. H., and Hughes, C. W., Arch. Surg., *100*:646, 1970.)

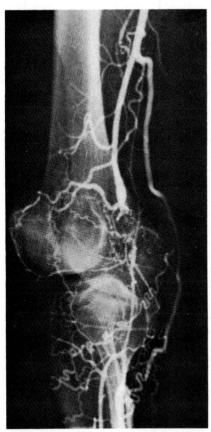

Figure 24–20. Collateral circulation can bypass a popliteal artery occlusion, as illustrated by this angiogram. (Strandness, D. E., Jr., and Bell, J. W., Ann. Surg., *161*(Suppl.):1, 1965.)

construction—a localized stenosis of the area of anastomosis, producing serious intermittent claudication—is shown in Figure 24–21. Reconstruction was successfully accomplished using an autogenous saphenous vein graft.

There are fewer statistics regarding the amputation rate in many civilian series. Brewer and associates (1969) described excellent results for treatment of simple popliteal artery perforations in 5 of 16 patients. In an additional five patients with more extensive injuries who would most likely otherwise have required an amputation, they felt that the results of their reconstructive procedures were gratifying. Extensive injuries from shotgun wounds led to amputations in two of their patients. Both had functioning vein grafts at the time of the amputations, and graft patency was demonstrated in one patient by an arteriogram seven days following injury (Fig. 24–22).

Ischemic time from injury to restoration of blood flow through the popliteal artery has been considered of varied importance. Brewer and associates (1969) found that 13 of the 16 patients in their series had established flow return within the first 12 hours. They did not feel that success or failure in their study correlated well with the ischemic time per se. These authors performed a successful vein interposition graft in a popliteal artery injured during a dislocation of the knee four days prior to the operation.

TABLE 24–8. POPLITEAL ARTERY REPAIR—CIVILIAN EXPERIENCE IN NASHVILLE*

Saphenous vein graft	10
End-to-end anastomosis	9
Lateral suture	2
Thrombectomy	2
Bovine graft	1
Teflon graft	1

There was one ligation and one primary amputation to complete the series of 27 injuries.

*Modified from Conkle, D. M., Richie, R. E., Sawyers, J. L., and Scott, H. W., Jr., Arch. Surg. *110*:1351, 1975. Copyright 1975, American Medical Association.

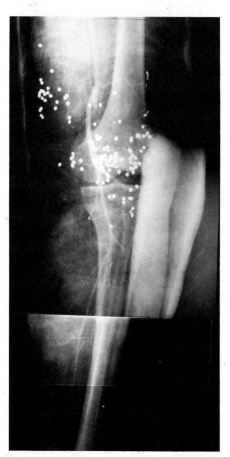

Figure 24–22. An arteriogram seven days after injury of the popliteal artery in a 20 year old patient with a shotgun wound. Vein bypass and tibial arteries were open, but amputation was necessary for extensive muscle necrosis. The "ischemic time" was 12 hours. The open graft remained through the 11 days until the above-the-knee amputation was required. (Brewer, P. L., Schramel, R. J., Menendez, C. V., and Creech, O., Jr., Am. J. Surg., *118*:36, 1969.)

In a report by Drapanas and associates (1970), nearly a 43 per cent amputation rate was found, with 6 out of a total of 14 popliteal artery injuries resulting in amputation. Conkle and associates (1975) used autogenous saphenous vein graft repairs and end-to-end anastomosis with nearly equal frequency in their Nashville experience (Table 24–8). Among the 15 successful procedures, 13 involved end-to-end anastomosis or saphenous vein grafts. Twelve of their 27 patients required amputations, for an amputation rate of about 44 per cent. They had better results with penetrating injuries (85 per cent, or 11 of 13) than with those caused by blunt trauma (29 per cent, or 4 of 14). All eight patients with associated long bone fractures, two of five with dislocations and all four with massive soft tissue damage required amputations. Nine of 20 popliteal veins were repaired, and seven of these nine were in salvaged limbs. Mattox (1975) reported an amputation rate of 23.5 per cent at Houston's Ben Taub Hospital among 65 patients with popliteal artery injuries. Hardy and co-workers (1975) used end-to-end anastomosis in the majority of their 19 popliteal arterial repairs—11 cases. They also used three saphenous vein grafts, two Teflon prostheses and one lateral repair. The two remaining cases in which ligation was used both resulted in amputation. Their overall amputation rate was about 30 per cent. Bole and co-workers (1976) had only one amputation among 12 patients with popliteal arterial trauma treated in New York City during 1968 to 1973. There was a pat-

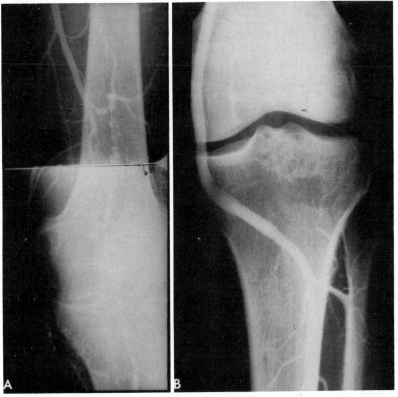

Figure 24–23. (A) Thrombosis of the popliteal artery with good collateral circulation around the knee and reconstitution of the distal popliteal artery. The patient had been wounded by a bullet in Algeria in 1957, and the severed popliteal artery was treated by "intubation" with a polyethylene catheter which remained patent for only 15 days. A clinically recognized thrombosis of the tube was confirmed 12 years later. (B) Successful vein bypass graft of the popliteal artery in 1969 gave the patient relief of his intermittent claudication. (Courtesy Le Professeur Agrege D. Rignault, Paris.)

ent vein graft bridging a popliteal arterial defect; however, amputation was required for sepsis.

Eger and colleagues (1971) proposed use of a temporary shunt to reduce ischemic time in the operating room. A year later these authors reported a series of 10 popliteal arterial injuries in their experience in Israel where the temporary shunt was used in which only one amputation was necessary—an amputation rate of 10 per cent. Rignault (1974) described the treatment of vascular injuries by "intubation" with a polyethylene catheter during the Algerian War in the late 1950's and early 1960's (Fig. 24–23). He noted that the amputation rate after intubation was about 41 per cent—5 amputations among 12 popliteal arterial injuries—compared to a higher amputation rate of nearly 70 per cent after attempted surgical repair of the popliteal artery.

Their current feeling was that intubation was "better than repair when done by surgeons non-trained in vascular surgery." Nevertheless, this situation is less likely to occur at the present time, and it is undoubtedly better to evacuate the patient to a definitive surgical center for arterial repair.

FOLLOW-UP

One late complication after reconstruction—a localized stenosis of the area of anastomosis, producing serious intermittent claudication—is shown in Figure 24–21. Reconstruction was successfully done with an autogenous saphenous vein graft. Successful repairs have been verified, however, in the follow-up through the Vietnam Vascular Registry (Fig. 24–24).

Brewer and associates (1969) reported some relatively long follow-up of their series. A patent interposed saphenous vein graft was demonstrated by arteriography in one patient 4½ years after injury (Fig. 24–25).

Trauma to the popliteal artery remains an enigma when management of these injuries is compared to that of other peripheral arterial injuries. Extensive tissue wounds with massive destruction of veins, nerves and bone have been contributing factors. Some enthusiastic inexperienced surgeons have attempted to reconstruct the arterial supply in a hopelessly damaged extremity. Acute venous insufficiency has contributed significantly to amputation rates in popliteal artery injuries. There is a need for both clinical and experimental evaluations to determine the incidence and relative importance of these factors.

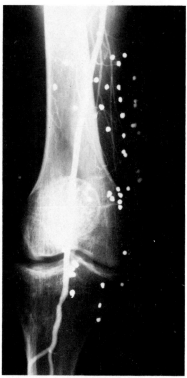

Figure 24–25. This angiogram demonstrates a patent interposed saphenous vein graft 4½ years after repair of the popliteal arterial injury. (Brewer, P. L., Schramel, R. J., Menendez, C. V., and Creech, O., Jr., Am. J. Surg., *118*:36, 1969.)

SPECIFIC PROBLEMS ASSOCIATED WITH POPLITEAL ARTERY INJURIES

1. Relatively high amputation rate.

2. Obtaining adequate debridement when the tendency might be to preserve more tissue than is indicated.

3. High failure rate associated with attempts to reconstitute the distal popliteal artery when the bifurcation has been involved.

4. Delayed recognition of a popliteal artery injury associated with a fracture or knee dislocation.

5. Acute venous insufficiency after successful popliteal artery reconstruction when irreparable damage to the popliteal and saphenous veins exist.

6. Associated unstable fractures.

7. Popliteal artery reconstruction despite massive soft tissue, osseous and nerve damage in the distal extremity.

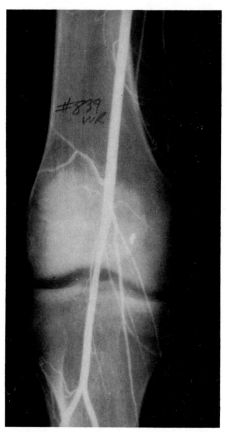

Figure 24–24. Angiography corroborated the clinical impression of a successful end-to-end anastomosis of the midpopliteal artery (offending fragment is adjacent to artery). Minimal narrowing was evident in this follow-up study 4½ months after repair. (Vietnam Vascular Registry #839, NMR.)

CHAPTER 25

ANTERIOR TIBIAL, POSTERIOR TIBIAL AND PERONEAL ARTERY INJURIES

Trauma to the anterior tibial, posterior tibial and peroneal arteries frequently has been overlooked or only given brief mention in numerous studies covering both military and civilian experience in managing acute arterial trauma. On the other hand, slightly more than one-fifth of the acute arterial injuries reported to DeBakey and Simeone (1946) in their World War II report of American casualties involved the tibial arteries (Table 25–1). In the majority of the civilian reports, the incidence has been approximately two to three per cent of all the acute arterial injuries.

TABLE 25–1. INCIDENCE OF TIBIAL ARTERY INJURIES*

	AUTHOR	TOTAL ARTERIES	TIBIAL	PER CENT
War Series				
WWI	Makins (1919)	1202	138	11.5
WW II	DeBakey and Simeone (1946)	2471	598	21.8
Koream	Hughes (1958)	304	–	–
Vietnam	Rich et al. (1970A)	1000	–	–
Civilian Series				
Houston	Morris et al. (1960)	220	5	2.3
Atlanta	Ferguson et al. (1961)	200	3	1.5
Denver	Owens (1963)	70	1	1.4
Detroit	Smith et al. (1963)	61	5	8.2
Dallas	Patman et al. (1964)	271	10	3.7
Los Angeles	Treiman et al. (1966)	159	–	–
St. Louis	Dillard et al. (1968)	85	–	–
New Orleans	Drapanas et al. (1970)	226	7	3.1
Dallas	Perry et al. (1971)†	508	12	2.4
Detroit	Smith et al. (1974)	127	5	3.9
Denver	Kelly and Eiseman (1975)	116	3	2.6
New York	Bole et al. (1976)	126	4	3.2

*Includes anterior tibial, posterior tibial and peroneal arteries.
† This is a sequential study including the earlier report by Patman et al., 1964.

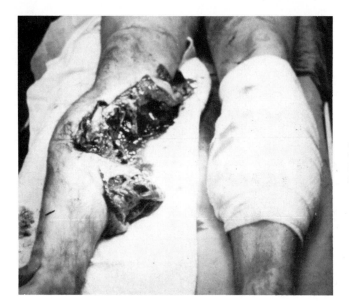

Figure 25–1. Massive soft tissue loss and comminuted fractures associated with tibial arterial trauma contribute to an increased amputation rate. (N.M.R., 2nd Surgical Hospital, 1966.)

Bernheim (1920) stated that, in his World War I experience, one vessel whose injury always gave trouble was the peroneal artery. He mentioned that it was remarkable how many times they found this injury, and that it was difficult to secure because of the position and the retraction of the artery.

Although any one of the three arteries frequently can be ligated independently without the development of significant distal ischemia, repair should be done when feasible. Hartsuck and colleagues (1972) emphasized the value of arterial reconstruction in five patients with injuries of the three major branches of the popliteal artery. On the other hand, if an amputation is required following tibial artery trauma, associated fractures and massive soft tissue destruction frequently are major contributing factors preventing limb salvage (Fig. 25–1).

SURGICAL ANATOMY

There is some controversy regarding the anatomy of the distal popliteal artery and its branches (see Chap. 24). A true trifurcation with the anterior tibial, posterior tibial and peroneal arteries all originating at the same level is unusual.

The anterior tibial artery commonly originates at the bifurcation of the popliteal, at the lower border of the popliteus muscle, and passes forward through the interosseous membrane between the tibia and fibula to the anterior surface of the leg (Fig. 25–2). In the upper portion it lies close to the medial side of the neck of the fibula. It descends on the anterior surface of the interosseous membrane in the direction of the tibia until, in its lower part, it lies on the tibia. It terminates on the front of the ankle joint, where it becomes more superficial and is named the dorsalis pedis artery. The anterior tibial artery courses its entire length through a relatively unyielding anterior compartment. It is covered in the upper two-thirds by muscles and fascia and in the lower third by skin, fascia and the transverse crural and cruciate ligaments. The anterior tibial artery is accompanied by a pair of venae comitantes. The deep peroneal nerve is lateral to the artery in the upper leg (Fig. 25–3).

The posterior tibial artery is usually the direct continuation of the popliteal beyond the origin of the anterior tibial at the lower border of the popliteus muscle. It extends downward in an oblique fashion until it lies behind the tibia. In its lower part it courses midway between the medial malleolus and the medial process of the calcaneal tuberosity and terminates by dividing into the medial and lateral plantar arteries (Fig. 25–2). It is covered throughout most of its course by the transverse fascia of the leg, which separates it from the gastrocnemius and soleus muscles. It is accompanied

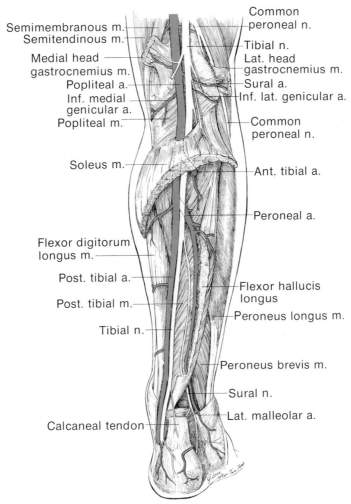

Semimembranous m.
Semitendinous m.
Medial head gastrocnemius m.
Popliteal a.
Inf. medial genicular a.
Popliteal m.
Soleus m.
Flexor digitorum longus m.
Post. tibial a.
Post. tibial m.
Tibial n.
Calcaneal tendon

Common peroneal n.
Tibial n.
Lat. head gastrocnemius m.
Sural a.
Inf. lat. genicular a.
Common peroneal n.
Ant. tibial a.
Peroneal a.
Flexor hallucis longus
Peroneus longus m.
Peroneus brevis m.
Sural n.
Lat. malleolar a.

Figure 25–2. Artist's conception of the distal popliteal artery and the origin of the anterior tibial, posterior tibial and peroneal trunks. Continuation of the anterior tibial artery after it passes through the interosseous membrane can be seen in Figure 25–3. The close proximity of the tibial nerve and its branches is emphasized.

by the posterior tibial nerve and by venae comitantes.

The peroneal artery usually originates from the posterior tibial artery at a variable distance below the origin of the anterior tibial (Fig. 25–2). It is the largest branch of the posterior tibial and usually arises about 2.5 cm below the origin of the posterior tibial. It runs downward in an oblique, lateral direction under the soleus muscle to the fibula, descends parallel to it, and emerges just above the ankle joint from beneath the flexor hallucis longus muscle. Distally it passes behind the inferior tibiofibular joint and terminates in a number of

lateral calcanean branches. It is accompanied by venae comitantes. According to Strandness (1969), many of the possible variations in the peroneal artery can easily be explained if this artery is regarded as the terminal branch of the popliteal artery with the tibial arteries as side branches.

The collateral circulation involving the three arteries is important. First, there is a reciprocal relationship at the ankle level, where the peroneal artery may produce the dorsalis pedis artery via a large perforating branch or may replace the lower posterior tibial artery through a communicating branch. Both the anterior and posterior

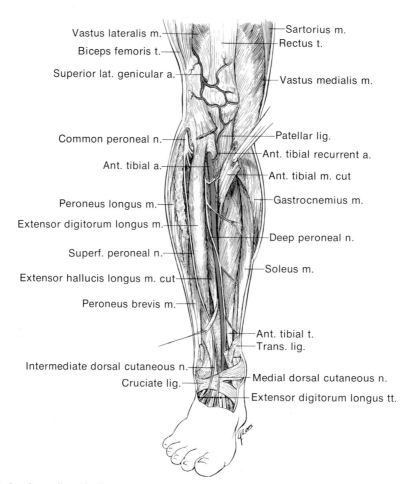

Figure 25–3. As outlined in Figure 25–2, the anterior continuation of the anterior tibial artery after it perforates the interosseous membrane is shown. On the dorsum of the foot, this artery becomes the dorsalis pedis artery. There is an important structure, the deep peroneal nerve, which is in close proximity to the distal two-thirds of the anterior tibial artery.

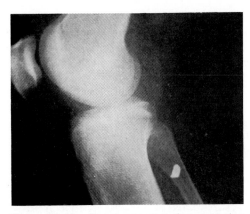

Figure 25–10. Roentgenogram demonstrating a bullet which embolized after the patient sustained a gunshot wound of the chest, with penetration of the descending aorta. Because the patient developed a cold, pulseless right leg, exploration was carried out, and the bullet was found in the proximal posterior tibial artery. (Thomas, T. V., Surg. Gynecol. Obstet., *125*:997, 1967.)

tibial and the peroneal arteries. It is frequently possible to distinguish between collateral flow and direct flow through a patent proximal tibial artery.

SURGICAL TREATMENT

Hemorrhage can be controlled by pressure in the majority of tibial artery injuries. Tourniquets are usually not warranted because the potential complications from their use outweigh any advantage. Fractures must be stabilized, adequate débridement performed and the usual supportive measures instituted.

Proximal arterial control can be obtained through a posterior approach, similar to that used in approaching the popliteal artery, by extending the incision distally between the gastrocnemius heads into the body of the soleus muscle (Fig. 25–11). A medial approach can also be used to expose the origin of the three vessels, making a longitudinal incision medial to the tibia similar to that used in femoropopliteal reconstruction for occlusive disease of the distal popliteal artery.

The posterior tibial and peroneal arteries can be followed distally once they are identified through either of these two approaches. Lower in the leg, it is possible to expose the posterior tibial artery beneath

the skin adjacent to the medial malleolus, and the artery can then be traced proximally. Similar approaches can be used at the ankle level for the anterior tibial and peroneal arteries. Because the anterior tibial artery lies anterior to the interosseous membrane, the greater length of this artery should be approached through a longitudinal incision over the anterior compartment or through the bed of the fibula, particularly if the fibula is removed at the time of fasciotomy.

Because of the small size of the anterior tibial, posterior tibial and peroneal arteries,

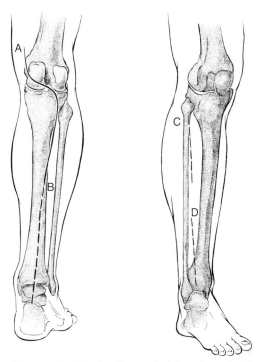

Figure 25–11. An S-type incision through the popliteal fossa can be utilized to expose the distal popliteal, the origin of the anterior tibial and the origin of the posterior tibial and peroneal arteries (A). Additional details concerning the popliteal artery can be found in Chapter 24. A continuation of this incision, splitting the middle of the body of the soleus muscle, can provide distal exposure of the posterior tibial and peroneal arteries (B). At the ankle level, a separate incision can be made over the distal posterior tibial artery just above and posterior to the medial malleolus. Separate incisions can be made for exposure of the anterior tibial artery after it passes through the interosseous membrane for the more proximal portion (C) or for the more distal segment of the artery (D). In specific situations, removal of a portion or all of the fibula may expedite adequate exposure of the anterior tibial artery.

reconstruction is frequently not feasible with extensive injuries. However, if there is a small laceration or defect, end-to-end anastomosis may be performed easily and successfully. If time and the patient's condition will permit, reconstruction with a saphenous vein graft should be considered. A portion of the distal saphenous vein may be selected at the knee level or below to match the size of the tibial vessels. If more than one of the three arteries has been injured and it is necessary to ligate one or two, then greater effort must be made to repair the remaining one or two arteries. Presently there is no place for prosthetic material in repairing these small vessels. Whether small vein patches are used in repairs is a matter of preference, but end-to-end anastomoses are usually acceptable (Fig. 25–12).

As recently as 1965, O'Neill and Killen emphasized that little attention had been given to small vessel repair, such as that of the posterior tibial artery, which might determine limb loss or salvage. They described the case of a 41 year old male with an accidental self-inflicted gunshot wound of the lower extremity which disrupted the posterior tibial artery. The arterial defect was successfully replaced with an 8-cm length of autogenous greater saphenous vein (Fig. 25–13). Heparinization during the operation and the administration of antibiotics are important adjuncts in the management. Hartsuck and colleagues (1972) emphasized the value of placing the anastomoses of the vein bypass graft, through separate incisions if necessary, above and below the site of arterial injury when performing tibial artery repairs in contaminated wounds with soft tissue loss. In a tibial artery repair, either by end-to-end anastomosis or by autogenous vein graft repair, the repair must be covered with viable soft tissue, preferably viable muscle.

An aggressive approach should be utilized in managing fractures that are associated with large hematomas or distal ischemia. Reluctance to explore the tibial arteries may result in amputation.

Fasciotomy often will be accomplished at the time of exploration of the tibial arteries. Adequate fasciotomy is frequently necessary, particularly when there is associated venous injury and delay in the repair. Concomitant venous injuries should be repaired whenever possible. This is particularly important if a lateral venous repair can be accomplished, because the incidence of patency is highest following this type of repair. Great care should be taken to preserve the ipsilateral superficial venous system, particularly if it is necessary to ligate concomitant injuries of the deep venous system.

Cohen and associates (1969) emphasized

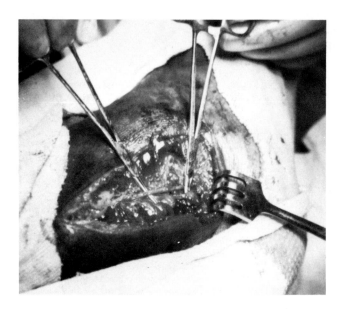

Figure 25–12. Repair of tibial arteries should be accomplished when possible, particularly when more than one of the three arteries is traumatized and when the injury occurs in the larger, proximal portion. This operative photograph shows a successful end-to-end anastomosis of the distal posterior tibial artery at the ankle. (N.M.R., 2nd Surgical Hospital, 1966.)

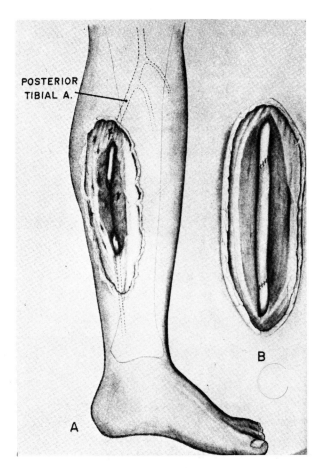

Figure 25–13. Artist's conception of the extent of a shotgun blast injury of the lower extremity (A). Reconstruction of the posterior tibial artery using an autogenous saphenous vein graft was possible (B). (O'Neill, J. A., and Killen, D. A., Ann. Surg., *162*:218, 1965.)

the problem of small vessel injuries associated with calf wounds. They presented the case of a 21 year old helicopter pilot who sustained multiple fragments from a rocket-propelled grenade in Vietnam. The right lower extremity had 10 to 15 small fragment wounds. Repair of both the superficial femoral artery and vein was accomplished but the calf was not explored. There was a dorsalis pedis pulse but no posterior tibial pulse. On the fifth postoperative day, there was hemorrhage of approximately 500 ml of blood from the calf. The patient was returned to the operating room and the posterior calf was explored. The posterior tibial artery was found to be divided and bleeding into the muscle. The artery was ligated and the limb continued to be viable. This is a good example of delayed hemorrhage from unsuspected and overlooked arterial disruption below the popliteal artery. Although ligation was selected in this case, in the absence of infection repair may be indicated.

Intraoperative angiography can be of value in determining distal patency following tibial artery repair and should be available.

POSTOPERATIVE CARE

The supportive measurements usual for the patient with lower extremity injury are important. Particular attention should be given to the development of any edema or to any change in the neurologic status of the lower extremity. If fasciotomies were not performed at operation, it may be necessary to perform them in the early postoperative period.

The ultrasonic sounding device (Doppler) can be quite valuable in determining the flow distal to the repair of any of these three arteries. In most situations this would preclude the necessity for performing postoperative angiograms. These adjunctive measures are only supportive in the early

TABLE 25–2. INCIDENCE OF LOSS OF LIMB WITH LIGATION FOLLOWING INJURY OF THE POSTERIOR TIBIAL ARTERY*

REFERENCE	DATE	INJURY POST. TIBIAL ARTERY ALONE		INJURY POST. AND ANT. TIBIAL ARTERIES	
		Cases	Amputations	Cases	Amputations
Makins	1919	97	9	7	2
Bradford et al.	1946	–	–	8	7
DeBakey and Simeone	1946	265	36	92	64
Smith	1947	7†	4	5	2
Jahnke and Seeley	1953	9	3	3	0
Ziperman	1954	20	4	4	2
Total		398	56 (14.1%)	119	77 (64.7%)

*Adapted from O'Neill, J. A., Jr., and Killen, D. A., Ann. Surg., *162*:218, 1965.
†Includes only patients with injury of upper portion of posterior tibial artery.

postoperative period when clinical evaluation of viability of the extremity is most important.

As with other peripheral arterial injuries, when there is an absence of infection, delayed primary closure of the wound four to seven days later is frequently possible.

COMPLICATIONS

Thrombosis of the relatively small repaired artery is frequent. Although the statistics remain incomplete from our own experience in the Vietnam Vascular Registry and Clinic, the clinical impression of repair thrombosis often has been made in follow-up. If thrombosis involves only one injured artery and two other arteries are patent, the significance is unimportant and often probably not recognized.

Other complications include infection and possible disruption of the suture line with resultant hemorrhage. Particularly in a contaminated wound, ligation of the artery would be the safest approach in managing this problem.

RESULTS

In the World War II series, DeBakey and Simeone (1946) reported an amputation rate of 13.5 per cent after posterior tibial artery ligation, 8.5 per cent after anterior tibial artery ligation and 69.3 per cent after ligation of both tibial branches. According to a review in 1965 by O'Neill and Killen,

from previous war experience, there was an average amputation of 14 per cent following ligation of the posterior tibial artery (Table 25–2). The amputation rate was greatly increased to approximately 65 per cent following ligation of both anterior and posterior tibial arteries. These authors emphasized that there was no information concerning morbidity in limbs which survived posterior tibial ligation either alone or combined with anterior tibial ligation.

Although the statistics from Vietnam remain incomplete in the Registry, nearly one-fourth of the anterior tibial artery injuries were repaired (Table 25–3). There were a total of 151 repairs among 670 injuries in which identification of the method of management was possible, which represented a repair rate of 22.5 per cent. Slightly more than three-fourths of all the injuries were ligated. Because there are 1107 tibial artery injuries that have been documented in the Registry, with the possibility that there will even be a small increase in this total number as the statistics from the Registry are completed, the total experience is not yet available.

TABLE 25–3. TIBIAL ARTERY TRAUMA*

ARTERY	TOTAL	REPAIR	LIGATED
Posterior Tibial	415	90 (21.7%)	325 (78.3%)
Anterior Tibial	218	53 (24.3%)	165 (75.7%)
Peroneal	37	8 (21.6%)	29 (78.4%)
Total	670	151 (22.5%)	519 (77.5%)

*These are incomplete statistics from the Vietnam Vascular Registry representing 60.5 per cent of 1107 tibial artery injuries which have been documented.

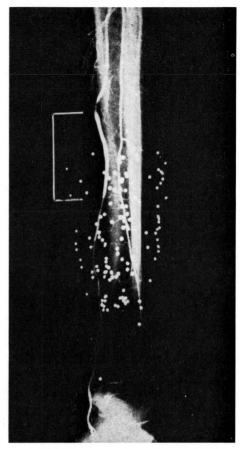

Figure 25–14. This postoperative angiogram, taken 78 days after an autogenous saphenous vein graft repair of the posterior tibial artery, demonstrates patency of the vein graft indicated by the bracket (see Fig. 25–13). (O'Neill, J. A., and Killen, D. A., Ann. Surg., *162*:218, 1965.)

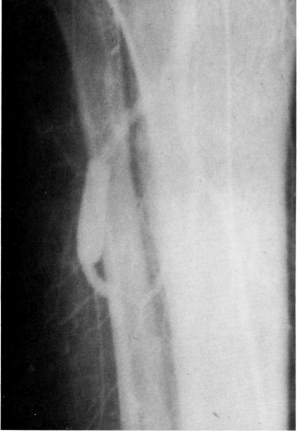

Figure 25–15. This postoperative angiogram demonstrates a disparity in size of the autogenous greater saphenous vein graft used to repair the anterior tibial artery. The ultimate fate of this repair in the long term follow-up is of particular interest. (Vietnam Vascular Registry.)

Smith and co-authors (1963) reported that one of the only two amputations occurring in their civilian experience involved both the anterior and posterior tibial vessels. Among 18 instances of ligation of radial, ulnar and tibial arteries in their series of 136 arterial injuries reported from Houston prior to July 31, 1956, by Morris and co-workers (1957), there were only two amputations, one of which followed ligation of one posterior tibial artery.

Ortner and colleagues (1961) recommended further efforts to repair small vessel injuries in an attempt to improve limb salvage. They cited the fact that Jahnke and Seeley noted from the Korean experience in 1953 that there was an amputation rate of 11.6 per cent for 43 injuries of minor vessels, which was higher than the amputation rate for several major arterial injuries.

Hartsuck and colleagues (1972) reported five tibial artery repairs; in four an autogenous saphenous vein was used, while in one end-to-end anastomosis was used. Two of their patients had good long term function without edema when it was possible to preserve the ipsilateral saphenous vein, even though the deep venous system was ligated. On the other hand, they found edema a prominent feature when deep venous interruption was associated with an ischemic time greater than five hours.

FOLLOW-UP

In a late evaluation of the patient with a shotgun blast of the lower extremity described earlier in this chapter (Fig. 25–13), O'Neill and Killen (1965) found the vein graft patent on angiography 2½ months later (Fig. 25–14). In a personal communication from these authors, it was learned that a strong pulse remained distal to the repair site seven years later.

In the Peripheral Vascular Surgery Clinic at Walter Reed General Hospital, numerous asymptomatic patients have been seen who have had ligation of one of the tibial arteries. Ankle pressures and plethysmographic tracings frequently have been unaltered by the division of one of the three branches. Although routine angiographic studies have not been done in the postoperative period, the discrepancy in size of one greater saphenous vein graft used to repair an anterior tibial artery can be demonstrated in Figure 25–15. Long term changes in this graft will be of particular interest.

CHAPTER 26

REFLECTIONS AND PROJECTIONS

We should not rest content with the work of our predecessors, or assume that it has proved everything conclusively; on the contrary it should serve only as a stimulus to further investigation.

Ambroise Paré

This quote from the translated review by Billroth on studies on the nature and treatment of gunshot wounds emphasizes the historical development and current status of vascular surgery. While some might say that all the principles of vascular surgery are established and accepted by the vast majority of surgeons, we must not lose sight of the need for continued analysis of results and continued investigation to solve the problems that remain.

Problems do remain. As a prime example, the "ideal conduit" still has not been discovered. A substitute conduit for both the arterial and venous systems is greatly needed. A conduit of varied size in diameter and length that would be an acceptable biologic substitute will always be needed in the repair of traumatized arteries and veins. While some might argue that the ravages of atherosclerosis can be greatly helped by drug therapy and other conservative medical regimens in the foreseeable future, the increasing incidence of injured arteries and veins, in civil life as well as on the battlefield, accentuates the importance of the need for a substitute vascular conduit. Many materials have been investigated, both clinically and under laboratory conditions. At Walter

Reed Army Institute of Research, an assortment of grafts and prostheses has been utilized in the venous system without universal success. The problem remains more significant in the repair of injured veins than of injured arteries.

Considering that the Nobel Prize in Medicine was awarded to Carrel in 1912 based in part on his contributions to vascular surgery, including the reconstruction of arteries and veins, this might be an additional stimulus to the serious investigator in search of the "ideal conduit." A major factor in this remaining problem in vascular surgery has been the obvious paucity of long term follow-up studies of vascular repairs.

The importance of long term follow-up of patients with vascular injuries cannot be overemphasized. This would be true of both patients who have had successful repair and those in whom repair failed or was not possible. In the former group, periodic evaluation of the function of the repair should be carried out. There is early documentation of the value of providing details of vascular cases with appropriate follow-up information. Although arterial aneurysms previously had been treated by proximal ligation, excision, or the Matas

563

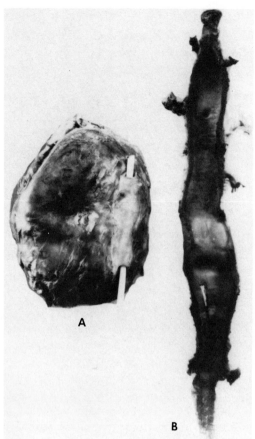

Figure 26–1. The value of adequate documentation and follow-up of vascular cases was demonstrated early by Pringle. (A) An excised popliteal aneurysm is shown, and (B) the vein graft specimen obtained years later at post mortem. Pringle reported his work in 1913, when he modified the method of Carrel and Guthrie in excising an aneurysm of the popliteal artery by re-establishing continuity with an autogenous saphenous vein graft. (Photograph obtained from and used with permission of the Royal College of Surgeons of Edinburgh.)

repair from within the sac, Pringle (1913) developed a modification of the method used by Carrel and Guthrie in excising an aneurysm of the popliteal artery and re-establishing continuity with an autogenous saphenous vein graft. Both the resected popliteal aneurysm and the vein graft specimen were obtained years later post mortem, and the findings are shown in Figure 26–1.

Goodman (1918), in describing his experience at the No. 1 (Presbyterian U.S.A.) General Hospital in France during World War I, reported a successful closure with continuous silk suture of 5 mm longitudinal openings in both the popliteal artery and vein in one patient with a shell fragment. However, the patient was followed for only nine days before being transferred to the Base Hospital. Goodman reported: "An attempt to obtain further information covering the case is now underway and will be embodied in a subsequent report." If there was any further follow-up information obtained or reported, it became obscured in the available literature. At least this military surgeon recognized the importance of obtaining long term follow-up information to thoroughly evaluate his method of managing vascular trauma.

In the classic report by DeBakey and Simeone (1946) from the American experience in World War II, early patency of a venous graft in the arterial system was demonstrated angiographically (Fig. 26–2). Although considerable time and effort were expended following World War II in an attempt to provide additional long term follow-up information, the results of this effort are not generally available. Individual follow-up has been possible in a random way for some patients, such as in the case of an acute, femoral arteriovenous fistula that was repaired shortly after D-Day in Normandy on June 16, 1944 (Boyden, 1970). This was an unusual case because it involved the successful repair of both the common femoral artery and the common femoral vein in a combat zone at a time when ligation of vascular injuries was the accepted principle. Unfortunately, when it was possible more than 26 years later to obtain follow-up data on this patient, it was learned that hemorrhage occurred in the left inguinal wound after the patient was evacuated to a General Hospital in England. Ligation of both the common femoral artery and the common femoral vein was required. Additional follow-up was not possible because the patient died of tuberculosis approximately 16 months after receiving the wound.

The importance of a well-documented past medical history covering previous vascular trauma was emphasized in the long term follow-up of a 50 year old former United States Army officer who entered the Peripheral Vascular Surgery Clinic at Walter Reed General Hospital for evalua-

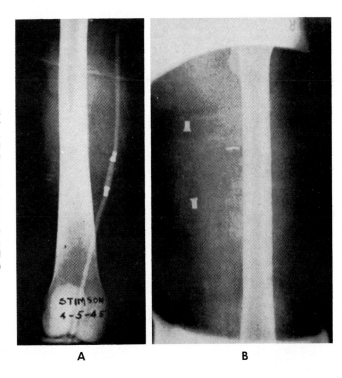

Figure 26–2. (A) This arteriogram was performed three and one-half weeks after a nonsuture anastomosis of the superficial femoral artery. There is patency of the anastomosis and no evidence of undue ballooning of the vein segment. The operation was performed at the 8th Evacuation Hospital during World War II. (B) This roentgenogram of a successful nonsuture anastomosis of the superficial femoral artery shows the extent of the defect bridged by the position of the Vitallium tubes. (DeBakey, M. E., and Simeone, F. A., Ann. Surg., *123*:534, 1946.)

A   B

tion to rule out cerebrovascular ischemia. The patient had complained of several episodes of visual disturbance and weakness of his left hand during the past year. The patient knew that he had had a ligation of "some of the arteries in his neck" during World War II. An angiogram of the aortic arch and its major branches was obtained to determine the amount of arterial flow to the brain. This study demonstrated no identifiable right common carotid artery or its branches, and there was no late retrograde filling of the right internal carotid artery. A copy of part of his old military medical records was finally obtained and it was revealed that he had sustained a fragment wound of the right side of the neck on January 19, 1945 on Saipan when an ammunition dump exploded. Although only debridement was necessary at first, approximately six months later ligation of the right common internal and external carotid arteries was necessary. In subsequent follow-up through the Vascular Clinic, the patient has had no significant problems.

Murray (1952) stated approximately 25 years ago that the fate of venous grafts in the arterial system had been under considerable discussion. However, he felt that these venous grafts would continue to function without complications for a long period of time. He reported that he had removed a venous graft that had functioned in the carotid artery of a dog for nine years. Although the graft was slightly larger than the adjacent artery and there was some arteriosclerotic change in one area, it continued to function well. There are some reports of good results without aneurysmal formation in utilizing an adjacent vein, such as the femoral vein next to the common femoral artery as documented by Murray (1952), but the greater saphenous vein still appears to be the best arterial substitute present at this time, particularly for major arteries of the extremities.

The outstanding documentation of the American experience during the Korean Conflict by Hughes, Jahnke, Spencer and others has provided an opportunity for long term follow-up. Figure 26–3 is an angiogram of a patient followed up after 19 years with a patent interposition greater saphenous vein in the proximal right superficial femoral artery. The establishment of a Vascular Registry and Blood Flow Laboratory at Walter Reed General Hospital in 1966 has provided an opportunity for long term follow-up of former combat casualties

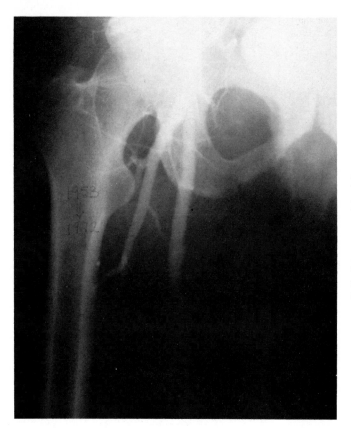

Figure 26–3. This long term follow-up femoral angiogram demonstrates patency of an interposition autogenous greater saphenous vein used to repair the proximal right superficial femoral artery. The follow-up period extended from 1953 until the patient was evaluated at Walter Reed General Hospital in 1972 (19 years). This is one of the longest known follow-ups and represents the continued effort to provide this type of data for former combat casualties from the Korean Conflict. (NMR, W.R.G.H., 1972.)

who sustained vascular injuries. In the early efforts of the Vietnam Vascular Registry, the problems of obtaining long term follow-up of patients who had vascular injuries in Vietnam were illustrated by an attempt to follow those listed in Fisher's report (1967) of 108 vascular injuries. After an intensive investigation at the time of organization of statistics for the preliminary report for the Vietnam Vascular Registry, which was more than two years after Fisher's data was given to the Registry, it was possible to find only 60 of his patients whose postoperative period and convalescence could be completely evaluated. This represents slightly more than 50 per cent of the patients of the original study. In subsequent years, however, the long term follow-up percentage has continued to improve.

What is the long term fate of the autogenous greater saphenous vein used as an interposed segmental graft in the arterial system? Most surgeons continue to believe that the long term patency is excellent. However, few recognize the development of aneurysmal changes in these grafts. The

long term follow-up effort in the Vietnam Vascular Registry has continued to demonstrate an increasing number of patients with these changes. The true significance and the actual percentage of these changes remain unknown. This does, however, emphasize the great need for continued long term follow-up studies. This complication of fusiform aneurysmal dilatation of an autogenous greater saphenous interposition segment used for repair of an injured artery was first brought to our attention by Carrasquilla and Weaver (1972) when they reported on the follow-up of a 22 year old Marine who had originally been wounded and treated in Vietnam. Figure 26–4 demonstrates the findings. With the accumulation of approximately 150 follow-up angiograms of Vietnam casualties, with the range in time from months to years, the number of recognized aneurysmal dilatation of these venous interposition grafts is in the range of 6 per cent.

It is often not practical or economically feasible to routinely obtain follow-up angiograms, particularly in asymptomatic pa-

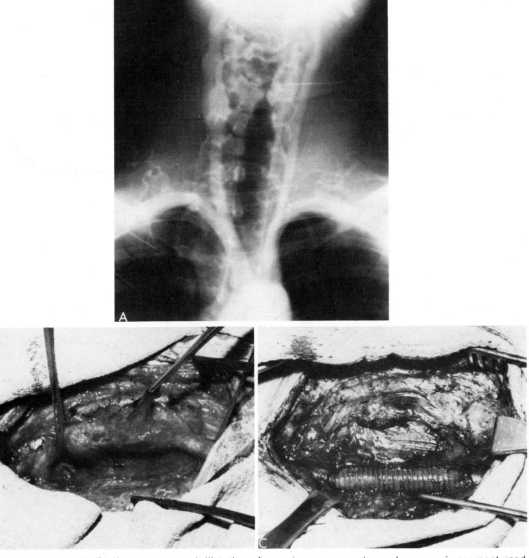

Figure 26–4. (A) Fusiform aneurysmal dilatation of an autogenous greater saphenous vein segment used as an interposition graft in the right common carotid artery of a Vietnam casualty is demonstrated angiographically. (B) The operative photograph demonstrates the dilated segment of saphenous vein. (C) Arterial reconstruction was completed with a Dacron prosthesis. (Carrasquilla, C., and Weaver, A. W., Vasc. Surg., 6:66, 1972.)

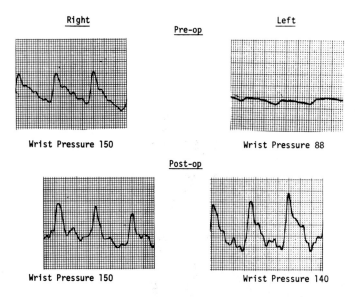

Right   Left

Pre-op

Wrist Pressure 150   Wrist Pressure 88

Post-op

Wrist Pressure 150   Wrist Pressure 140

Figure 26–5. The long term follow-up through the Vietnam Vascular Registry includes the recording of wrist pressures and Doppler ultrasonic tracings. The two tracings at the top show the comparison of the right side and the abnormal left side, where occlusion of the repair of the left brachial artery with a saphenous vein graft had occurred in 1969. The two lower tracings show the change after reconstruction of the left brachial artery with a new segment of autogenous greater saphenous vein. There is considerable improvement in the wrist pressure and Doppler tracing on the left. (NMR, W.R.G.H., 1973.)

tients. The long term follow-up through the Vietnam Vascular Registry relies to a great extent on the noninvasive approach through the Blood Flow Laboratory. Figure 26–5 demonstrates this type of follow-up, utilizing the measurement of wrist pressures and obtaining tracings with the Doppler ultrasound method. Unfortunately, aneurysmal changes in venous grafts in the arterial system cannot be detected in this manner. B-mode ultrasonography has been tested to augment this information; however, data remains fragmentary and unsatisfactory.

The continued challenge that remains in the management of patients with vascular injuries is exemplified by the questions and problems involving the search for the "ideal conduit" for segmental replacement of injured arteries and veins. There are also many other aspects of the management of injured patients with vascular injuries that could be expanded. The management of concomitant fractures associated with vascular injuries, the use of fasciotomy in extremities with vascular injuries, and other associated considerations are among these factors. Moreover, there are a multitude of professional challenges that exist in unusual situations involving vascular trauma. The following is cited as an example. Kapp and colleagues (1973) stated that they could find only four cases of intravascular metallic fragment embolization to the cerebral circulation. To their surgical review they

added the report of two patients who were treated by the 24th Evacuation Hospital in the Republic of South Vietnam. Because of the unusual problem, some details of one of these cases follow:

A 19 year old American soldier received a fragment wound of the right side of the neck from a grenade explosion, associated with immediate onset of weakness of the left side of his body. An exploration of his neck was carried out and showed no evidence of vascular trauma. Three days after wounding, the patient was transferred to the 24th Evacuation Hospital where he showed slight improvement of his left-sided weakness.

Roentgenograms of the skull showed a small, jagged, metallic fragment, and an arteriogram revealed that the fragment was lodged at the origin of the middle cerebral artery, completely occluding the middle cerebral artery and projecting into the carotid artery (Fig. 26–6).

It was also thought that there was thrombus formation around the fragment. Six days following injury, the right internal carotid artery, the anterior cerebral artery and the middle cerebral artery were exposed through a right frontotemporal craniotomy. After applying temporary vascular clamps, the fragment was removed without difficulty through a longitudinal arteriotomy in the internal carotid artery. A thrombus was also extracted from the middle cerebral artery. An arteriorrhaphy was performed, with some initial spasm at the repair site. In the postoperative period the patient's neurologic status improved. An arteriogram performed on the 25th postoperative

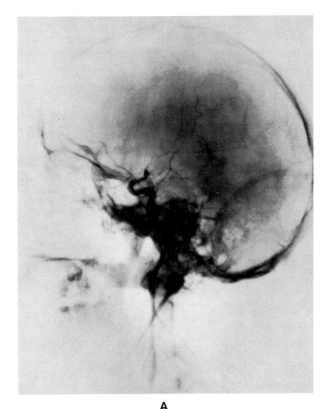

A

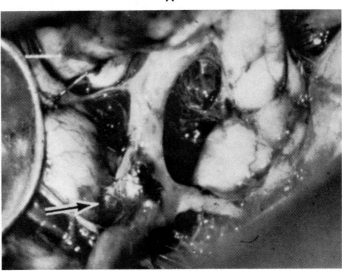

B

Figure 26–6. (A) Reports of migration of intravascular metallic fragments have been rare. This right caro-tid angiogram demonstrates an intra-arterial metal fragment at the intracranial bifurcation of the carotid artery in a 19 year old soldier who received a fragment wound on the right side of the neck from a grenade explosion. (B) This operative photograph taken at the 24th Evacuation Hospital in Vietnam shows an intra-arterial fragment with extreme thinning of the wall of the artery overlying the fragment at the origin of the middle cerebral artery. (Kapp, J. P., Gielchinsky, I., and Jelsma, R., J. Trauma, *13*:256, 1973.)

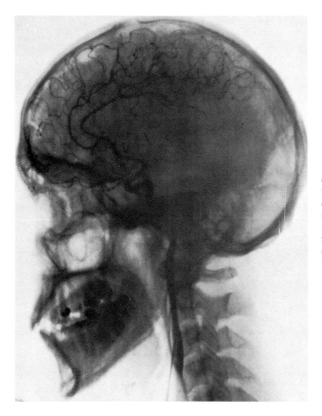

Figure 26–7. This angiogram performed 25 days after removal of the intra-arterial metallic fragment shown in Figure 26–6A and B demonstrates patency of the carotid artery, a patent anterior cerebral artery that is larger than normal, and thrombosis of the origin of the middle cerebral artery. (Kapp, J. P., Gielchinsky, I., and Jelsma, R., J. Trauma, *13*:256, 1973.)

day revealed that the carotid artery was patent and without stenosis or aneurysmal formation (Fig. 26–7). The middle cerebral artery was thrombosed at its origin, but its branches filled readily via collateral channels with a large patent right anterior cerebral artery.

These authors outlined the possible problems that might occur when a metallic fragment lodges in a cerebral vessel:

1. Neurologic defect secondary to arterial occlusion and infarction.

2. Proximal and distal propagation of thrombus, which could extend the infarcted area.

3. Erosion with hemorrhage.

4. Infection, arteritis, and then abscess formation or meningitis.

5. Infection with mycotic aneurysm formation and probable subsequent rupture.

They emphasized that one of their main concerns was the possibility of erosion through the small, thin-walled artery caused by pulsatile motion of the fragment. They also stressed the importance of maintaining a high index of suspicion in patients with neurologic symptoms who have wounds of the neck and chest.

International exchange of information is important in the treatment of patients with vascular trauma. In some parts of the world, specific vascular injuries are seen infrequently. Occasionally, the etiology of the vascular trauma, such as avulsion of the femoral vessels by a bull's horn in the bullring in Mexico or in Spain, may be unique to a certain region or country. Nevertheless, the common goal of all surgeons to provide the best medical care possible creates a desirable situation for exchange of data and experience among surgeons in all parts of the world who have an interest in the management of vascular injuries. Language difficulties can often be overcome through personal exchange and translation of scientific articles. An example of this is the personal exchange that took place with Dr. Peter Maurer in Munich in 1973. Mack, Sherer and Maurer (1973) described the treatment of 154 patients with vascular injuries in Munich between January 1965 and December 1971. They found

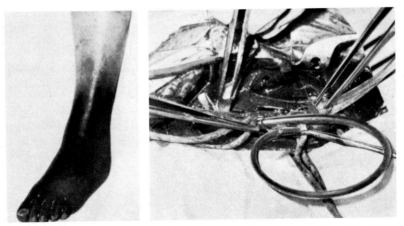

Figure 26–8. Temporary intraluminal arterial shunts have been used in Munich, Germany, as shown above, to reduce the ischemic time, to diminish thrombosis in the peripheral venous system, and to allow repair of concomitant lacerated veins for major arterial repair. This use of the temporary intraluminal arterial shunt in the management of acute arterial injuries is somewhat unique in that it was not documented in the United States during the same time period between 1965 and 1971). (Mack, D., Scherer, H., and Maurer, P., Mschr. Unfallheilk., 76:217, 1973.)

that 80 per cent or 129 of their patients had suffered additional trauma, including fractures, trauma to the head, and rupture of abdominal organs. Also, 60 per cent of their patients had had vascular injuries in association with concomitant fractures. They found angiography to be of great value in diagnosing the vascular injury. One relatively unique aspect of their management, in contrast to the management of arterial injuries in the United States during the same time period, was re-establishing arterial flow by temporary intraluminal shunts (Fig. 26–8). They felt that this reduced ischemic time, diminished thrombosis in the peripheral venous system and allowed repair of lacerated veins before arterial repair was instituted. They were successful in restoring circulation in 75.8 per cent of their patients; 12.6 per cent showed remaining symptoms secondary to complications associated with vascular injuries, and their amputation rate was 4.2 per cent.

Recently in the United States, Weinstein and Golding utilized temporary external silastic arterial and venous shunts in replanting a traumatically amputated upper extremity in a ten year old boy who was involved in an automobile accident (Fig. 26–9). The level of the incomplete traumatic amputation was at the upper third of the arm, with only a posterior skin bridge intact. These authors emphasized that early

arterial perfusion decreased the total anoxic time. The challenge persists with unusual and complex injuries such as this, and the varied and unique additions to the surgeon's armamentarium that might assist in obtaining satisfactory results should be known and understood.

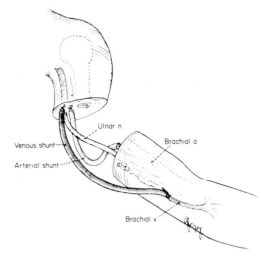

Figure 26–9. This diagrammatic drawing demonstrates the use of temporary external silastic arterial and venous shunts during replantation of a traumatically amputated upper extremity in a ten year old boy involved in an automobile accident. The shunts, which were 20 cm long and 2.5 mm in internal diameter, reduced the anoxic time during replantation of the upper extremity. (Weinstein, M. H. and Golding, A. L., J. Trauma, 15:912, 1975.)

The following quote by Carleton Math-ewson, Jr. (1956) in the discussion of the paper by Morris and associates (1957) is most apropos:

Unfortunately in many quarters these lessons so well emphasized during the stress of world conflict have been neglected in the complacency of civilian life. It is important, therefore, that we reemphasize the seriousness of vascular injury and, where possible, stress the favorable circum-stances that present themselves in civilian life with the successful primary repair of injured vessels.

We would be remiss if we did not gain something positive from an experience with as many negative aspects as the American involvement in Southeast Asia between 1965 and 1972. The Vietnam Vascular Registry provides a unique opportunity for long term follow-up of thousands of young men with vascular repairs. The challenge remains and the potential is great.

REFERENCES

Abbe, R.: The Surgery of the Hand. N.Y. Med. J., Jan. 13, 1894.

Abbott, W. M., and Darling, R. C.: Axillary Artery Aneurysms Secondary to Crutch Trauma. Am. J. Surg., *125*:515, 1973.

Agnew, D., II: The Principles and Practice of Surgery. H. P. Lippincott and Company, Philadelphia, 1878.

Allen, T. W., Reul, G. J., Morton, J. R., and Beall, A. C., Jr.: Surgical Management of Aortic Trauma. J. Trauma, *12*:862, 1972.

Amato, J. J., Vanecko, R. M., Yao, S. T., and Weinberg, M., Jr.: Emergency Approach to the Subclavian and Innominate Vessels. Ann. Thorac. Surg., *8*:537, 1969.

Amato, J. J., Billy, L. J., Gruber, R. P., Lawson, N. S., and Rich, N. M.: Vascular Injuries: An Experimental Study of High and Low Velocity Missile Wounds. Arch. Surg., *101*:167, 1970.

Amato, J. J., Rich, N. M., Billy, L. J., Gruber, R. P., and Lawson, N. S.: High Velocity Arterial Injury: A Study of the Mechanism of Injury. J. Trauma, *11*:412, 1971.

Amato, J. J., and Rich, N. M.: Temporary Cavity Effect in Blood Vessel Injury by High Velocity Missiles. J. Cardiovasc. Surg., *13*:147, 1972.

Amato, J. J., Billy, L. J., Lawson, N. S., and Rich, N. M.: High Velocity Missile Injury. An Experimental Study of the Retentive Forces of Tissue. Am. J. Surg., *127*:454, 1974.

Amine, A. R. C., and Sugar, O.: Repair of Severed Brachial Plexus: A Plea to Emergency Room Physicians. J.A.M.A., *235*:1039, 1976.

Annandale, T.: Traumatic Popliteal Arterio-venous Aneurism Treated Successfully by Ligature of the Popliteal Artery and Vein. Lancet, *1*:568, 1875.

Anthopoulos, L. P., Johnson, J. B., and Spellman, M.: Arteriovenous Fistula in Multiple Saccular Arterial Aneurysms of a Finger, Following Childhood Human Bite. Angiology, *16*:89, 1965.

Antyllus: Oribasius *4*:52 (Daremberg Edition). Cited by Osler in Lancet, *1*:949, 1915.

Archambault, R., Archambault, H. A., and Mizeres, N. J.: Rupture of the Thoroacromial Artery and Anterior Dislocation of the Shoulder. Am. J. Surg., *97*:782, 1959.

Arom, K̃. V., Richardson, J. D., Webb, G., Grover, F. L., and Trinkle, J. K.: Subxyphoid Pericardial Window in Patients With Suspected Traumatic Pericardial Tamponade. Ann. Thorac. Surg., *23*:545, 1977.

Aronstam, E. M., Strader, L. D., Geiger, J. P., and Gomex, A. C.: Traumatic Left Ventricular Aneurysms. Thorac. Cardiovasc. Surg., *59*:239, 1970.

Asfaw, I., and Arbulu, A.: Penetrating Wounds of the Pericardium and Heart. Surg. Clin. North Am., *57*:37, 1977.

Ashbell, T. S., Kleinert, H. E., and Kutz, J. E.: Vascular Injuries About the Elbow. Clin. Orth., *50*:107, 1967.

Aufranc, O. E., Jones, W. N., and Stewart, W. G., Jr.: Common Fracture with Unusal Associated Vascular Injury. J.A.M.A., *191*:1073, 1965.

Ayella, R. J., Hankins, J. R., Turney, S. Z., and Cowley, R. A.: Ruptured Thoracic Aorta Due to Blunt Trauma. J. Trauma, *17*:199, 1977.

Baek, S., Brown, R. S., and Shoemaker, W. C.: Cardiac Tamponade Following Wound Tract Injection. J. Trauma, *13*:85, 1973.

Bailey, H. (Ed.): Wounds of the Neck. *In* Surgery of Modern Warfare. E. & S. Livingston, Ltd., Edinburgh, 1944.

Baird, R. J., and Doran, M. L.: The False Aneurysm. Can. Med. Assoc. J., *91*:281, 1964.

Ballance, C.: The Surgery of the Heart (Bradshaw Lecture). Lancet, *1*:1, 1920.

Barcia, P. J., Nelson, T. G., and Whelan, T. J., Jr.: Importance of Venous Occlusion in Arterial Repair Failure: An Experimental Study. Ann. Surg., *175*:223, 1972.

Baret, A. C., DeLong, R. P., Tukanowicz, S. A., and Blakemore, W. S.: Transfixation of the Aorta Accompanied by a Browne-Séquard Syndrome: Report of a Case. J. Thorac. Surg., *35*:359, 1958.

Barker, N. W., and Hines, E. A., Jr.: Arterial Occlusion in the Hands and Fingers Associated With Repeated Occupational Trauma. Proc. Staff Meet. Mayo Clin., *19*:345, 1944.

Bassett, F. H., and Hauck, W. S., Jr.: False Aneurysm of Profunda Femoris Artery After Subtrochanteric Osteotomy and Nail-plate Fixation. J. Bone Joint Surg., *46-A*:583, 1964.

Bassett, F. H., and Silver, D.: Arterial Injury Associated with Fractures. Arch. Surg., *92*:13, 1966.

Beall, A. C., Jr.: Penetrating Wounds of the Aorta. Am. J. Surg., *99*:770, 1960.

Beall, A. C., Jr., Ochsner, J. L., Morris, G. C., Cooley, D. A., and DeBakey, M. E.: Penetrating Wounds to the Heart. J. Trauma, *1*:195, 1961.

Beall, A. C., Jr., Morris, G. C., Jr., and Cooley, D. A.: Temporary Cardiopulmonary Bypass in the Management of Penetrating Wounds of the Heart. Surgery, *52*:330, 1962.

Beall, A. C., Harrington, O. B., Crawford, E. S., and DeBakey, M. E.: Surgical Management of Traumatic Arteriovenous Aneurysms. Am. J. Surg., *106*:610, 1963A.

Beall, A. C., Shirkey, A. L., and DeBakey, M. E.: Penetrating Wounds of the Carotid Arteries. J. Trauma, *3*:276, 1963B.

Beall, A. C., Jr., Diethrich, E. B., Morris, G. C., Jr., and DeBakey, M. E.: Surgical Management of Vascular Trauma. Surg. Clin. North Am., *36*:1001, 1966A.

Beall, A. C., Jr., Diethrich, E. B., Crawford, H. W., Cooley, D. A., and DeBakey, M. E.: Surgical Management of Penetrating Cardiac Injuries. Am. J. Surg., *112*:686, 1966B.

Beall, A. C., Jr., Dietrich, E. B., Cooley, D. A., and DeBakey, M. E.: Surgical Treatment of Penetrating Cardiovascular Trauma. South Med. J., *60*:698, 1967.

Beall, A. C., Jr., Arbergast, N. R., Ripepi, A. C., Bricker, D. L., Diethrich, E. B., Hallman, G. L., Cooley, D. A., and DeBakey, M. E.: Aortic Laceration Due to Rapid Deceleration. Arch. Surg., *98*:595, 1969.

Beall, A. C., Jr., Gasior, R. M., and Bricker, D. L.: Gunshot Wounds of the Heart: Changing Patterns of Surgical Management. Ann. Thorac. Surg., *11*:523, 1971.

Beall, A. C., Jr., Patrick, T. A., Okies, J. E., Bricker, D. L., and DeBakey, M. E.: Penetrating Wounds of the Heart: Changing Patterns of Surgical Management. J. Trauma, *12*:468, 1972.

Beattie, E. J., Jr., and Greer, D.: Laceration of the Aorta: Case Report of Successful Repair Forty-Eight Hours After Injury. J. Thorac. Surg., *23*:293, 1952.

Beattie, W. M., Oldham, J. B., and Ross, J. A.: Superior Thyroid Arteriovenous Aneurysm. Br. J. Surg., *48*:456, 1961.

Beatty, R. A.: Dissecting Hematoma of the Internal Carotid Artery Following Chiropractic Cervical Manipulation. J. Trauma, *17*:248, 1977.

Beck, C. S.: Wounds of the Heart: The Technique of Suture. Arch. Surg., *13*:205, 1926.

Beck, C. S.: Further Observations on Stab Wounds of the Heart. Ann. Surg., *115*:698, 1942.

Beebe, H. G. (Ed.): Complications in Vascular Surgery. J. B. Lippincott Company, Philadelphia, 1973.

Bell, D., and Cockshott, W. P.: Angiography of Traumatic Arterio-venous Fistulae. Clin. Radiol., *16*:241, 1965.

Bell, J.: Principles of Surgery. Vol. I, Discourse 9. 1801, p. 404.

Ben Hur, N., Gemer, M., and Milwidsky, H.: Perforating Injury of the Heart Caused by a Nail Fired From a Studgun. J. Trauma, *84*:850, 1964.

Bennett, J. E.: Expanding Forearm Hematoma After Apparent Minor Injury. Plastic Reconstr. Surg., *36*:322, 1965.

Benvenuto, R., Rodman, F. S. B., Gilmour, J., Phillips, A. F., and Callagham, J. C.: Composite Venous Grafts for Replacement of the Superior Vena Cava. Arch. Surg., *89*:100, 1962.

Bergan, F.: Traumatic Intimal Rupture of the Popliteal Artery with Acute Ischemia of the Limb in Cases with Supracondylar Fractures of the Femur. J. Cardiovasc. Surg., *4*:300, 1963.

Bergan, J. J., Conn, J., Jr., and Trippel, O. H.: Severe Ischemia of the Hand. Ann. Surg., *173*:301, 1971.

Bergan, J. J., Dean, R. H., and Yao, J. S. T.: Vascular Injuries in Pelvic Cancer Surgery. Am. J. Obstet. Gynecol., *124*:562, 1976.

Bergentz, S. E., Hansson, L. O., and Norback, B.: Surgical Management of Complications to Arterial Puncture. Ann. Surg., *164*:1021, 1966.

Bernheim, B. M.: Surgery of the Vascular System. J. B. Lippincott Company, Publishers, 1913.

Bernheim, B. M.: Blood Vessel Surgery in War. Surg. Gynecol. Obstet., *30*:564, 1920.

Bickham, W. S.: Arteriovenous Aneurism. Ann. Surg., *39*:767, 1904.

Billings, K. J., Nasca, R. J., and Griffin, H. A.: Traumatic Arteriovenous Fistula with Spontaneous Closure. J. Trauma, *13*:741, 1973.

Billroth, T. (1858): Historical Studies on the Nature and Treatment of Gunshot Wounds From the 15th Century to the Present Time. Translation by C. P. Rhoads. *In* Yale J. Biol. Med., *4*:16, 1931.

Billroth, T. (1875): Cited in Ballance, C.: The Surgery of the Heart (Bradshaw Lecture). Lancet, *1*:1, 1920.

Billroth, T. (1883): Cited in Beck, C. S.: Wounds of the Heart: The Technique of Suture. Arch. Surg., *13*:205, 1926.

Billy, L. J., Amato, J. J., and Rich, N. M.: Aortic Injuries in Vietnam. Surgery, *70*:385, 1971.

Binkley, F. M., and Wylie, E. J.: A New Technique for Obliteration of Cerebrovascular Arteriovenous Fistulae. Arch. Surg., *106*:524, 1973.

Birkeland, I. W., and Taylor, T. K. F.: Major Vascular Injuries in Lumbar Disc Surgery. J. Bone Joint Surg., *51B*:4, 1969.

Bizer, L.: Peripheral Vascular Injuries in the Vietnam War. Arch. Surg., *98*:165, 1969.

Blackwell, T. L., and Whelan, T. J.: Arteriovenous Fistula as a Complication of Gastrectomy. Am. J. Surg., *109*:197, 1965.

Blaisdell, F. W.: Discussion in Buscaglia et al.: Penetrating Abdominal Vascular Injuries. Arch. Surg., *99*:764, 1969.

Blakemore, A. H., and Lord, J. E., Jr.: A Non-sutured Method of Blood Vessel Anastomosis. Ann. Surg., *121*:435, 1945.

Blakemore, A. H., Lord, J. W., Jr., and Stefko, P. L.: The Severed Primary Artery in the War Wounded. Surgery, *12*:488, 1942.

Blalock, A.: Successful Suture of a Wound of the Ascending Aorta. J.A.M.A., *103*:1617, 1934.

Blalock, A., and Ravitch, M. M.: A Consideration of the Non-operative Treatment of Cardiac Tamponade Resulting From Wounds to the Heart. Surgery, *14*:157, 1943.

Bland, E. F., and Beebe, G. W.: Missiles in the Heart: A Twenty Year Follow-Up Report of World War II Cases. N. Engl. J. Med., *274*:1039, 1966.

Bloom, J. D., Mozersky, D. J., Buckley, C. G., and Hagood, C. O., Jr.: Defective Limb Growth as a Complication of Catheterization of the Femoral Artery. Surg. Gynecol. Obstet., *138*:524, 1974.

Boerhaave, H.: Cited in Elkin, 1941. Aphorismi de Cognoscendis et Curandis Morbis (Aphorism 170), 1709.

Bolanowki, P. J. P., Swaminatham, A. P., and Neville, W. E.: Aggressive Surgical Management of Penetrating Cardiac Injuries. J. Thorac. Cardiovasc. Surg., *66*:52, 1973.

Bolasny, B. L., and Killen, D. A.: Surgical Management of Arterial Injury Secondary to Angiography. Ann. Surg., *174*:962, 1971.

Bole, P. V., Purdy, R. T., Munda, R. T., Moallem, S., Devanesan, J., and Clauss, R. H.: Civilian Arterial Injuries. Ann. Surg., *183*:13, 1976A.

Bole, P. V., Munda, R., Purdy, R. T., Lande, A., Gomez, R., Clauss, R. H., Kazarian, K. K., and Mersheimer, W. L.: Traumatic Pseudo-aneurysms: A Review of 32 Cases. J. Trauma, *16*:63, 1976B. Although the title states 32 cases, the series consists of 23 patients with 23 pseudo-aneurysms.

Borja, A. R., and Lansing, A. M.: Traumatic Rupture of the Heart: A Case Successfully Treated. Ann. Surg., *171*:438, 1970A.

Borja, A. R., and Lansing, A. M.: Thrombosis of the Abdominal Aorta Caused by Blunt Trauma. J. Trauma, *10*:399, 1970B.

Bosher, L. H., and Freed, T. A.: The Surgical Treatment of Traumatic Rupture or Avulsion of the Innominate Artery. J. Thorac. Cardiovasc. Surg., *54*:732, 1967.

Boyd, D. P., and Farha, G. J.: Arteriovenous Fistula in Isolated Vascular Injuries Secondary to Intervertebral Disc Surgery. Ann. Surg., *161*:524, 1965.

Boyden, A. M.: Personal Communication, 1970.

Bradham, G. B., Nunn, D. B., and Brailsford, L. E.: Successful Repair of a Bullet Wound of the Abdominal Aorta. Ann. Surg., *155*:86, 1962.

Bradley, E. L., III: Management of Penetrating Carotid Injuries: An Alternative Approach. J. Trauma, *13*:248, 1973.

Brandt, R. L., Foley, W. J., Fink, G. H., and Regan, W. J.: Mechanism of Perforation of the Heart with Production of Hydropericardium by Venous Catheter and Its Prevention. Am. J. Surg., *119*:311, 1970.

Branham, H. H.: Aneurismal Varix of the Femoral Artery and Vein Following a Gunshot Wound. Int. J. Surg., *3*:250, 1890.

Brantigan, C. O.: Delayed Major Vessel Hemorrhage Following Tracheostomy. J. Trauma, *13*:235, 1973.

Brener, B. J., and Couch, N. P.: Peripheral Arterial Complications of Left Heart Catheterization and Their Management. Am. J. Surg., *125*:521, 1973.

Brewer, L. A., III: Wounds of the Chest in War and Peace. Ann. Thorac. Surg., *7*:387, 1969.

Brewer, L. A., III, and Carter, R.: Wounds of the Great Vessels of the Thorax. Diagnosis and Surgical Approach in 24 Cases. Am. J. Surg., *114*:340, 1967A.

Brewer, L. A., III, and Carter, R.: Elective Cardiac Arrest in the Management of Massively Bleeding Heart Wounds. J.A.M.A., *200*:1023, 1967B.

Brewer, L. A., III, and Carter, R.: A Rational Treatment of Small and Large Wounds of the Heart. Surg. Gynecol. Obstet., *126*:977, 1968.

Brewer, P. L., Schramel, R. J., Menendez, C. V., and Creech, O., Jr.: Injuries of the Popliteal Artery: A Report of 16 Cases. Am. J. Surg., *118*:36, 1969.

Bricker, D. L., Noon, G. P., Beall, A. C., Jr., and DeBakey, M. E.: Vascular Injuries of the Thoracic Outlet. J. Trauma, *10*:1, 1970A.

Bricker, D. L., Beall, A. C., Jr., and DeBakey, M. E.: The Differential Response to Infection of Autogenous Vein Versus Dacron Arterial Prostheses. Chest, *58*:566, 1970B.

Bricker, D. L., Morton, J. R., Okies, J. E., and Beall, A. C., Jr.: Surgical Management of Injuries to the Vena Cava: Changing Patterns of Injury and Newer Techniques of Repair. J. Trauma, *11*:725, 1971.

Brisbin, R. L., Geib, P. O., and Eiseman, B.: Secondary Disruption of Vascular Repair Following War Wounds. Arch. Surg., *99*:787, 1969.

Brittain, R. S., Marchioro, T. L., Hermann, G., Waddell, W. R., and Starzel, E. E.: Accidental Hepatic Artery Ligation in Humans. Am. J. Surg., *107*:822, 1964.

Broca (1762): Cited in Murphy, J. B., 1897.

Brooks, A. L., and Fowler, S. B.: Axillary Artery Thrombosis After Prolonged Use of Crutches. J. Bone Joint Surg., *46A*:863, 1964.

Brown, A. J.: The Surgery of Hieronymus Brunschwig. Surg. Gynecol. Obstet., *38*:133, 1924.

Brown, R. S., Boyd, D. R., Matsuda, T., and Lowe, R. J.: Temporary Internal Vascular Shunt for Retrohepatic Vena Cava Injury. J. Trauma, *11*:736, 1971.

Brunschwig, H. (1497): Cited in Schwartz, 1958, and Brown, 1924.

Bryant, M. F., Jr., Lazenby, W. D., and Howard, J. M.: Experimental Replacement of Short Segment of Veins. Arch. Surg., *76*:289, 1958.

Buchman, R. J., Thomas, P. A., Jr., and Park, B.: Carotid Artery Injuries: Follow-Up of 15 Patients Treated in Vietnam. Angiology, *23*:97, 1972.

Buckner, F., Lyons, C., and Perkins, R.: Management of Lacerations of the Great Vessels of the Upper Thorax and Base of the Neck. Surg. Gynecol. Obstet., *107*:135, 1958.

Burnett, H. F., Parnell, C. L., Williams, G. D., and Campbell, G. S.: Peripheral Arterial Injuries: A Reassessment. Ann. Surg., *183*:701, 1976.

Burns, G. R., and Sherman, R. T.: Trauma of the Abdominal Aorta and Inferior Vena Cava. Am. Surg., *38*:303, 1972.

Burrell, H. L.: Ligature of the Innominate Artery With a Report of a Case. Trans. Am. Soc. A., *13*:291, 1895.

Buscaglia, L. C., Blaisdell, F. W., and Lim, R. C.: Penetrating Abdominal Vascular Injuries. Arch. Surg., *99*:764, 1969.

Callander, C. L.: Study of Arterio-venous Fistula With An Analysis of 447 Cases. Johns Hopkins Hosp. Rev., *19*:259, 1920.

Cameron, H. S., Laird, J. J., and Carroll, S. E.: False Aneurysms Complicating Closed Fractures. J. Trauma, *12*:67, 1972.

Cappelen, A.: Vulnus cordis, sutur of hjrtet. Nor. Mag. f. Laegevidensk., *11*:285, 1896.

Carlsson, E., and Silander, T.: Rupture of the Subclavian and Innominate Artery Due to Nonpenetrating Trauma of the Chest. Acta Chir. Scand., *125*:294, 1963.

Carrasquilla, C., and Weaver, A. W.: Aneurysm of the Saphenous Graft to the Common Carotid Artery. Vasc. Surg., *6*:66, 1972.

Carrasquilla, C., Wilson, R. F., Walt, A. J., and Arbulu, A.: Gunshot Wounds of the Heart. Ann. Thorac. Surg., *13*:208, 1972.

Carrel, A.: La Technique Opératorie des Anastomoses Vasculaires et la Transplantation des Viscéres. Lyon Medical, *98*:859, 1902.

Carrel, A.: Results of Transplantation of Blood Vessels, Organs and Limbs. J.A.M.A., *51*:1662, 1908.

Carrel, A., and Guthrie, C. C.: Uniterminal and Biterminal Venous Transplantations. Surg. Gynecol. Obstet., *2*:266, 1906.

Cerino, M., McGraw, J. Y., and Luke, J. C.: Autogenous Vein Graft Replacement of Thrombosed Deep Veins. Experimental Approach to the Treatment of the Post Phlebitic Syndrome. Surgery, *55*:123, 1964.

Chandler, J. G., and Knapp, R. W.: Early Definitive Treatment of Vascular Injures in the Vietnam Conflict. J.A.M.A., *202*:960, 1967.

Chase, M. D., and Schwartz, S. I.: Suture Anastomosis of Small Arteries. Surg. Gynecol. Obstet., *117*:214, 1963.

Cheek, R. C., Pope, J. C., Smith, H. F., Britt, L. G., and Pate, J. W.: Diagnosis and Management of Major Vascular Injuries: A Review of 200 Operative Cases. Am. Surg., *41*:755, 1975.

Ciaravella, J. M., Ochsner, J. L., and Mills, N. L.: Traumatic Avulsion of the Innominate Artery: A Case Report and Literature Review. J. Trauma, *16*:751, 1976.

Clermont, G.: Suture Laterale et Circulaire des Veines. Presse Med., *1*:229, 1901.

Cohen, A., Baldwin, J. N., and Grant, R. N.: Problems in the Management of Battlefield Vascular Injuries. Am. J. Surg., *118*:526, 1969.

Cohen, A., Brief, D., and Mathewson, C., Jr.: Carotid Artery Injuries: An Analysis of 85 Cases. Am. J. Surg., *210*, 1970.

Coley, R. W. (Translation for Fleming, J.): Case of Rupture of the Carotid Artery and Wound of Several of Its Branches Successfully Treated by Tying Off the Common Trunk of the Carotid Itself. Med. Chir. J (Lond.), *3*:2, 1817.

Collins, H. A., and Jacobs, J. K.: Acute Arterial Injuries Due to Blunt Trauma. J. Bone Joint Surg., *43-A*:193, 1961.

Collins, R. E., and Douglass, F. M.: Small Vein Anastomosis With and Without Operative Microscope: A Comparative Study. Arch. Surg., *88*:740, 1964.

Conkle, D. M., Richie, R. E., Sawyers, J. L., and Scott, W. H., Jr.: Surgical Treatment of Popliteal Artery Injuries. Arch. Surg., *110*:1351, 1975.

Conn, J., Jr., Trippel, O. H., and Bergan, J. J.: A New Atraumatic Aortic Occluder. Surgery, *64*:1158, 1968.

Conn, J. H., Hardy, J. D., Chavez, C. M., and Fain, W. R.: Challenging Arterial Injuries. J. Trauma, *11*:167, 1971.

Connolly, J.: Management of Fractures Associated with Arterial Injuries. Am. J. Surg., *120*:331, 1970.

Connolly, J., Williams, E., and Whittaker, D.: The Influence of Fracture Stabilization on the

Outcome of Arterial Repair in Combined Fracture-Arterial Injuries. Surg. Forum, *20*:450, 1969.

Connolly, J. F., Whittaker, D., and Williams, E.: Femoral and Tibial Fractures Combined with Injuries to the Femoral or Popliteal Artery. J. Bone Joint Surg., *53-A*:56, 1971.

Cook, F. W., and Haller, J. A., Jr.: Penetrating Injuries of the Subclavian Vessels Associated with Venous Complications. Ann. Surg., *155*:370, 1962.

Cooley, D. A., Dunn, J. R., Brockman, H. L., and DeBakey, M. E.: Treatment of Penetrating Wounds of the Heart: Experimental and Clinical Observations. Surgery, *37*:882, 1955.

Cooper, B.: Wounds in Arteries and Traumatic Aneurysms. Guy's Hosp. Rep., *8*:195, 1853.

Cooper, E. S.: Aneurism of the Right Carotid and Subclavian Arteries. Am. J. Med. Sci., *38*:395, 1859.

Couves, C. M., Lumpkin, M. B., and Howard, J. M.: Arterial Injuries Due to Blunt—Nonpenetrating—Trauma; Experiences with 15 Patients. Can. J. Surg., *1*:197, 1958.

Cranley, J. J., and Krause, R. J.: Injury to the Axillary Artery Following Anterior Dislocation of the Shoulder. Am. J. Surg., *95*:524, 1958.

Creech, O., Jr.: Acute Arterial Injuries. Postgrad. Med., *29*:581, 1961.

Creech, O., Jr., Gantt, J., and Wren, H.: Traumatic Arteriovenous Fistula at Unusual Sites. Ann. Surg., *161*:908, 1965.

Crissey, M. M., and Bernstein, E. F.: Delayed Presentation of Carotid Intimal Tear Following Blunt Craniocervical Trauma. Surgery, *75*:543, 1974.

Dainko, E. A.: Complications of the Use of the Fogarty Balloon Catheter. Arch. Surg., *105*:79, 1972.

Dale, W. A.: Chronic Iliofemoral Venous Occlusion Including Seven Cases of Cross-over Vein Grafting. Surgery, *59*:117, 1966.

Dale, W. A. (Ed.): Management of Arterial Occlusive Disease (National Conference on Management of Arterial Occlusive Disease, Nashville, 1970). Year Book Medical Publishers, Inc., Chicago, 1971.

Dameron, T. B., Jr.: False Aneurysm of Femoral Profundus Artery Resulting From Internal-Fixation Device (Screw). J. Bone Joint Surg., *46A*:577, 1964.

Davie, J. C., and Coxe, W.: Occlusive Disease of the Carotid Artery in Children. Arch. Neurol., *17*:313, 1967.

Davis (1834): Cited in Straus, R.: Pulmonary Embolism Caused by a Lead Bullet Following a Gunshot Wound of the Abdomen. Arch. Path., *33*:63, 1942.

DeBakey, M. E., and Simeone, F. A.: Battle Injuries of Arteries in World War II: An Analysis of 2,471 Cases. Ann. Surg., *123*:534, 1946.

DeBakey, M. E., and Elkin, D. C. (1955): *In* Elkin, D. C., and DeBakey, M. E., 1955.

DeBakey, M. E., Cooley, D. A., Morris, G. C., and Collins, H.: Arteriovenous Fistula Involving the Abdominal Aorta. Ann. Surg., *147*:646, 1958.

DeBakey, M. E., Beall, A. C., Jr., and Wukasch, D. C.: Recent Developments in Vascular Surgery with Particular Reference to Orthopedics. Am. J. Surg., *109*:134, 1965.

DeMuth, W. E., Jr., Baue, A. E., and Odom, J. A., Jr.: Contusions of the Heart. J. Trauma, *7*:443, 1967.

De Nayer, P., Jaumin, P., and Linard, D.: Lesions Osteo-Articulaires des Membres Compliquees de Traumatismes Vasculaires. Acta Chir. Belg., *72*:427, 1973.

DeSaussure, R. L.: Vascular Injury Coincident to Disc Surgery. J. Neurosurg., *16*:222, 1959.

DesForges, O., Ridder, W. P., and Lenoci, R. J.: Successful Suture of Ruptured Myocardium After Nonpenetrating Injury. N. Engl. J. Med., *252*:567, 1955.

de Takats, G.: Vascular Surgery in the War. War Medicine, *3*:291, 1943.

de Takats, G.: Vascular Surgery. W. B. Saunders Company, Philadelphia, 1959.

de Takats, G.: Symptoms and Signs of Peripheral Arterial Disease. Med. Clin. North Am., *46*:647, 1962.

de Takats, G., and Fowler, E. F.: Trauma to the Arteriosclerotic Limb. J. Trauma, *4*:47, 1963.

de Takats, G., and Pirani, C. L.: Aneurysms: General Considerations. Angiology, *5*:173, 1954.

Dillard, B. M., Nelson, D. L., and Norman, H. G., Jr.: Review of 85 Traumatic Arterial Injuries. Surgery, *63*:391, 1968.

Dillard, B. M., and Staple, T. W.: Bullet Embolism from the Aortic Arch to the Popliteal Artery. Arch. Surg., *98*:326, 1969.

Dimond, F. C., Jr., and Rich, N. M.: M–16 Wounds in Vietnam. J. Trauma, *7*:618, 1967.

Diveley, W. L., Daniel, R. A., Jr., and Scott, H. W., Jr.: Surgical Management of Penetrating Injuries of the Ascending Aorta and Aortic Arch. J. Thorac. Cardiovasc. Surg., *41*:23, 1961.

DiVincenti, F. C., and Weber, B. B.: Traumatic Carotid Artery Injuries in Civilian Practice. Am. J. Surg., *40*:277, 1974.

Dixon, R. G., and McEwan, P.: Notes on a Case of Penetrating Wound of the Heart. Br. Med. J., *1*:755, 1916.

Dörfler, J.: Uber Arteriennaht. Beitr. Klin. Chir., *25*:781, 1889.

Dosios, T. J., Magovern, G. J., Gay, T. C., and Joyner, C. R.: Cardiac Tamponade Complicating Pericutaneous Catheterization of Subclavian Vein. Surgery, *78*:261, 1975.

Doty, D. B., Treiman, R. L., Rothschild, P. D., Gaspar, M. R., et al.: Prevention of Gangrene Due to Fractures. Surg. Gynecol. Obstet., *125*:284, 1967.

Drapanas, T., Hewitt, R. L., Weichert, R. F., and Smith, A. D.: Civilian Vascular Injuries: A Critical Appraisal of Three Decades of Management. Ann. Surg., *172*:351, 1970.

Dshanelidze, II: Manuskript Petrograd, 1922 (Cited in Lilianthal, H., 1926).

Dubinsky, M. B.: Suture of the Abdominal Aorta. Khirurigica, *4*:71, 1944.

Earle, A. S., Horsley, J. S., Villavicencio, J. L., and Warren, R.: Replacement of Venous Defects by Venous Autografts. Arch. Surg., *80*:119, 1960.

Eastcott, H. H. G.: The Management of Arterial Injuries. J. Bone Joint Surg., *47B*:394, 1965.

Eastcott, H. H. G.: Arterial Surgery. J. B. Lippincott Company, Philadelphia, 1969.

Eck, N. V.: K. voprosu o perevyazkie vorotnois veni. Predvaritelnoye soobshtshjenye (Ligature of the Portal Vein). Voen. Med. J., St. Petersburg, *130*(2):1–2, 1877.

Edmundson, E.: Transfixion of the Aorta (by Arrow). Br. J. Surg., *23*:869, 1936.

Edwards, W. S., and Lyons, C.: Traumatic Arterial Spasm and Thrombosis. Ann. Surg., *140*:318, 1954.

Eger, M., Golcman, L., Goldstein, A., and Hirsch, M.: The Use of a Temporary Shunt in the Management of Arterial Vascular Injuries. Surg. Gynecol. Obstet., *132*:67, 1971.

Eger, M., Golcman, L., Schmidt, B., and Hirsch, M.: Problems in the Management of Popliteal Artery Injuries. Surg. Gynecol. Obstet., *134*:921, 1972.

Eger, M., Golcman, L., Trok, G., and Hirsch, M.: Inadvertent Arterial Stripping in the Lower Limb: Problems of Management. Surgery, *73*:23, 1973.

Eisenbrey, A. B.: Arteriovenous Aneurysm of the Superficial Femoral Vessels. J.A.M.A., *61*:2155, 1913.

Elkin, D. C.: The Diagnosis and Treatment of Cardiac Trauma. Ann. Surg., *114*:169, 1941.

Elkin, D. C.: Vascular Injuries of Warfare. Ann. Surg., *120*:284, 1944A.

Elkin, D. C.: Wounds of the Heart. Ann. Surg., *120*:817, 1944B.

Elkin, D. C.: Arteriovenous Aneurysm. Surg. Gynecol. Obstet., *80*:217, 1945.

Elkin, D. C.: Traumatic Aneurysm: The Matas Operation—Fifty-Seven Years After. Surg. Gynecol. Obstet., *82*:1, 1946.

Elkin, D. C. (1955): *In* Elkin, D. C., and DeBakey, M. E.: Vascular Surgery. U.S. Government Printing Office, Washington, D.C., 1955.

Elkin, D. C., and Banner, E. A.: Arteriovenous Aneurysms Following Surgical Operations. J.A.M.A., *131*:1117, 1946.

Elkin, D. C., and DeBakey, M. E.: Vascular Surgery. Office of the Surgeon General, Department of the Army, Washington, D.C., 1955.

Elkin, D. C., and Harris, M. H.: Arteriovenous Aneurysm of the Vertebral Vessels. Ann. Surg., *124*:934, 1946.

Elkin, D. C., and Shumacker, H. B., Jr.: *In* Elkin, D. C., and DeBakey, M. E. (Eds.): Vascular Surgery in World War II. U.S. Government Printing Office, Washington, D.C., 1955.

Elkin, D. C., and Woodhall, B.: Combined Vascular and Nerve Injuries of Warfare. Ann. Surg., *119*:411, 1944.

Elliot, J. A.: Acute Arterial Occlusion; An Unusual Cause. Surgery, *39*:825, 1956.

Ellis, J.: Case of Gunshot Wound, Attended with Secondary Hemorrhage in Which Both Carotid Arteries Were Tied at an Interval of Four and a Half Days. N.Y. J. Med., *5*:187, 1845.

Engleman, R. M., Clements, J. M., and Herrmann, J. B.: Stab Wounds and Traumatic False Aneurysms in the Extremities. J. Trauma, *9*:77, 1969.

Ernst, C. B., and Kaufer, H.: Fibulectomy-Fasciotomy: An Important Adjunct in the Management of Lower Extremity Arterial Trauma. J. Trauma, *11*:365, 1971.

Erskine, J. M.: Case Report: A True Traumatic Aneurysm of the Radial Artery at the Wrist Successfully Treated by Resection and Arterial Repair. J. Trauma, *4*:630, 1964.

Eshaghy, B., Loeb, H. S., Miller, S. E., Scanlon, P. J., Towne, W. D., and Gunnar, R. M.: Mediastinal and Retropharyngeal Hemorrhage: A Complication of Cardiac Catheterization. J.A.M.A., *226*:427, 1973.

Esmarch, F.: The Surgeons Handbook of the Treatment of the Wounded in War. L. W. Schmidt, New York, 1878.

Espada, R., Whisennand, H. H., Mattox, K. L., and Beall, A. C., Jr.: Surgical Management of Penetrating Injuries to the Coronary Arteries. Surgery, *78*:755, 1975.

Evans, W. E., and Bernhard, V. M.: Tibial Artery Bypass for Ischemia Resulting From Fractures. J. Trauma, *11*:999, 1971.

Fallah-Nejad, M., Wallace, H. W., Su, C. C., Kutty, A. C., and Blakemore, W. S.: Unusual Manifestations of Penetrating Cardiac Injuries. Arch. Surg., *110*:1357, 1975.

Fallon, G., and Thomford, N. R.: False Aneurysm of the Superficial Femoral Artery Associated Wtih Fracture of the Femur. Angiology, *21*:120, 1970.

Falor, W. H., Hansel, J. R., and Williams, G. B.: Gangrene of the Hand: A Complication of Radial Artery Cannulation. J. Trauma, *16*:713, 1976.

Feller, I., and Woodburne, R. T.: Surgical Anatomy of the Abdominal Aorta. Ann. Surg., *154*:239, 1961.

Ferguson, I. A., Sr., Byrd, W. M., and McAfee, D. K.: Experiences in the Management of Arterial Injuries. Ann. Surg., *153*:980, 1961.

Ferguson, W. M.: Arterio-venous Aneurysm Following Osteotomy for Genu valgum. Lancet, *1*:532, 1914.

Fish, G. D., Jr., and Hockhauser, M.: Laceration of the Popliteal Artery Due to Blunt Trauma. Am. J. Surg., *94*:651, 1957.

Fisher, G. W.: Acute arterial injuries treated by the United States Army Medical Service in Vietnam, 1965–1966. J. Trauma, *7*:844, 1967.

Fisher, R. D., and Rienhoff, W. F., III: Subclavian Artery Laceration Resulting from Fractured First Rib. J. Trauma, *6*:579, 1966.

Fitchett, V. H., Pomerantz, M., Butsch, D. W., Simon, R., and Eiseman, B.: Penetrating Wounds of the Neck. Arch. Surg., *99*:307, 1969.

Fitts, C. T., Barnett, L. T., Webb, C. M., Sexton, J., and Yarbrough, D. R., III: Perforating Wounds of the Heart Caused by Central Venous Catheters. J. Trauma, *10*:764, 1970.

Fleming, J. (1803): Case of Rupture of the Carotid Artery and Wound of Several of Its Branches Successfully Treated by Tying Off the Common Trunk of the Carotid Itself. (Translated by R. W. Coley.) Med. Chir. J. (Lond.), *3*:2, 1817.

Fleming, J. F. R., and Petrie, D.: Traumatic Thrombosis of the Internal Carotid Artery with Delayed Hemiplegia. Can. J. Surg., *11*:166, 1968.

Flint, L. M., Snyder, W. H., Perry, M. O., and Shires, G. T.: Management of Major Vascular Injuries in the Base of the Neck: An 11-Year Experience with 146 Cases. Arch. Surg., *106*:407, 1973.

Fogarty, T. J., and Cranley, J. J.: Catheter Technique for Arterial Embolectomy. Ann. Surg., *161*:325, 1965.

Fogarty, T. J., Cranley, J. J., Krause, R. J., Strasser, E. S., and Hafner, C. D.: A Method for Extraction of Arterial Emboli and Thrombi. Surg. Gynecol. Obstet., *116*:241, 1963.

Fomon, J. J., and Warren, W. D.: Late Complications of Peripheral Arterial Injuries. Arch. Surg., *91*:610, 1965.

Foramitti, K. (1909): Cited in Foramitti: Wien. Klin. Wschr., *25*:957, 1910.

Foramitti, K.: Cited in Rea et al.: Coronary Artery Lacerations: An Analysis of 22 Patients. Ann. Thorac. Surg., *7*:518, 1969. Wien. Klin. Wschr., *25*:957, 1910.

Foster, J. H., Carter, J. W., Grahamm, C. P., Jr., and Edwards, W. H.: Arterial Injury Secondary to the Use of the Fogarty Catheter. Ann. Surg., *171*:971, 1970.

Fraser, G. A.: Closed Traumatic Rupture of Common Femoral Artery. Ann. Surg., *161*:539, 1965.

Freeark, R. J.: Role of Angiography in the Management of Multiple Injuries. Surg. Gynecol. Obstet., *128*:745, 1969.

Freeman, N. E.: Secondary Hemorrhage Arising From Gunshot Wounds of the Peripheral Blood Vessels. Ann. Surg., *122*:631, 1945.

Freeman, N. E.: Arterial Repair in the Treatment of Aneurysms and Arteriovenous Fistulae; A Report of 18 Successful Restorations. Ann. Surg., *124*:888, 1946.

Freeman, N. E., and Shumacker, H. B., Jr. (1955): Cited in Elkin, D. C., and DeBakey, M. E.: Vascular Surgery. U.S. Government Printing Office, Washington, D.C., 1955.

Fromm, S. H., Carrasquilla, C., and Lucas, C.: The Management of Gunshot Wounds of the Aorta. Arch. Surg., *101*:388, 1970.

Frouin, A.: Sur la sutre des vaisseaux. Presse Med., *16*:233, 1908.

Fu, W. R.: Angiography of Trauma. Charles C Thomas, Publisher, Springfield, Ill., 1972.

Fullen, W. D., Hunt, J., and Altemeier, W. A.: The Clinical Spectrum of Penetrating Injury to the Superior Mesenteric Arterial Circulation. J. Trauma, *12*:656, 1972.

Furman, S., Vijaynagar, R., Rosenbaum, R., McMullen, M., and Scher, D. J. W.: Lethal Sequelae of Intra-aortic Balloon Rupture. Surgery, *69*:121, 1971.

Gardner, C.: Traumatic vasospasm and its complications. Am. J. Surg., *83*:468, 1952.

Gardner, W. J., and Storer, J.: The Use of the G Suit in Control of Intra-abdominal Bleeding. Surg. Gynecol. Obstet., *123*:792, 1966.

Gaspar, M. R., and Hare, R. R.: Gangrene Due to Intra-arterial Injection of Drugs by Drug Addicts. Surgery, *72*:573, 1972.

Gaspar, M. R., and Treiman, R. L.: The Management of Injuries to Major Veins. Am. J. Surg., *100*:171, 1960.

Gaspar, M. R., Treiman, R. L., Payne, J. H., Rothschild, P. D., and Gaspard, D. J.: Principles of Treatment and Special Problems in Vascular Trauma. Surg. Clin. North Am., *48*:1355, 1968.

Gaspard, D. J., and Gaspar, M. R.: Arteriovenous Fistula After Fogarty Catheter Thrombectomy. Arch. Surg., *105*:90, 1972.

Geer, T. M.: Personal Communication, 1972.

Geer, T. M., and Rich, N. M.: Cardiac Trauma in Vietnam: Unpublished Data in the Vietnam Vascular Registry, 1972.

Geis, W. P., Johnson, C. F., Zajtchuk, R., and Kittle, C. F.: Extrapericardial (Mediastinal) Cardiac Tamponade. Arch. Surg., *100*:305, 1970.

Gensoul (1883): Cited in Simeone et al.: On the Question of Ligation of the Concomitant Vein When a Major Artery Is Interrupted. Surgery, *29*:932, 1951.

Gensoul: Note sur les Blessés Reçus á l'Hôtel Dieu de Lyon, Pendant les Troubles de 1831. Gaz. Méd. Paris, 1883, p. 297.

Gerbode, F., Holman, E., Dickenson, E. H., and Spencer, F. C.: Arteriovenous Fistulas and Arterial Aneurysms: The Repair of Major Arteries Injured in Warfare, and the Treatment of an Arterial Aneurysm with a Vein Graft Inlay. Surgery, *32*:259, 1952.

Gerlock, A. J., Thal, E. R., and Snyder, W. H., III: Venography and Penetrating Injuries of the Extremities. Am. J. Roentgenol. Radium Ther. Nucl. Med., *126*:1023, 1976.

Gibson, J. M. C.: Rupture of the Axillary Artery. J. Bone Joint Surg., *44B*:114, 1962.

Gielchinsky, I., and McNamara, J. J.: Cardiac Wounds at a Military Evacuation Hospital in Vietnam: A Review of One Year's Experience. J. Thorac. Cardiovasc. Surg., *60*:603, 1970.

Gielchinsky, I., and McNamara, J. J.: Flechette Wounds of the Heart. Surgery, *69*:229, 1971.

Gluck, T.: Ueber Zwei Fälle von Aortenaneurysmen Nebst Bemerkungen Uber die Naht der Blutgefässe. Arch. Klin. Chir., *28*:548, 1883.

Goldman, L. I., Maier, W. P., Drezner, A. D., and Rosemond, G. P.: Another Complication of Subclavian Puncture: Arterial Laceration. J.A.M.A., *217*:78, 1971.

Gomes, M. M. R., and Bernatz, P. E.: Arteriovenous Fistulas: A Review and 10 Year Experience at the Mayo Clinic. Mayo Clin. Proc., *45*:81, 1970.

Goodman, C.: Suture of Blood Vessel From Projectiles of War. Surg. Gynecol. Obstet., *27*:528, 1918.

Gorman, J. F.: Combat Wounds of the Popliteal Artery. Ann. Surg., *168*:974, 1968.

Gorman, J. F.: Combat Arterial Trauma. Analysis of 106 Limb-Threatening Injuries. Arch. Surg., *98*:160, 1969.

Goyanes, J.: Neuvos trabajos de chirurgia vascular: Substitution plastica de las arterias por las venas, o arterio-plastia venosa, aplicado, como neuvo metodo, al traitamiento de los aneurismas. El Siglo Med., *53*:561, 1906.

Grablowsky, O. M., Weichert, R. F., III, Goff, J. B., and Schlegel, J. U.: Renal Artery Thrombosis Following Blunt Trauma: Report of Four Cases. Surgery, *67*:895, 1970.

Greenfield, L. J., and Ebert, P. A.: Technical Considerations in the Management of Axillobrachial Arterial Injuries. J. Trauma, *7*:606, 1967.

Greenough, J.: Operations on Innominate Artery. Report of a Successful Ligation. Arch. Surg., *19*:1484, 1929.

Griswold, R. A., and Drye, J. C.: Cardiac Wounds. Ann. Surg., *139*:783, 1954.

Griswold, R. A., and Maguire, C. H.: Penetrating Wounds of the Heart in Pericardium. Surg. Gynecol. Obstet., *74*:406, 1942.

Gryska, P. F.: Major Vascular Injuries; Principles in Management in Selected Cases of Arterial and Venous Injuries. N. Engl. J. Med., *266*:381, 1962.

Guerriero, W. G., Carlton, C. E., Jr., Scott, R., Jr., and Beall, A. C., Jr.: Renal Pedical Injuries. J. Trauma, *11*:53, 1971.

Guilfoil, P. H., and Christiansen, T.: An Unusual Vascular Complication of Fractured Clavicle. J.A.M.A., *200*:178, 1967.

Gurdjian, E. S., Hardy, W. G., Lindner, D. W., and Thomas, L. M.: Closed Cervical Cranial Trauma, Associated With Involvement of Carotid and Vertebral Arteries. J. Neurosurg., *20*:418, 1963.

Guthrie, C. C.: Blood Vessel Surgery. Edward Arnold & Company, London, 1912.

Guthrie, G. J.: Diseases and Injuries of Arteries. 1830.

Guthrie, G. J.: On Gun Shot Wounds of the Extremities, Requiring the Different Operations of Amputation with Their After Treatment. Longman and others, London, 1815.

Haas, L., and Staple, T.: Arterial Injuries Associated with Fractures of the Proximal Tibia Following Blunt Trauma. South. Med. J., *62*:1439, 1969.

Haimovici, H.: History of Arterial Grafting. J. Cardiovasc. Surg., *4*:152, 1963.

Haimovici, H. H., Hoffert, B. W., Zinicola, N., and Steinman, C.: An Experimental and Clinical Evaluation of Grafts in the Venous System. Surg. Gynecol. Obstet., *131*:1173, 1970.

Haller, J. A.: Bullet Transection of Both Carotid Arteries: Immediate Repair with Recovery. Am. J. Surg., *103*:532, 1962.

Hallowell (1759): Cited by Lambert: Extract of a Letter from Mr. Lambert, Surgeon at Newcastle upon Tyne, to Dr. Hunter, giving an account of a new method of treating an aneurysm. Med. Obser. Inq. (Lond.), Ch. 30, p. 360, 1762.

Halsted, W.: Ligation of the First Portion of the Left Subclavian Artery and Excision of a Sub-clavico-axillary Aneurysm. Bull. Johns Hopkins Hosp., *3*:93, 1892.

Halsted, W. S.: The Effect of Ligation of the Common Iliac Artery on the Circulation and Function of the Lower Extremity. Report of a Cure of Iliofemoral Aneurism by the Application of an Aluminum Band to the Vessel. Bull. Johns Hopkins Hosp., *23*:191, 1912.

Halsted, W.: Discussion in Bernheim, B. M.: The Ideal Operation for Aneurism of the Extremity. Report of a Case. Bull. Johns Hopkins Hosp., *27*:93, 1916.

Halsted, W. S.: Ligation of the Left Subclavian Artery in its First Portion. Bull. Johns Hopkins Hosp., *21*:1, 1924.

Handsaker, G.: An Ordeal in a Snowdrift. The Evening Star, Washington, D.C., Monday, June 14, 1971.

Harbison, S. P.: Major Vascular Complication of Intervertebral Disc Surgery. Ann. Surg., *140*:342, 1954.

Hardin, C. A.: Bypass Saphenous Grafts for the Relief of Venous Obstruction of the Extremity. Surg. Gynecol. Obstet., *115*:709, 1962.

Hardy, J. D., and Timmis, H. H.: Repair of Intracardiac Gunshot Injuries: Report of Three Cases. Ann. Surg., *169*:906, 1969.

Hardy, J. D., and Williams, R. D.: Penetrating Heart Wounds. Analysis of 12 Consecutive Cases Without Mortality. Ann. Surg., *166*:228, 1967.

Hardy, J. D., Raju, S., Neely, W. A., and Berry, D. W.: Aortic and Other Arterial Injuries. Ann. Surg., *181*:640, 1975.

Harken, D. E.: Foreign Bodies in and in Relation to the Thoracic Blood Vessels and Heart. Surg. Gynecol. Obstet., *13*:117, 1946.

Harken, D. E., and Williams, A. C.: Foreign Bodies in and in Relation to the Thoracic Blood Vessels and Heart. Am. J. Surg., *72*:80, 1946.

Harken, D. E., and Zoll, P. M.: Foreign Bodies in and in Relation to the Thoracic Blood Vessels and Heart. Am. Heart J., *32*:1, 1946.

Harris, J. D.: A Case of Arteriovenous Fistula Following Closed Fracture of Tibia and Fibula. Br. J. Surg., *50*:774, 1963.

Hart, R. J., Jr., and Gregoratos, G.: Ventricular Septal Defects Caused by Stab Wounds: Report of Two Cases. Milit. Med., *139*:289, 1974.

Hartsuck, J. M., Moreland, H. J., and Williams, G. R.: Surgical Management of Vascular Trauma Distal to the Popliteal Artery. Arch. Surg., *105*:937, 1972.

Harvey, E. N., and McMillen, J. H.: An Experimental Study of Shock Waves Resulting From the Impact of High Velocity Missiles on Animal Tissue. J. Exp. Med., *85*:321, 1947.

Harvey, E. N., Butler, E. G., McMillen, J. H., and Puckett, W. O.: Mechanism of Wounding. War Med., *8*:91, 1945.

Harvey, E. N., Korr, I. M., Oster, G., and McMillen, J. H.: Secondary Damage in Wounding Due to Pressure Changes Accompanying the Passage of High Velocity Missiles. Surgery, *21*:218, 1947.

Heaton, L. D., Hughes, C. W., Rosegay, H., Fisher, G. W., and Feighny, R. E.: Military Surgical Practices of the United States Army in Vietnam. Year Book Medical Publishers, Inc., Chicago, 1966.

Heidenhain, L.: Über Naht von Arterienwunden. Centralbl. Chir., *22*:1113, 1895.

Herget, C. H.: Wound Ballistics. *In* Bowers, W. B. (Ed.): Surgery of Trauma. J. B. Lippincott & Company, Philadelphia, 1956.

Herlyn, K. E.: Erfahrungen auf dem Gebiete von Aneurysmen und Arteriovenosen Fisteln. Atti della Prima Riunione Internacionale de Angio-Cardio-Chirurgia. Casa Edetrice "Mellon" Milano, 1951.

Hermreck, A. S., Sifers, T. M., Reckling, S. W., Asher, M. A., and Hardin, C. A.: Traumatic Vascular Injuries: Methods and Results of Repair. Am. J. Surg., *128*:813, 1974.

Hershey, F. B.: Secondary Repair of Arterial Injuries. Am. Surg., *27*:33, 1961.

Hershey, F. B., and Spencer, A. D.: Surgical Repair of Civilian Arterial Injuries. Arch. Surg., *80*:953, 1960.

Hershey, F. B., and Spencer, A. D.: Autogenous Vein Grafts for Repair of Arterial Injuries. Arch. Surg., *86*:836, 1963.

Hertzer, N. R.: Peripheral Atheromatous Embolization Following Blunt Abdominal Trauma. Surgery, *82*:244, 1977.

Hewitt, R. L.: Technical Considerations in Acute Military Vascular Injuries of the Extremities. Milit. Med., *134*:617, 1969.

Hewitt, R. L., and Collins, D. J.: Acute Arteriovenous Fistulas in War Injuries. Ann. Surg., *169*:447, 1969.

Hewitt, R. L., Collins, D. J., and Hamit, H. F.: Arterial Injuries at a Surgical Hospital in Vietnam. Arch. Surg., *98*:313, 1969.

Hewitt, R. L., and Grablowsky, O. M.: Acute Traumatic Dissecting Aneurysm of the Abdominal Aorta. Ann. Surg., *171*:160, 1970.

Hewitt, R. L., Smith, A. D., Jr., Weichert, R. F., and Drapanas, T.: Penetrating Cardiac Injuries: Current Trends in Management. Arch. Surg., *101*:683, 1970.

Hewitt, R. L., Smith, A. D., and Drapanas, T.: Acute Traumatic Arteriovenous Fistulas. J. Trauma, *13*:901, 1973.

Hewitt, R. L., Smith, A. D., Becker, M. L., Lindsey, E. S., Dowling, J. B., and Drapanas, T.: Penetrating Vascular Injuries of the Thoracic Outlet. Surgery, *76*:715, 1974.

Hiebert, C. A., and Gregory, F. J.: Bullet Embolism From the Head to the Heart. J.A.M.A., *229*:442, 1974.

Hiertonn, T., and Rybeck, B. (Eds.): Traumatic Arterial Lesions. Försvarets Forskningsanstalt, Stockholm, 1968.

Hirsch, B. (1881): *In* Guthrie, C. C.: Blood Vessel Surgery. Edward Arnold & Company, London, 1912.

Hirsch, E. F.: *In* Discussion of Rich, N. M., et al.: J. Trauma, *11*:463, 1971.

Hobson, R. W., II, Croom, R. D., and Swan, K. G.: Hemodynamics of the Distal Arteriovenous Fistula in Venous Reconstruction. J. Surg. Res., *4*:483, 1973A.

Hobson, R. W., Howard, E. W., Wright, C. B., Collins, G. J., and Rich, N. M.: Hemodynamics of Canine Femoral Venous Ligation: Significance in Combined Arterial and Venous Injuries. Surgery, *74*:824, 1973B.

Hobson, R. W., II, Wright, C. B., Rich, N. M., and Collins, G. J., Jr.: Assessment of Colonic Ischemia During Aortic Surgery by Doppler Ultrasound. J. Surg. Res., *20*:231, 1976.

Hohf, R. P.: Arterial Injuries Occurring During Orthopedic Operations. Clin. Orthop., *28*:21, 1963.

Holman, E.: The Physiology of an Arteriovenous Fistula. Arch. Surg., 7:64, 1923.

Holman, E.: Arteriovenous Aneurysms: Abnormal Communication Between the Arterial and Venous Circulations. The MacMillan Company, New York, 1937.

Holman, E.: Clinical and Experimental Observations on Arteriovenous Fistulae. Ann. Surg., *112*:840, 1940.

Holman, E.: War Injuries to Arteries and Their Treatment. Surg. Gynecol. Obstet., *75*:183, 1942.

Holman, E.: Contributions to Cardiovascular Physiology Gleaned From Clinical and Experimental Observations of Abnormal Arteriovenous Communications. J. Cardiovasc. Surg., *3*:48, 1962.

Holman, E.: Abnormal Arteriovenous Communications: Great Variability of Effects With Particular Reference to Delayed Development of Cardiac Failure. Circulation, *32*:1001, 1965.

Holman, E.: Abnormal Arteriovenous Communications: Peripheral and Intracardiac, Acquired and Congenital. 2nd ed. Charles C Thomas, Publisher, Springfield, Ill., 1968.

Holman, E.: Sir William Osler and William Stewart Halsted — Two Contrasting Personalities. Pharos AOA, *34*:134, 1971.

Holzer, C. E., Jr.: Gunshot Wound Involving the Abdominal Artery. Surgery, *23*:645, 1948.

Hoover, N. W.: Injuries of the Popliteal Artery Associated With Fractures and Dislocations. Surg. Clin. North Am., *41*:1099, 1961.

Horsely, V.: The Destructive Effects of Small Projectiles. Nature, *50*:106, 1894.

Horsley, J. S.: Surgery of the Blood Vessels. C. V. Mosby Company, St. Louis, Mo., 1915.

Hughes, C. W.: Acute Vascular Trauma in Korean War Casualties: An Analysis of 180 Cases. Surg. Gynecol. Obstet., *99*:91, 1954A.

Hughes, C. W.: Use of Intra-aortic Balloon Catheter Tamponade for Controlling Intra-abdominal Hemorrhage in Man. Surgery, *36*:65, 1954B.

Hughes, C. W.: The Primary Repair of Wounds of Major Arteries. Ann. Surg., *141*:297, 1955.

Hughes, C. W.: Arterial Repair During the Korean War. Ann. Surg., *147*:555, 1958A.

Hughes, C. W.: Vascular Injuries in the Orthopedic Patient. J. Bone Joint Surg., *40A*:1271, 1958B.

Hughes, C. W.: Vascular Surgery in the Armed Forces. Milit. Med., *124*:30, 1959.

Hughes, C. W., and Bowers, W. F.: Traumatic Lesions of Peripheral Vessels. Charles C Thomas, Publisher, Springfield, Ill., 1961.

Hughes, C. W., and Jahnke, E. J., Jr.: The Surgery of Traumatic Arteriovenous Fistulas and Aneurysms: A Five Year Follow-Up Study of 215 Lesions. Ann. Surg., *148*:790, 1958.

Hughes, C. W., and Rich, N. M.: The Management of Vascular Injuries. South. Med. Bull., *57*:36, 1969.

Huguier (1848): Cited by Horsely: The Destructive Effects of Small Projectiles. Nature, *50*:106, 1894.

Huguier: Anévrisme ratérioso-veineux de l'artère fémorale gauche. Bull. Soc. Chir. Paris, *ii*:106, 1852.

Hull, D. A., and Hyde, C. L.: Arterial Injuries in Civilian Practice. J. Ken. Med. Assoc., *65*:975, 1967.

Hunt, T. K., Blaisdell, W., and Okimoto, J.: Vascular Injuries of the Base of the Neck. Arch. Surg., *98*:586, 1969.

Hunt, T. K., Leeds, F. H., Wanebo, H. J., and Blaisdell, F. W.: Arteriovenous Fistulas of Major Vessels of the Abdomen. J. Trauma, *2*:483, 1971.

Hunter, J. (1786): Cited in Power, D-Arcy: Hunter's Operation for the Cure of Aneurysm. Brit. J. Surg., *17*:193, 1929.

Hunter, J.: A Treatise on the Blood, Inflammation and Gunshot Wounds. George Nicol, London, 1794.

Hunter, W.: The History of an Aneurysm of the Aorta, With Some Remarks on Aneurysms in General. Med. Obs. Soc. Phys. Lond., *1*:323, 1757.

Hunter, W.: Further Observations Upon a Particular Species of Aneurysm. Med. Obs. Soc. Phys. Lond., *2*:390, 1762.

Hurwitt, E. S., and Seidenberg, B.: Rupture of the Heart During Cardiac Massage. Ann. Surg., *137*:115, 1953.

Hurwitt, E. S., and Seidenberg, B.: The Nonoperative Management of Two Cases of Catheter Perforation of the Aorta. Am. J. Surg., *110*:452, 1965.

Ikard, R., and Merendino, K. A.: Accidental Excision of the Superior Mesenteric Artery. Surg. Clin. North Am., 50:1075, 1970.

Imamoglu, K., Read, R. C., and Huebl, H. C.: Cervicomediastinal Vascular Injuries. Surgery, 61:274, 1967.

Inahara, T.: Arterial Injuries of the Upper Extremity. Surgery, 51:605, 1962.

Inui, F. K., Shannon, J., and Howard, J. M.: Arterial Injuries in the Korean Conflict. Surgery, 37:850, 1955.

Isaacs, J. P.: Sixty Penetrating Wounds of the Heart. Clinical and Experimental Oservations. In Blalock, A.: Recent Advances in Surgery. Surgery, 45:696, 1959.

Isaacs, J. P., Swanson, H. S., and Smith, R. A.: Transient Childhood Strokes From Internal Carotid Stenosis. J.A.M.A., 207:859, 1969.

Israel: Cited in Murphy, J. B.: Resection of Arteries and Veins Injured in Continuity—End-to-End Suture—Experimental Clinical Research. Med. Rec., 51:73, 1897.

Jahnke, E. J., Jr.: The Surgery of Acute Vascular Injuries. Milit. Surg., 112:249, 1953.

Jahnke, E. J., Jr.: Late Structural and Functional Results of Arterial Injuries Primarily Repaired. Surgery, 43:175, 1958.

Jahnke, E. J., Jr., and Howard, J. M.: Primary Repair of Major Arterial Wounds. Arch. Surg., 66:646, 1953.

Jahnke, E. J., Jr., and Seeley, S. F.: Acute Vascular Injuries in the Korean War: An Analysis of 77 Consecutive Cases. Ann. Surg., 138:158, 1953.

Jahnke, E. J., Jr., Hughes, C. W., and Howard, J. M.: The Rationale of Arterial Repair on the Battlefield. Am. J. Surg., 87:396, 1954.

Jarstfer, B. S., and Rich, N. M.: The Challenge of Arteriovenous Fistula Formation Following Disk Surgery: A Collective Review. J. Trauma, 16:726, 1976.

Jassinowsky, A.: Die Arteriennhat: Eine Experimentelle Studie. Inaug. Diss. Dorpat., 1889.

Javid, H.: Vascular Injuries of the Neck. Clin. Orth., 28:70, 1963.

Jensen: Ueber circulare Gefassutur. Arch. Klin. Chir., 69:938, 1903.

Jensen, A. R.: Bullet Wound of the Abdominal Aorta With Survival. J. Fla. Med. Assoc., 49:656, 1963.

Jeresaty, R. M., and Liss, J. P.: Effects of Brachial Artery Catheterization on Arterial Pulse and Blood Pressure in 203 Patients. Am. Heart J., 76:481, 1968.

Jernigan, W. R., and Gardner, W. C.: Carotid Artery Injuries Due to Closed Cervical Trauma. J. Trauma, 11:429, 1971.

Johns, T. N. P.: A Comparison of Suture and Non-suture Methods for the Anastomosis of Veins. Surg. Gynecol. Obstet., 84:939, 1947.

Johnson, G., Jr., and Blythe, W. B.: Hemodynamic Effects of Arteriovenous Shunts Used for Hemodialysis. Ann. Surg., 171:715, 1970.

Johnson, G. W., and Lowry, J. H.: Rupture of the Axillary Artery Complicating Anterior Dislocation of the Shoulder. J. Bone Joint Surg., 44-B:116, 1962.

Johnson, G., Jr., Peters, R. M., and Dart, C. H., Jr.: A Study of Cardiac Vein Negative Pressure in Arterio-venous Fistula. Surg. Gynecol. Obstet., 124:82, 1967.

Johnson, V., and Eiseman, B.: Evaluation of Arteriovenous Shunts to Maintain Patency of Venous Autograft. Am. J. Surg., 118:915, 1969.

Jones, E. W., and Helmsworth, J.: Penetrating Wounds of the Heart: Thirty Years' Experience. Arch. Surg., 96:671, 1968.

Jones, J. W., Hewitt, R. L., and Drapanas, T.: Cardiac Contusion: A Capricious Syndrome. Ann. Surg., 181:567, 1975.

Kakkar, V. V.: The Cephalic Vein as a Peripheral Vascular Graft. Surg. Gynecol. Obstet., 128:551, 1969.

Kakos, G. S., Williams, T. E., Jr., Kilman, J. W., and Klassen, K. P.: Traumatic Left Ventricular Aneurysms After Penetrating Chest Injury. Ann. Surg., 174:202, 1971.

Kapp, J. P., Gielchinsky, I., and Jelsma, R.: Metallic Fragment Embolization to the Cerebral Circulation. J. Trauma, 13:256, 1973.

Kay, J. K., Dykstra, P. C., and Tsuji, H. K.: Retrograde Ilio-aortic Dissection: A Complication of Common Femoral Arterial Perfusion During Open-Heart Surgery. Am. J. Surg., 3:464, 1966.

Kelly, G. L., and Eiseman, B.: Civilian Vascular Injuries. J. Trauma, 15(6):507, 1975.

Kemmerer, W. T., Eckert, W. G., Gathright, J. B., Reemtsma, K., and Creech, O., Jr.: Patterns of Thoracic Injuries in Fatal Traffic Accidents. J. Trauma, 1:595, 1961.

Kennedy, J. C.: Complete Dislocations of the Knee. J. Bone Joint Surg., 41-B:878, 1959.

Kennedy, J. C.: Complete Dislocation of the Knee Joint. J. Bone Joint Surg., 45A:889, 1963.

Keynes, G. (Ed.): The Apologie and Treatise of Ambroise Paré. University of Chicago, Chicago, 1952.

Kilburn, P., Sweeney, J. G., and Silk, F. F.: Three Cases of Compound Posterior Dislocation of the Elbow With Rupture of the Brachial Artery. J. Bone Joint Surg., 44-B:119, 1962.

Killen, D. A.: Injury of the Superior Mesenteric Vessel Secondary to Non-penetrating Abdominal Trauma. Am. Surg., 30:306, 1964.

Kinmonth, J. B.: A Report on the Physiology and Relief of Traumatic Arterial Spasm. Br. Med. J.,
    1:59, 1952.
Kirkup, J. R.: Major Arterial Injury Complicating Fracture of the Femoral Shaft. J. Bone Joint Surg.,
    45-B:337, 1963.
Kleinert, H. E.: Homograft Patch Repair of Bullet Wounds of the Aorta: Experimental Study and
    Report of a Case. Arch. Surg., *76*:811, 1958.
Kleinert, H. E.: Vascular Diseases. Unpublished Paper, 1972.
Kleinert, H. E., and Kasdan, M. L.: Restoration of Blood Flow in Upper Extremity Injuries. J.
    Trauma, *3*:461, 1963.
Kleinert, H. E., Kasdan, M. L., and Romero, J. L.: Restoration of Blood Flow in Upper Extremity
    Injuries. J. Trauma, *3*:461, 1963A.
Kleinert, H. E., Kasdan, M. L., and Romero, J. L.: Small Blood Vessel Anastomosis for Salvage of
    Severely Injured Upper Extremity. J. Bone Joint Surg. *45A*:788, 1963B.
Kleinert, H. E., and Volianitis, G. J.: Thrombosis of the Palmar Arch and Its Tributaries: Etiology
    and Newer Concepts in Treatment. J. Trauma, *5*:447, 1965.
Kleinert, H. E., Burget, G. C., Morgan, J. A., Kutz, J. E., and Atasoy, E.: Aneurysms of the Hand.
    Arch. Surg., *106*:554, 1973.
Kleinsasser, L. J.: The Removal of a Wire Lodged in the Interventricular Septum of the Heart.
    Surgery, *50*:500, 1961.
Kline, D. G., and Hackett, E. R.: Reappraisal of Timing for Exploration of Civilian Peripheral Nerve
    Injuries. Surgery, *78*:54,.1975.
Klingensmith, W., Oles, P., and Martinez, H.: Fractures with Associated Blood Vessel Injury. Am. J.
    Surg., *110*:849, 1965A.
Klingensmith, W., Oles, P., and Martinez, H.: Arterial Injuries Associated with Dislocation of the
    Knee or Fracture of the Lower Femur. Surg. Gynecol. Obstet., *120*:961, 1965B.
Kootstra, G., Schipper, J. J., Klasen, H. J., and Binnendijk, B.: Femoral Shaft Fracture with Injury of
    the Superficial Femoral Artery in Civilian Accidents. Surg. Gynecol. Obstet., *142*:399, 1976.
Kornblith, B. A.: Gunshot Wound Through the Abdominal Aorta. Ann. Surg., *113*:637, 1941.
Krauss, M.: Studies in Wound Ballistics. Temporary Cavity Effects in Soft Tissues. Milit. Med.,
    120:221, 1957.
Krosnick, A.: Death Due to Migration of the Ball From an Aortic-valve Prosthesis. J.A.M.A.,
    191:1083, 1965.
Kuiper, D. H.: Cardiac Tamponade and Death in a Patient Receiving Total Parenteral Nutrition.
    J.A.M.A., *230*:877, 1974.
Kümmel: Über Circuläre Naht der Gefässe. Munch. Med. Wschr., *46*:1398, 1899.
La Garde, L. A.: Report of the Surgeon General of the Army to the Secretary of War. U.S.
    Government Printing Office, Washington, D.C., 1893.
La Garde, L. A.: Gunshot Injuries (How They Are Inflicted, Their Complications and Treatment).
    William Wood & Company, New York, 1916.
Lai, M. D., Hoffman, H. B., and Adamkiewicz, J. J.: Dissecting Aneurysm of Internal Carotid Artery
    After Non-penetrating Neck Injury. Acta Radiol. Diag., *5*:290, 1966.
Lambert (1759, 1761): Letter to Dr. Hunter. Cited in Lambert, 1762.
Lambert: Extract of a Letter from Mr. Lambert, Surgeon at Newcastle upon Tyne, to Dr. Hunter;
    Giving an Account of a New Method of Treating an Aneurysm. Med. Observ. Inq. (Lond.), Ch.
    30, p. 360, 1762.
Langenbeck, B.: Beitrage Zur Chirurgischen Pathologie der Venen. Arch. Klin. Chir., *1*:1, 1861.
Langley, G. F.: Gunshot Wound of the Innominate Artery. Brit. Med. J., *2*:711, 1943.
Larrey, D. J.: Sur une blessure du pericorde suivie d'hydropericarde. Bull. Sci. Med., *6*:1, 1810.
Larrey, D. J.: Clin. Chir. Paris, *2*:284, 1829.
Lavenson, G. S., Jr., Rich, N. M., and Baugh, J. H.: Value of Ultrasonic Flow Detector in the
    Management of Peripheral Vascular Disease. Am. J. Surg., *120*:522, 1970.
Lavenson, G. S., Jr., Rich, N. M., and Strandness, D. E., Jr.: Ultrasonic Flow Detector Value in the
    Management of Combat Incurred Vascular Injuries. Arch. Surg., *103*:644, 1971.
Lawrence, K. B., Shefts, L. M., and McDaniel, J. R.: Wounds of Common Carotid Arteries: Report of
    17 Cases From World War II. Am. J. Surg., *76*:29, 1948.
Lawton, R. L., Rossi, N. P., and Funk, D. C.: Intracardiac Perforation. Arch. Surg., *98*:213, 1969.
Learmonth, J. R.: An Unusual Type of Arteriovenous Communication. Br. J. Surg., *32*:321,
    1945.
Learmonth, J. R.: Vascular Injuries in War. Roy. Soc. Med., *39*:488, 1946.
Learmonth, J.: Combined Neuro-vascular Lesions. Acta Chir. Scand., *104*:93, 1952–53.
Lee, H. and Beale, L. S.: On the Repair of Arteries and Veins after Injury. Trans. Med.-Chir. Soc.,
    50:477, 1865.
Lemos, P. C. P., Okumura, M., Azevedo, A. C., Paula, W. D., and Zerbini, E. J.: Cardiac Wounds:
    Experience Based on a Series of 120 Operated Cases. J. Cardiovasc. Surg., *17*:1, 1976.
Lester, J.: Arteriovenous Fistula After Percutaneous Vertebral Angiography. Acta Radiol. Diag.,
    5:337, 1966.
LeVeen, H. H., and Cerruti, M. M.: Surgery of Large Inaccessible Arteriovenous Fistulas. Ann.
    Surg., *158*:258, 1963.

Levin, P. M., Rich, N. M., and Hutton, J. E., Jr.: The Role of Collateral Circulation in Arterial Injuries. Arch. Surg., *102*:392, 1971A.

Levin, P. M., Rich, N. M., Hutton, J. E., Jr., Barker, W. F., and Zeller, J. A.: The Role of Arteriovenous Shunts in Venous Reconstruction. Am. J. Surg., *122*:183, 1971B.

Levitsky, S., James, P. M., Anderson, R. W., and Hardeway, R. M., II: Vascular Trauma in Vietnam Battle Casualties: An Analysis of 55 Consecutive Cases. Ann. Surg., *168*:831, 1968.

Lewis, T.: The Adjustment of Blood Flow to the Affected Limb in Arteriovenous Fistula. Clin. Sci., *4*:277, 1940.

Lewtas, J.: Traumatic Subclavian Aneurysm; Ligature of Innominate Carotid Arteries; Recovery. Br. Med. J., *2*:312, 1889.

Lexer, E.: Die Ideale Operation des Arteriellen und des Arteriell-Venosen Aneurysma. Arch. Klin. Chir., *83*:459, 1907.

Lichtenstein, M. E.: Acute Injuries Involving the Large Blood Vessels in the Neck. Surg. Gynecol. Obstet., *85*:165, 1947.

Liddicoat, J. E., Bekassy, S. M., Daniell, M. B., and DeBakey, M. E.: Inadvertent Femoral Artery "Stripping": Surgical Management. Surgery, *77*:318, 1975.

Lilienthal, H.: Thoracic Surgery: The Surgical Treatment of Thoracic Disease. W. B. Saunders Company, Philadelphia, 1926.

Lim, R. C., Jr., Trunkey, D. D., and Blaisdell, F. W.: Acute Abdominal Aortic Injury: An Analysis of Operative and Postoperative Management. Arch. Surg., *109*:706, 1974.

Linberg, E. J.: Bullet Wound of the Thoracic Aorta with Survival. Maryland State Med. J., *8*:285, 1959.

Lindskog, G. E.: The Surgery of the Innominate Artery. N. Engl. J. Med., *235*:71, 1946.

Lindskog, G. E., Liebow, A. A., and Glenn, W. W. L.: Thoracic and Cardiovascular Surgery With Related Pathology. Appleton-Century-Crofts, New York, 1962.

Linton, R. R.: Injuries to Major Arteries and Their Treatment. N.Y. J. Med., *49*:2039, 1949.

Linton, R. R.: Arterial Injuries Associated With Fractures of the Extremity. J. Bone Joint Surg., *46A*:575, 1964.

Lipscomb, P. R., and Burleson, R. J.: Vascular and Neural Complications in the Supracondylar Fractures of the Humerus in Children. J. Bone Joint Surg., *37A*:487, 1955.

Little, J. M., and Ferguson, D. A.: The Incidence of Hypothenar Hammer Syndrome. Arch. Surg., *105*:684, 1972.

Lloyd, J. T.: Traumatic Peripheral Aneurysms. Am. J. Surg., *93*:755, 1957.

Loello, F. V., and Nunn, D. B.: False Aneurysm of the Inferior Epigastric Artery as a Complication of Abdominal Retention Sutures. Surgery, *74*:460, 1973.

Lord, J. W., Jr., Stone, P. W., Clouthier, W. A., and Breidenbach, L.: Major Blood Vessel Injury During Elective Surgery. Arch. Surg., *77*:282, 1958.

Lord, R. S. A., Ehrenfeld, W. K., and Wylie, E. J.: Arterial Injury from the Fogarty Catheter. Med. J. Aust., *2*:70, 1968.

Lord, R. S. A., and Irana, C. N.: Assessment of Arterial Injury in Limb Trauma. J. Trauma, *14*:1042, 1974.

Love, C. R., and Evans, S. S.: Gunshot Wound of the Abdominal Aorta and Anoxic Cardiac Arrest: Report of a Survival. Ann. Surg., *158*:131, 1963.

Lowen, H. J., Fink, S. A., and Helpern, M.: Transfixion of the Heart by Embedded Ice Pick Blade with Eight Months' Survival. Circulation, Vol. II, September, 1950.

Lucas, R. J., Tumacder, O., and Wilson, G. S.: Hepatic Artery Occlusion Following Hepatic Artery Catheterization. Ann. Surg., *173*:238, 1971.

Ludewig, R. M., and Wangensteen, S. L.: Aortic Bleeding and the Effect of External Counter Pressure. Surg. Gynecol. Obstet., *128*:252, 1969.

Luke, J. C.: Arterial Trauma. J. Cardiovasc. Surg., *3*:165, 1962.

Lumpkin, M. B., Logan, W. D., Couves, C. M., and Howard, J. M.: Arteriography as an Aid in the Diagnosis and Localization of Acute Arterial Injuries. Ann. Surg., *147*:353, 1958.

Lyons, C., and Perkins, R.: Cardiac Stab Wounds. Am. Surg., *23*:507, 1957.

McCann, W. J.: Successful Repair of a Stab Wound of the Ascending Aorta. N.Y. State J. Med., *58*:3177, 1958.

McCormack, L. J., Cauldwell, E. W., and Anson, B. J.: Brachial and Antebrachial Arterial Patterns: A Study of 750 Extremities. Surg. Gynecol. Obstet., *96*:43, 1953.

McDonald, E. J., Jr., Goodman, P. C., and Winestock, D. T.: The Clinical Indications for Arteriography and Trauma to the Extremity: A Review of 114 Cases. Radiology, *116*:45, 1975.

McDonough, J. J., and Altemeier, W. A.: Subclavian Venous Thrombosis Secondary to Indwelling Catheters. Surg. Gynecol. Obstet., *133*:397, 1971.

McGough, E. C., Helfrich, L. R., and Hughes, R. K.: Traumatic Intimal Prolapse of the Common Carotid Artery. Am. J. Surg., *123*:724, 1972.

McKenzie, A. D., and Sinclair, A. M.: Axillary Artery Occlusion Complicating Shoulder Dislocation: A Report of Two Cases. Ann. Surg., *148*:139, 1958.

MacLachlin, A. D., Carroll, S. E., Meades, G. E., and Amacher, A. L.: Valve Replacement in the Recanalized Incompetent Superficial Femoral Vein in Dogs. Ann. Surg., *162*:446, 1965.

MacLean, L. D.: The Diagnosis and Treatment of Arterial Injuries. Can. Med. Assoc. J., *88*:1091, 1963.

MacLean, L. D., Flam, R. S., and Petersen, D. H.: Diagnosis and Treatment of Arterial Injuries. Minn. Med., *44*:133, 1961.

McNamara, J. J., Brief, D. K., Beasley, W., and Wright, J. K.: Vascular Injury in Vietnam Combat Casualties: Results of Treatment at the 24th Evacuation Hospital, 1 July 1967 to 12 August 1969. Ann. Surg., *178*:143, 1973A.

McNamara, J. J., Brief, D. K., Stremple, J. F., and Wright, J. K.: Management of Fractures With Associated Arterial Injury in Combat Casualties. J. Trauma, *13*:17, 1973B.

Makin, G. S., Howard, J. M., and Green, R. L.: Arterial Injuries Complicating Fractures and Dislocations: The Necessity for a More Aggressive Approach. Surgery, *59*:203, 1966.

Makins, G.: Blessures des Vaisseaux. Comptes-Rendus Conférence Chirurgicale Inter-Alliée Pour L'Étude des Plaies de Guerre, 17 May 1917. Arch. Méd. Pharm. Mil., *68*:341, 1917.

Makins, G. H.: Gunshot Injuries to the Blood Vessels. John Wright and Sons, Ltd., Bristol, England, 1919.

Malt, R. A., and McKhann, C. F.: A Report on Replantation of Severed Arms. J.A.M.A., *189*:716, 1964.

Malt, R. A., Remensnyder, J. P., and Harris, W. H.: Long Term Utility of Replanted Arms. Ann. Surg., *176*:334, 1972.

Mandelbaum, I., and Kalsbeck, J. E.: Extrinsic Compression of Internal Carotid Artery. Ann. Surg., *171*:434, 1970.

Manlove, G. H., Quattlebaum, F. W., Flom, R. S., and LaFave, J. W.: Gunshot Wounds of the Abdominal Aorta. Am. J. Surg., *99*:941, 1960.

Mansberger, A. R., and Linberg, E. J.: First Rib Resection for Distal Exposure of Subclavian Vessels. Surg. Gynecol. Obstet., *120*:579, 1965.

Matas, R.: Traumatic Aneurism of the Left Brachial Artery; . . . Incision and Partial Excision of Sac; Recovery. Phila. Med. News, *53*:462, 1888.

Matas, R.: Traumatisms and Traumatic Aneurysms of the Vertebral Artery and Their Surgical Treatment. Ann. Surg., *18*:477, 1893.

Matas, R.: Traumatic Arterio-venous Aneurisms of the Subclavian Vessels, With an Analytical Study of Fifteen Reported Cases, Including One Operated. Trans. Am. Surg. Assoc., *xix*:237, 1901.

Matas, R.: An Operation for Radical Cure of Aneurism Based on Arteriorrhaphy. Ann. Surg., *37*:161, 1903.

Matas, R.: Recent Advances in the Technique of Thoracotomy and Pericardiotomy for Wounds of the Heart. South. Med. J., *1*:75, 1908A.

Matas, R.: *In* Keen's Surgery. Vol. V. W. B. Saunders Company, Philadelphia, 1908B.

Matas, R.: Testing the Efficiency of the Collateral Circulation as a Preliminary to the Occlusion of the Great Surgical Arteries. Ann. Surg., *53*:1, 1911.

Matas, R.: The Suture as Applied to a Surgical Cure of Aneurysm. Trans. Seventeenth Int. Cong. (Lond.), Aug., 1913.

Matas, R.: Testing the Efficiency of the Collateral Circulation as a Preliminary to the Occlusion of the Great Surgical Arteries. J.A.M.A., *68*:1441, 1914.

Matas, R.: Endo-aneurismorrhaphy. I. Statistics of Operation of Endo-aneurismorrhaphy. II. Personal Experiences and Observations on the Treatment of Arteriovenous Aneurisms by the Intrasaccular Method of Suture; with Special References to the Transvenous Route. Surg. Gynecol. Obstet., *30*:456, 1920.

Matas, R.: Military Surgery of the Vascular System. *In* Keen's Surgery. Vol. VII. W. B. Saunders Company, Philadelphia, 1921.

Mathewson, C.: Discussion. Am. J. Surg., *47*:484, 1940.

Mathur, A. P., Pochaczevsky, R., Levotitz, B. S., and Feraru, F.: Fogarty Balloon Catheter for Removal of Catheter Fragment in Subclavian Vein. J.A.M.A., *217*:481, 1971.

Matloff, D. B., and Morton, J. H.: Acute Trauma to the Subclavian Arteries. Am. J. Surg., *115*:675, 1968.

Mattox, K. E.: Discussion in Conckle et al.: Surgical Treatment of Popliteal Artery Injuries. Arch. Surg., *110*:1331, 1975.

Mattox, K. L., Beall, A. C., Jr., Jordan, G. L., and DeBakey, M. E.: Cardiorrhaphy in the Emergency Center. J. Thorac. Cardiovasc. Surg., *68*:886, 1974.

May, A. G., Lipchik, E. O., and DeWeese, J. A.: Repair of Hepatic and Superior Mesenteric Artery Injury: Patency Demonstrated by Arteriography. Ann. Surg., *162*:869, 1965.

Mengoli, L. R.: Aneurysmorrhaphy of the Internal Carotid Artery Utilizing Intraluminal Distal Control. Am. J. Surg., *117*:397, 1969.

Meyer, J. A., Neville, J. F., Jr., and Hansen, W. G.: Traumatic Rupture of the Aorta in a Child. J.A.M.A., *208*:527, 1969.

Meyer, T. L., Jr., and Slager, R. F.: False Aneurysm Following Subtrochanteric Osteotomy. J. Bone Joint Surg., *46A*:581, 1964.

Miller, D. S.: Gangrene From Arterial Injuries Associated With Fractures and Dislocations of the Leg in the Young and in Adults With Normal Circulation. Am. J. Surg., *93*:367, 1957.

Miller, D. S., and Freeark, R.: Injuries to the Popliteal Artery Among the Young. Am. J. Surg., *104*:633, 1962.

Miller, H. H., and Welch, C. S.: Quantitative Studies on Time Factor in Arterial Injuries. Ann. Surg., *130*:428, 1949.

Monson, D. O., Saletta, J. D., and Freeark, R. J.: Carotid-vertebral Trauma. J. Trauma, *9*:987, 1969.

Montgomery, M. L.: Effect of Therapeutic Venous Ligation on Blood Flow in Cases of Arterial Occlusion. Proc. Soc. Exp. Biol. Med., *27*:178, 1929.

Moore, C. A., and Cohen, A.: Combined Arterial, Venous and Ureteral Injury Complicating Lumbar Disc Surgery. Am. J. Surg., *115*:574, 1968.

Moore, C. H., Wolma, F. J., Brown, R. W., and Derrick, J. R.: Vascular Trauma, A Review of 250 Cases. Am. J. Surg., *122*:576, 1971.

Moore, H. G., Nyhus, L. M., Kanar, E. A., and Harkins, H. N.: Gunshot Wounds of the Major Arteries: An Experimental Study with Clinical Implications. Surg. Gynecol. Obstet., *98*:129, 1954.

Moore, T. C.: Acute Arterial Obstruction Due to the Traumatic Circumferential Intimal Fracture. Ann. Surg., *118*:111, 1958.

Morris, G. C., Jr., Creech, O., Jr., and DeBakey, M. E.: Acute Arterial Injuries in Civilian Practice. Am. J. Surg., *93*:565, 1957.

Morris, G. C., Jr., Beall, A. C., Jr., Roof, W. R., and DeBakey, M. E.: Surgical Experience with 220 Acute Arterial Injuries in Civilian Practice. Am. J. Surg., *99*:775, 1960A.

Morris, G. C., Jr., Beall, A. C., Jr., Berry, W. B., Feste, J., and DeBakey, M. E.: Anatomical Studies of the Distal Popliteal Artery and Its Branches. Surg. Forum, *10*:398, 1960B.

Morton, J. H., Southgate, W. A., and DeWeese, J. A.: Arterial Injuries of the Extremities. Surg. Gynecol. Obstet., *123*:611, 1966.

Morton, J. R., and Crawford, E. S.: Bilateral Traumatic Renal Artery Thrombosis. Ann. Surg., *176*:62, 1972.

Morton, J. R., Reul, G. J., Arbegast, N. R., Okies, J. E., and Beall, A. C., Jr.: Bullet Embolus to the Right Ventricle: Report of Three Cases. Am. J. Surg., *122*:584, 1971.

Motsay, G. J., Manlove, C., and Perry, J. F.: Major Venous Injury With Pelvic Fracture. J. Trauma, *9*:343, 1969.

Mott, V.: Reflections on Securing in a Ligature the Arteria Innominata. Med. Surg., *1*:9, 1918.

Moure, P.: Les Greffes Vasculaires. Paris, Doin, 1914.

Mourin (1914): Cited in Moure, P.: Les Greffes Vasculaires, 1914.

Mufti, M. A., LaGuerre, J. N., Pochazevsky, R., Kassner, E. G., Richter, R. M., and Levowitz, B. S.: Diagnostic Value of Hematoma in Penetrating Arterial Wounds of the Extremities. Arch. Surg., *101*:562, 1970.

Mulder, D. G., and Grollman, J. H., Jr.: Traumatic Disruption of the Thoracic Aorta: Diagnostic and Surgical Considerations. Am. J. Surg., *118*:311, 1969.

Muller, W. H., Jr., and Goodwin, W. E.: Renal Arteriovenous Fistula Following Nephrectomy. Ann. Surg., *144*:240, 1956.

Murphy, J. B. (1896): Cited in Murphy, 1897.

Murphy, J. B.: Resection of Arteries and Veins Injured in Continuity – End-to-End Suture – Experimental and Clinical Research. Med. Rec., *51*:73, 1897.

Murphy, J. B.: Myositis. J.A.M.A., *63*:1249, 1914.

Murray, D. S.: Post Traumatic Thrombosis of the Internal Carotid and Vertebral Arteries After Non-penetrating Injuries of the Neck. Br. J. Surg., *44*:556, 1957.

Murray, G. D. W.: Heparin in Thrombosis and Embolism. Br. J. Surg., *27*:567, 1940.

Murray, G.: Surgical Repair of Injuries to Main Arteries. Am. J. Surg., *83*:480, 1952.

Murray, G., and Janes, J. M.: Prevention of Acute Failure of Circulation Following Injuries to Large Arteries: Experiments With Glass Cannulae Kept Patent by Administration of Heparin. Lancet, *1*:6, 1940.

Muscatello (1890): Cited in Murphy, 1897.

Mustard, W. T., and Bull, C.: A Reliable Method for Relief of Traumatic Vascular Spasm. Ann. Surg., *155*:339, 1962.

Myers, W. O., Lawton, B. R., and Sautter, R. D.: An Operation for Tracheal-Innominate Artery Fistula. Arch. Surg., *105*:269, 1972.

Naclerio, E. A.: Penetrating Wounds of the Heart: Experience with 249 Patients. Dis. Chest, *46*:1, 1964.

Nakano, J., and DeSchryver, C.: Effects of Arteriovenous Fistula on Systemic and Pulmonary Circulations. Am. J. Physiol., *207*:1319, 1964.

Natali, J., Lacombe, M., Bruchou, P., and Vinardi, G.: Les Traumatismes Artériels Vus Tardivement Conduite à Tenir En Leur Présence. Presse Med., *72*:2273, 1964.

Natali, J., Maraval, M., Kieffer, E., and Petrovic, P.: Fractures of a Clavicle and Injuries of the Subclavian Artery: Report of 10 Cases. J. Cardiovasc. Surg., *16*:541, 1975.

Neely, W. A., Hardy, J. D., and Artz, C. P.: Arterial Injuries in Civilian Practice: A Current Reappraisal With Analysis of 43 Cases. J. Trauma, *1*:424, 1961.

Ngu, V. A., and Konstam, P. G.: Traumatic Dissecting Aneurysm of the Abdominal Aorta. Br. J. Surg., 52:981, 1965.

Nguyen, L. Q., and Lewin, J. R.: Angiographic Demonstration of Fistula Between Abdominal Aorta and Thoracic Duct. J.A.M.A., 211:499, 1970.

Nicholas, G. G., and DeMuth, W. E., Jr.: Long-term Results of Brachial Thrombectomy Following Cardiac Catheterization. Ann. Surg., 183:436, 1976.

Nicoladoni, C.: Phlebarteriectasie der Rechten Oberen Extremitat. Arch. Klin. Chir., 18:252, 1875.

Nolan, B.: Vascular Injuries. J. Roy. Coll. Surg., 13:72, 1968.

Noon, G. P.: In Discussion of Buscaglia, L. C., Blaisdell, F. W., and Lim, R. C., Jr.: Arch Surg., 99:764, 1969.

Noon, G. P., Boulafendis, D., and Beall, A. C., Jr.: Rupture of the Heart Secondary to Blunt Trauma. J. Trauma, 11:122, 1971.

Norris, G.: Varicose Aneurysm at the Bend of the Arm: Ligature of the Artery Above and Below the Sac; Secondary Hemorrhages With a Return of the Aneurysm Thrill on the Tenth Day; Cure. Am. J. Med. Sci., 5:17, 1843.

Norton, L. W., and Spencer, F. C.: Long-term comparison of vein patch with direct suture. Arch. Surg., 89:1083, 1964.

Noth, P. H.: Electrocardiographic Patterns in Penetrating Wounds of the Heart. Am. Heart J., 32:713, 1946.

Odom, C. B.: Causes of Amputations of Battle Injuries With Emphasis on Vascular Injuries. Surgery, 19:562, 1946.

Ogilvie, W. H.: War Surgery in Africa. Br. J. Surg., 31:313, 1944.

O'Neill, J. A., Jr., and Killen, D. A.: Autogenous Vein Graft for Repair of Acute Tibial Artery Injury. Ann. Surg., 162:218, 1965.

Ortner, A. B., Berg, H. F., and Lebendiger, A.: Limb Salvage Through Small-vessel Surgery. Arch. Surg., 83:102, 1961.

Osler, W.: Case of Arterio-venous Aneurysm of the Axillary Artery and Vein of 14 Years Duration. Ann. Surg., 17:37, 1893.

Osler, W.: Report of a Case of Arteriovenous Aneurism of the Thigh. Johns Hopkins Hosp. Bull., 16:119, 1905.

Osler, W.: An Arterio-venous Aneurysm of the Axillary Vessels of 30 Years Duration. Lancet, 2:1248, 1913.

Osler, W.: Remarks on Arteriovenous Aneurysm. Lancet, 1:949, 1915.

Ouchi, H., Ohara, I., and Kijima, M.: Intraluminal Protrusion of Completely Disrupted Intima: An Unusual Form of Acute Arterial Injury. Surgery, 57:220, 1965.

Overbeck, W., Gruenagel, H. H., and Krauss, H.: Eisensplitterverletzung der intraprikardialen Aorta. Thoraxchirurgie, 16:274, 1968.

Owens, J. C.: The Management of Arterial Trauma. Surg. Clin. North Am., 43:371, 1963.

Pagenstecher, A. H.: Cited in Rea et al.: Coronary Artery Lacerations: An Analysis of 22 Patients. Ann. Thor. Surg., 7:518, 1969.

Paget, S.: The Surgery of the Chest. John Wright and Company, London, 1896.

Palma, E. C., and Esperon, R.: Vein Transplants and Graft in the Surgical Treatment of the Post-phlebitic Syndrome. J. Cardiovasc. Surg., 1:94, 1960.

Paré, A. (1546): The Apologie and Treatise of Amboise Paré Containing the Voyages Made Into Diverse Places With Many of His Writings Upon Surgery. Edited by G. Keynes. The University of Chicago Press, Chicago, 1952.

Parmley, L. F., Jr., Orbison, J. A., Hughes, C. W., and Mattingly, T. W.: Acquired Arteriovenous Fistulas Complicated by Endarteritis and Endocarditis Lenta Due to *Streptococcus faecalis*. N. Engl. J. Med., 250:305, 1954.

Parmley, L. F., Mattingly, T. W., and Manion, W. C.: Penetrating Wounds of the Heart and Aorta. Circulation, 17:953, 1958A.

Parmley, L. F., Manion, W. L., and Mattingly, T. W.: Nonpenetrating Traumatic Injury of the Heart. Circulation, 18:371, 1958B.

Parmley, L. F., Mattingly, T. W., Manion, W. C., and Jahnke, E. J.: Nonpenetrating Traumatic Injury of the Aorta. Circulation, 17:1086, 1958C.

Pate, J. W., and Richardson, R. L., Jr.: Penetrating Wounds of Cardiac Valves. J.A.M.A., 207:309, 1969.

Pate, J. W., and Wilson, H.: Arterial Injuries of the Base of the Neck. Arch. Surg., 89:1106, 1964.

Pate, J. W., Sherman, R. T., Jackson, T., and Wilson, H.: Cardiac Failure Following Traumatic Arteriovenous Fistula: A Report of 14 Cases. J. Trauma, 5:398, 1965.

Patman, R. D., Poulos, E., and Shires, T. C.: The Management of Civilian Arterial Injuries. Surg. Gynecol. Obstet., 118:725, 1964.

Patman, R. D., and Thompson, J. E.: Fasciotomy in Peripheral Vascular Surgery. Arch. Surg., 101:663, 1970.

Paton, B. C., Elliott, D. P., Taubman, J. O., and Owens, J. C.: Acute Treatment of Traumatic Aortic Rupture. J. Trauma, 11:1, 1971.

Patterson, F. P., and Morton, K. S.: The Cause of Death in Fractures of the Pelvis: With a Note on Treatment by Ligation of the Hypogastric (Internal Iliac) Artery. J. Trauma, *13*:849, 1973.

Patterson, R. H., Burns, W. A., and Jannotta, F. S.: Rupture of the Thoracic Aorta: Complication of Resuscitation. J.A.M.A., *226*:197, 1973.

Penn, I.: The Vascular Complications of Fractures of the Clavicle. J. Trauma, *4*:819, 1964.

Pennington, D. G., and Dranpanas, T.: Acute Post-traumatic Coarctation of the Abdominal Aorta. Surgery, *78*:538, 1975.

Perdue, G. D., Jr., and Smith, R. B.: Intra-abdominal Vascular Injury. Surgery, *64*:562, 1968.

Perkins, R., and Elchos, T.: Stab Wound of the Aortic Arch. Ann. Surg., *147*:83, 1958.

Perry, M. O. (1974): Closing Remarks in Thal et al.: Management of Carotid Artery Injuries. Surgery, *76*:955, 1974.

Perry, M. O., Thal, E. R., and Shires, G. T.: Management of Arterial Injuries. Ann. Surg., *173*:403, 1971.

Petit-Dutaillis, D., Janet, H.: Thiébaut, F., and Guillaumat, L.: Effets d'une Inversion Circulatoire par Anastomose Carotido-jugulaire sur une Hémiplégie Droit avec Aphasie due à une Thrombose de la Carotide Interne d'Origine Inconnue Chez un Adolescent de 13 Ans. Rev. Neurol., *81*:75, 1949.

Petrovsky, B. V., and Milinov, O. B.: "Arterialization" and "Venization" of Vessels Involved in Traumatic Arteriovenous Fistulae: Aetology and Pathogenesis (An Experimental Study). J. Cardiovasc. Surg., *8*:396, 1967.

Pick, T. P.: On Partial Rupture of Arteries from External Violence. St. George's Hosp. Rep. (Lond.), *6*:161, 1873.

Pick, T. P.: A Clinical Lecture of a Case of Arterio-venous Aneurysm. Lond. Med. Times Gaz., *2*:677, 1883.

Pitner, S. E.: Carotid Thrombosis Due to Intraoral Trauma: An Unusual Complication of a Common Childhood Accident. N. Engl. J. Med., *274*:764, 1966.

Piwnica, A. H., Chetochine, F., Soyer, R., and Winckler, C. L.: Traumatic Rupture of the Aortic Arch With Disinsertion of the Innominate Artery. J. Thorac. Cardiovasc. Surg., *61*:246, 1971.

Pomerantz, M., and Hutchison, D.: Traumatic Wounds of the Heart. J. Trauma, *9*:135, 1969.

Pontius, G. V., Kilbourne, B. C., and Paul, E. G.: Non-penetrating Abdominal Trauma. Arch. Surg., *72*:800, 1957.

Pool, E. H.: The Medical Department of the United States Army in the World War. Vol. II. U.S. Government Printing Office, Washington, D.C., 1927.

Porter, W. B., and Bigger, I. A.: Stab Wounds of the Heart and Great Vessels: A Study of Seventeen Cases. Trans. Am. Clin. Assoc., *54*:96, 1939.

Postempski, P.: La Sutura dei Vasi Sanguigni. Arch. Soc. Ital. Chir. Roma, *3*:391, 1886.

Pouyanne, H., Arne, L., Loiseau, P., and Mouton, L.: Considerations Sur Deux Cas de Thrombose de la Carotide Interne Chez l'Enfant. Rev. Neurol., *97*:525, 1957.

Power, D-Arcy: Hunter's Operation for the Cure of Aneurysm. Br. J. Surg., *17*:193, 1929.

Pratt, G. H.: Importance of a Knowledge of Vascular Surgery in World War II. Am. J. Surg., *56*:335, 1942.

Preston, A. P.: Arterial Injuries of Warfare: Complications and Management. Surgery, *20*:786, 1946.

Pridgen, W. R., and Jacobs, J. K.: Postoperative Arteriovenous Fistula. Surgery, *51*:205, 1962.

Pritchard, D. A., Maloney, J. D., Barnhorst, D. A., and Spittell, J. A., Jr.: Traumatic Popliteal Arteriovenous Fistulas. Arch. Surg., *112*:849, 1977.

Puckett, W. O.: The Wounding Effect of Small High Velocity Fragments As Revealed by High Speed Radiography. J. Elisha Mitchell Sci. Soc., *62*:59, 1946.

Quast, D. C., Shirkey, A. L., Fitzgerald, J. B., Beall, A. C., Jr., and DeBakey, M. E.: Surgical Correction of Injuries of the Vena Cava: An Analysis of Sixty-One Cases. J. Trauma, *5*:1, 1965.

Rabinowitz, R., and Goldfarb, D.: Surgical Treatment of Axillosubclavian Venous Thrombosis: A Case Report. Surgery, *70*:703, 1971.

Ransdell, H. T., and Glass, H., Jr.: Gunshot Wounds of the Heart: A Review of 20 Cases. Am. J. Surg., *999*:788, 1960.

Ransohoff, J. L.: Arteriovenous Aneurysm of the Superior Thyroid Artery and Vein. Surg. Gynecol. Obstet., *61*:816, 1935.

Razek, M. S. A., Mnaymneh, W., and Yacoubian, H. D.: Injuries of Peripheral Arteries With Associated Bone and Soft Tissue Injuries. J. Trauma, *13*:907, 1973.

Rea, W. J., Sugg, W. L., Wilson, L. C., Webb, W. R., and Ecker, R. R.: Coronary Artery Lacerations: An Analysis of 22 Patients. Ann. Thorac. Surg., *7*:518, 1969.

Rehn, L.: Ueber Penetrirende Herzwunden und Herznalt. Arch. Klin. Chir., *55*:315, 1897.

Reid, M. R.: The Effect of Arteriovenous Fistula upon the Heart and Blood Vessels: An Experiment and Clinical Study. Bull. Johns Hopkins Hosp., *31*:43, 1920.

Reid, M. R.: Abnormal Arteriovenous Communications. Acquired and Congenital. II. The Origin and Nature of Arteriovenous Aneurysms, Cirsoid Aneurysms and Simple Angiomas. Arch. Surg. (Chicago), *10*:996, 1925.

Reid, M. R., and McGuire, J.: Arteriovenous Aneurysm. Ann. Surg., *108*:643, 1938.

Reynolds, B. M., and Balsano, N. A.: Venography in Pelvic Fractures: A Clinical Evaluation. Ann. Surg., *173*:104, 1971.

Rhodes, G. R., Cox, C. B., and Silver, D.: Arteriovenous Fistula and False Aneurysm as the Cause of Consumption Coagulopathy. Surgery, *73*:535, 1973.

Rich, N. M.: Vietnam Missile Wounds Evaluated in 750 Patients. Milit. Med., *133*:9, 1968A.

Rich, N. M.: Wounding Power of Various Ammunition. Res. Physiol., *14*:72, 1968B.

Rich, N. M.: Missile Wound Evaluation at the 2nd Surgical Hospital in Vietnam. *In* Georjiade, N. M. (Ed.): Plastic and Maxillofacial Trauma Symposium. Ch. 2, pp. 9–16. The C. V. Mosby Co., St. Louis, 1969.

Rich, N. M.: Vascular Trauma in Vietnam. J. Cardiovasc. Surg., *11*:368, 1970.

Rich, N. M.: Surgery for Arterial Trauma. *In* Dale, W. A. (Ed.): Management of Arterial Occlusive Disease. Ch. 14. Year Book Medical Publishers, Inc., Chicago, 1971.

Rich, N. M.: Complications of Operations for Vascular Trauma, Arteriovenous Fistulas and False Aneurysms. *In* Beebee, H. G.: Complications in Vascular Surgery. Ch. 5. J. B. Lippincott and Co., Philadelphia, 1973A.

Rich, N. M.,: Vascular Trauma. Surg. Clin. North Am., *53*:1367, 1973B.

Rich, N. M.: Vascular Injuries. *In* Whelan, T. J., Jr. (Ed. in Chief): Emergency War Surgery: NATO Handbook. Ch. 13. U.S. Government Printing Office, Washington, D.C., 1975A.

Rich, N. M.: Weapons and Wounds (Editorial). J. Trauma, *15*:464, 1975B.

Rich, N. M., and Hobson, R. W., II: Historical Background of Repair of Venous Injuries. *In* Witkin, E., et al. (eds.): Venous Diseases, Medical and Surgical Management. Mouton, The Hague, Netherlands, 1974.

Rich, N. M., and Hobson, R. W., II: Trauma to the Venous System. *In* Swan, K. G., et al. (Eds.): Symposium on Venous Surgery in the Lower Extremity. Warren H. Green Publishers, Inc., St. Louis, 1975A.

Rich, N. M., and Hobson, R. W., II: Venous Trauma: Emphasis for Repair Is Indicated. J. Cardiovasc. Surg. Special Issue: *571*, 1975B.

Rich, N. M., and Hughes, C. W.: Vietnam Vascular Registry: A Preliminary Report. Surgery, *65*:218, 1969.

Rich, N. M., and Hughes, C. W.: The Fate of Prosthetic Material Used to Repair Vascular Injuries in Contaminated Wounds. J. Trauma, *12*:459, 1972A.

Rich, N. M., and Hughes, C. W.: Fifty Years Progress in Vascular Surgery. ACS Bull., *57*:35, 1972B.

Rich, N. M., and Sullivan, W. G.: Clinical Recanalization of an Autogenous Vein Graft in the Popliteal Vein. J. Trauma, *12*:919, 1972.

Rich, N. M., Johnson, E. V., and Dimond, F. C., Jr.: Wounding Power of Missiles Used in the Republic of Vietnam. J.A.M.A., *157*:1967.

Rich, N. M., Baugh, J. H., and Hughes, C. W.: Popliteal Artery Injuries in Vietnam. Am. J. Surg., *118*:531, 1969A.

Rich, N. M., Clarke, J. S., and Baugh, J. H.: Successful Repair of a Traumatic Aneurysm of the Abdominal Aorta. Surgery, *66*:492, 1969B.

Rich, N. M., Manion, W. C., and Hughes, C. W.: Surgical and Pathological Evaluation of Vascular Injuries in Vietnam. J. Trauma, *9*:279, 1969C.

Rich, N. M., Baugh, J. H., and Hughes, C. W.: Acute Arterial Injuries in Vietnam: 1,000 Cases. J. Trauma, *10*:359, 1970A.

Rich, N. M., Hughes, C. W., and Baugh, J. H.: Management of Venous Injuries. Ann. Surg., *171*: 724, 1970B.

Rich, N. M., Baugh, J. H., and Hughes, C. W.: The Significance of Complications Associated with Vascular Repairs Performed in Vietnam. Arch. Surg., *100*:646, 1970C.

Rich, N. M., Metz, C. W., Jr., Hutton, J. E., Jr., Baugh, J. H., and Hughes, C. W.: Internal Versus External Fixation of Fractures with Concomitant Vascular Injuries in Vietnam. J. Trauma, *11*:463, 1971A.

Rich, N. M., Amato, J. J., and Billy, L. J.: Arterial Thrombosis Secondary to Temporary Cavitation. Surg. Digest, *6*:12, 1971B.

Rich, N. M., Hobson, R. W., II, Jarstfer, B. S., and Geer, T. M.: Subclavian artery trauma. J. Trauma, *13*:485, 1973.

Rich, N. M., Hobson, R. W., II, Wright, C. B., and Fedde, C. W.: Repair of Lower Extremity Venous Trauma: A More Aggressive Approach Required. J. Trauma, *14*:639, 1974A.

Rich, N. M., Jarstfer, B. S., and Geer, T. M.: Popliteal Artery Repair Failure: Causes and Possible Prevention. J. Cardiovasc. Surg., *15*:340, 1974B.

Rich, N. M., Hobson, R. W., II, and Fedde, C. W.: Vascular Trauma Secondary to Diagnostic and Therapeutic Procedures. Am. J. Surg., *128*:715, 1974C.

Rich, N. M., Jarstfer, B. S., and Geer, T. M.: Concomitant Popliteal and Venous Trauma. *In* Swan, K. G., et al. (Eds.): Symposium on Venous Surgery in the Lower Extremity. Warren H. Green Publishers, Inc., St. Louis, 1975A.

Rich, N. M., Hobson, R. W., II, Fedde, C. W., and Collins, C. J., Jr.: Common Femoral Arterial Trauma. J. Trauma, *15*:628, 1975B.

Rich, N. M., Hobson, R. W., II, and Collins, G. J., Jr.: Elective Vascular Reconstruction Following Trauma. Am. J. Surg., *130*:712, 1975C.

Rich, N. M., Hobson, R. W., II, and Collins, G. J., Jr.: Traumatic Arteriovenous Fistulas and False Aneurysms: A Review of 558 Lesions. Surgery, *78*:817, 1975D.

Rich, N. M., Levin, P. M., and Hutton, J. E., Jr.: Effect of Distal Arteriovenous Fistulas on Venous Graft Patency. *In* Swan, K. G., et al. (Eds.): Symposium on Venous Surgery in the Lower Extremity. Warren H. Green Publishers, Inc., St. Louis, 1975E.

Rich, N. M., Hobson, R. W., II. Wright, C. B., and Swan, K. G.: Techniques of Venous Repair. *In* Swan, K. G., et al. (Eds.): Symposium on Venous Surgery in the Lower Extremity. Warren H. Green Publishers, Inc., St. Louis, 1975F.

Rich, N. M., Hobson, R. W., II, Collins, G. J., Jr., and Andersen, C. A.: The Effect of Acute Popliteal Venous Interruption. Ann. Surg., *183*:365, 1976.

Rich, N. M., Collins, G. J., Jr., Andersen, C. A., and McDonald, P. T.: Autogenous Venous Interposition Grafts in Repair of Major Venous Injuries. J. Trauma, *17*:512, 1977A.

Rich, N. M., Collins, G. J., Jr., Andersen, C. A., and McDonald, P. T.: Venous Trauma: Successful Venous Reconstruction Remains an Interesting Challenge. Am. J. Surg.: *134*:226, 1977B.

Rich, N. M., Collins, G. J., Jr., Hobson, R. W., II, Andersen, C. A., and McDonald, P. T.: Carotid-Axillary Bypass: Clinical and Experimental Evaluation. Am. J. Surg., *134*: 1977C.

Richards, A. J., Lamis, P. A., Rogers, J. P., Jr., and Bradham, G. B.: Laceration of Abdominal Aorta and Study of Intact Abdominal Wall as Tamponade: Report of Survival and Literature Review. Ann. Surg., *164*:321, 1966.

Ricks, R. K., Howell, J. F., Beall, A. C., Jr., and DeBakey, M. E.: Gunshot Wounds of the Heart: A Review of 31 Cases. Surgery, *57*:787, 1965.

Rignault, D.: Personal Communication, 1974.

Risley, T. S., and McClerkin, W. W.: Bullet Transection of Both Carotid Arteries: Delayed Repair With Recovery. Am. J. Surg., *121*:385, 1971.

Rittenhouse, E. A., Dillard, D. H., Winterschild, L. C., and Merendino, K. A.: Traumatic Rupture of the Thoracic Aorta: A Review of the Literature and a Report of Five Cases With Attention to Special Problems in Early Management. Ann. Surg., *170*:87, 1969.

Rob, C. G.: A History of Arterial Surgery. Arch. Surg., *105*:821, 1972.

Rob, C. G., and Battle, S.: Arteriovenous Fistula Following the Use of the Fogarty Balloon Catheter. Arch. Surg., *102*:144, 1971.

Rob, C. G., and Standeven, A.: Closed Traumatic Lesions of the Axillary and Brachial Arteries. Lancet, *1*:597, London, 1956.

Roberson, G.: Combined Stab Wound of the Aorta and Vena Cava of the Abdomen. Arch. Surg., *95*:12, 1967.

Rojas, R. H., Levitsky, S., and Stansel, H. C.: An Evaluation of Acute Traumatic Subclavian Steal Syndrome. J. Thorac. Cardiovasc. Surg., *51*:113, 1966.

Romanoff, H., and Goldberger, S.: Major Peripheral Vein Injuries. Vasc. Surg., *10*:157, 1976.

Roper, B. A., and Provan, J. L.: Late Thrombosis of the Femoral Artery Complicating Fracture of the Femur. J. Bone Joint Surg., *47-B*:510, 1965.

Rosensweig, J., and Simon, M. A.: Traumatic Aneurysm of the Axillary Artery: A Golf Hazard. Can. Med. Assoc. J., *93*:165, 1965.

Rosenthal, J. J., Gaspar, M. R., Gjerdrum, T. C., and Newman, J.: Vascular Injuries Associated With Fractures of the Femur. Arch. Surg., *110*:494, 1975.

Rubio, P. A., Reul, G. J., Jr., Beall, A. C., Jr., Jordan, G. L., Jr., and DeBakey, M. E.: Acute Carotid Artery Injury: 25 Years Experience. J. Trauma, *14*:967, 1974.

Rutherford, R. B.: Discussion in Buscaglia et al.: Penetrating Abdominal Vascular Injuries. Arch. Surg., *99*:764, 1969.

Rybeck, B.: Missile Wounding and Hemodynamic Effects of Energy Absorption. Acta Chir. Scand. (Suppl.), *450*:1, 1974.

Saaman, H. A.: The Hazards of Radial Artery Pressure Monitoring. J. Cardiovasc. Surg., *12*:342, 1971.

Sabanyeff (1896): Cited in Murphy, J. B.: Resection of Arteries and Veins Injured in Continuity—End-to-End Suture—Experimental and Clinical Research. Med. Rec., *51*:73, 1897.

Sachatello, C. R., Ernst, C. B., and Griffen, W. O., Jr.: The Acute Ischemic Upper Extremity: Selected Management. Surgery, *76*:1002, 1974.

Sako, Y., and Varco, R. L.: Arteriovenous Fistula: Results of Management of Congenital and Acquired Forms, Blood Flow Measurements, and Observations on Proximal Arterial Degeneration. Surgery, *67*:40, 1970.

Saletta, J. D., and Freeark, R. J.: The Partially Severed Artery. Arch. Surg., *97*:198, 1968.

Saletta, J. D., and Freeark, R. J.: Vascular Injuries Associated With Fractures. Orthop. Clin. North Am., *1*:93, 1970.

Saletta, J. D., and Freeark, R. J.: Injuries to the Profunda Femoris Artery. J. Trauma, *12*:778, 1972.

Samson, P. C.: Two Unusual Cases of War Wounds of the Heart. Surgery, *20*:373, 1946.

Samson, P. C.: Battle Wounds and Injuries of the Heart and Pericardium: Experiences in Forward Hospitals. Ann. Surg., *127*:1127, 1948.

Sauerbach, F.: Chirurgie der Brustorgane. Berlin, Gottingen, 1925. Cited in Fallah-Nejad et al., 1975.

Schaff, H. V., and Brawley, R. K.: Operative management of penetrating vascular injuries of the thoracic outlet. Surgery, *82*:182, 1977.

Schede, M.: Zur Frage von der Jodoformvergiftung. Zentralb. Chir. Beil, *9*:33, 1882.

Schenk, W. G., Jr., Bahn, R. A., Cordell, A., and Stephens, J. G.: The Regional Hemodynamics of Acute Experimental Arteriovenous Fistulas. Surg. Gynecol. Obstet., *105*:733, 1957.

Schenk, W. G., Jr., Martin, J. W., Leslie, M. B., and Portin, B. A.: The Regional Hemodynamics of Chronic Arteriovenous Fistulas. Surg. Gynecol. Obstet., *110*:44, 1960.

Schramek, A., and Hashmonai, M.: Distal Arteriovenous Fistula for the Prevention of Occlusion of Venous Interposition Grafts to Veins. J. Cardiovasc. Surg., *15*:392, 1974.

Schramek, A., Hashmonai, M., Farbstein, J., and Adler, O.: Reconstructive Surgery in Major Vein Injuries in the Extremities. J. Trauma, *15*:816, 1975.

Schwartz, A. M.: The Historical Development of Methods of Hemostasis. Surgery, *44*:604, 1958.

Schwartz, D. L., and Haller, J. A., Jr.: Open Anterior Hip Dislocation with Femoral Vessel Transection in a Child. J. Trauma, *14*:1054, 1974.

Schwartz, M. L., Fisher, R., Sako, Y., Castaneda, A. R., Grage, T. B., and Nicoloff, D. M.: Post-traumatic Aneurysms of the Thoracic Aorta. Surgery, *78*:589, 1975.

Scott, R.: Aspects of Military Surgery. Injury, *2*:116, 1970.

Seeley, S. F.: Vascular Surgery at Walter Reed Army Hospital. U.S. Armed Forces Med. J., *V*:8, 1954.

Seeley, S. F., Hughes, C. W., Cooke, F. N., and Elkin, D. C.: Traumatic Arteriovenous Fistulas and Aneurysms in War Wounded. Am. J. Surg., *83*:471, 1952.

Seeley, S. F., Hughes, C. W., and Jahnke, E. J., Jr.: Surgery of the Popliteal Artery. Ann. Surg., *138*:712, 1953.

Seeley, S. F., Hughes, C. W., and Jahnke, E. J., Jr.: Major Vessel Damage in Lumbar Disc Operation. Surgery, *35*:421, 1954.

Seidenberg, B., and Hurwitt, E. S.: Retrograde Femoral—Seldinger—Aortography: Surgical Complications in Twenty-Six Cases. Ann. Surg., *163*:221, 1966.

Sencert, L.: Les Blessures des Vaisseaux. Masson & Cie, Paris, 1917.

Sencert, L.: *In* Burghard, F. F. (Ed.): Wounds of the Vessels. University of London Press, London, 1918.

Sethi, G. K., and Scott, S. M.: Subclavian Artery Laceration Due to Migration of a Hagie Pin. Surgery, *80*:644, 1976.

Shepard, G. H., Rich, N. M., and Dimond, F. C., Jr.: Punji Stick Wounds: Experience with 342 Wounds in 324 Patients in Vietnam. Ann. Surg., *166*:902, 1967.

Sher, M. H.: Principles in the Management of Arterial Injuries Associated With Fracture/Dislocation. Ann. Surg., *182*:630, 1975.

Shoemaker, W. C., Carey, J. S., Yao, S. T., Mohr, P. A., et al.: Hemodynamic Alterations in Acute Cardiac Tamponade After Penetrating Injuries of the Heart. Surgery, *67*:754, 1970.

Shoemaker, W. C., Carey, J. S., and Yao, S. T.: Hemodynamic Monitoring for Physiologic Evaluation, Diagnosis, and Therapy of Acute Hemopericardial Tamponade from Penetrating Wounds. J. Trauma, *13*:36, 1973.

Shrock, T., Blaisdell, F. W., and Mathewson, C., Jr.: Management of Blunt Trauma to the Liver and Hepatic Veins. Arch. Surg., *96*:698, 1968.

Shuck, J. M., and Trump, D. S.: Non-penetrating Abdominal Trauma With Injuries to Blood Vessels. Am. Surg., *27*:693, 1961.

Shuck, J. M., Omer, J. E., Jr., and Lewis, C. E., Jr.: Arterial Obstruction Due to Intimal Disruption in Extremity Fractures. J. Trauma, *12*:481, 1972.

Shumacker, H. B., Jr.: Incisions in Surgery of Aneurysms: With Special Reference to Exploration in the Antecubital and Popliteal Fossae. Ann. Surg., *124*:586, 1946.

Shumacker, H. B., Jr.: Surgical Cure of Innominate Aneurysm. Report of a Case With Comments on the Applicability of Surgical Measures. Surgery, *22*:729, 1947A.

Shumacker, H. B., Jr.: Resection of the Clavicle With Particular Reference to the Use of Bone Chips in the Periosteal Bed. Surg. Gynecol. Obstet., *84*:245, 1947B.

Shumacker, H. B., Jr.: The Problem of Maintaining the Continuity of the Artery in the Surgery of Aneurysms and Arteriovenous Fistulae: Notes on the Development and Clinical Application of Methods of Arterial Suture. Ann. Surg., *127*:207, 1948A.

Shumacker, H. B., Jr.: Operative Exposure of the Blood Vessels in the Superior Anterior Mediastinum. Am. Surg., *127*:464, 1948B.

Shumacker, H. B., Jr.: Arterial Aneurysms and Arteriovenous Fistulas. Spontaneous Problems. Cures in Surgery. *In* Elkin, D. C., and DeBakey, M. E. (Eds.): World War II, Vascular Surgery. U.S. Government Printing Office, Office of the Surgeon General, Department of the Army, Washington, D.C., 1955, pp. 361–374.

Shumacker, H. B., Jr.: Arterial Suture Techniques and Grafts; Past, Present and Future. Surgery, *66*:419, 1969.

Shumacker, H. B., Jr., and Carter, K. L.: Arteriovenous Fistulas and False Aneurysms in Military Personnel. Surgery, *20*:9, 1946.

Shumacker, H. B., Jr., and Stahl, N. M.: A Study of the Cardiac Frontal Area in Patients With Arteriovenous Fistulas. Surgery, *26*:928, 1949.

Shumacker, H. B., Jr., and Stokes, G. E.: Studies of Combined Vascular and Neurologic Injuries. Ann. Surg., *132*:386, 1950.

Shumacker, H. B., Jr., and Wayson, E. E.: Spontaneous Cure of Aneurysms and Arteriovenous Fistulas, With Some Notes on Intrasaccular Thrombosis. Am. J. Surg., *79*:532, 1950.

Siegel, R. E.: Galen on Surgery of the Pericardium: An Early Record of Therapy Based on Anatomical and Experimental Studies. Am. J. Cardiol., *26*:524, 1970.

Sigel, B., Popky, G. L., Wagner, D. K., Boland, J. P., Mapp, E. M., and Feigl, P.: Comparison of Clinical and Doppler Ultrasound Evaluation of Confirmed Lower Extremity Venous Disease. Surgery, *64*:332, 1968.

Silen, W., and Spieker, D.: Fatal Hemorrhage from the Innominate Artery After Tracheostomy. Ann. Surg., *162*:1005, 1965.

Simeone, F. A., Grillo, H. C., and Rundle, F.: On the Question of Ligation of the Concomitant Vein When a Major Artery Is Interrupted. Surgery, *29*:932, 1951.

Singh, I., and Gorman, J. F.: Vascular Injuries in Closed Fractures Near Junction of Middle and Lower Thirds of Tibia. J. Trauma, *12*:592, 1972.

Skinner, D. G.: Traumatic Renal Artery Thrombosis: A Successful Thrombectomy and Revascularization. Ann. Surg., *177*:264, 1973.

Sloop, R. D., and Robertson, K. A.: Non-penetrating Trauma of the Abdominal Aorta With Partial Vessel Occlusion: Report of Two Cases. Am. Surg., *41*:555, 1975.

Smith, K., Ben-Menachem, B., Duke, J. H., and Hill, G. L.: The Superior Gluteal: An Artery at Risk in Blunt Pelvic Trauma. J. Trauma, *16*:273, 1976.

Smith, L. L., Foran, R., and Gaspar, M. R.: Acute Arterial Injuries of the Upper Extremity. Am. J. Surg., *106*:144, 1963.

Smith, R. F., Szilagyi, D. E., and Pfeifer, J. R.: A Study of Arterial Trauma. Arch. Surg., *86*:825, 1963.

Smith, R. F., Szilagyi, D. E., and Elliott, J. P., Jr.: Fracture of Long Bones With Arterial Injury Due to Blunt Trauma. Arch. Surg., *99*:315, 1969.

Smith, R. F., Elliott, J. P., Hageman, J. H., et al.: Acute Penetrating Arterial Injuries of the Neck and Limbs. Arch. Surg., *109*:198, 1974.

Smith, V. N., Hughes, C. W., Sapp, O., Joy, R. J. T., and Mattingly, T. W.: High Output Circulatory Failure Due to Arteriovenous Fistula Complication of Intervertebral Disc Surgery. AMA Arch. Int. Med., *100*:833, 1957.

Soubbotitch, V.: Military Experiences of Traumatic Aneurysms. Lancet, *2*:720, 1913.

Spencer, A. D.: The Reliability of Signs of Peripheral Vascular Injury. Surg. Gynecol. Obstet., *114*:490, 1962.

Spencer, F. C.: The Use of Optical Magnification in Coronary Bypass Grafting. J. Thorac. Cardiovasc. Surg., 1970.

Spencer, F. C.: *In* Schwartz, S. I., et al. (Eds.): Principles of Surgery. McGraw-Hill Book Company, New York, 1974.

Spencer, F. C., and Grewe, R. V.: The Management of Acute Arterial Injuries in Battle Casualties. Ann. Surg., *141*:304, 1955.

Spencer, F. C., and Tompkins, R. K.: Management of Acute Arterial Injuries. Postgrad. Med., *28*:476, 1960.

Spencer, F. C., Guerin, P. F., Blake, H. A., and Bahnson, H. T.: A Report of 15 Patients With Traumatic Rupture of the Thoracic Aorta. J. Thor. Cardiovasc. Surg., *41*:1, 1961.

Stallone, R. J., Ecker, R. R., and Samson, P. C.: Management of Major Acute Thoracic Vascular Injuries. Am. J. Surg., *128*:262, 1974.

Stanley-Brown, E. G.: Cited in Hughes, C. S.: Arterial Repair During the Korean War. Ann. Surg., *147*:555, 1958.

Steenburg, R. W., and Ravitch, M. M.: Cervico-Thoracic Approach for Subclavian Vessel Injury From Compound Fracture of the Clavicle: Considerations of Subclavian-Axillary Exposures. Ann. Surg., *157*:839, 1963.

Steichen, F. M., Dargan, E. L., Efron, G., Pearlman, D. M., and Weil, P. H.: A Created Approach to the Management of Penetrating Wounds of the Heart. Arch. Surg., *103*:574, 1971.

Stein, A. H., Jr.: Arterial Injury in Orthopaedic Surgery. J. Bone Joint Surg., *38A*:669, 1956.

Stein, L., Shubin, H., and Weil, M. H.: Recognition in Management of Pericardial Tamponade. J.A.M.A., *225*:503, 1973.

Stein, R. E., Bono, J., Korn, J., and Wolff, W. I.: Axillary Artery Injury in Closed Fracture of the Neck of the Scapular: A Case Report. J. Trauma, *11*:528, 1971.

Stelzner, V. F., and Horatz, K.: Correction of Gunshot Wounds of Extrapericardial Ascending Aorta. Thoraxchirurgie, *10*:632, 1963.

Stemmer, E. A., Oliver, C., Carey, J. P., and Connolly, J. E.: Fatal Complications of Tracheotomy. Am. J. Surg., *131*:288, 1976.

Stewart, F. T.: Arteriovenous Aneurism Treated by Angeiography (Angeiorrhaphy). Abb. Surg., 57:574, 1913.

Stich, R.: Ueber Gefaess und Organ Transplantationen Mittelst Gefaessnaht. Ergeon Chir. Orth., 1:1, 1910.

Stokes, J. M., and McAfee, C. A.: Increasing Limb Survival in Vascular Injury With Fracture. J. Trauma, 5:162, 1965.

Stone, H. H., Oxford, W. M., and Austin, J. T.: Penetrating Wounds of the Abdominal Aorta. South. Med. J., 66:1351, 1973.

Stone, W.: Observations on the Treatment of Wounded Arteries, With Cases. New Orleans Med. Surg. J., 2:168, 1857.

Strandness, D. E., Jr.: Collateral Circulation in Clinical Surgery. W. B. Saunders Co., Philadelphia, 1969.

Strandness, D. E., Jr., and Bell, J. W.: Peripheral Vascular Disease: Diagnosis and Objective Evaluation Using a Mercury Strain Gauge. Ann. Surg., 161(Supplement):1, 1965.

Straus, R.: Pulmonary Embolism Caused by a Lead Bullet Following a Gunshot Wound of the Abdomen. Arch. Pathol., 33:63, 1942.

Sturm, J. T., Strate, R. G., Mowlem, A., Quattlebaum, F. W., and Perry, J. F., Jr.: Blunt Trauma to the Subclavian Artery. Surg. Gynecol. Obstet., 138:915, 1974.

Sturm, J. T., Perry, J. F., Jr., and Cass, A. S.: Renal Artery and Vein Injury Following Blunt Trauma. Ann. Surg., 182:696, 1975.

Sugg, W. L., Rea, W. J., Ecker, R. R., et al.: Penetrating Wounds of the Heart: An Analysis of 459 Cases. J. Thorac. Cardiovasc. Surg., 56:531, 1968.

Sullivan, M. F.: Rupture of the Brachial Artery from Posterior Dislocation of the Elbow Treated by Vein Graft. Br. J. Surg., 58:470, 1971.

Sullivan, M. J., Smalley, R., and Banowsky, L. H.: Renal Artery Occlusion Secondary to Blunt Abdominal Trauma. J. Trauma, 12:509, 1972.

Sullivan, W. G., Thornton, F. G., Baker, L. H., LaPlante, E. S., and Cohen, A.: Early Influence of Popliteal Vein Repair in the Treatment of Popliteal Vessel Injuries. Am. J. Surg., 122:528, 1971.

Summerall, C. P., Lee, W. J., Jr., and Boone, J. A.: Intracardiac Shunts After Penetrating Wounds of the Heart. N. Engl. J. Med., 272:240, 1965.

Svane, H., and Ottosen, T.: Traumatic Vascular Lesions. J. Cardiovasc. Surg., 4:303, 1963.

Swan, K. G., Hobson, R. W., II, Reynolds, D. G., Rich, N. M., and Wright, C. B. (Eds.): Venous Surgery in the Lower Extremities. Warren H. Green Publishers, Inc., St. Louis, 1975.

Sweetman, W. R.: Subclavian Steal Syndrome Following Trauma: Case Report. Am. Surg., 31:463, 1965.

Symbas, P. N., Pourhamidi, A., and Levin, J. M.: Traumatic Rupture of the Aortic Arch Between the Left Common Carotid and Left Subclavian Arteries and Avulsion of the Left Subclavian Artery. Ann. Surg., 170:152, 1969.

Symbas, P. N., and Sehdeva, J. S.: Penetrating Wounds of the Thoracic Aorta. Ann. Surg., 171:441, 1970.

Symbas, P. N., Tyras, D. H., Ware, R. E., and Diroio, D. A.: Traumatic Rupture of the Aorta. Ann. Surg., 178:6, 1973.

Symbas, P. N., Kourias, E., Tyras, D. H., and Hatcher, C. R., Jr.: Penetrating Wounds of Great Vessels. Ann. Surg., 179:757, 1974.

Symbas, P. N., Harlaftis, N., and Waldo, W. J.: Penetrating Cardiac Wounds: A Comparison of Different Therapeutic Methods. Ann. Surg., 183:377, 1976.

Symonds, F. C., Garnes, A. L., Porter, V., and Crikelair, G. F.: Pitfalls in the Management of Penetrating Injuries of the Forearm. J. Trauma, 11:47, 1971.

Szentpetery, S., and Lower, R. R.: Changing Concepts in the Treatment of Penetrating Cardiac Injuries. J. Trauma, 17:457, 1977.

Szilagyi, D. E.: Discussion on "Choice of Vascular Graft Material for Patients." *In* Wesolowski, S. A., and Dennis, C. (Eds.): Fundamentals of Vascular Grafting. McGraw-Hill Book Co., New York, 1963, pp. 397–419.

Tassi, A. A., and Davies, A. L.: Pericardial Tamponade Due to Penetrating Fragment Wounds of the Heart. Am. J. Surg., 118:535, 1969.

Taylor, T. K. F., and Wardill, J. C.: Successful Primary Repair of Rupture of the Popliteal Artery in Association with Compound Dislocation of the Knee-joint. Br. Surg., 51:163, 1964.

Tector, A. J., Reuben, C. F., Hoffman, J. F., Gelfand, E. T., Keelan, M., and Worman, L.: Coronary Artery Wounds Treated With Saphenous Vein Bypass Grafts. J.A.M.A., 225:282, 1973.

Tector, A. J., Worman, L. W., Romer, J. F., De Cock, D. G., and Lepley, D.: Unusual Injury to the Aortic Arch: A Case Report. J. Thorac. Cardiovasc. Surg., 67:547, 1974.

Thal, E. R., Snyder, M. H., III, Hays, R. J., and Perry, M. O.: Management of Carotid Artery Injuries. Surgery, 76:955, 1974.

Thio, R. T.: False Aneurysm of the Ulnar Artery After Surgery Employing a Tourniquet. Am. J. Surg., 123:604, 1972.

Thomas, C. S., Jr., Carter, J. W., and Lowder, S. C.: Pericardial Tamponade from Central Venous Catheters. Arch. Surg., 98:217, 1969.

Thomas, H. S.: Personal Communication, 1972.

Thomas, T. V.: Management of Cardiac and Intrathoracic Great Vessel Injuries. Surg. Gynecol. Obstet., *125*:997, 1967.

Thomford, N. R., Curtiss, P. H., and Marable, S. A.: Injuries of the Iliac and Femoral Arteries Associated With Blunt Skeletal Trauma. J. Trauma, *9*:126, 1969.

Tilney, N. L., and McLamb, J. R.: Leg Trauma With Posterior Tibial Artery Tear. J. Trauma, *7*:807, 1967.

Tipton, W. W., and D'Ambrosia, R. D.: Vascular Impairment as a Result of Fracture-Dislocation of the Ankle. J. Trauma, *15*:524, 1975.

Toivio, I., and Karlsson, B.: Treatment of Ischemia of Extremity Caused by a Shotgun Blast. Ann. Med. Milit. Fenn., *4*:159, 1975.

Tomatis, L. A., Doornobs, F. A., and Beard, J. A.: Circumferential Intimal Tear of the Aorta With Complete Occlusion Due to Blunt Trauma. J. Trauma, *8*:1096, 1968.

Towne, J. B., Delbert, D. N., and Smith, J. W.: Thrombosis of the Internal Carotid Artery Following Blunt Cervical Trauma. Arch. Surg., *104*:565, 1972.

Travers, B. (1816): Cited in Travers, B., and Cooper, A.: On Wounds and Ligature of Veins. Surgical Essays (Lond.), *1*:243, 1818.

Travers, B., and Cooper, A.: On Wounds and Ligature of Veins. Surgical Essays (Lond.), *1*:243, 1818.

Treiman, R. L., Doty, D., and Gaspar, M. R.: Acute Vascular Trauma. A Fifteen-Year Study. Am. J. Surg., *111*:469, 1966.

Trimble, C.: Arterial Bullet Embolism Following Thoracic Gunshot Wounds. Ann. Surg., *168*:911, 1968.

Trinkle, J. K.: Personal Communication, 1977.

Trinkle, J. K., Marcos, J., Grover, F. L., and Cuello, L. M.: Management of the Wounded Heart. Ann. Thorac. Surg., *17*:230, 1974.

Trueblood, H. W., Wuerflein, R. D., and Angell, W. W.: Blunt Trauma Rupture of the Heart. Ann. Surg., *177*:66, 1973.

Tuffier, M.: Contemporary French Surgery. Br. J. Surg., *3*:100, 1915.

Turney, S.: Personal Communication, 1967.

Ulvestad, L. E.: Repair of Laceration of Superior Mesenteric Artery Acquired by Non-penetrating Injury to the Abdomen. Ann. Surg., *140*:752, 1954.

Utley, J. R., Singer, M. M., Roe, B. B., Fraser, D. B., and Dedo, H. H.: Definitive Management of Innominate Artery Hemorrhage Complicating Tracheostomy. J.A.M.A., *220*:557, 1972.

Valle, A. R.: War Injuries of Heart and Mediastinum. Arch. Surg., *70*:398, 1955.

Vollmar, J.: Surgical Experience With 197 Traumatic Arterial Lesions (1953–66). *In* Hiertonn, T., and Rybeck, B. (Eds.): Traumatic Arterial Lesions. Försvarets Forskningsanstalt, Stockholm, 1968.

Vollmar, J.: Bone Fracture and Vascular Lesion. Lang. Arch. Chir., *339*:473, 1975.

Vollmar, J., and Krumhaar, D.: Surgical Experience With 200 Traumatic Arteriovenous Fistulae. *In* Hiertonn, T., and Rybeck, B. (Eds.): Traumatic Arterial Lesions. Försvarets Forskningsanstalt, Stockholm, 1968.

von Horach, C.: Die Gefässnaht. Allg. Wien. Med. Ztg., *33*:263, 1888.

Von Zoege-Manteuffel (1895a): Cited in Murphy, J. B.: Resection of Arteries and Veins Injured in Continuity—End-to-End Suture—Experimental and Clinical Research. Med. Rec., *51*:73, 1897.

Von Zoege-Manteuffel: Demonstration Eines Praparates von Aneurysma arteriovenosum ossificans der Art femoralis profunda. Verhandl. Dtsch. Ges. Chir., *i*:167, 1895b.

Waddell, W. G., Vogelfanger, I. J., Prudhomme, P., Ram, J. D., Beattie, W. G., and Ewing, J. D.: Venous Valve Transplantation. Arch. Surg., *88*:5, 1964.

Waibel, P. T., and Ludin, H.: Unusual Sources of Peripheral Arterial Embolization. Arch. Surg., *92*:105, 1966.

Walker, A. G., and Walker, R. M.: Traumatic Thrombosis of the Aorta. Br. Med. J., *1*:1514, 1961.

Ward, P. A., and Suzuki, A.: Gunshot Wound of the Heart With Peripheral Embolization. J. Thorac. Cardiovasc. Surg., *68*:440, 1974.

Warren, R.: Report to the Surgeon General. Department of the Army, Washington, D.C., April, 1952.

Watson, N. W., and Rushmer, R. F.: Ultrasonic Blood Flowmeter Transducers. Proc. San Diego Sympos. Biomed. Engineer, *3*:87, 1963.

Watson, W. L., and Silverstone, S. M.: Ligature of the Common Carotid Artery in Cancer of the Head and Neck. Ann. Surg., *109*:1, 1939.

Weber, T. R., Dent, T. L., Lindenauer, S. M., Allen, E., Weatherbee, L., Spencer, H. H., and Gleich, M. S.: Viable Vein Graft Preservation. J. Surg. Res., *18*:247, 1975.

Weiland, A., Robinson, H., and Futrell, J. W.: External Stabilization of a Replanted Upper Extremity: Case Report. J. Trauma, *16*:239, 1976.

Weinstein, M. H., and Golding, A. L.: Temporary External Shunt Bypass in the Traumatically Amputated Upper Extremity. J. Trauma, *15*:912, 1975.